SEVENTH EDITION

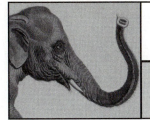

APPLETON & LANGE

REVIEW

OBSTETRICS & GYNECOLOGY

Louis A. Vontver, MD, MEd, FACOG
Professor Emeritus
Director, Division of Education
Department of Obstetrics and Gynecology
University of Washington School of Medicine
Seattle, Washington

Victor Y. Fujimoto, MD, FACOG
Director
UCSF In Vitro Fertilization Program
University of California, San Francisco
San Francisco, California

Gretchen M. Lentz, MD, FACOG
Assistant Professor, Division of Women's Health
Associate Director, Women's Health Care Center
Department of Obstetrics and Gynecology
University of Washington School of Medicine
Seattle, Washington

Sharon Phelan, MD
Professor
Department of Obstetrics and Gynecology
University of Alabama
Birmingham, Alabama

Vern Katz, MD
Clinic Associate Professor
Oregon Health Sciences University
Medical Director, Perinatal Services
Sacred Heart Medical Center
Eugene, Oregon

Lisa Lepine, MD, FACOG
Atlanta Minimally Invasive Gynecological Surgery
Center
Piedmont Hospital
Atlanta, Georgia

Roger Smith, MD
Professor and Director of Ambulatory Care
Residency Director
University of Missouri
Kansas City–Truman Medical Center
Kansas City, Missouri

Appleton & Lange/McGraw-Hill
Medical Publishing Division

New York   Chicago   San Francisco   Lisbon   London   Madrid   Mexico City   Milan
New Delhi   San Juan   Seoul   Singapore   Sydney   Toronto

Appleton & Lange Review of Obstetrics & Gynecology, Seventh Edition

Copyright © 2003, 2000 by The **McGraw-Hill Companies**, Inc. All Rights reserved. Printed in the United States of America. Except as permitted under the United States Copyright Act of 1976, no part of this publication may be reproduced or distributed in any form or by any means, or stored in a data base or retrieval system, without the prior written permission of the publisher.

1234567890 CUSCUS 09876543

ISBN 0-07-138649-1

This book was set in Palatino by Rainbow Graphics.
The editors were Catherine A. Johnson and John M. Morriss.
The production supervisor was Lisa Mendez.
The cover designer was Aimee Nordin.

Von Hoffmann, Inc., was printer and binder.

This book is printed on acid-free paper.

Library of Congress Cataloging-in-Publication Data

Appleton & Lange review of obstetrics & gynecology.—7ed./Louis A. Vontver ... [et al.]
      p. ; cm
   Rev. ed of: Appleton & Lange's review of obstetrics & gynecology / Louis A.
Vontver ... [et al.]. 6th ed. c2000.
   Includes bibliographical references.
   ISBN 0-07-138649-1 (alk. paper)
   1. Gynecology—Examinations, questions, etc. 2. Obstetrics—Examinations, questions,
ets. I. Title: Appleton and Lange review of obstetrics and gynecology. II. Title: Review
of obstetrics & gynecology. III. Title: Review of obstretrics and gynecology. IV. Vontver,
Louis A. V. Appleton & Lange's review of obstetrics and gynecology.
   [DNLM: 1. Genital Diseases, Female—Examination Questions. 2.
Obstetrics—Examination Questions. WP 18.2 A649 2002]
   RG111.V66 2002
   618'.076—dc21
                                                                2002033813
INTERNATIONAL EDITION ISBN 0-07-121217-5
Copyright © 2003. Exclusive rights by the McGraw-Hill Companies, Inc. for manufacture and export. This book cannot be re-exported from the country to which it is consigned by McGraw-Hill. The International Edition is not available in North America.

Contents

Introduction iv

Abbreviations xi

USMLE Step 2 Laboratory Values xiii

1. Anatomy 1

   Answers and Explanations 11

2. Histology and Pathology 25

   Answers and Explanations 32

3. Embryology 41

   Answers and Explanations 46

4. Genetics and Teratology 53

   Answers and Explanations 61

5. Physiology of Reproduction 69

   Answers and Explanations 79

6. Maternal Physiology During Pregnancy 91

   Answers and Explanations 99

7. Placental, Fetal, and Newborn Physiology 107

   Answers and Explanations 114

8. Prenatal Care 121

   Answers and Explanations 129

9. Diseases Complicating Pregnancy 139

   Answers and Explanations 156

10. **Normal Labor and Delivery** 169

　　Answers and Explanations 178

11. **Abnormal Labor and Delivery** 187

　　Answers and Explanations 197

12. **Operative Obstetrics** 205

　　Answers and Explanations 214

13. **Puerperium** 221

　　Answers and Explanations 227

14. **Newborn Assessment and Care** 233

　　Answers and Explanations 239

15. **Infertility** 245

　　Answers and Explanations 251

16. **Clinical Endocrinology** 259

　　Answers and Explanations 266

17. **Contraception** 275

　　Answers and Explanations 280

18. **Gynecology: Common Lesions of the Vulva, Vagina, Cervix, and Uterus;
　　Gynecologic Pain Syndromes; Imaging in Obstetrics and Gynecology** 289

　　Answers and Explanations 296

19. **Pelvic Floor Dysfunction: Genital Prolapse and Urogynecology** 305

　　Answers and Explanations 313

20. **The Pelvic Mass** 321

　　Answers and Explanations 327

21. **Gynecologic Oncology: Premalignant and Malignant Diseases of the Lower Genital Tract—
　　Vulva, Vagina, and Cervix** 333

　　Answers and Explanations 341

22. **Gynecologic Oncology: Upper Genital Tract Malignancies** 349

　　Answers and Explanations 365

23. **Breast Cancer** 385

   Answers and Explanations 390

24. **Gynecologic Oncology: Chemotherapy and Radiation Therapy in the Treatment
   of Malignancies of the Female Genital Tract** 395

   Answers and Explanations 400

25. **Infectious Diseases in Obstetrics and Gynecology** 405

   Answers and Explanations 415

26. **Special Topics in Gynecology: Pediatric and Adolescent Gynecology, Sexual Abuse,
   Medical Ethics, and Medical–Legal Considerations** 425

   Answers and Explanations 425

27. **Primary Health Care for Women** 433

   Answers and Explanations 440

28. **Practice Test** 447

   Answers and Explanations 467

References 483

Introduction

Education is the kindling of a flame, not the filling of a vessel.

—*Socrates*

The seventh edition of this book has been written, as were the prior editions, to be a study aid for self-examination and review in the field of obstetrics and gynecology. Each chapter has been updated with new questions written to keep pace with new information, which is continually being discovered. The questions are designed to review many topics, which are also covered in tests such as the USMLE Step 2. The questions are written in styles similar to those utilized in that examination. An answer is given for each question along with a comment that amplifies and/or explains the answer. This reinforces your knowledge and provides feedback to guide further study.

Proven knowledge and feedback help create interest and motivation that makes learning exciting. Interest and motivation also produces and accelerates the habit of lifelong learning, which is necessary to keep abreast of any changing and dynamic field. We hope that using this review will help you consolidate your knowledge, evaluate your capabilities, and motivate you to continually expand your horizons to levels far beyond this study aid.

THE UNITED STATES MEDICAL LICENSING EXAMINATION, STEP 2

The USMLE Step 2 is a computerized examination consisting of approximately 400 questions testing your knowledge in the clinical sciences. It contains multiple-choice questions organized within three dimensions: 1. System, 2. Process, and 3. Organizational Level. Although each dimension is weighted, the projected percentage for each is subject to change from exam to exam. The application materials illustrate the percentage breakout and offer a detailed content outline to aid you in your review.

Question Format

The style and presentation of the questions have been fully revised to conform with the USMLE. This will enable readers to familiarize themselves with the types of questions to be expected and practice answering questions in each format.

Each of the chapters contains multiple-choice questions (or "items"). Most of these are one best answer–single item questions, some are one best answer–matching sets, and some are comparison–matching set questions and some are Pick-N in which more than one answer is correct. In some cases, a group of two or three questions may be related to one situation. In addition, some questions have illustrations (graphs, x-rays, tables, or line drawings) that require understanding and interpretation. Moreover, each question may be categorized at one of three levels of difficulty depending on the level of skill needed to answer it: rote memory, a clear understanding of the problem, or both understanding and judgment. Since the USMLE seems to prefer questions requiring judgment and critical thinking, we have attempted to emphasize these questions.

One Best Answer–Single Item Question. The majority of the questions are posed in the A-type, or "one best answer–single item" format. This is the most popular question format in most exams. It generally consists of a brief statement, followed by four or five options of which only ONE is entirely correct. The options on the USMLE are lettered A, B, C, D, and E. Although the format for this question type is straightforward, these questions can be difficult because some of the distractors may be partially correct. The instructions you will see for this type of question will generally appear as below:

DIRECTIONS: Each of the numbered items or incomplete statements in this section is followed by answers or by completions of the statement. Select the ONE lettered answer or completion that is BEST in each case.

The following is an example of this question type:

1. An obese 21-year-old woman complains of increased growth of coarse hair on her lip, chin, chest, and abdomen. She also notes menstrual irregularity with long periods of amenorrhea. The most likely cause is

    (A) polycystic ovary disease

    (B) an ovarian tumor

    (C) an adrenal tumor

    (D) Cushing's disease

    (E) familial hirsutism

In the question above, the key word is "most." Although ovarian tumors, adrenal tumors, and Cushing's disease are causes of hirsutism (described in the stem of the question), polycystic ovary disease is a much more common cause. Familial hirsutism is not associated with the menstrual irregularities mentioned. Thus, the most likely cause of the manifestations described can only be "(A) polycystic ovary disease."

STRATEGIES FOR ANSWERING ONE BEST ANSWER— SINGLE ITEM QUESTIONS

1. Remember that only one choice can be the correct answer.
2. Read the question carefully to be sure that you understand what is being asked.
3. Quickly read each choice for familiarity. (This important step is often not done by test takers.)
4. Go back and consider each choice individually.
5. If a choice is partially correct, tentatively consider it to be incorrect. (This step will help you eliminate choices and increase your odds of choosing the correct answer.)
6. Consider the remaining choices and select the one you think is the answer. At this point, you may want to quickly scan the item to be sure you understand the question and your answer.
7. If you do not know the answer, make an educated guess. Your score is based on the number of correct answers, not the number you get incorrect. **Do not leave any blanks.**
8. The actual examination is timed for an average of 50 seconds per question. It is important to be thorough to understand the questions, but it is equally important for you to keep moving.

One Best Answer–Matching Set Questions. This format presents lettered options followed by several items related to a common topic. The directions you will generally see for this type of question are as follows:

DIRECTIONS (Questions 2 through 4): Each set of matching questions in this section consists of a list of 4 to 26 lettered options followed by several numbered items. For each item, select the ONE best lettered option that is most closely associated with it. Each lettered heading may be selected once, more than once, or not at all.

Below is an example of this type of question:

For each adverse drug reaction listed below, select the antibiotic with which it is most closely associated.

    (A) tetracycline

    (B) chloramphenicol

    (C) clindamycin

    (D) cefotaxime

    (E) gentamicin

2. Bone marrow suppression

3. Pseudomembranous enterocolitis

4. Acute fatty necrosis of liver

Note that unlike the single-item questions, the choices in the matching sets *precede* the actual questions. However, as with the single-item questions, only one choice can be correct for a given question.

STRATEGIES FOR ANSWERING ONE BEST ANSWER–MATCHING SET QUESTIONS

1. Remember that the lettered choices are followed by the numbered questions.
2. As with single-item questions, only one answer will be correct for each item.
3. Quickly read each choice for familiarity.
4. Read the question carefully to be sure that you understand what is being asked.
5. Go back and consider each choice individually.
6. If a choice is partially correct for a particular item, tentatively consider it to be incorrect. (This step will help you eliminate choices and increase your odds of choosing the correct answer.)
7. Consider the remaining choices and select the one you think is the answer.
8. If you do not know the answer, make an educated guess. Your score is based on the number of correct answers, not the number you get incorrect. **Do not leave any blanks.**
9. Again, the actual examination allows an average of 50 seconds per question.

Extended One Best Answer–Matching/Choosing Questions. The USMLE Step 2 uses a new type of matching question that is similar to the one above, but can contain up to 26 lettered options followed by several items. The directions you will see for this type of question will generally read the same as the ones listed for the best answer–matching sets since this is another version of the same question. An example of this type of question is:

(A) sarcoidosis
(B) tuberculosis
(C) histoplasmosis
(D) coccidiomycosis
(E) amyloidosis
(F) bacterial pneumonia
(G) mesothelioma
(H) carcinoma
(I) fibrosing alveolitis
(J) silicosis

627. A right lower lobectomy specimen contains a solitary 1.2-cm diameter solid nodule. The center of the nodule is fibrous. The periphery has granulomatous inflammation. With special stains, multiple 2 to 5 μm budding yeasts are evident within the nodule. Acid-fast stains are negative.

628. A left upper lobectomy specimen is received containing a 4.6-cm nodule with central cystic degeneration. Microscopically, the nodule is composed of anaplastic squamous cells. Similar abnormal cells are seen in a concomitant biopsy of a hilar lymph node.

629. After a long history of multiple myeloma, a 67-year-old male is noted to have abundant acellular eosinophilic deposits around the pulmonary microvasculature at autopsy. A Congo red special stain demonstrates apple green birefringence.

630. A large pleural-based lesion is found on chest x-ray of an asbestos worker. Electron microscopy of the biopsy shows abundant long microvilli.

Note that, like other matching sets, the lettered options are listed first.

STRATEGIES FOR ANSWERING EXTENDED ONE BEST ANSWER–MATCHING/CHOOSING QUESTIONS

1. Read the lettered options through first.
2. Work with one item at a time.
3. Read the item through, then go back to the options and consider each choice individually.
4. As with the other question types, if the choice is partially correct, tentatively consider it to be incorrect.
5. Consider the remaining choices and select the answer.
6. Remember to make a selection for each item.
7. Again, the test allows for 50 seconds per item.

Pick N–More Than One Answer This format mimics the single best answer format, but contains more than one correct answer. These questions are identifiable by their stem, "Which three of the following . . ." Correct answers can range from two to four. The directions you will generally see for this type of question are as follows:

DIRECTIONS (Questions 1 through 3): Each of the numbered items or incomplete statements in this section is followed by answers or by completions of the statement. Select the answers or completions that may apply.

Below is an example of this type of question:

Which three of the following contraindications would you mention when discussing reasons to use caudal anesthesia in your laboring patient?

  (A) pilonidal sinus
  (B) thrombocytopenia
  (C) maternal heart disease
  (D) anticoagulant therapy
  (E) premature labor

STRATEGIES FOR ANSWERING PICK-N QUESTIONS

1. Remember that one or more answer or completions will be correct, the questions will state how many answers or completions are correct and therefore should be selected.
2. Read the question carefully so that you understand what is being asked.
3. Read each answer or completion individually and decide if it is correct or incorrect.
4. Select the number of correct answers or completions that you are asked to select.
5. Remember that the test allows for approximately 50 seconds per question.

Practice Test At the end of the book we have included a practice test that contains randomly ordered questions of all styles covering all the topics. This test is designed to more closely approximate the form of the USMLE Step 2 examination. An answer and comment section follows the practice test, and relates to the questions contained in it.

Answers and Explanations In each of the sections of this book, the question sections are followed by a section containing the answers and explanations. This section (1) tells you the answer to each question; (2) gives you an explanation/review of why the answer is correct, background information on the subject matter, and why the other answers are incorrect. We encourage you to use this section as a basis for further study and understanding.

If you choose the correct answer to a question, you can then read the explanation (1) for reinforcement and (2) to add to your knowledge about the subject matter (remember that the explanations may tell not only why the answer is correct, but also why the other choices are incorrect). **If you choose the wrong answer** to a question, you can read the explanation for a learning/reviewing discussion of the material in the question.

SPECIFIC INFORMATION ON THE STEP 2 EXAMINATION

The official source of all information with respect to the United States Medical Licensing Examination Step 2 is the National Board of Medical Examiners (NBME), 3930 Chestnut Street, Philadelphia, PA 19104 (www.nbme.org). Established in 1915, the NBME is a voluntary, nonprofit, independent organization whose sole function is the design, implementation, distribution, and processing of a vast bank of question items, certifying examinations, and evaluative services in the professional medical field.

Please contact the NBME with all questions related to eligibility, scoring, and physical conditions of the examination.

Abbreviations

ABH: A and B are blood antigens; H is the substrate from which they are formed.
ACTH: adrenocorticotropic hormone
ADH: antidiuretic hormone
AFP: alpha$_1$ fetoprotein
AP: anteroposterior
ATN: acute tubular necrosis

B: basophils
BMR: basal metabolic rate
BP: blood pressure
BSO: bilateral salpingo-oophorectomy
BSU: Bartholin, Skene's, and urethral glands

CAH: congenital adrenal hyperplasia
CHD: congenital heart disease
CHF: congestive heart failure
CIN: cervical intraepithelial neoplasia
CNS: central nervous system
CP: cerebral palsy
CPD: cephalic disproportion
CSF: cerebrospinal fluid
CST: contraction stress test

D&C: dilation and curettage
DES: diethylstilbestrol
DHEA: dehydroepiandrosterone
DHEAS: dehydroepiandrosterone sulfate
DIC: disseminated intravascular coagulation

E: eosinophils
E^3: estriol
EDC: estimated date of confinement
ESR: erythrocyte sedimentation rate
EUA: examination under anesthesia

5-FU: 5-fluorouracil
FHTs: fetal heart tones

FIGLU: formiminoglutamic acid
FIGO: International Federation of Gynecology and Obstetrics
FSH: follicle-stimulating hormone
FTA: fluorescent treponemal antibody (test)

G6 PD: glucose-6-dehydrogenase deficiency
GH: growth hormone
GI: gastrointestinal
GU: genitourinary

Hb A: adult hemoglobin
Hb F: fetal hemoglobin
HCG: human chorionic gonadotropin
HCS: human chorionic somatomammotropin
Hct: hematocrit
H & E: hematoxylin and eosin (stain)
HLA: histocompatibility locus antigen
HPF: hepatic plasma flow
HPV: human papilloma virus

ICSH: interstitial-cell stimulating hormone
INH: isonicotinoylhydrazine
IRDS: infant respiratory distress syndrome
IVP: intravenous pyelogram

KUB: kidneys, ureters, & bladder

L: lymphocytes
LE: lupus erythematosus
LH: luteinizing hormone
LHRH: luteinizing hormone–releasing hormone
LMP: last menstrual period
LMT: left mentotransverse
LOA: left occipito-anterior
LOP: left occiput posterior
LOT: left occiput transverse
L/S: lecithin/sphingomyelin

LSB: left sternal border
LST: left sacrotransverse

M: monocytes
MCH: mean corpuscular hemoglobin
MCHC: mean corpuscular hemoglobin concentration
MCV: mean corpuscular volume
MeV: mega electron volt
MF: menstrual formula
MI: maturation index
MIF: müllerian-inhibiting factor
mm: muscles
MMK: Marshall–Marchetti–Krantz procedure

NST: nonstress test

OA: occipito-anterior
OCT: oxytocin challenge test
OD: optical density
OP: occiput posterior
OR: operating room

P: plasma cells
PAS: para-aminosalicylic acid

PBI: protein-bound iodine
PG: prostaglandin
PID: pelvic inflammatory disease
PIF: prolactin-inhibiting factor
PKU: phenylketonuria

ROP: right occipitoposterior

SGOT: serum glutamic-oxaloacetic transaminase
SLE: systemic lupus erythematosus
SRT: sacrum right transverse
SS: sickle cell anemia

TAH: total abdominal hysterectomy
TB: tuberculosis
TNM: tumor, node, metastasis
TRH: thyrotropin-releasing hormone
TSH: thyroid-stimulating hormone

UA: urinalysis
UPD: urinary production (rate)
UTI: urinary tract infection

WBC: white blood cell count

USMLE Step 2 Laboratory Values
*Included in the Biochemical Profile (SMA-12)

	REFERENCE RANGE	SI REFERENCE INTERVALS
BLOOD, PLASMA, SERUM		
Follicle-stimulating hormone, serum/plasma	Male: 4–25 mIU/mL	4–25 U/L
	Female: premenopause 4–30 mIU/mL	4–30 U/L
	Midcycle peak 10–90 mIU/mL	10–90 U/L
	Postmenopause 40–250 mIU/mL	40–250 U/L
Gases, arterial blood (room air)		
pH	7.35–7.45	[H^+] 36–44 nmol/L
P_{CO_2}	33–45 mm Hg	4.4–5.9 kPa
P_{O_2}	75–105 mm Hg	10.0–14.0 kPa
*Glucose, serum	Fasting: 70–110 mg/dL	3.8–6.1 mmol/L
	2-h postprandial: < 120 mg/dL	< 6.6 mmol/L
Luteinizing hormone, serum/plasma	Male: 6–23 mIU/mL	6–23 U/L
	Female: follicular phase 5–30 mIU/mL	5–30 U/L
	Midcycle 75–150 mIU/mL	75–150 U/L
	Postmenopause 30–200 mIU/mL	30–200 U/L
Prolactin, serum (hPRL)	< 20 ng/mL	< 20 µg/L
*Proteins, serum		
Total (recumbent)	6.0–7.8 g/dL	60–78 g/L
Albumin	3.5–5.5 g/dL	35–55 g/L
Globulin	2.3–3.5 g/dL	23–35 g/L
Thyroid-stimulating hormone, serum or plasma	0.5–5.0 µU/mL	0.5–5.0 mU/L
Thyroidal iodine (^{123}I) uptake	8–30% of administered dose/24 h	0.08–0.30/24 h
Thyroxine (T_4), serum	5–12 µg/dL	64–155 nmol/L
Triglycerides, serum	35–160 mg/dL	0.4–1.81 mmol/L
Triiodothyronine (T_3), serum (RIA)	115–190 ng/dL	1.8–2.9 nmol/L
Triiodothyronine (T_3) resin uptake	25–35%	0.25–0.35
*Urea nitrogen, serum (BUN)	7–18 mg/dL	1.2–3.0 mmol urea/L
*Uric acid, serum	3.0–8.2 mg/dL	0.18–0.48 mmol/L
HEMATOLOGIC		
Bleeding time template	2–7 minutes	2–7 minutes
Erythrocyte count	Male: 4.3–5.9 million/mm³	4.3–5.9 × 10¹²/L
	Female: 3.5–5.5 million/mm³	3.3–5.5 × 10¹²/L
Erythrocyte sedimentation rate (Westergren)	Male: 0–15 mm/h	0–15 mm/h
	Female: 0–20 mm/h	0–20 mm/h
Hematocrit	Male: 41–53%	0.41–0.53
	Female: 36–46%	0.36–0.46
Hemoglobin A_{1C}	≤ 6%	≤ 0.06%
Hemoglobin, blood	Male: 13.5–17.5 g/dL	2.09–2.71 mmol/L
	Female: 12.0–16.0 g/dL	1.86–2.48 mmol/L
Hemoglobin, plasma	1–4 mg/dL	0.16–0.62 mmol/L
Leukocyte count and differential		
Leukocyte count	4,500–11,000/mm³	4.5–11.0 × 10⁹/L
Segmented neutrophils	54–62%	0.54–0.62
Band forms	3–5%	0.03–0.05
Eosinophils	1–3%	0.01–0.03
Basophils	0–0.75%	0–0.0075
Lymphocytes	25–33%	0.25–0.33
Monocytes	3–7%	0.03–0.07
Mean corpuscular hemoglobin	25.4–34.6 pg/cell	0.39–0.54 fmol/cell
Mean corpuscular hemoglobin concentration	31–36% Hb/cell	4.81–5.58 mmol Hb/L
Mean corpuscular volume	80–100 µm³	80–100 fl
Partial thromboplastin time (activated)	25–35 seconds	25–35 seconds
Platelet count	150,000–400,000/mm³	150–400 × 10⁹/L
Prothrombin time	11–15 seconds	11–15 seconds
Reticulocyte count	0.5–1.5% of red cells	0.005–0.015
Thrombin time	< 2 seconds deviation from control	< 2 seconds deviation from control
Volume		
Plasma	Male: 25–43 mL/kg	0.025–0.043 L/kg
	Female: 28–45 mL/kg	0.028–0.045 L/kg
Red cell	Male: 20–36 mL/kg	0.020–0.036 L/kg
	Female: 19–31 mL/kg	0.019–0.031 L/kg

CHAPTER 1

Anatomy
Questions

DIRECTIONS (Questions 1 through 54): Each of the numbered items or incomplete statements in this section is followed by answers or by completions of the statement. Select the ONE lettered answer or completion that is BEST in each case.

1. Most adult females have a pelvic inlet that would be classified as which of the following Caldwell–Moloy types?

    (A) android
    (B) platypelloid
    (C) anthropoid
    (D) gynecoid
    (E) triangular

2. Hernias may occur beneath the thickened lower margin of a fascial aponeurosis extending from the pubic tubercle to the anterior superior iliac spine. This thickened fascia is the

    (A) inguinal ligament
    (B) Cooper's ligament
    (C) linea alba
    (D) posterior rectus sheath
    (E) round ligament

3. If the inguinal canal in an adult female was surgically opened, which of the following structures would normally be found?

    (A) a cyst of the canal of Nuck
    (B) Gartner's duct cyst
    (C) Cooper's ligament
    (D) the round ligament and the ilioinguinal nerve
    (E) the pyramidalis muscle

4. Which option includes all of the bones that make up the pelvis?

    (A) trochanter, hip socket, ischium, sacrum, and pubis
    (B) ilium, ischium, pubis, sacrum, and coccyx
    (C) ilium, ischium, and pubis
    (D) sacrum, ischium, ilium, and pubis
    (E) trochanter, sacrum, coccyx, ilium, and pubis

5. Which of the following bears the weight of a seated human?

    (A) the rami of the ischium
    (B) the levator ani muscle and the coccygeus muscle
    (C) the ileum
    (D) the pubis
    (E) the ischial tuberosities

6. In the female, the true pelvis anatomically

    (A) has an oval outlet
    (B) has three defining planes, an inlet, a midplane, and an outlet
    (C) has an inlet made up of a double triangle
    (D) is completely formed by two fused bones
    (E) lies between the wings of the paired ileum

7. The sacrum is the most posterior bone of the pelvis and

    (A) is formed from 11 or 12 small fused vertebrae
    (B) has an uppermost anterior portion called the obstetrical conjugate
    (C) has a concave pelvic surface in women
    (D) is separated from the vertebrae that make up the coccyx by a highly mobile sacrococcygeal joint
    (E) is most often the limiting factor in determining the size of the pelvic outlet

8. The portion of the pelvis lying above the linea terminalis has little effect on a woman's ability to deliver a baby vaginally. This portion is called the

    (A) true pelvis
    (B) midplane
    (C) outlet
    (D) false pelvis
    (E) sacrum

9. The plane from the sacral promontory to the inner posterior surface of the pubic symphysis is an important dimension for normal delivery. It is referred to as the

    (A) true conjugate
    (B) obstetric conjugate
    (C) diagonal conjugate
    (D) bi-ischial diameter
    (E) oblique diameter

10. During an operation, a midline incision was made at an anatomic location 2 cm below the umbilicus. Which of the following lists (in order) the layers of the anterior abdominal wall as they would be incised or separated?

    (A) skin, subcutaneous fat, superficial fascia (Camper's), deep fascia (Scarpa's), fascial muscle cover (anterior rectus sheath), rectus muscle, a deep fascial muscle cover (posterior rectus sheath), preperitoneal fat, and peritoneum
    (B) skin, subcutaneous fat, superficial fascia (Scarpa's), deep fascia (Camper's), fas-cial muscle covering (anterior abdominal sheath), transverse abdominal muscle, a deep fascial muscle cover (posterior rectus sheath), preperitoneal fat, and peritoneum
    (C) skin, subcutaneous fat, superficial fascia (Camper's), deep fascia (Scarpa's), fascial muscle cover (anterior rectus sheath), rectus muscle, a deep fascial muscle cover (posterior rectus sheath), peritoneum, and preperitoneal fat
    (D) skin, subcutaneous fat, superficial fascia (Scarpa's), deep fascia (Camper's), fascial muscle cover (anterior rectus sheath), rectus muscle, a deep fascial muscle cover (posterior rectus sheath), preperitoneal fat, and peritoneum
    (E) skin, subcutaneous fat, superficial fascia (Camper's), deep fascia (Scarpa's), fascial muscle cover (anterior rectus sheath), transverse abdominal muscle, a deep fascial muscle covering (posterior rectus sheath), preperitoneal fat, and peritoneum

11. The diagonal conjugate can be measured clinically to help predict ability to deliver a baby vaginally. In the normal pelvis it should be at least

    (A) 6 cm
    (B) 8.5 cm
    (C) 10 cm
    (D) 12 cm
    (E) 14 cm

12. The joint between the two pubic bones is called the

    (A) sacroiliac joint
    (B) pubic symphysis
    (C) sacrococcygeal joint
    (D) piriformis
    (E) intervertebral joint

13. Which of the following statements applies to the outlet of the true pelvis?

    (A) It begins at the iliopectineal line.
    (B) It is the most cephalad of the three planes.

(C) It is gynecoid in shape.

(D) It has lateral walls.

(E) It consists of anterior and posterior tri-angles.

14. Of the following, the best definition of per-ineum is

(A) the entire area between the thighs from the symphysis to the coccyx, bounded caudally by the skin and cephalad by the levator muscles of the pelvic diaphragm

(B) the anus and perianal area

(C) the superficial skin layer of the vulva

(D) the tendon joining the muscles deep to the external genitalia

(E) the complex of the bulbocavernosus, is-chiocavernosus, and transverse perineal muscles

15. What is the usual shape of the escutcheon in the female?

(A) diamond-shaped

(B) triangular

(C) oval

(D) circular

(E) heart-shaped

16. Where do the Bartholin's glands ducts open?

(A) into the midline of the posterior fourchette

(B) bilaterally, beneath the urethra

(C) bilaterally, on the inner surface of the labia majora

(D) bilaterally, into the posterior vaginal vestibule

(E) bilaterally, approximately 1 cm lateral to the clitoris

17. Myrtiform caruncles are

(A) circumferential nodules in the areola of the breast

(B) healing Bartholin cysts

(C) remnants of the wolffian duct

(D) remnants of the hymen

(E) remnants of the müllerian duct

18. The major nerve supply to the clitoris is from the

(A) lumbar spinal nerve

(B) pudendal nerve

(C) femoral nerve

(D) ilioinguinal nerve

(E) anterior gluteal nerve

19. Which of the following is a muscle of the ex-ternal genitalia?

(A) the gluteus

(B) the sartorious

(C) the superficial transverse perineal

(D) the deep transverse perineal

(E) the levator ani

20. Which of the following is NOT a function of the vagina?

(A) It connects the internal and external gen-italia.

(B) It maintains a flat (closed) lumen during normal activities.

(C) It actively secretes serous fluid.

(D) It distends during sexual arousal.

21. In the uterus of a normal female infant, the cervix, isthmus, and fundus have what rela-tionship?

(A) The cervix is larger than the fundus.

(B) The isthmus is longer than either the cervix or the fundus.

(C) They are all of equal size.

(D) The fundus is the largest portion.

22. Nabothian cysts result from

(A) wolffian duct remnants

(B) blockage of crypts in the uterine cervix that are lined with columnar epithelium

(C) squamous cell debris that causes cervical irritation

(D) carcinoma

(E) paramesonephric remnants

23. The uterine corpus is composed mainly of

(A) fibrous tissue

(B) estrogen receptors

(C) muscle tissue

(D) elastic tissue

24. The uterus and adnexa have some relatively fixed anatomic characteristics that can be noted on pelvic examination or laparoscopic observation. Which of the following characteristics would you most likely find in a normal patient?

(A) anteflexion of the uterus

(B) ovaries caudad to the cervix

(C) round ligaments attached to the uterus posterior to the insertion of the fallopian tubes

(D) immobility of the uterus

25. Of the following ligaments, those providing the most support to the uterus (in terms of preventing prolapse) are the

(A) broad ligaments

(B) infundibulopelvic ligaments

(C) utero-ovarian ligaments

(D) cardinal ligaments

26. The fallopian tube has which of the following characteristics?

(A) It is a conduit from the peritoneal space to the uterine cavity.

(B) It is found in the utero-ovarian ligament.

(C) It has five separate parts.

(D) It is attached to the ipsilateral ovary by the mesosalpinx.

(E) It is entirely extraperitoneal.

27. In the female, the urogenital diaphragm

(A) includes the fascial covering of the deep transverse perineal muscle

(B) encloses the ischiorectal fossa

(C) is synonymous with the pelvic diaphragm

(D) is located in the anal triangle

(E) envelops the Bartholin's gland

28. The levator ani is

(A) the superficial muscular sling of the pelvis

(B) a tripartite muscle of the pelvic floor penetrated by the urethra, vagina, and rectum

(C) made up of the bulbocavernosus, the ischiocavernosus, and the superficial transverse perineal muscle

(D) a three-part muscle that abducts the thighs

(E) part of the deep transverse perineal muscle

29. The pelvic diaphragm is

(A) made up mainly by the coccygeus

(B) covered on one side by fascia and on the other by peritoneum

(C) innervated by L2,3,4

(D) synonymous with the pelvic floor

30. When performing a hysterectomy, the surgeon must be aware that at its closest position to the cervix, the ureter is normally separated from the cervix by which of the following distances?

(A) 0.5 mm

(B) 1.2 mm

(C) 12 mm

(D) 3 cm

(E) 5 cm

31. In its course through the pelvis, the ureter passes

(A) anterior to the internal iliac and uterine arteries

(B) posterior to the iliac artery and anterior to the uterine artery

(C) anterior to the uterine artery and posterior to the iliac artery

(D) posterior to the uterine artery and medial to the iliac artery

(E) posterior to the uterine artery and posterior to the hypogastric artery

32. The female urethra has which of the following characteristics?

    (A) It is a hollow, multilayered tube 7 to 10 cm long.
    (B) It joins with the bladder at the level of the midtrigone.
    (C) There is a true anatomic sphincter within the urethra.
    (D) The upper two thirds of the urethra is integrated with the anterior vaginal wall.
    (E) The intrinsic "increased" resting tone of the urethra provides part of the continence mechanism for urinary control.

33. The upper two thirds of the vagina is innervated by

    (A) sympathetic fibers from the presacral nerve and parasympathetic fibers from the hypogastric plexus
    (B) the pudendal nerve
    (C) the clitoral nerve
    (D) the genitofemoral nerve

34. The dural space in the spinal canal ends at approximately _____, whereas the spinal cord ends at approximately _____.

    (A) T10, T8
    (B) L2, T10
    (C) L5, T12
    (D) S2, L2
    (E) S5, S2

35. The blood supply of the vagina is from which of the following arteries?

    (A) internal pudendal
    (B) superior hemorrhoidal
    (C) inferior mesenteric
    (D) superior vesical

36. The lymphatic drainage of the vulva is primarily directed to the

    (A) inguinal and pelvic lymph nodes
    (B) para-aortic nodes
    (C) obturator nodes
    (D) femoral nodes

37. Where is Cloquet's node found?

    (A) superficial inguinal area
    (B) superficial femoral area
    (C) deep inguinal area
    (D) external iliac area

38. The main arterial blood supply to the vulva is the

    (A) pudendal
    (B) inferior hemorrhoidal
    (C) ilioinguinal
    (D) femoral
    (E) inferior hypogastric

39. The normal term placenta in the human is

    (A) approximately 10 cm in diameter
    (B) approximately 8 cm thick
    (C) about one sixth the weight of the term infant (400 to 600 g)
    (D) derived from fetal tissues only

40. Which of the following statements about the term placenta is accurate?

    (A) Elevated septae divide the placenta into its cotyledons.
    (B) The fetal side of the placenta will be irregular, deep red, and beefy
    (C) The maternal side will be shiny and smooth.
    (D) The villous surface (portion for exchange) may measure up to 12 m^2.

41. The chorion laeve is

    (A) the site of chorionic implantation
    (B) the cluster of chorionic villi next to the decidua basalis
    (C) maternal decidual formation
    (D) the chorion, denuded of villi

42. Which of the following is consistent with the general anatomy of the female breast?

    (A) The breast contains only glandular and ductal tissue.
    (B) Each breast consists of two conical lobes.
    (C) Each lobe in the breast consists of a group of lobules.
    (D) About 20 to 25% of a normal breast is fat.
    (E) Alveoli decrease in size and number during pregnancy.

43. The tail of Spence is

    (A) a phrase describing the overhanging characteristic of pendulous breasts
    (B) the area of darkened color found underneath the breast in obese women, usually resulting from chronic pressure
    (C) a fungal rash found on the chest wall that presents in a "tail-like" pattern
    (D) a triangular tongue-shaped portion of breast tissue that extends superiorly toward the axilla
    (E) a book about obstetric and gynecologic infections

44. The deep perineal space in women contains the

    (A) superficial transverse perineal muscle
    (B) ischiocavernosus muscle
    (C) bulbocavernosus muscle
    (D) deep transverse perineal muscle
    (E) levator ani muscle

45. The superficial perineal space contains which of the following?

    (A) hood of the clitoris
    (B) deep transverse perineal muscle
    (C) ischiocavernosus muscle
    (D) internal anal sphincter
    (E) levator ani muscle

46. The space of Retzius refers to which of the following?

    (A) potential retropubic space anterior to the bladder and posterior to the pubis
    (B) the narrow cul-de-sac between the anterior surface of the body of the uterus and the upper surface of the bladder
    (C) peritoneum on the body of the posterior uterus that extends down to cover the posterior vaginal fornix and upward from there to overlie the rectum
    (D) personal space needed by Retzius for emotional comfort
    (E) the space directly beneath the symphysis pubis between the descending pubic rami

47. You are performing an ultrasound examination on a patient who is being considered to undergo in vitro fertilization. In order to harvest oocytes, the reproductive endocrinologist must be able to identify the position of the patient's ovaries by ultrasound scanning. Which of the following statements is true regarding ovum retrieval?

    (A) Distortion of the normal pelvic anatomy by prior endometriosis or pelvic infection will make the collection of oocytes impossible.
    (B) A retroverted uterus or an enlarged uterus (size greater than 7 to 8 weeks' gestation) often makes ovum retrieval easier because the uterine corpus will push the ovaries down into the posterior cul-de-sac.
    (C) Despite changes in pelvic anatomy due to disease processes or adhesions, the ovaries can generally be visualized on ultrasound examination as overlying the iliac vessels on either side of the pelvis.
    (D) Only in rare cases of extreme abnormalities in the pelvis are oocytes retrieved transvaginally using a needle aspiration with ultrasound guidance.

48. A patient develops a neurologic disease that destroys components of S2,3,4 bilaterally. What clinical manifestation would you expect the patient to have as a result?

    (A) inability to abduct her thigh
    (B) rectal incontinence
    (C) painless menses
    (D) labor without pain

49. A 56-year-old woman comes to your office for a yearly examination. During physical examination, you notice that her left breast has a 2-cm area of retraction in the upper-outer quadrant that can be seen by simple inspection. What is the most likely diagnosis?

   (A) Mondor's disease

   (B) benign fibroadenoma

   (C) fibrocystic change

   (D) breast cancer

50. A woman who is 32 weeks' pregnant comes in complaining of lumps in her breasts. These lumps are multiple in number and on inspection are within the areola. By palpation they seem to be uniform in size, nontender, and soft. What is the most likely diagnosis?

   (A) Mondor's disease

   (B) Montgomery's follicles

   (C) inflammatory breast carcinoma

   (D) fibrocystic breast changes

   (E) lactiferous deciduosis of pregnancy

51. During mastectomy surgery, which of the following complications is most likely?

   (A) necrosis of the breast from ligation of an intercostal artery in the supra-areolar area

   (B) massive hemorrhage from an injury to the brachial plexus

   (C) damage to the long thoracic nerve (nerve of Bell), resulting in a "winged" scapula

   (D) spread of tumor into the contralateral breast from medial dissection of the involved breast

52. A 33-year-old infertility patient has incapacitating midline dysmenorrhea. Hormonal management has been unsuccessful and she gets no relief from analgesics, yet she wishes to retain her uterus in hope of becoming pregnant. A presacral neurectomy, removing the nerve directly adherent to the concavity of the sacrum (the presacral nerve), may be performed for relief of midline pain. What is the most common serious intraoperative complication of this operation?

   (A) accidental ligation of the inferior mesenteric artery, resulting in bowel necrosis

   (B) ureteral injury

   (C) hemorrhage from the internal iliac artery

   (D) bowel and bladder dysfunction

   (E) hemorrhage from the middle sacral artery or veins

53. A woman has a radical hysterectomy and pelvic lymphadenectomy for Stage I carcinoma of the cervix. After surgery she complains that she cannot adduct her left leg and there is an absence of sensation on the medial aspect of her left thigh. How could you explain this anatomically?

   (A) injury to the obturator nerve

   (B) femoral nerve injury

   (C) hematoma in the pouch of Douglas

   (D) injury to the uterosacral nerve

54. During delivery of a first twin a very tight nuchal cord is reduced from the baby's neck by clamping and dividing it. After this, the second twin (as yet unborn) develops severe fetal distress. Of the following, what is the most likely mechanism for the distress in the second twin?

   (A) a twin-to-twin transfusion before birth

   (B) the second twin may no longer be connected to its placenta

   (C) placenta previa in the second twin

   (D) amniotic fluid embolism

DIRECTIONS (Questions 55 and 56): Each of the numbered items or incomplete statements in this section is followed by answers or by completions of the statement. Select the answers or completions that may apply.

55. Which four of the following ligaments are attached to the uterus?

   (A) uterosacral

   (B) broad

   (C) round

   (D) cardinal

   (E) Cooper's

56. The pelvic peritoneum covers which four of the following?

(A) fimbria of the fallopian tube

(B) uterine fundus

(C) round ligament

(D) uterorectal pouch of Douglas

(E) uterosacral ligament

DIRECTIONS (Questions 57 through 92): Each set of questions in this section consists of a list of lettered options followed by several numbered items. For each numbered item, select the ONE lettered option that is most closely associated with it. Each lettered option may be selected once, more than once, or not at all.

Questions 57 through 60

Ligaments of the pelvis are important for their attachment and support. They are often used in the surgical repair of pelvic relaxation.

(A) a thick band of fibers filling the angle created by the pubic rami

(B) passes from the anterior superior iliac spine to the pubic tubercle

(C) triangular and extends from the lateral border of the sacrum to the ischial spine

(D) attaches to the crest of the ilium and the posterior iliac spines superiorly with an inferior attachment to the ischial tuberosity

57. Sacrospinous ligament

58. Sacrotuberous ligament

59. Ilioinguinal ligament

60. Arcuate ligament

Questions 61 through 66

(A) obturator foramen

(B) greater sciatic foramen

(C) lesser sciatic foramen

(D) sacrospinous ligament

(E) pudendal (Alcock's) canal

(F) sacral foramina

61. The piriformis muscle, gluteal vessels, and posterior femoral cutaneous nerves pass through this structure.

62. Formed by the superior and inferior pubic rami and covered by a central membrane through which a nerve, artery, and vein pass.

63. The internal pudendal vessels and pudendal nerve exit the pelvis but then re-enter through this structure.

64. Divides and demarcates the greater and lesser sciatic foramen.

65. Has four anterior and four posterior openings through which small nerves pass.

66. A sheath of fascia on the lateral wall of the ischiorectal fossa containing vessels and nerve.

Questions 67 through 71

(A) male pelvis

(B) female pelvis

67. Parallel sidewalls and a round inlet.

68. The bones are comparatively lighter, shorter, less dense, more pliable, and less tightly connected.

69. The joints are larger and less mobile.

70. The sacrum is wider and shorter and the pubic arch broader.

71. The internal diameters are generally 0.5 to 2.5 cm smaller.

Questions 72 through 77

(A) anterior hypogastric nerve (T12)

(B) posterior iliac nerve (T12–L1)

(C) ilioinguinal nerve (L1)

(D) genitofemoral nerve (L1–2)

(E) the pudendal nerve (S2,3,4)

(F) terminal branch of the pudendal nerve

72. Mons veneris and anterior labia majora

73. Gluteal area

74. Anterior and medial labia majora

75. Deep labial structures

76. Main innervation of the labia

77. Clitoris

Questions 78 through 84

   (A) Battledore placenta
   (B) bipartite placenta
   (C) circumvallate placenta
   (D) multiple-pregnancy placenta
   (E) placenta accreta
   (F) placenta previa
   (G) succenturiate lobe

78. A small central chorionic plate surrounded by a thick whitish ring, associated with increased rates of perinatal bleeding and fetal death

79. An accessory cotyledon

80. Divided into two lobes

81. Umbilical cord inserted at the placental margin

82. Placenta abnormally adherent to the myometrium

83. Placenta covers the cervical os

84. May be two distinct entities or fused

Questions 85 through 89

   (A) midline incision
   (B) Pfannenstiel incision
   (C) Maylard incision
   (D) Cherny incision
   (E) paramedian incision

85. Opens the abdomen through the linea alba and can be extended from the symphysis pubis to the xiphoid without dividing the muscles of the abdomen.

86. Divides all layers of the lower abdominal wall transversely, including the muscles.

87. A transverse incision caudal to the rectus muscles, dividing the fascial attachment of the rectus to the symphysis but not dividing the muscles.

88. The skin is incised lateral to the anatomic midline, while the rectus sheath and muscles are divided in the anatomic midline.

89. A low transverse incision extended downward and through the anterior rectus fascia, with the anterior rectus sheath separated from the underlying muscles, from the pubis to near the level of the umbilicus.

Questions 90 to 92

For each of the following postoperative patients with areas of skin anesthesia, pain, and/or muscle weakness, select the most likely cause.

   (A) electrolyte imbalance
   (B) obturator nerve injury
   (C) pudendal nerve injury
   (D) femoral nerve injury
   (E) disruption of peripheral (skin) nerves
   (F) ilioinguinal nerve injury
   (G) spinal cord injury
   (H) sciatic nerve injury
   (I) diabetes

90. A 56-year-old white woman who had paravaginal suspension and Burch procedure 2 days ago complains of pain over the right mons pubis, right labia, and right medial thigh.

91. A 36-year-old patient who underwent a total abdominal hysterectomy for uterine fibroids complains of weakness of her left leg and numbness of her left anterior medial thigh.

92. A patient, following a pelvic lymphadenectomy for cervical cancer, complains of some numbness in the medial thigh. On examination, she is found to have full range of motion of her leg, but weakness to adduction.

Answers and Explanations

1. **(D)** Most pelvises in U.S. women are gynecoid, but they may be of a mixed type (for instance, having a gynecoid forepelvis and an anthropoid posterior pelvis). The obstetrician has to judge the capacity of the pelvis on the basis of its total configuration, including midplane and outlet capacities, and always in relation to the size and position of the fetus.

2. **(A)** From the pubic tubercle to the anterior superior iliac spine, the thickened lower margin of the fascial aponeurosis forms the inguinal ligament. This aponeurosis of the external oblique muscle fuses with its counterpart from the opposite side and with the underlying internal oblique fascia. Cooper's ligament is a thickening of fascia along the pubic bone. The linea alba is in the midline and the round ligament attaches to the uterus.

3. **(D)** The superficial inguinal ring is just cephalad to the pubic tubercle, and just lateral to it the deep inguinal ring passes through the transversalis fascia. The connection of these rings forms the inguinal canal. The round ligament, the ilioinguinal nerve, and the processus vaginalis pass out of the abdomen through this canal (as does the spermatic cord in the male). Gartner's ducts are found in the lateral walls of the vagina. One would not normally find a cyst of the processus vaginalis (cyst of the canal of Nuck).

4. **(B)** The pelvis surrounds the birth passage, provides attachment for muscles and fascia, and includes the ilium, ischium, pubis, sacrum, and coccyx. The ilium, the ischium, and the pubic bone compose the innominate bone.

5. **(E)** The ischial tuberosities bear the weight of a seated human. The ischium serves as an attachment for the obturator internus muscle, which in turn forms the attachment of the levator ani muscle.

6. **(B)** The true pelvis has three planes: inlet, midplane, and outlet. It is made up of the paired ileum, ischium, and pubic bones, and the single sacrum and coccyx. The true pelvis is caudad to the false pelvis, which lies between the paired ileum wings. Its inlet is usually gynecoid.

7. **(C)** The sacrum is formed from five or six fused vertebrae. The uppermost anterior portion is called the promontory or sacral promontory. The obstetrical conjugate is the clinical term applied to an estimate of the anterior–posterior adequacy of the pelvic inlet. The pelvic surface of the sacrum is concave, thus facilitating internal and external rotation of the fetus during delivery. The distalmost portion of the sacrum is fused with the three to five vertebrae that make up the coccyx. The sacrococcygeal junction is relatively inflexible, and as a result may be broken at the time of vaginal birth, resulting in severe coccydynia (pain) in some cases. The sacrum seldom obstructs delivery unless it is flat, rather than concave.

8. **(D)** The false pelvis or pelvis major lies

above the linea terminalis. It seldom affects obstetric management, and measurements of the iliac crest flare do not usually aid in determining the size of the true pelvis. An important measurable indicator of the size of the true pelvis is the interspinous diameter.

9. **(B)** The obstetric conjugate is the shortest line from the inside of the symphysis to the most prominent point on the front two segments of the sacrum. It defines what is often the smallest diameter of the pelvic inlet. It should be estimated during clinical examination (pelvimetry) and considered whenever evaluating a pelvis for possible cephalopelvic disproportion, especially during abnormalities of labor. It differs from the true conjugate, which is measured from the top of the symphysis, and also from the diagonal conjugate, which is measured clinically from the bottom of the symphysis to the sacral promontory. The bi-ischial diameter is on the pelvic outlet.

10. **(A)** Layers at the midline of the abdominal wall, 2 cm below the umbilicus, that would be incised or separated are: skin, subcutaneous fat, superficial fascia (Camper's), deep fascia (Scarpa's), and the fascial muscle coverings (anterior rectus sheath). The rectus muscles would be separated and the deep fascial layer (posterior rectus sheath), preperitoneal fat, and peritoneum would be incised. The posterior rectus sheath is only present cephalad to the arcuate line. Camper's is the most superficial fascia and transversus abdominal muscle would not be found in the midline (see Figure 1–1).

11. **(D)** The diagonal conjugate is the most important clinical measurement in pelvimetry. It is used not only to estimate the size of the pelvic inlet but also as a factor in determining the pelvic type and overall pelvic size. Twelve centimeters is usually adequate to allow delivery of a normal-sized infant if the position is good and the rest of the pelvis is also normal.

12. **(B)** The joint between the two pubic bones is the pubic symphysis. It is not a stable joint. Joints between the bones of the pelvis, such as the sacroiliac and sacrococcygeal joints, are called synarthroses. They have limited motion but do become more mobile and even separate a bit during pregnancy. The relaxation is attributed to the hormone relaxin. The piriformis is a muscle.

13. **(E)** The true pelvis in the female is a cylindrical canal with parallel sidewalls, formed by the symphysis and pubic bones anteriorly: the pubic rami and ischium laterally, and the sacrum and coccyx posteriorly. The plane of its outlet is shaped like an irregular diamond consisting of an anterior triangle and a posterior triangle. The anterior triangle is bounded by the symphysis and pubic rami (pubic arch) and the posterior triangle by the ischial tuberosities, sacrotuberous ligaments, and the coccyx (see Figure 1–2).

14. **(A)** The perineum is a term that has been used to describe the entire area between the thighs from the symphysis to the coccyx, bounded inferiorly by the skin and superiorly by the levator muscles of the pelvic diaphragm.

15. **(B)** The escutcheon, or configuration of the pubic hair on the mons veneris and lower abdomen, is generally an inverted triangle in the female. It is considered a secondary sex characteristic. The male pattern (a diamond shape extending upward toward the umbilicus) may exist in 25% of women. Sometimes a male-pattern escutcheon in the female may be associated with increased levels of androgens.

16. **(D)** The vestibule is an area enclosed by the labia minora. Bartholin's glands, sometimes called the major vestibular glands, open into the posterior vestibule. These glands are prone to infection with resulting occlusion of the ducts and the formation of grossly enlarged tender cysts.

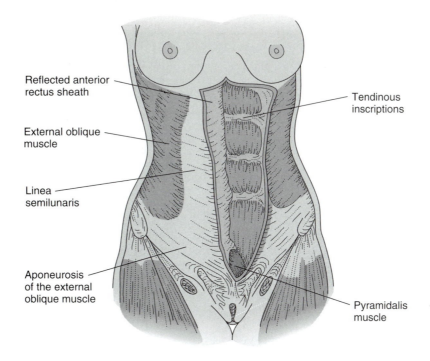

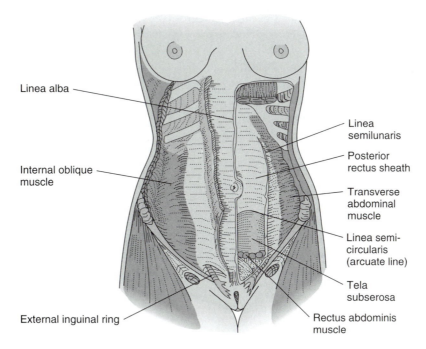

Figure 1–1. Abdominal wall musculature.
(Reproduced, with permission, from DeCherney AH, Nathan L. *Current Obstetric and Gynecologic Diagnosis and Treatment,* 9th ed. New York: McGraw-Hill, 2003.)

17. **(D)** The hymen is a membrane that may cover all or part of the vaginal opening just above the vestibule. It may vary from being only small integumental remnants (known as myrtiform caruncles), to being perforated with one or many openings of various sizes, to being completely closed (imperforate hymen) and require surgical intervention to al-

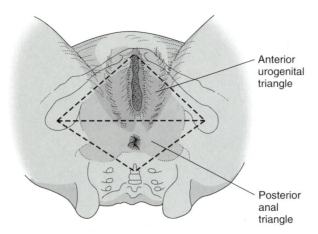

Figure 1–2. Urogenital and anal triangles. (Reproduced, with permission, from DeCherney AH, Nathan L. *Current Obstetric and Gynecologic Diagnosis and Treatment,* 9th ed. New York: McGraw-Hill, 2003.)

low menstruum to drain. The presence of myrtiform caruncles are not pathognomonic of prior vaginal penetration (e.g., intercourse or childbirth). They are of no pathologic significance.

18. **(B)** The clitoris consists of two crura, a short body, and the glans clitoris with overlying skin called the prepuce. It is attached to the pubic bone by a suspensory ligament. Within the shaft are corpora cavernosa consisting of erectile tissue (loose in structure) that engorges with blood, causing erection and enlargement (two times usual size) during sexual excitement. The clitoris and prepuce are the primary areas of erotic stimulation in most women. The prepuce has the most innervation, which usually comes from a terminal branch of the pudendal nerve in most women. Some women, however, have alternate innervations and, in a few, innervation is sparse.

19. **(C)** The muscles of the external genitalia are the ischiocavernosus, bulbocavernosus, superficial transverse perineal, and external anal sphincter. The paired bulbocavernosus muscles surround the distal vagina and vestibule on each side. The muscle originates on the perineal body and inserts into the fibrous tissue dorsal to the clitoris. It surrounds the crura of the clitoris and with the

ischiocavernosus muscle contributes to the voluntary urethral sphincter, but it is not a sphincter. The ischiocavernosus muscle takes origin from the ischial tuberosity and inferior ischial ramus and inserts under the pubic symphysis on each side. Each clitoral crura is covered by the ipsilateral ischiocavernosus muscle. Contraction of these muscles allows arterial blood to flow into the body of the clitoris but inhibits venous outflow, thereby maintaining clitoral erection.

The superficial transverse perineal muscle is a muscle of the external genitalia and arises from the ischial tuberosity and inferior ischial ramus. It inserts into the central tendon between the posterior vagina and anterior rectum, referred to as the perineal body. The perineal body serves as a central connection for all the superficial muscles of the external genitalia and also for the muscles of the anus and anal canal. The deep transverse perineal, the levators, and the gluteus muscles are deep to the external genitalia and the sartorious is a muscle of the thigh (see Figure 1–3).

20. **(C)** The vagina is lined by squamous epithelium, which excretes lubricating fluid. It does not actively secrete but it does distend during sexual arousal. It is a 7- to 10-cm canal connecting the internal and external genitalia as it passes from the vestibule to the uterine cervix. It is a hollow, distensible, fibromuscular tube with the apex (vault) having an H-shaped lumen and the external opening being flattened in the dorsal–ventral dimension. The body of the vaginal tube is flat in its normal resting state. The lower one quarter lies in close proximity to the rectum posteriorly, separated only by the anal sphincter and perineal body. Its axis in the midportion is nearly parallel to the lower sacrum. Here it is surrounded and supported by fibers of the bulbocavernosus, posterior levator ani muscles, and the rectovaginal septum.

The upper portion of the vagina bulges outward to form what are referred to as fornices (anterior, posterior, and lateral) at the point where it joins the cervix. The posterior wall is approximately 2 cm longer than the

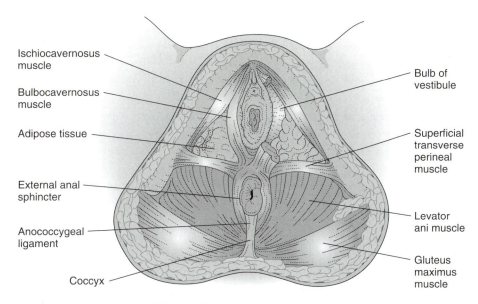

Figure 1–3. Inferior pelvic musculature.
(Reproduced, with permission, from DeCherney AH, Nathan L. *Current Obstetric and Gynecologic Diagnosis and Treatment,* 9th ed. New York: McGraw-Hill, 2003.)

anterior wall. The posterior fornix is adjacent to the peritoneal pouch (posterior cul-de-sac, retrouterine space, or pouch of Douglas) directly behind the uterus.

21. **(A)** The size of the cervix and corpus changes with age and hormonal status; so does the ratio of cervix to corpus. The infant uterus is only 2.5 to 3 cm in total length, and the cervix is larger than the corpus. With aging, the size of the uterus changes, as does the ratio of cervix to corpus length. The normal adult uterus is 7 to 10 cm long.

22. **(B)** Nabothian cysts are also called retention cysts because they are full of mucus from the blocked crypts. They are benign and need no specific therapy. Their appearance is characteristic both grossly and through the colposcope. Seldom is there any need for biopsy.

23. **(C)** The uterus has a body (corpus), composed mainly of smooth muscle, and a cervix, composed mainly of connective and elastic tissues, that are joined by a transitional portion (isthmus). It is an estrogen-dependent organ measuring about 7.5 cm long by 5 cm in width, with a 4-cm anterior-to-posterior diameter. After puberty the

uterus weighs about 50 g in the nullipara and 70 g in the multipara. It lies between the bladder anteriorly and the pouch of Douglas in front of the rectum posteriorly, with the cervical portion extending from the intraperitoneal area into the vagina. The opening at the distal tip of the cervix is called the external os. It is connected by the cervical canal to the internal os, which is located just below the endometrial cavity.

24. **(A)** The cervix protrudes into the fornix of the vagina, and the ovaries are intraperitoneal; therefore, they are found cephalad to the cervix. The round ligaments are attached to the uterus anterior to the attachment of the fallopian tubes. Anteflexion implies a sharp angle between the cervix and the fundus of the uterus, which is bent anteriorly. This is a common position of the uterus, though it can also be midposition or retroflexed. These are all normal positions of the uterus. It is important to recognize which way the uterine body is flexed so that you do not perforate the lower uterine segment while sounding or dilating the cervix. The uterus is normally mobile and if it is not, adhesions or tumor may be present.

25. (D) The cardinal ligaments are also called the transverse cervical ligaments, or Mackenrodt's ligaments, and are considered part of the uterosacral ligament complex. These ligaments serve as the major support for the apex of the vagina and are severed at the time of hysterectomy. Once divided at hysterectomy, vaginal vault prolapse becomes more likely. The broad ligaments are mainly peritoneum and the round ligaments mainly muscle. Neither provide much support.

26. (A) Fallopian tubes are a conduit from the peritoneal to the uterine cavity. Each tube is covered by peritoneum and consists of three layers: serosa, muscularis, and mucosa. They traverse the superior portion of the broad ligament attached by a mesentery (mesosalpinx). It has four distinct areas in its 8- to 12-cm length: the portion that runs through the uterine wall (interstitial or cornual portion), the portion immediately adjacent to the uterus (isthmic portion), the midportion of the tube (ampulla), and the distal portion containing the fingerlike fimbriae that sweep the ovum into the infundibulum of the tube. The fimbriae are intraperitoneal. The tubal lumen becomes increasingly more complex as it approaches the ovary. In tubal reanastomoses, the greatest success is attained when isthmic–isthmic or isthmic–ampullary regions can be reapproximated. The longest of the fimbriae (the fimbriae ovarica) is attached to the ovary.

27. (A) The urogenital diaphragm is immediately deep to the muscles of the external genitalia. It consists of a tough fibrous fascial membrane inferiorly, covering the triangular area under the pubic arch and extending posteriorly to the ischial tuberosities. It is penetrated by the urethra and vagina in the female. Just cephalad to this fascia are the deep transverse perineal muscle and the urethral sphincter mechanism. The superior fascia of the urogenital diaphragm is attached tightly to these muscles and is just caudad to the levator ani muscle. The urogenital diaphragm supplies support for the anterior vagina, urethra, and trigone of the bladder. The area en-compassing the urogenital diaphragm and the superficial and deep perineal spaces is referred to as the urogenital triangle.

28–29. (28-B, 29-D) The pelvic diaphragm (also called the pelvic floor) is made up of the levator ani muscle, which has three portions (iliococcygeus, pubococcygeus, puborectalis), and the coccygeus. It is connected to the pelvic sidewall by its attachment to the obturator internus muscle at the arcus tendineus. The pelvic diaphragm provides support and closure for the intraperitoneal cavity caudally just as the thoracic diaphragm provides closure in the cephalad direction. It is covered by fascia on both sides and innervated from S2,3,4. The potential spaces through which the vagina, urethra, and rectum pass are the possible sites of pelvic prolapse (see Figure 1–4).

30. (C) A surgeon has a little more than a 1-cm space between the cervix and the ureter when performing a hysterectomy. Just lateral to the cervix is a high-risk area for injury to the ureter during gynecologic surgery. The importance of dissecting away the bladder, staying close to the cervix, and not placing clamps too far laterally or inserting wide sutures is apparent. At times it is necessary to dissect enough to allow visualization of both ureters prior to ligation of the uterine arteries.

31. (D) One can remember the ureter's distal course posterior to the uterine artery by recalling that "water runs under the bridge." Do not confuse the uterine artery–ureteral relationship with the iliac artery–ureteral relationship. In the pelvis the ureter is always anterior and medial to the iliac arteries. The position of the ureter in relation to the uterine artery makes it particularly vulnerable at the time of hysterectomy.

32. (E) The urethra is a hollow, multilayered tube, 2.5 to 5 cm long in the female, as opposed to being about 20 cm long in the male. It connects the bladder with the outside world. The proximal portion begins at the

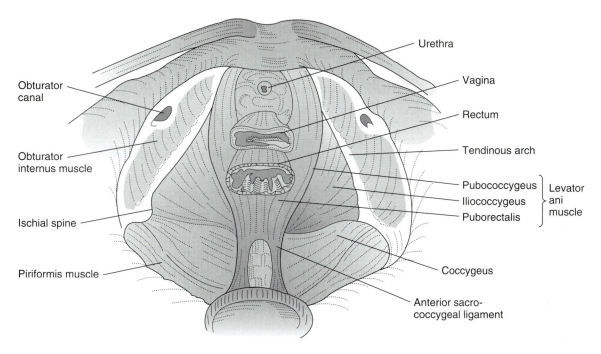

Figure 1–4.

junction of the bladder base at the lowest portion of the trigone. It contains a functional sphincter mechanism but not a true anatomic sphincter. It has a higher intrinsic resting pressure than the bladder in normal women, thus helping to maintain continence. The lower two thirds of the urethra is just anterior to the anterior vaginal wall.

33. **(A)** The upper two thirds of the vagina is largely innervated by sympathetic fibers from the presacral nerve (which originates from the sympathetic nerve trunks T11 to L2) after it divides into the hypogastric plexus and parasympathetic fibers from the hypogastric plexus and pelvic splanchnic nerves. The upper vagina has few touch or pain fibers. The lower one third of the vagina has both pain and touch fibers, carried by afferent autonomic fibers in the same plexuses, and is very sensitive to stimulation.

34. **(D)** The spinal cord ends within the dura at about L2. The dural space ends at about S2. The filum terminal and cauda equina extend within the dura for some distance after the spinal cord ends. Caudal anesthesia inter-

cepts the spinal nerves after they emerge from the dural space. When giving spinal anesthesia, one should recognize that one usually enters the subarachnoid space at or below the termination of the spinal cord. The cauda equina extends for some distance within the dura. This relationship allows for effective anesthesia and analgesia with minimal risk of injury to the spinal cord.

35. **(A)** The arterial supply of the vagina comes from the internal pudendal, cervicovaginal branch of the uterine artery, inferior vesical, and middle hemorrhoidal arteries. Venous drainage of the vagina is accomplished through an extensive plexus rather than through well-defined channels. The same is true of the surrounding venous drainage of the bladder. The lymphatic drainage is such that the superior portion of the vagina (along with the cervix) drains into the external iliac nodes, the middle portion into the internal iliac nodes, and the lower third mainly into the superficial inguinal nodes and internal iliac nodes (like the vulva). The vagina is richly supplied with blood and lymphatics.

36. **(A)** The lymphatic drainage of the vulva has a superficial component (draining the anterior two thirds of the vulva) and a deep drainage system (draining the posterior one third of the vulva). The superficial drainage is to the superficial inguinal lymph nodes, and the deep drainage is to the deep inguinal nodes, external iliac, and femoral nodes. The posterior aspects of the labia may drain to the lymphatic plexus surrounding the rectum. These anatomic relationships for lymphatic drainage are of great significance in the treatment of vulvar cancers.

37. **(C)** Cloquet's lymph node is the first deep inguinal lymph node that is quite constant in location medial to the femoral vein. It is the sentinel node (first deep lymph node encountered) in the dissection done during radical vulvectomy. If it is free of tumor on frozen section, many feel dissection of the ipsilateral deep pelvic lymph nodes is not necessary.

38. **(A)** The major blood supply to the vulva is from the internal pudendal or its branches, the inferior hemorrhoidal and perineal. Some is provided by the external pudendal artery, which is from the femoral. There is good collateral circulation to the vulva, and either the hypogastric or pudendal artery can be occluded on either side without compromise to the vulva. The pelvic circulation provides communication so that right- and left-sided vessels may provide accessory flow to the contralateral side.

39. **(C)** The normal placenta is a reddish, rounded, and discoid organ about 15 to 20 cm in diameter and about 2 to 4 cm thick. It weighs about one sixth of what the term infant does. About 80% of the placenta is fetal in origin and 20% maternal in origin (decidua basalis, remnants of blood vessels).

40. **(D)** Irregular grooves, not elevated septae, separate the placenta into its cotyledons. The maternal side of the placenta at birth will be irregular, deep red, and beefy. The fetal side will be shiny and smooth with the membranes identifiable and large vessels (branches of the fetal umbilical vessels) traversing its surface. The villous surface (portion for exchange) may measure up to 12 m².

41. **(D)** Chorion laeve is the proper designation of the chorionic membranes at term. The chorion frondosum refers to the shaggy placental membranes with obvious villi that are seen early in gestation. Chorion laeve means "bald chorion."

42. **(C)** The breast contains glandular and ductal tissue, fibrous stroma binding the individual lobes together, and fatty tissue within and between the lobes. Each breast consists of 12 to 20 conical lobes, with the base of the lobe resting on the ribs and the apex under the areola. Each lobe consists of a group of lobules and many lactiferous ducts. The ducts unite to form a major duct that drains each lobe. Alveoli increase in size and number during pregnancy, preparing for lactation with secretion of milk proteins and lipid. About 80 to 85% of a normal breast is fat.

43. **(D)** The tail of Spence is the eponym given to the triangular, tail-shaped tongue of breast tissue that extends into the axilla. It ends in close apposition to the axillary lymph nodes, blood vessels, and nerves.

44. **(D)** The deep perineal space contains the deep transverse perineal muscle with its fascia, which is called the urogenital diaphragm. It is part of the main supporting structure of the pelvic organs and provides a sphincter action for the urethra. The deep transverse perineal muscle is in the deep perineal space and the levator ani is part of the pelvic diaphragm, which is further cephalad (see Figure 1–5).

45. **(C)** The superficial perineal space contains the ischiocavernosus muscle. Other contents are the bulbocavernosus and superficial transverse perineal muscles, Bartholin's glands, and bulbs of the vestibule.

46. **(A)** The prevesical or retropubic space (space of Retzius) is a potential space that is crossed

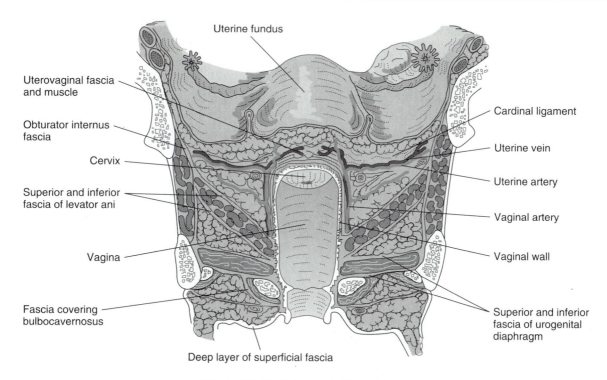

Figure 1–5. Fascial support of the pelvis.
(Reproduced, with permission, from DeCherney AH, Nathan L. *Current Obstetric and Gynecologic Diagnosis and Treatment,* 9th ed. New York: McGraw-Hill, 2003.)

by the transverse vesical fold. It lies anterior to the bladder and behind the pubis. It is generally closed (except when artificially opened during retropubic surgery to restore urinary incontinence). It contains mainly retropubic areolar tissue, fat, and large veins. The narrow cul-de-sac between the anterior surface of the body of the uterus and the upper surface of the bladder is the prevesical space or anterior cul-de-sac. The posterior cul-de-sac (or pouch of Douglas) refers to the evagination created by the peritoneum on the body of the posterior uterus that extends down to cover the posterior vaginal fornix and upward from there to overlie the rectum. The posterior vaginal fornix is the thin structure between the abdominal and vaginal cavities and makes a clinically useful axis to the peritoneal cavity through the vagina (to aspirate blood or pus for diagnosis or therapy on it). The posterior vaginal fornix with its mucosa, thin muscle wall, and serosa is the only structure between the abdominal and vaginal cavities and makes a clinically useful access to the peritoneal cavity through the vagina (to

aspirate blood or pus for diagnosis or therapy).

47. **(C)** Reproductive endocrinologists generally use a needle to aspirate the ovarian follicles to obtain oocytes. This is most commonly done as an office procedure under ultrasound guidance. The technique of aspiration is generally unaffected by previous pelvic disease. In fact, the ovary that is immobilized by pelvic adhesions may be an easier target to hit than one that is freely mobile. Since the ovaries are anatomically below the uterine corpus and just above the cul-de-sac, transvaginal aspiration is the method of choice for most clinicians. On routine scanning for ovarian position, the ovaries almost always are found to overlie the great vessels of the pelvis. These vessels are therefore used as a landmark during pelvic scanning.

48. **(B)** The S2,3,4 innervation, if damaged at the level of the spinal cord, is most likely to produce incontinence of bladder or bowel. The patient may also have decreased vulvar sen-

sation. Uterine pain with labor or menses is mediated by the sympathetic and parasympathetic system.

49. **(D)** The deep surface of the breast lies on the fascia covering the chest muscles. The fascia of the chest is condensed into many bands (Cooper's ligaments) that support the breast in its normal position on the chest wall. It is the distortion of these ligaments caused by infiltrative tumors that results in the "dimpling" appearance of the breast associated with malignancy. At age 56, the most likely cause of this is cancer. Fibroadenomas are usually found in younger women, and neither fibrocystic change nor fibroadenomas usually cause significant dimpling (see Figure 1–6). Mondor's disease is a residual of venous thrombophlebitis of the breast; it is rare.

50. **(B)** These multiple, small, elevated nodules, beneath which lie the sebaceous glands, are called Montgomery's follicles. The glands are responsible for lubrication of the areola. They may hypertrophy markedly in pregnancy. The small openings of the lactiferous ducts are situated on the nipple.

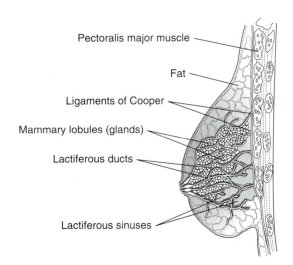

Pectoralis major muscle

Fat

Ligaments of Cooper

Mammary lobules (glands)

Lactiferous ducts

Lactiferous sinuses

Figure 1–6. Sagittal section of the female breast. (Reproduced, with permission, from DeCherney AH, Nathan L. *Current Obstetric and Gynecologic Diagnosis and Treatment*, 9th ed. New York: McGraw-Hill, 2003.)

51. **(C)** The blood supply of the breast consists of several sources, including the internal thoracic artery, anterior intercostal arteries, pectoral arteries, external mammary arteries, and other perforating branches. The upper breast has a much greater blood supply than the lower breast. The brachial plexus is a group of nerves; cutting one may cause neurologic damage but not hemorrhage. Injury to the long thoracic nerve does happen—fortunately, in less than 2% of cases. Unilateral mastectomy does not increase the risk of cancer in the other breast any more than the increased risk due to having the unilateral cancer in the first place.

52. **(E)** The middle sacral artery is a direct terminal branch of the aorta. It is often encountered during dissection of the presacral space. Bleeding is difficult to control, because these vessels are firmly attached directly over the hollow of the sacrum, and sacral veins may retract into the bone. The inferior mesenteric artery, the internal iliac artery, and the ureter are all far away from the site of resection.

53. **(A)** The injury is to the obturator nerve, which has both a sensory component on the medial thigh and a motor component to adduct the leg. At the time of the lymphadenectomy, the obturator nerve is often exposed. Just below it in the obturator space are many venous plexuses. If bleeding becomes active in this area, efforts to control it could damage the obturator nerve. This same type of nerve injury can also happen in pregnancy secondary to its compression by the fetus against the pelvic floor.

54. **(B)** In this case placenta previa can be ruled out because the first twin has already been delivered through the cervix. If there had been a severe twin–twin transfusion, it would be unlikely to manifest itself at this time in the pregnancy. An amniotic fluid embolism does not affect the fetus but rather the mother. That leaves us with a cord accident. Using our knowledge of the placenta, we know that there may be one placenta or two,

but we know that both babies have their own umbilical cord. However, the cord wrapped around the neck of the first twin might belong to the second twin!

55. **(A, B, C, D)** The main ligaments for uterine support are the thickened caudal portion of the broad ligament, called the cardinal and the uterosacral ligaments. The round ligament does not provide much physical support. Division of these ligaments at the time of hysterectomy may predispose to vaginal prolapse. Cooper's ligaments, which are not attached to the uterus, demonstrate one of the problems with anatomic eponyms, as ligaments with the same name are found in the breast.

56. **(B, C, D, E)** Most pelvic structures are retroperitoneal. However, the ostia of the tubes open into the peritoneal cavity, creating a communication between the peritoneal cavity and the external environment via the vagina, uterus, and tubes. This may also serve as a portal of entry for bacteria, which can cause pelvic inflammatory disease.

57–60. **(57-C, 58-D, 59-B, 60-A)** The sacrospinous ligament is triangular and extends from the lateral border of the sacrum to the ischial spine. It is a common landmark in gynecologic (vaginal-suspension operations) and obstetric operations (as a marker both for the midpelvis and for the administration of regional anesthesia). The sacrotuberous ligament attaches superiorly to the posterior crest of the ilium, the posterior iliac spines, and the lateral posterior aspect of the lower sacrum. The inferior attachment is the ischial tuberosity. The ilioinguinal ligament passes from the anterior superior iliac spine to the pubic tubercle. These ligaments are very firm in the nonpregnant patient but in the pregnant patient will soften in response to the hormone relaxin, as will the symphysis and sacroiliac joints. The arcuate ligament is connective tissue that fills the space below the pubic arch (see Figure 1–7).

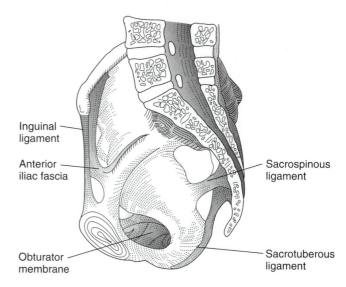

Figure 1–7. Pelvic ligaments.
(Reproduced, with permission, from DeCherney AH, Nathan L. *Current Obstetric and Gynecologic Diagnosis and Treatment,* 9th ed. New York: McGraw-Hill, 2003.)

61–66. **(61-B, 62-A, 63-C, 64-D, 65-F, 66-E)** The superior and inferior pubic rami form the obturator foramen, covered by the obturator membrane with an opening (obturator canal) through which the obturator nerve, artery, and vein pass. The sacrospinous ligament divides and demarcates the greater and lesser sciatic foramina. The piriformis muscle and gluteal vessels pass out of the pelvis into the thigh through the greater sciatic foramen. The sciatic nerve and posterior femoral cutaneous nerves also pass through it. The internal pudendal vessels and pudendal nerve leave the pelvis through the greater sciatic foramen and then enter the perineal region by passing through the lesser sciatic foramen. The obturator internus muscle and its corresponding nerve also pass out of the pelvis through the lesser sciatic foramen. The sacrum has four anterior foramina through which the sacral nerves (S1–4) pass and four posterior foramina through which the small posterior rami of these same nerves pass. The pudendal canal (Alcock's canal) is a sheath of fascia on the lateral wall of the ischiorectal fossa containing the pudendal vessels and nerve.

67–71. (67-B, 68-B, 69-A, 70-B, 71-A) The pelvises of the male and female differ significantly. The pelvis in the female has parallel sidewalls and a round (gynecoid) outlet. The bones are lighter, shorter, less dense, more pliable, and less tightly connected. The joints are smaller and more mobile. The sacrum is wider and shorter and the pubic arch broader. The diameters are generally 0.5 to 2.5 cm larger. These differences facilitate childbirth. Assessment of the pelvic size at prenatal and intrapartum examinations is done by assessing these measurements (clinical pelvimetry). When asked to compare the two types of pelves anatomically, remember that the female pelvis will have those structural characteristics that aid in giving birth.

72–77. (72-A, 73-B, 74-C, 75-D, 76-E, 77-F) The anterior hypogastric nerve (T12) supplies the mons veneris and the anterior labia majora, often with branches of the ilioinguinal and genitofemoral nerve. The posterior iliac nerve supplies the gluteal area. The ilioinguinal nerve supplies the anterior and medial labia majora. The genitofemoral nerve supplies the deep labial structures. The sacral plexus (S2,3,4), largely via the pudendal nerve, supplies the middle and posterior labia. The clitoris is supplied by the terminal branch of the pudendal nerve (see Figure 1–8). There is significant overlap in the perineal nerve distribution.

78–84. (78-C, 79-G, 80-B, 81-A, 82-E, 83-F, 84-D) The placenta can have many configurations. It may be small and constricted by an amniotic ring (circumvallate placenta), which predisposes to prematurity, bleeding, and early delivery. Older multiparas seem to have this predisposition. The succenturiate lobe is an accessory cotyledon. It may not deliver with the rest of the placenta and in such a case can cause significant postpartum hemorrhage. Whoever delivers a baby should therefore carefully inspect for large vessels that seem to run off the edge of the placenta, which suggests the possibility of an accessory lobe.

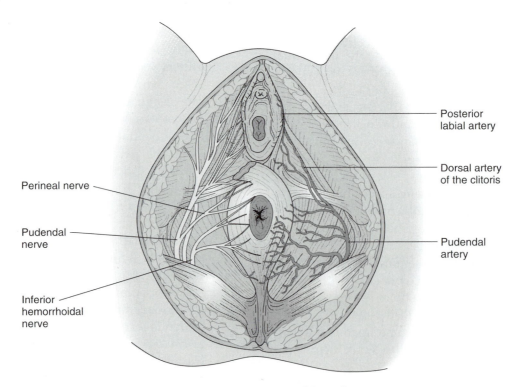

Perineal nerve

Pudendal nerve

Inferior hemorrhoidal nerve

Posterior labial artery

Dorsal artery of the clitoris

Pudendal artery

Figure 1–8. Arteries and nerves of the perineum.
(Reproduced, with permission, from DeCherney AH, Nathan L. *Current Obstetric and Gynecologic Diagnosis and Treatment*, 9th ed. New York: McGraw-Hill, 2003.)

The bipartite placenta, on the other hand, has two more or less equal portions connected by membranes and large vessels: retention of either half can cause major hemorrhage. The Battledore placenta (or marginal insertion of the cord) has a cord that inserts on the edge of the placenta. Placenta accreta (meaning firmly attached) forms when the decidual layer is incompletely developed and firm attachment occurs to the underlying myometrium. Percreta is even more firmly implanted, and increta means the placenta has grown completely through the myometrium. Previous surgery, grand multiparity, prior cesarean section, and placenta previa all predispose to abnormally firm placental adherence. Sometimes hysterectomy is necessary to stop the bleeding from these placental abnormalities. Multiple pregnancy placentas can be single, connected, or even separate.

85–89. **(85-A, 86-C, 87-D, 88-E, 89-B)** During surgery a number of incisions are used. The midline incision opens the abdomen through the linea alba and can be extended from the symphysis pubis to the xiphoid without dividing the muscles of the abdomen. Its advantage is roominess. The Pfannenstiel incision is a low transverse incision extended downward and through the anterior rectus fascia. The anterior rectus sheath is then separated from the underlying muscles to near the level of the umbilicus. The abdominal muscles are then bluntly separated in the midline to allow access to the abdominal cavity. Its advantage is cosmetic. The Maylard incision divides all layers of the lower abdominal wall transversely, including the muscles. The Cherney incision is a transverse incision caudal to the rectus muscles dividing the fascial attachment of the rectus to the symphysis but not dividing the muscles. The latter two combine roominess with cosmetic

result. The paramedian incision is chosen in order to open the skin and the rectus sheath so that the suture lines will not overlap. This was at one time thought to increase the strength and improve the healing of the wound. Probably neither is true. Other abdominal incisions can be used, but those described are the most commonly used in gynecology. The type of incision is chosen in order to provide adequate access and visualization of the surgical site; provide the best result in terms of healing, both in terms of incisional strength and decreasing possible infection; and provide the best cosmetic result.

90. **(F)** The ilioinguinal nerve passes medially to the inguinal ligament and supplies the mons pubis, labia, and medial thigh. Entrapment of the nerve during surgical procedures for incontinence may result in pain over these areas. The pain may occur immediately or within a few days.

91. **(D)** The femoral nerve rises from L2–4 and supplies motor fibers to the quadriceps and sensation to the anterior and medial thigh. The nerve may be compressed by abdominal retractor blades that have impinged on the psoas muscle where the nerve perforates. The nerve can also undergo stretch injury from hip flexion or abduction during vaginal procedures. Either of these can result in pain or numbness or paresthesias over the anterior and medial thigh, as well as weakness of the quadriceps, causing inability to raise the knee and therefore affecting gait.

92. **(B)** Iatrogenic injury to the obturator nerve can cause sensory defects over the medial thigh. As it supplies the medial muscles of the thigh, injury may cause a decrease in ability to adduct. Fortunately, the injury is often transitory or easily compensated.

Histology and Pathology
Questions

93. A pathology report of a vulvar biopsy is returned to you. The epithelium is described as acanthotic. This means

    (A) there is a hyperplasia of keratinocytes in the prickle cell layer (stratum spinosum) thickening the epidermis
    (B) there is increased thickening of the superficial layers of the epidermis
    (C) there are many nucleated cells on the surface of the lesion
    (D) the area of the biopsy is likely to have a clinically "thin" appearance
    (E) the biopsy was likely taken from an area of ulceration

94. Histologically, the labium minus differs from the labium majus in that

    (A) the skin of the labium minus is usually thicker than the skin of the labium majus
    (B) the labium majus normally forms keratin pearls
    (C) the labium minus lacks hair follicles
    (D) adipose tissue is present within the labium minus
    (E) the labium minus does not attach to the fascia of the vulva

95. Which of the following would be most abnormal to find on a biopsy of the vagina in an adult woman?

    (A) bacteria
    (B) a small (3-mm) cyst lined by simple cuboidal epithelium
    (C) a thin keratin layer
    (D) a 3-mm-thick epithelial layer

96. Near the external os of the cervix there is normally a transition from columnar epithelium to

    (A) keratinized epithelium
    (B) squamous epithelium
    (C) transitional epithelium
    (D) cuboidal epithelium
    (E) cervical erosion

97. During routine examination, an asymptomatic multiparous patient is found to have a raised 1-cm cyst on her cervix. The area is biopsied, and clear mucus is extruded. Histologic examination of the specimen shows a cleft of flattened columnar or cuboidal-type cells. This clinical picture would be most compatible with

    (A) herpes cervicitis
    (B) varicella infection
    (C) cervical intraepithelial neoplasia
    (D) Nabothian cyst
    (E) cervical adenosis

98. On a cytologic specimen, herpesvirus infection may be suspected (if not diagnosed) from the presence of

    (A) intranuclear inclusion bodies
    (B) intracytoplasmic inclusions
    (C) copious glassy cytoplasm
    (D) Donovan bodies
    (E) multiple round nucleoli

99. Figure 2–1 illustrates three groups of cells. From their appearance, which would you consider to be most dysplastic?

    (A) group A
    (B) group B
    (C) group C
    (D) groups B and C are equally dysplastic

100. In cytopathology, which of the following changes in cells can be mistaken for malignancy?

    (A) degeneration
    (B) regeneration
    (C) inflammation

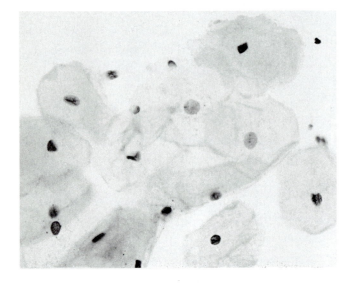

A

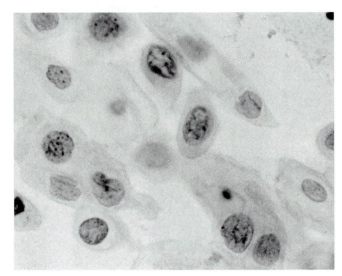

B

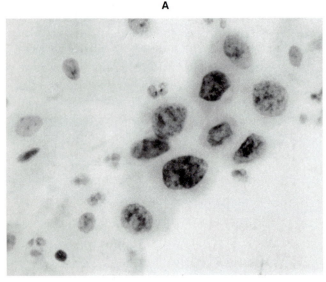

C

Figure 2–1. Cell types.
(Reproduced, with permission, from Stenchever, MA, et al. *Comprehensive Gynecology,* 4th ed. St. Louis, MO: Mosby, 2001: 860, 861, 863.)

(D) atrophy

(E) all of the above

101. During the menstrual cycle the histologic appearance of the endometrium will change significantly. During the first half of the menstrual cycle, the endometrium becomes thicker and rebuilds largely in response to _____. In the second half of the cycle the endometrial arteries become spiraled in appearance, the glands produce vacuoles, and the endometrium becomes more compact. This is in response to _____.

(A) progesterone, estrogen

(B) follicle-stimulating hormone (FSH), luteinizing hormone (LH)

(C) estrogen, progesterone

(D) LH, FSH

(E) gonadotropin-releasing hormone (GnRH), prolactin

102. Endometrium can be "dated" by using which histologic features?

(A) number of arteries per unit surface area in the endometrium

(B) thickness of the endometrium, appearance of the glands, and stromal edema

(C) amount of mucus within the glands

(D) amount of hemorrhage within the glands

(E) width and ciliation of the endometrial glands and the eosinophilic coloration of the basalis

103. Marked cellular atypism, glandular proliferation, and significant mitotic activity of endometrial glands during pregnancy constitute the phenomenon known as

(A) hidradenoma

(B) microcystic glandular hyperplasia

(C) Arias–Stella reaction

(D) Schiller–Duvall bodies

(E) adenomatoid change

104. The term *decidualization* means

(A) derived from cytotrophoblast

(B) derived from syncytiotrophoblast

(C) small, dark-staining cells found in the endometrium during pregnancy

(D) endometrial cells that are proliferating

(E) a response of cells to progesterone

105. The histology of adenomyosis shows

(A) the metaplastic change of glandular epithelium to muscle fibers in the uterus

(B) the same pattern and location as endometriosis

(C) the presence of endometrial glands and stroma deep within uterine muscle

(D) a premalignant change of the endometrium

(E) a premalignant change of the uterine muscle

106. Which of the following best describes leiomyoma of the uterus?

(A) a soft, interdigitating mass of the uterine wall

(B) a premalignant papule of the uterine wall

(C) a rapidly dividing necrotic malignancy

(D) a rounded, smooth, firm, and well-circumscribed mass

(E) erythematous, tender, and hereditary

107. Which of the following is the best description of endometrial hyperplasia?

(A) endometrial glands scattered throughout an atrophic-appearing uterine muscle

(B) increased number of glands with a piling up of their cells and decreased intervening stroma

(C) tightly spiraled endometrial glands with eosinophilic cytoplasm surrounding the arterioles

(D) tortuous glands with a loose, edematous stroma

(E) endometrial glands surrounding a fibrovascular stroma, often with a characteristic central blood vessel

108. The normal lining of the fallopian tube is

   (A) squamous epithelium
   (B) transitional epithelium
   (C) cuboidal epithelium
   (D) columnar epithelium with cilia
   (E) fibrous connective tissue

109. The main purpose of the cilia and mucus in the fallopian tube is to

   (A) transport ova toward the uterus
   (B) transport sperm toward the ovary
   (C) remove the outer coating of the sperm
   (D) remove bacteria from sperm prior to entry into the peritoneal cavity
   (E) stimulate the zygote to divide

110. If an ovary from a menstruating woman was bivalved, the correct layers from the surface to the center would be

   (A) medulla, cortex, germinal epithelium
   (B) cortex, germinal epithelium, medulla
   (C) germinal epithelium, medulla, cortex
   (D) cortex, medulla, germinal epithelium
   (E) germinal epithelium, cortex, medulla

111. The ovaries are covered by a thin layer of epithelium called germinal epithelium. It is called germinal epithelium because

   (A) the germ cells arise from it during fetal life
   (B) it produces germ cells throughout menstrual life
   (C) it protects the ova from bacteria
   (D) at one time it was thought to produce germ cells
   (E) it is made up of germ cells

112. The correct order of cell layers surrounding an ovarian follicle from the oocyte outward is

   (A) zona pellucida, granulosa, theca interna
   (B) granulosa, theca interna, zona pellucida
   (C) theca interna, zona pellucida, granulosa
   (D) theca interna, granulosa, zona pellucida
   (E) zona pellucida, theca interna, granulosa

113. Most of the ovarian follicles that begin to develop at each cycle

   (A) develop and ovulate at sometime during the person's life
   (B) continue to grow, forming follicle cysts
   (C) undergo atresia
   (D) remain to continue their development in the next cycle
   (E) regress to primordial follicles

114. Which of the following ovarian tumors is thought to be derived from the ovarian germinal epithelium?

   (A) dysgerminoma
   (B) fibroma
   (C) theca cell
   (D) endometrioid
   (E) teratoma

115. An involuted corpus luteum becomes a hyalinized mass known as a

   (A) corpus delicti
   (B) corpus granulosa
   (C) graafian follicles
   (D) corpus atretica
   (E) corpus albicans

116. Luteinization refers to the process whereby

   (A) the granulosa cells turn red
   (B) mature granulosa and the theca interna cells become epithelioid and form a corpus luteum
   (C) the ovarian stroma undergoes adipose degeneration prior to ovulation
   (D) the nonovulated follicles undergo fatty degeneration
   (E) none of the above

117. An ovary is removed for frozen section pathologic examination. The ovary is enlarged, with small surface excrescences. Pathologic examination reveals numerous cysts lined by serous epithelium with six to eight cell layers piled on top of one another to form the cyst walls. The cells show marked cytologic atypia, and nests of similar cells are

present in the ovarian stroma. Round laminated calcium bodies are also seen. This histologic description indicates a diagnosis of

(A) normal proliferative phase follicle
(B) corpus luteum cyst
(C) ovarian endometriosis
(D) borderline ovarian carcinoma
(E) cystadenocarcinoma

118. Histologically, an ovarian teratoma is determined to be benign or malignant by the presence of

(A) squamous cells
(B) all three germ cell lines
(C) immature fetal-like cells
(D) neural ectoderm
(E) an ovarian capsule

119. The breast is best described as a/an

(A) female genital organ
(B) modified sweat gland
(C) specialized sex gland
(D) endodermal swelling
(E) endocrine organ

120. Dimpling of the skin of the breast should alert one to the possibility of

(A) pregnancy
(B) weight gain
(C) aging
(D) fibrocystic disease
(E) carcinoma

121. Histologic examination of the normal breast from a postmenopausal woman as compared to the breast from a premenopausal woman would show which of the following?

(A) a decrease in the number and size of acinar glands and ductal elements, with decreased density of the breast parenchyma
(B) an increase in breast size and turgidity because of an increase in the density of the parenchyma

(C) increase in number and size of acinar cells and a widening of the ductal lumens
(D) significant atrophy of the adipose tissue of the breast with little change in the actual breast parenchyma
(E) no significant change in histology

122. The most common pathologic type of breast cancer is

(A) ductal
(B) lobular
(C) Paget's
(D) inflammatory
(E) adenoid cystic

123. Medullary, colloid (mucinous), tubular, and papillary carcinoma of the breast are subtypes of which pathologic type of breast cancer?

(A) ductal
(B) lobular
(C) carcinoma in situ
(D) sarcomatous
(E) Paget's

124. A breast biopsy on a 35-year-old woman shows "atypical epithelial hyperplasia confined within the biopsy site," which means

(A) her biopsy is benign, and she is at no risk for cancer of the breast in the future
(B) her biopsy is benign, but she is at increased risk for developing breast cancer in the future
(C) her biopsy is definitely premalignant, and bilateral prophylactic subcutaneous mastectomy is indicated
(D) her biopsy is malignant, and she will need to undergo radiation therapy but no further surgery since the lump has been removed
(E) her biopsy is malignant, and she should undergo radical mastectomy and sampling of the axillary lymph nodes

125. A 37-year-old woman complains of a painful lump in her breast. The lump is removed, and microscopic examination of the mass shows "microscopic cysts, papillomatosis, fibrosis, and ductal hyperplasia." Which of the following is the most likely diagnosis?

    (A) benign intraductal papilloma
    (B) endometriosis of the breast
    (C) fibrocystic changes
    (D) lobular carcinoma in situ
    (E) infiltrating ductal carcinoma

126. An asymptomatic 24-year-old college student is found to have a 4-cm, very firm mass in her breast that she has not previously noticed. The mass is mobile, smooth, and non-tender in the upper, outer quadrant of her breast. An excision biopsy is performed and shows "a well-circumscribed, fibrous lesion with glands interspersed throughout the body of the tumor." Which of the following is the most likely diagnosis?

    (A) cystosarcoma phyllodes
    (B) macromastia
    (C) mastitis
    (D) fat necrosis
    (E) fibroadenoma

127. Which of the following statements is TRUE?

    (A) Both decidua and trophoblast are of maternal origin.
    (B) Neither decidua nor trophoblast is of maternal origin.
    (C) Decidua is of fetal origin.
    (D) Trophoblast is of maternal origin.
    (E) Decidua is of maternal origin.

128. In the normal placenta, which of the following form after 2 months?

    (A) primary and secondary villi
    (B) a chorionic plate
    (C) syncytium
    (D) septation of the basal plate
    (E) cotyledons

129. As a placenta ages, which of the following changes occur?

    (A) villous branching decreases
    (B) the number of capillaries decreases
    (C) cytotrophoblast decreases
    (D) fibrin is cleared from the intervillous space

130. Histologic grading of a hydatidiform mole

    (A) permits great precision in predicting its future behavior
    (B) is of little use because the individual case prognosis cannot be predicted
    (C) enables one to predict invasion but not embolic metastases
    (D) enables one to predict embolic metastases but not invasion
    (E) enables one to estimate the level of human chorionic gonadotropin (hCG) produced by the tumor

131. Which of the following pathologic features is most helpful in distinguishing complete hydatidiform mole from normal placenta?

    (A) trophoblastic proliferation
    (B) absence of blood vessels
    (C) hydropic degeneration of villi
    (D) cellular atypia
    (E) sex chromatin positivity

DIRECTIONS (Questions 132 and 133): Each of the numbered items or incomplete statements in this section is followed by answers or by completions of the statement. Select the answers or completions that may apply.

132. Biopsy of a vulvar lesion would be most likely to include which four of the following structures?

    (A) epidermis
    (B) papillary dermis
    (C) reticular dermis
    (D) subcutaneous tissue
    (E) deep fascia

133. The histologic composition of the breast would include which four of the following tissue types?

   (A) glands

   (B) ducts

   (C) fibrous stroma

   (D) fat

   (E) skeletal muscle

DIRECTIONS (Questions 134 through 142): Each set of questions in this section consists of a list of lettered options followed by several numbered items. For each numbered item, select the ONE lettered option that is most closely associated with it. Each lettered option may be selected once, more than once, or not at all.

Questions 134 through 137

   (A) molluscum contagiosum

   (B) vulvar intraepithelial neoplasia

   (C) lichen sclerosis

   (D) condyloma acuminata

134. Grossly, a raised lesion of the vulva with an irregular appearance. Histologic section shows a papilliform shape to the epithelium. The section is acanthotic, with increased keratin and parakeratosis. The surface is irregular and spiked in appearance.

135. Found in an intertriginous area. Appears as a waxy, raised papule with an umbilicated center. Microscopically, there are eosinophilic inclusions in a central cistern within a raised lesion.

136. A thin, white epithelium. Microscopically, it has a thin epidermis, with flattened rete pegs and a dense hyaline appearance in the dermis. The dermis has a distinct lack of cellularity.

137. A discrete lesion that is slightly raised and can be white or pigmented. The microscopic appearance shows cellular disorganization, with a loss of epithelial cell stratification. There is increased cellular density and variation in cell size with numerous mitotic figures.

Questions 138 through 140

   (A) metaplasia

   (B) cervical intraepithelial neoplasia (CIN)

   (C) acanthosis

   (D) hyperkeratosis

   (E) dyskaryosis

138. A large nuclear:cytoplasmic (N/C) ratio

139. Transformation of areas of columnar cells to squamous cells

140. A term that describes cellular maturation defects of the cervical epithelium

Questions 141 and 142

   (A) isoimmunization

   (B) maternal alpha-thalassemia

   (C) maternal parvovirus

   (D) placenta angioma

   (E) cystic adenomatoid malformation of the fetal lung

   (F) fetal congenital heart disease

   (G) fetal nephrotic syndrome

   (H) fetal cardiac arrhythmia

141. A mother has hydramnios and positive Ro (SSA) and La (SSB) antibodies.

142. A mother had a slight rash, low-grade fever, and red cheeks for several days approximately 3 weeks ago. She now is well, but has developed a rapidly enlarging uterus at 30 weeks' gestation.

Answers and Explanations

93. **(A)** Acanthosis is found with syphilis, lichen planus, venereal warts, and cancer, as well as other conditions. Clinically, it refers to a hyperplasia of keratinocytes, causing a thickening of the prickle layer of the epidermis, which clinically appears as a diffusely thickened or localized plaque. Thickening of the superficial horny layer of the skin is called hyperkeratosis. The presence of nucleated surface cells is called parakeratosis. Thinning or atrophy means fewer cells and cell layers present. Ulceration means there is absence of epithelium.

94. **(C)** The labia differ in that the labia majora have hair follicles and many sweat glands and the labia minora have no hair follicles and few sweat glands. The skin of the labia majora is thicker in most instances and it has subcutaneous fat. Both attach to underlying vulvar fascia.

95. **(C)** Keratin is not normally present in the vagina. It can occur in response to chronic irritation or infection. Many kinds of bacteria are present in the vagina as normal vaginal flora and may be seen on a biopsy. As long as they are confined to the surface, they are probably a normal variant. A 3-mm cyst lined by cuboidal epithelium is likely to be a remnant of the wolffian duct (Gartner's duct cyst). They are common. Endocervical-type mucus-secreting glands may also be found in the vagina. If present, they are called vaginal adenosis. They are more common in women whose mothers were exposed to DES (diethylstilbestrol) during their pregnancy. The stratified squamous epithelium lining in the vagina is usually no more than 3 mm in thickness. For various lesions that may be found in the vagina, see Figure 2–2.

96. **(B)** The cervix is covered with glandular epithelium in childhood. The cervical epithelium will undergo change (metaplasia) as it is exposed to estrogen. The columnar epithelium is replaced by squamous epithelium. The area that changes is called the transformation zone, and the leading edge of the area of change is the squamocolumnar junction. Squamous changes are thought to begin at the squamocolumnar junction where active metaplasia is occurring. This area must be sampled by a Pap smear, and it must be completely seen with a colposcope, or biopsied during diagnostic procedures to evaluate abnormal Pap smears.

97. **(D)** Nabothian cysts occur when a cleft of columnar endocervical cells becomes walled off by epidermidization, entrapping mucous secretions. They are common and benign and are usually recognized visually. Rarely, it may be necessary to biopsy them for identification. This cyst is found on the surface of the cervix, in contrast to the histologically similar Gartner's duct cyst (wolffian duct remnant) found deep within the stroma of the cervix. Cervical intraepithelial neoplasia is not cystic. Herpes may cause vesicles but they are thin, last a short time before rupture, and contain serous fluid. Cervical adenosis is made up of columnar glandular epithelium but is not a cyst.

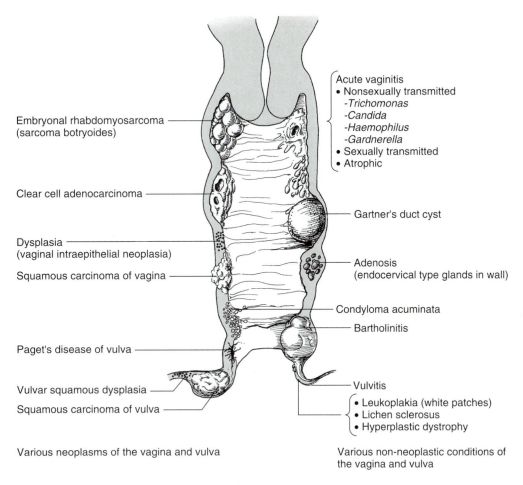

Embryonal rhabdomyosarcoma
(sarcoma botryoides)

Clear cell adenocarcinoma

Dysplasia
(vaginal intraepithelial neoplasia)

Squamous carcinoma of vagina

Paget's disease of vulva

Vulvar squamous dysplasia

Squamous carcinoma of vulva

Acute vaginitis
• Nonsexually transmitted
 -*Trichomonas*
 -*Candida*
 -*Haemophilus*
 -*Gardnerella*
• Sexually transmitted
• Atrophic

Gartner's duct cyst

Adenosis
(endocervical type glands in wall)

Condyloma acuminata

Bartholinitis

Vulvitis
• Leukoplakia (white patches)
• Lichen sclerosus
• Hyperplastic dystrophy

Various neoplasms of the vagina and vulva

Various non-neoplastic conditions of
the vagina and vulva

Figure 2–2.

98. (A) Intranuclear inclusion bodies, irregular nucleoli, and multinuclei are characteristic of herpes simplex virus. These findings are sometimes detected by biopsy or Tzanck staining of a cytologic smear, or sometimes with routine Pap smear (50% sensitivity). Donovan bodies are found with granuloma inguinale and sulfur granules with actinomyces.

99. (C) This group of cells shows a high nuclear:cytoplasmic ratio and nuclear hyperchromatism. It is therefore the most dysplastic appearing. Group A demonstrates mild dysplasia. Group B demonstrates moderate dysplasia.

100. (E) Degeneration, regeneration, inflammation, and atrophy can all result in changes that mimic malignancy, such as loss of cyto-

plasm, irregular or hyperchromatic nuclei, or angular nucleoli.

101. (C) In the first half of the menstrual cycle the endometrium is influenced by estrogen. The endometrium develops from its basal layer (basalis). Estrogen makes the lining proliferate (hence, the proliferative phase). At midcycle, estrogen production continues, but with ovulation, progesterone is also produced, which causes coiling of the endometrial arteries and compaction of the endometrium. Progesterone also causes endometrial glands to secrete (hence, secretory phase). While it is true that gonadotropins (GnRH, FSH, and LH) serve as signals for this process, they have little direct effect on endometrium. In the normal postmenopausal woman gonadotropins are elevated, but the endometrium does not change because no estrogen or progesterone is produced (see Figure 2–3).

102. **(B)** The endometrium can be "dated"; in other words, histologic examination of the endometrium allows determination of when during the menstrual cycle the biopsy was taken. The proliferative phase can be divided into early, mid, or late proliferative based on the thickness (or length) of the glands and the number of mitoses present. The secretory phase can be divided into the day of the menstrual cycle using the glandular secretions and stromal edema. The histology of the secretory phase is read as days 14 through 28, usually using only even-numbered days. The presence of subnuclear vacuoles indicates day 16. Supranuclear vacuoles indicate day 18. By day 21 or 22 stromal edema appears. By day 24 the arteries are tightly coiled and decidualization occurs around blood vessels in the stroma. By day 26 neutrophils appear in the endometrium, and day 28 shows necrosis and hemorrhage (see Figure 2–3).

103. **(C)** The Arias–Stella reaction in the endometrium is found in about 25% of pregnancies. Because of the atypism, mitoses, and proliferation, it has been mistaken for adenocarcinoma or endometriosis. The patient's pregnancy should always be conveyed to the pathologist, as this information will influence the interpretation of the changes seen. If this change were seen in a dilation and curettage (D&C) specimen and there were no placental villi, one should think about ectopic pregnancy.

104. **(E)** Decidualization is a characteristic of the endometrium of the pregnant uterus. It is a response of maternal cells to progesterone. However, decidualization may be used to describe any change due to progesterone, including the eosinophilic proliferation around arterioles after ovulation.

105. **(C)** Adenomyosis is a condition in which endometrial glands and stroma are found within the myometrium on histologic examination. These structures must be one or more

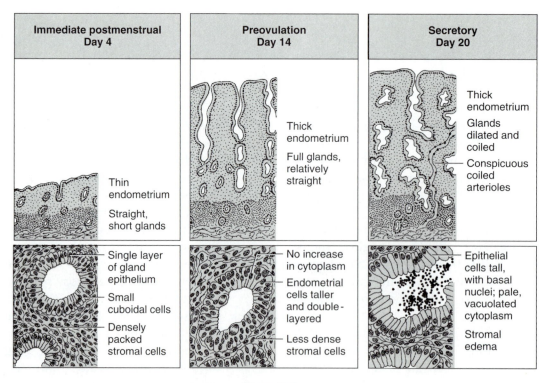

Immediate postmenstrual Day 4	Preovulation Day 14	Secretory Day 20

Thin endometrium

Straight, short glands

Thick endometrium

Full glands, relatively straight

Thick endometrium

Glands dilated and coiled

Conspicuous coiled arterioles

Single layer of gland epithelium

Small cuboidal cells

Densely packed stromal cells

No increase in cytoplasm

Endometrial cells taller and double-layered

Less dense stromal cells

Epithelial cells tall, with basal nuclei; pale, vacuolated cytoplasm

Stromal edema

Figure 2–3.

low-power microscopic fields below the surface. It is not malignant. Endometrial glands do not undergo metaplasia to muscle, nor does muscle undergo metaplasia to glands. Endometriosis is the term that refers to ectopic endometrium in any location outside the uterus. Adenomyosis used to be referred to as endometriosis interna.

106. **(D)** Leiomyomas are common benign neoplasms of uterine smooth muscle. They are usually discrete, very firm, smooth masses that are tan in color. They are found most commonly attached to the uterus, though they can occur at other sites. They are also called fibroids, fibromyoma, myomas, and other colloquial terms. They are not premalignant and are rarely tender or inflamed. Most patients who have them are asymptomatic.

107. **(B)** Endometrial hyperplasia is a condition with increased numbers of endometrial glands and a decrease (but not an absence) in the amount of intervening stroma. The cells lining the glands also build up and overlap (see Figure 2–4). Hyperplasia with atypical cells is often a precursor to endometrial carcinoma. Distractor C is a description of decidualization. Distractor D describes secretory endometrium, and E is a description of an endometrial polyp.

108. **(D)** Each portion of the female genital tract has a characteristic epithelial lining. The fallopian tube is lined by ciliated columnar epithelium. Many of the tubal cells appear ciliated, while others are secretory or absorptive. The cilia and mucus facilitate egg transport.

109. **(A)** The cilia facilitate the movement of the ova toward the midtube and into the uterus after fertilization. The sperm transports itself by its own swimming action. The cervical mucus is responsible for eliminating most of the bacteria before the sperm becomes intraperitoneal.

110. **(E)** The medulla is the central core of the ovary and is continuous with the hilum, where blood vessels and lymphatics gain entrance. The cortex is the outer layer, containing primary oocytes and stroma. The ovary is covered by a thin "germinal" epithelium, which is not derived from germ cells. It is derived from the peritoneum.

111. **(D)** Ova were thought to arise from this lining. Though we now recognize that they do not, the older terminology persists. Understanding this anomalous terminology is important in the classification of ovarian tumors.

112. **(A)** The oocyte is surrounded by the zona pellucida, the granulosa, and the theca. During each menstrual cycle, the follicles selected for ovulation grow until an egg is ovulated by erupting through the surface of the ovary surrounded by some of the follicle cells. If the early eggs are not surrounded by follicular cells to form primordial follicles, they resorb.

113. **(C)** Of the many follicles present at birth, only about 400 to 600 ever mature and extrude an ovum. Many become atretic and disappear without developing, and others that start to develop become atretic. Only a small proportion will ovulate, form a corpus luteum, and produce progesterone.

114. **(D)** There are three predominant histologic types of ovarian tissue. They are the serosa (germinal epithelium), germ cells, and stromal cells, which are divided into undifferen-

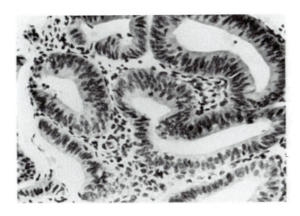

Figure 2–4.

tiated stroma and specialized stroma. Neoplasms may be derived from each of these histologic types. Other neoplasms may be metastatic to the ovary. Dysgerminoma and teratomas are derived from the germ cells, not from the germinal epithelium. Fibromas are derived from the stroma and granulosa thecal cell tumors from the specialized stroma. Germinal epithelium is a misnomer. It does not give rise to germ cells or tumors derived from germ cells. Epithelial tumors of the ovary (serous, mucinous, and endometrioid) derive from it. There may also be mixed forms of tumor, but they are rare.

115. **(E)** Corpora albicans are found in almost all normal ovaries during the menstrual age range. They are the site of previously active but now hyalinized corpora lutea.

116. **(B)** The cell layer surrounding the follicle (outside the granulosa) is called the theca. Cells closest to the granulosa are called the theca interna. These cells develop and convert their cytoplasm to become efficient producers of both estrogen and progesterone. Cholesterol is stored within them, imparting a yellow color. The whole structure is known as the corpus luteum. High levels of hCG as seen in multiple pregnancies or hydatidiform moles can stimulate abnormal luteinization and the production of many luteinized cysts (theca lutein cysts). These cysts can make the ovaries very large.

117. **(E)** In serous cystadenocarcinoma, more than three cell layers of stratification exist in the epithelial cell lining. The individual cells are atypical, and there is invasion of the ovarian stroma and/or protrusion from the capsule (excrescences). A borderline malignant tumor has three or fewer cells in the lining of the cyst and no evidence of invasion. It is the thickness of the lining, invasion, and atypia that makes the diagnosis of ovarian carcinoma. The calcifications are called psammoma bodies and are suggestive but not diagnostic of an ovarian malignancy (see Figure 2–5).

118. **(C)** Immature teratomas are malignant, containing embryonic-like tissues. Mature teratomas may contain all three germ lines but they may or may not be malignant. Mature teratomas can be malignant, usually because they have malignant elements of mature skin (squamous epithelium) and neural ectoderm. The neural tissue is most useful in grading the virulence of the tumor (those with large areas of neuroblast are most virulent).

119. **(B)** The breasts are glands of ectodermal origin and are classified as modified sweat glands. They are not exclusive to the female, being present in both sexes. Their major purpose is the production of milk for offspring. They are endocrine-dependent organs and do not produce hormones.

120. **(E)** The fascia of the superficial chest muscles become condensed into bands called Cooper's ligaments. These bands run from the base of the breast to the skin to provide support for the breast. Distortion of these bands by a tumor may cause dimpling of the skin overlying the breast. Such dimpling is considered a sign of malignancy.

121. **(A)** After menopause the breast undergoes involution. There is a decrease in the acinar and ductal elements and generalized atrophy. Parenchymal elements decrease and are replaced by fat, making the breast appear less dense on mammography.

122. **(A)** The pathologic types of breast cancer are identified by their histologic appearance. About 75% of breast cancers will arise from ductal epithelium. No other cell type in the breast accounts for more than 10% of pathologic types. The histologic subtype has less bearing on prognosis than stage of the cancer at treatment, which is the most important prognostic factor for survival.

123. **(A)** Most cancers of the breast originate from ductal epithelium and often are invasive at the time of diagnosis. The subtypes listed are all infiltrating ductal carcinoma with different architectural patterns.

Benign serous cystadenoma
• Single layer of epithelial cells
• No atypia

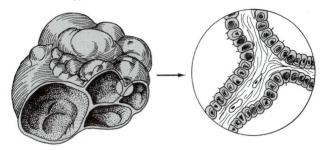

Serous tumor of low malignant potential
• Mild atypia
• Stratification of cells less than 3 layers deep

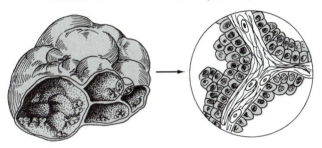

Malignant serous cystadenocarcinoma
• Stratified epithelium with marked cytologic atypia
• Invasion of stroma

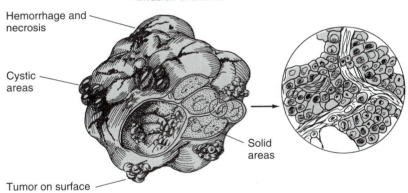

Hemorrhage and necrosis

Cystic areas

Solid areas

Tumor on surface

Figure 2–5.

124. **(B)** The biopsy showing atypical hyperplasia indicates a risk greater than the general population for developing breast cancer, but it is not a malignancy. It indicates a need for close surveillance, as approximately 8% of these women will develop breast cancer within 15 years. If other risk factors were present, such as two or more first-degree relatives with breast cancer or a previous carcinoma in the other breast, other plans or treatment modalities might be considered, but usually not on the basis of this biopsy result alone.

125. **(C)** Fibrocystic breast changes are common in women 30 to 50 years old and are often asymptomatic. When symptomatic, they often present as a painful mass that changes with menses. The histology may be impre-

cise, and these changes may represent a normal process in the breast. It is generally thought not to be a risk factor for most women (Figure 2–6).

126. **(E)** By definition, fibrous tissue and glands should be a fibroadenoma. It is most common in women younger than 35. It is generally asymptomatic and presents as a 1- to 5-cm mass. Local excision may or may not be necessary, depending on patient reliability. Cystosarcoma phyllodes is a type of fibroadenoma with a cellular stroma. It can grow quickly and may recur and act like a malignancy unless completely excised. Macromastia is simply large breasts. This may or may not be a problem for the patient. Mastitis is an infection of the breast almost always secondary to breast feeding. Fat necrosis is usually secondary to injury and may or may not produce a mass. It does not need treatment if the condition can be accurately identified.

127. **(E)** Decidua is maternal. Part of the decidua is sloughed (shed like decidual trees shed their leaves) with each period. Trophoblast is fetal in origin. The placenta contains maternal and fetal tissue in an immunologically privileged relationship.

128. **(D)** By analyzing the structure of the placenta microscopically, one can determine whether the pregnancy is early or late in gestation. The blastocyst implants about a week after fertilization and in the following 2 months, the trophoblast proliferates (with resultant syncytium formation); lacunae develop; and primary, secondary, and tertiary villi form, as do the chorionic plate and cotyledons. At 3 months or later, septa form between lobes.

129. **(C)** As the placenta ages, villous branching occurs and the number of capillaries increases. The cytotrophoblast becomes less prominent, and more fibrin is deposited. Some of these changes appear to improve, while others appear to inhibit the placenta's transport of the fetal nutrients. On the whole, the post-term placenta is likely to become suboptimal in its respiratory function, making frequent fetal surveillance imperative after it reaches term.

130. **(B)** The correlation between benign and malignant behavior of a mole and its histology is

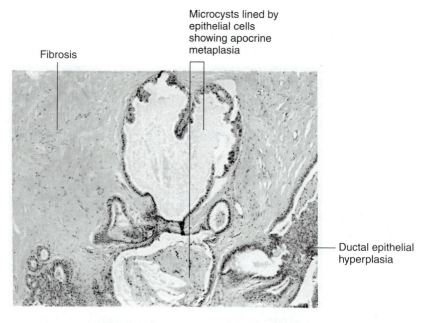

Figure 2–6. Fibrocystic changes in the breast.
(Reproduced, with permission, from Chandrasoma P, Taylor CR. *Concise Pathology,* 3rd ed. New York: McGraw-Hill, 2001.)

not strong. The titer of hCG is a much better predictor (tumor marker) than is histologic analysis.

131. **(B)** One of the distinctions between complete mole and normal placenta is the lack of blood vessels in the moles. In most cases, complete moles are 46,XX with euploidy and are therefore sex chromatin positive. One half of normal placentas are sex chromatin positive. Microscopically, moles have edematous villi (hydropic degeneration) and both moles and placentas have proliferating syncytiocytotrophoblast, although random mix of cyto- and syncytiotrophoblast is more common in moles. However, some placentas, especially of hydropic fetuses, can show this also. Cellular atypia is common in both normal and molar placentas.

132. **(A, B, C, D)** The vulva has an external covering of skin, which has the same structure as other skin. From the surface downward, these layers include epidermis, papillary dermis, reticular dermis, subcutaneous tissue, and deep fascia; the muscle fibers are found beneath the skin. Since vulvar lesions are superficial skin lesions in most cases, there would be no need for a biopsy to extend to the deep fascia.

133. **(A, B, C, D)** The adult female breast is made up of glands, ducts, a fibrous stroma, and fat, all arranged into lobules and lobes. As a woman gets older, relatively more fatty tissue accumulates in the breast. This change makes mammograms more effective in detecting abnormalities and easier to read. Skeletal muscle is deep to the breast tissue.

134. **(D)** Grossly, a condyloma is a raised white lesion of the vulva with an irregular appearance. Histologic section shows a papilliform shape to the epithelium. The section is acanthotic, with increased keratin and parakeratosis. The surface is irregular and spiked in appearance. This is a classic description of a wart.

135. **(A)** Molluscum contagiosum lesions appear as waxy, raised, dome-shaped papules with

an umbilicated center. Microscopically, there are eosinophilic inclusions contained in a central cistern of a raised lesion.

136. **(C)** Lichen sclerosis is a chronic lesion that is common on the vulva. It is often pruritic and has a smooth and atrophic appearance. The epidermis is usually thin and may have a significant keratin layer. Pathologic characteristics are a lack of rete pegs and a pink hyaline appearance with lack of cellularity in the dermis.

137. **(B)** Vulvar intraepithelial neoplasia can involve a small fraction or the entire thickness of the epithelium. It may appear as a discrete or diffuse lesion. It can be unifocal or multifocal. It may be white, red, brown, or black. Histologic sections will show a lack of normal differentiation of cells. Large basal cells are not confined to the basal-most layers but extend well up into the epithelium. Cellular density and mitotic activity is increased. Some of the mitoses may be abnormal. Multinucleation and nuclear hyperchromasia are common features.

138. **(B)** Dysplastic cells make up CIN. They have large, irregular nuclei and abnormal mitoses. They are also likely to be aneuploid. Gross clinical examination, however, will not reveal this.

139. **(A)** Squamous metaplasia is commonly found in cervical epithelium. It is a physiologic process by which squamous epithelium replaces columnar epithelium. Squamous metaplasia is found within the transformation zone of the uterine cervix (see Figure 2–7).

140. **(B)** Cervical intraepithelial neoplasia (CIN) is graded as I, II, or III. It refers to dysplastic cells with a defect in their nuclear:cytoplasmic ratio and chromatin abnormalities of the nucleus. These abnormally maturing cells may progress from CIN I to CIN II to CIN III as they encompass greater amounts of the epithelial thickness. CIN does not include specimens with any evidence of invasion below

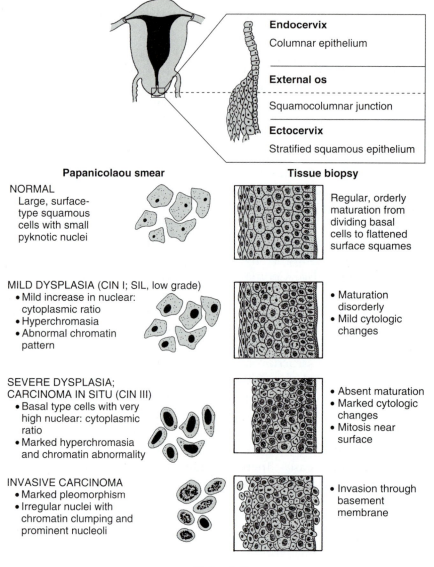

Figure 2–7.

the basement membrane. Such invasion denotes cancer, not a precursor (see Figure 2–7).

141. **(H)** Women who are positive for Ro (SSA) and La (SSB) often have infants with heart blocks, which can lead to hydrops. These antibodies, or systemic lupus erythematosus (SLE) antibodies can cross the placenta and cause fibrosis and inflammation of the fetal cardiac conducting system.

142. **(C)** Parvovirus (B19) infection of the mother is often mild and causes few symptoms, one of which is a red face—the slapped-cheek sign—along with low-grade fever, mild arthritis, and a faint rash on the trunk and extremities. The fetus may have a transient aplastic crisis with anemia and high-output congestive heart failure. It is diagnosed by testing for maternal immunoglobulin M (IgM) and immunoglobulin G (IgG) antibodies to parvovirus.

Embryology
Questions

DIRECTIONS (Questions 143 through 173): Each
of the numbered items or incomplete statements
in this section is followed by answers or by completions of the statement. Select the ONE lettered
answer or completion that is BEST in each case.

143. Meiosis differs from mitosis in several ways.
The major difference is that

    (A) meiosis is confined to germ cells,
    whereas mitosis occurs in all cells of the
    body throughout life
    (B) the end product of meiosis is a cell with
    a haploid number of chromosomes
    (C) in meiosis each germ cell undergoes a
    single reduction-division, whereas in
    mitosis there are two
    (D) meiosis occurs in one stage with separa-
    tion of sister chromosomes
    (E) in meiosis the cells become sex chro-
    matin positive from the genetic inactiva-
    tion of one half of the cellular material

144. The primitive streak

    (A) identifies the caudal end of the embryo
    (B) becomes the adult brain
    (C) is the beginning of the embryonic excre-
    tory system
    (D) becomes the cardiovascular system of
    the embryo
    (E) gives rise to primal urges

145. The stage of gestational development at
which endometrial implantation occurs is

    (A) eight-cell embryo
    (B) zygote
    (C) morula formation
    (D) blastocyst
    (E) embryonic disk

146. During growth of the embryo, the inner cell
mass is referred to as the embryonic disk.
This embryonic disk differentiates initially
into

    (A) decidua
    (B) cytotrophoblast
    (C) ectoderm and endoderm
    (D) syncytiotrophoblast
    (E) mesoderm

147. In spermatogenesis, the second meiotic division produces two daughter cells. In oogenesis, how many functional daughter cells are
produced after both meiotic stages are complete?

    (A) four
    (B) three
    (C) two
    (D) one

148. During fetal development, organogenesis,
with the exception of the brain, is completed
within

    (A) 2 weeks after ovulation
    (B) 8 weeks after ovulation
    (C) 16 weeks after ovulation
    (D) 24 weeks after ovulation
    (E) 36 weeks after ovulation

149. Fetal hematopoiesis first occurs in the

    (A) heart
    (B) liver
    (C) yolk sac
    (D) bone marrow
    (E) lymph nodes

150. The embryo and fetus form hemoglobin. The type(s) of hemoglobin formed is/are

    (A) Gower 1
    (B) hemoglobin A (HbA)
    (C) Gower 2
    (D) hemoglobin F (HbF)
    (E) all of the above

151. Three excretory systems form successively, with temporal overlap during the embryonic period. In order of development these are the

    (A) pronephros, mesonephros, metanephros
    (B) pronephros, metanephros, mesonephros
    (C) metanephros, pronephros, mesonephros
    (D) nephrogenic cord, pronephros, mesonephros
    (E) nephrogenic cord, pronephros, pronephric tubes

152. Which of the following best describes the function of the pronephros?

    (A) It begins the developmental sequence that forms the permanent excretory ducts and kidneys.
    (B) They are the primitive kidney and ureter that will mature to become the adult ureter.
    (C) They originate as part of the cervical somites.
    (D) They will serve as the fetal kidney until after birth.
    (E) They form the primitive kidney that will mature but do not form the primitive ureter. That function is from the mesonephros.

153. Genetic sex is determined

    (A) at ovulation
    (B) at conception

    (C) by the presence or absence of testosterone
    (D) in the absence of müllerian inhibiting factor
    (E) psychosocially after birth

154. The earliest morphologic indicators of sex appear at about how many weeks' gestation?

    (A) 4 to 5 weeks
    (B) 8 to 10 weeks
    (C) 12 to 14 weeks
    (D) 16 to 20 weeks
    (E) after 24 weeks

155. On the basis of Jost's classic experiments in the sexually indifferent mammalian embryo, the development of the müllerian and wolffian duct systems is dependent on which of the following dominant factors?

    (A) the presence of an ovary elaborating a "feminizing hormone"
    (B) the presence of a testis elaborating a "masculinizing hormone"
    (C) fetal gonadotropins
    (D) maternal gonadotropins
    (E) a combination of all the above

156. Under the influence of estrogen in the embryo/fetus

    (A) paramesonephric ducts regress
    (B) wolffian ducts regress
    (C) müllerian ducts begin development
    (D) the gonadal ridge undergoes feminization
    (E) none of the above

157. Germ cells arise in the

    (A) germinal epithelium of the gonad
    (B) endoderm of the primitive gut
    (C) müllerian duct
    (D) mesonephron
    (E) ovarian cortex

158. The maximal number of oogonia are found at what age?

(A) 1 month's gestational age
(B) 5 months' gestational age
(C) birth
(D) puberty
(E) 21 years of age

159. The paramesonephric ducts will form

(A) the prostatic utricle
(B) seminal vesicles
(C) oviducts, uterus, and upper vagina
(D) upper vagina only
(E) the ureters

160. At approximately 8 weeks' gestation the right and left paramesonephric ducts normally

(A) begin to form as an invagination of coelomic epithelium in the urogenital ridge
(B) form the ostium of the oviduct by canalization
(C) fuse in the medial aspects of their caudalmost portions to form a single cavity
(D) spiral onto each other and, by canalization, form a double cavity with a midline septum that will later resorb under the influence of estrogen

161. Vaginal epithelium and the fibromuscular wall of the vagina originate from which of the following, respectively?

(A) mesonephric duct and endoderm of the urogenital sinus
(B) mesonephric duct and the uterovaginal primordium
(C) endoderm of the urogenital sinus and the mesonephric duct
(D) endoderm of the urogenital sinus and the uterovaginal primordium
(E) endoderm of the urogenital sinus and the paramesonephric ducts.

162. The urogenital sinus is derived from

(A) invagination of the genital ridges
(B) proliferation of the hindgut
(C) partitioning of the endodermal cloaca
(D) a track developing in the genital mesoderm
(E) hyperplasia of the metanephros

163. The cloacal cavity is separated from the extraembryonic amniotic cavity by the

(A) genital ridges
(B) cloacal membrane
(C) urorectal bridge
(D) pouch of Douglas
(E) genital tubercle

164. From a developmental embryology viewpoint, the hymen most probably represents

(A) distal fusion of the paramesonephric (müllerian) ducts
(B) the septum that separated the vesicle portion of the urogenital sinus from the pelvic portion
(C) the mesenchyme of the greater vestibular glands
(D) remnants of the vaginal plate and sinusal (müllerian) tubercle

165. Formation of the external genitalia is most influenced by which of the following?

(A) genetic sex of the embryo
(B) a normal urogenital sinus
(C) the sperm fertilizing the egg (carrying a Y chromosome)
(D) the presence of fetal androgens
(E) maternal hormonal levels

166. One of the earliest distinctions between the external genitalia of the male and female embryo is the presence of

(A) scrotal testes
(B) a penile urethral groove
(C) a prepuce for the glans penis
(D) a urogenital sinus
(E) the labioscrotal swellings

167. The labia majora are homologous with the male

    (A) penis
    (B) testicle
    (C) foreskin
    (D) scrotum
    (E) gubernaculum testes

168. The female clitoris is homologous to the male

    (A) scrotum
    (B) frenulum
    (C) prostate
    (D) foreskin
    (E) penis

169. The absence of the vagina is common in

    (A) congenital adrenal hyperplasia in a female infant
    (B) Turner syndrome
    (C) association with an absent or rudimentary uterus
    (D) drug-induced fetal masculinization of a female infant
    (E) gonadal dysgenesis

170. Which of the following, if any, are the result of lack of fusion of the wolffian duct system?

    (A) septate vagina
    (B) absent vagina
    (C) double uterus
    (D) more than one of the above
    (E) none of the above

171. If germ cells fail to enter the developing genital ridge, which of the following may occur?

    (A) ovarian teratomas
    (B) ectopic pregnancy
    (C) ovarian choriocarcinoma
    (D) gonadal agenesis
    (E) testicular feminization

172. True hermaphrodites have

    (A) ovaries and testicular remnants
    (B) the absence of any müllerian tissue due to müllerian-inhibiting factor

    (C) 46,XY karyotype
    (D) ambiguous genitalia
    (E) none of the above

173. In the examination of the newborn infant with ambiguous genitalia, which of the following is true?

    (A) Gonads that are palpable in the lower inguinal canal are always testes.
    (B) The presence of descended gonads rules out high testosterone virilization in an otherwise normal female infant.
    (C) Pelvic ultrasound is not a helpful method of assessing a newborn with ambiguous genitalia.
    (D) The presence of a normal uterus rules out the possibility of dysgenetic testes.
    (E) None of the above

DIRECTIONS (Questions 174 through 176): Each of the numbered items or incomplete statements in this section is followed by answers or by completions of the statement. Select the answers or completions that may apply.

174. The mesonephros will form which four of the following?

    (A) part of the early vesicle trigone
    (B) Gartner's duct cysts in the female
    (C) male epididymis
    (D) upper one third of the vagina
    (E) ductus deferens
    (F) cervix
    (G) fallopian tubes

175. A proliferation of mesoderm in the cloaca will fold the wall of the cloaca into a partition called the urorectal septum. When this is accomplished, which four of the following will take place?

    (A) The single-chambered cloaca is now subdivided into the urogenital sinus and anorectal canal.
    (B) The junction of the cloacal membrane with the urorectal septum will become the perineum.

(C) The cloacal membrane will now differentiate into the urogenital membrane and the anal membrane.

(D) The urogenital sinus will form the proximal vagina and posterior bladder wall.

(E) The urorectal septum will form the anterior wall of the rectum.

176. Improper fusion of the paramesonephric ducts may result in which four of the following conditions?

(A) uterus didelphys
(B) bicornuate uterus with a rudimentary horn
(C) unicornuate uterus
(D) longitudinal vaginal septum
(E) female hypospadias
(F) Gartner's duct cysts

DIRECTIONS (Questions 177 through 186): Each set of questions in this section consists of a list of lettered options followed by several numbered items. For each numbered item, select the ONE lettered option that is most closely associated with it. Each lettered option may be selected once, more than once, or not at all.

Questions 177 through 181

(A) morula
(B) blastocele
(C) trophoblast
(D) embryo
(E) zygote

177. The name applied to the 16-cell mass that precedes the blastocyst

178. A fertilized ovum

179. The name applied to the cell capable of invading endometrium

180. The name applied to the products of conception from the third to the eighth week after ovulation

181. The name applied to the fluid-filled cavity formed during the course of early embryonic development

Questions 182 through 186

(A) anomalous partitioning of the cloaca
(B) results from incomplete canalization of the vaginal plate
(C) an abnormality in caudal fusion
(D) müllerian aplasia

182. A transverse vaginal septum

183. A longitudinal vaginal septum

184. Absent vagina

185. Imperforate hymen

186. Persistence of the urogenital sinus

Answers and Explanations

143. **(B)** Gametogenesis is the production of germ cells (egg and sperm). The major difference in gametogenesis is that cells undergoing meiosis are in a process whereby the number of chromosomes is reduced by half (a haploid number) the normal complement. In the two stages of meiosis, two successive cell divisions occur, each resulting in this haploid number of chromosomes. The first division occurs just before ovulation and is referred to as the reduction-division.

144. **(A)** The primitive streak forms on the caudal end of the embryonic disk. It becomes the mesenchyme that will differentiate into the connective tissue elements in later life. It will normally regress by the fourth week of embryonic life. If it does not, it may present as a sacrococcygeal tumor.

145. **(D)** It is important to recognize that implantation occurs 6 to 7 days after ovulation and that the embryo is actively growing during this time. Progestin-only contraceptives and the so-called "morning-after pill" probably prevent the implantation of a growing blastocyst by their effect on the endometrium during the days between fertilization and implantation. Zygote is a term for the single fertilized cell with two pronuclei present. An embryo divides to become eight cells during its transportation through the fallopian tube.

146. **(C)** The embryonic disk is formed from the inner cell mass of the blastocyst. It differentiates into the various cell layers that will form the embryo, first as a bilaminar disk (ectoderm and endoderm) and then a trilaminar disk (mesoderm added). The outer wall of the blastocyst forms the trophoblast, which will further differentiate into cytotrophoblast and syncytiotrophoblast (see Figure 3–1).

147. **(D)** In the case of oogenesis only one viable egg is produced. The other daughter cell (polar body) has an intact nucleus but sparse cytoplasm. A polar body is produced at both the first and second meiotic divisions. So a spermatogonium produces four sperm by the end of meiosis. Each oogonium produces one egg and two polar bodies.

148. **(B)** Fifty-six days' gestational age is generally accepted as ending the embryonic period. Prior to this time teratogens can cause severe defects, with partial to complete absence of organ structures, depending upon the stage of development when the teratogen was present. Beyond this time period fetal effects of teratogens are few.

149. **(C)** The yolk sac production of red blood cells rapidly declines and is absent after 3 months. The next site of hematopoiesis is the liver and finally the bone marrow. In times of severe anemia in the fetus or neonate, often these primitive tissues will again become hematopoietic. They produce red cells that are nucleated.

150. **(E)** These types all differ in the globin moiety and can be differentiated by electrophoresis. Fetal hemoglobin (HbF) has more oxygen-binding capacity than adult hemoglobin (HbA). Gower 1 and 2 are embryonic hemoglobins and the most primitive of human he-

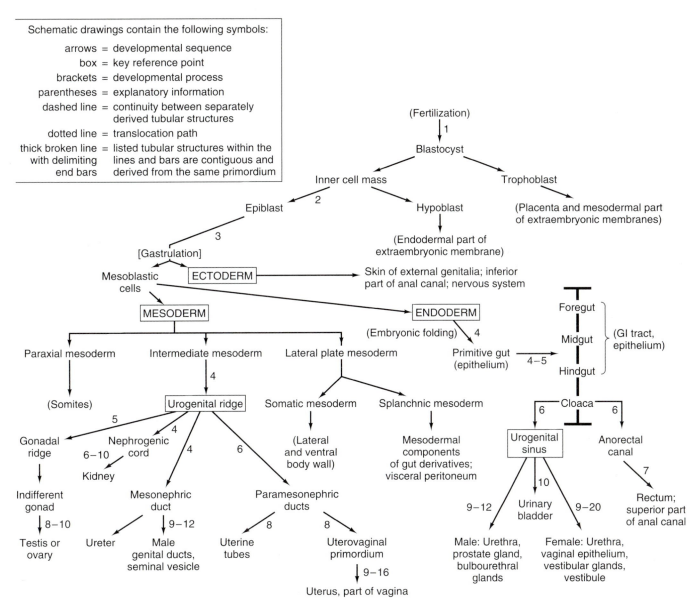

Schematic drawings contain the following symbols:

arrows = developmental sequence
box = key reference point
brackets = developmental process
parentheses = explanatory information
dashed line = continuity between separately derived tubular structures
dotted line = translocation path
thick broken line with delimiting end bars = listed tubular structures within the lines and bars are contiguous and derived from the same primordium

Figure 3–1. Embryonic development.
(Reproduced, with permission, from DeCherney AH, Nathan L. *Current Obstetric and Gynecologic Diagnosis and Treatment,* 9th ed. New York: McGraw-Hill, 2003).

moglobins. They are less efficient oxygen carriers than HbF.

151. **(A)** During development, the genital and urinary systems are closely associated. Primordial elements in the urinary system participate in the formation of genital structures. This overlap takes place between 4 and 12 weeks after fertilization. The first set of structures, the pronephroi, are rudimentary and nonfunctional. The pronephroi appear in human embryos early in the fourth week of gestation and subsequently degenerate. The

mesonephroi appear later in the fourth week and function temporarily as kidneys. The permanent kidneys arise from the metanephroi, the most caudal structures close to the cloaca. Development of the metanephros begins at about 5 weeks of gestation, with function occurring about 6 weeks later.

152. **(A)** The pronephric ducts grow caudally, and by week 5 of development they open into the lateral wall of the cloaca. The pronephroi degenerate by the end of the fourth week, but do initiate the events that will lead to the for-

mation of the adult kidney and collecting ducts.

153. **(B)** Genetic sex is determined at fertilization by the complement of sex chromosomes in the fertilizing sperm. If the sperm bears an X, a female is conceived. If it bears a Y, a male is conceived.

154. **(B)** In utero morphologic identification of sex is first possible at about 8–9 weeks' gestation. Before this time the gonad is referred to as the indifferent stage of development. When the genetic sex is expressed on the indifferent gonad, gonadal sex is expressed. The gonads develop from a thickened area of coelomic epithelium on the medial side of the mesonephros called the gonadal ridge. Testes differentiation occurs by the eighth week in males. In females, the ovaries develop by the tenth week.

155. **(B)** If embryonic genital tissue is allowed to differentiate without testosterone (androgen or masculinizing hormone), it does so as a female phenotype. Androgen is produced in the testes as is the anti-müllerian hormone (or müllerian-inhibiting factor). Müllerian-inhibiting factor (MIF) makes the female ducts regress. This concept is important to the understanding of intersex or ambiguous genitalia.

156. **(E)** Stimulation by testosterone causes the male mesonephric ducts (wolffian ducts) to differentiate. Anti-müllerian factor produced by the testes causes the müllerian (paramesonephric) ducts to regress. Absence of these hormones causes the müllerian ducts to persist and develop independent of the presence of estrogen. Genital sex is therefore determined by the presence or absence of androgen.

157. **(B)** Primordial germ cells are visible early in the fourth week among the endodermal cells of the wall of the yolk sac near the origin of the allantois. Migration of primordial germ cells (which will become ova) to the gonadal ridge occurs early in embryonic life (5 to 6 weeks). Germ cells migrate from the primitive yolk sac to the gonadal ridge by an unknown mechanism.

158. **(B)** An oogonium becomes an oocyte when it enters the first stage of meiosis. This occurs prior to birth. After birth there is a slow decrease in the number of oocytes. By menopause none can be found. By 5 months' gestation there is a maximum number of oocytes of about 4 to 7 million! At birth, the number of oocytes have decreased to 1 or 2 million. There continues to be attrition of oocytes during childhood so that by the onset of puberty less than 500,000 oocytes remain.

159. **(C)** The genital ducts (mesonephric or wolffian and paramesonephric or müllerian) are present in both sexes. The mesonephric ducts will become the male ducts and seminal vesicles. The female paramesonephros will form the oviducts, uterus, and upper two thirds of the vagina. The lining of these ducts becomes the epithelial lining of the adult structures. Muscle and connective tissue originate from the adjoining mesenchyme. The prostatic utricle and the appendix testis in the male may indeed be remnants of paramesonephric duct, but are not really formed by the ducts (see Figure 3–2).

160. **(C)** During the eighth week of gestation, well after invagination of coelomic epithelium in the urogenital ridge, the right and left paramesonephric (müllerian) ducts fuse medially in their caudal segments, forming a single cavity. This becomes the uterovaginal primordium and the unfused upper portions become the fallopian tubes. When this process is disordered, it results in anomalies of partial fusion.

161. **(D)** The vaginal epithelium is derived from the endoderm of the urogenital sinus while the fibromuscular wall of the vagina develops from the uterovaginal primordium. In the female, parts of the mesonephric duct persist as the duct of Gartner in the broad ligament along the lateral wall of the uterus. Occasionally, women may develop Gartner's duct cysts in the lateral vaginal walls. The paramesonephric duct develops into the uterus, fallopian tubes, broad ligament structures, and occasionally hydatid cysts of Morgagni.

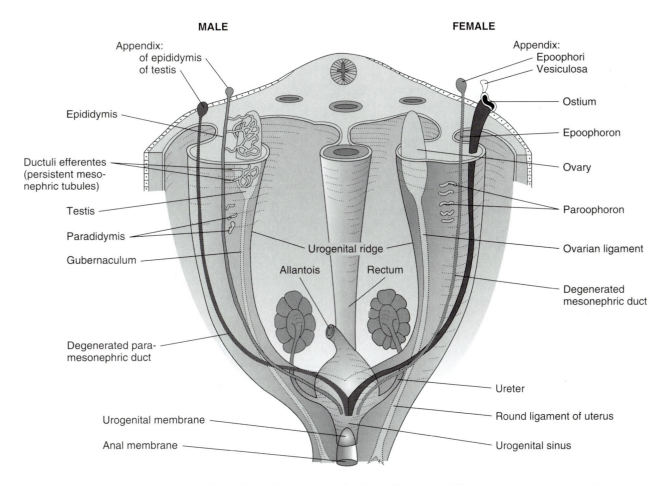

MALE

Appendix:
of epididymis
of testis

Epididymis

Ductuli efferentes
(persistent meso-
nephric tubules)

Testis

Paradidymis

Gubernaculum

Degenerated para-
mesonephric duct

Urogenital membrane

Anal membrane

Urogenital ridge

Allantois

Rectum

FEMALE

Appendix:
Epoophori
Vesiculosa

Ostium

Epoophoron

Ovary

Paroophoron

Ovarian ligament

Degenerated
mesonephric duct

Ureter

Round ligament of uterus

Urogenital sinus

Figure 3–2. Differentiation of male and female genitalia.
(Reproduced, with permission, from DeCherney AH, Nathan L. *Current Obstetric and Gynecologic Diagnosis and Treatment,* 9th ed.
New York: McGraw-Hill, 2003).

162. **(C)** The urogenital sinus is derived from partitioning of the endodermal-derived embryonic cloaca. It is the precursor to the urinary bladder and the genitalia in each sex. The cloaca is a pouch on the caudal end of the hindgut that was formed by folding of the caudal region of the embryonic disk.

163. **(B)** The cloacal membrane is composed of ectoderm and endoderm. It is the most caudal limit of the primitive gut and separates the cloacal cavity from the amniotic cavity. It is dorsal to the genital tubercle and separated from the rectum posteriorly by the urorectal septum.

164. **(D)** The urogenital sinus in the female forms the urinary bladder and the entire urethra, the distal vagina, the greater vestibular glands, and the hymen. The sinovaginal bulbs, two endodermal thickenings of the

pelvic portion of the urogenital sinus, fuse with uterovaginal primordium to form the distal vagina. The solid tissue mass at the end of the uterovaginal primordium is the vaginal plate. It will eventually canalize. Remnants of these two structures form the hymen.

165. **(D)** If androgens are not present, female genitalia will be formed, regardless of any of the other conditions being met. If the embryonal or fetal organs have an insensitivity to androgen (testicular feminization), female genitalia will form. In the presence of androgens (some forms of congenital adrenal hyperplasia), in spite of a 46,XX chromosomal makeup, male genitalia form.

166. **(B)** The urogenital sinus and labioscrotal folds are common to both sexes. The prepuce develops later, and scrotal testes develop

much later. A penile urethral groove can be recognized at 10 to 11 weeks' gestation or when the embryo is 50 mm long.

167. **(D)** In infants with ambiguous external genitalia, confusion may arise as to whether this rugated structure is a scrotal sac or a fused labia. The most common cause of ambiguous genitalia in the newborn is congenital adrenal hyperplasia (see Figure 3–3).

168. **(E)** The clitoris is a small, erectile body that responds to androgen stimulation with increased growth. Increasing clitoral size is one sign of virilism. Virilization can be caused by internal (adrenal or ovarian) androgens or by

androgenic substances such as some progestins that are ingested by the mother.

169. **(C)** The frequency of vaginal agenesis is about 0.025%. It is due to failure of the uterovaginal primordium to contact the urogenital sinus. The uterus is usually absent. Ovarian agenesis is rarely associated with vaginal agenesis. When the vagina is absent, the greater vestibular glands are still present in most cases. In müllerian aplasia, most of the vagina and uterus are absent. It is thought that 80 to 90% of individuals without a vagina have müllerian aplasia rather than atresia. One embryologic defect is apt to be associated with others. You should also look for abnor-

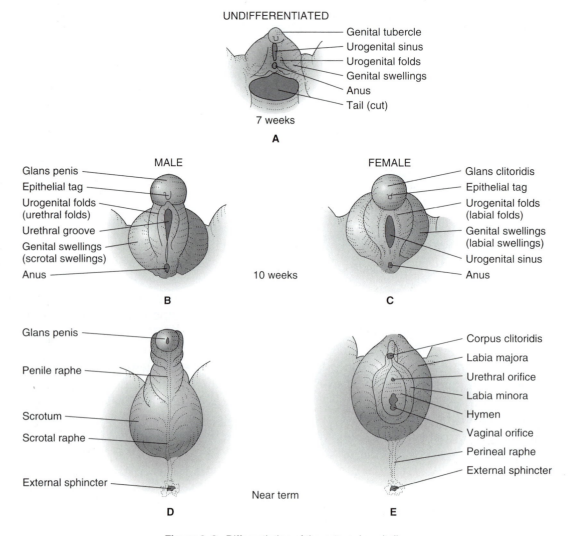

Figure 3–3. Differentiation of the external genitalia.
(Reproduced, with permission, from DeCherney AH, Nathan L. *Current Obstetric and Gynecologic Diagnosis and Treatment*, 9th ed. New York: McGraw-Hill, 2003).

malities of the urinary tract. In Turner syndrome, which is a form of gonadal dysgenesis, the uterus and vagina are present.

170. **(E)** The wolffian duct system makes up the male genital tract, and the failure of its development is normal in a female child. Uterine anomalies would generally result from a failure of fusion of the müllerian ducts.

171. **(D)** If germ cells do not reach the developing ovary, gonadoblastomas may form with 46, XY karyotype. The ovary does not develop normally. This lack of development is called gonadal dysgenesis.

172. **(D)** True hermaphroditism is characterized by ambiguous genitalia at birth. The gonads may be any combination of ovary, testis, or ovotestis. Interestingly, a testis or ovotestis is usually located on the right side. Müllerian structures are usually present on the side ipsilateral to an ovary or ovotestis. Most true hermaphrodites are 46,XX with no identifiable Y chromosome but rather small portions of the Y chromosome incorporated into their genome.

173. **(B)** The physical examination of the newborn with ambiguous genitalia may reveal gonads that are palpable in the scrotum or lower inguinal canal. These gonads may be testes or ovotestes. High circulating androgens in the female fetus are not sufficient to cause descent of normal ovaries and therefore descended gonads cannot be ovaries. Pelvic ultrasound is frequently useful in identifying müllerian structures while the presence of a normal uterus rules out the possibility of normal testicular tissue.

174. **(A, B, C, E)** The mesonephric ducts result in formation of part of the early trigone, the ductal diverticulum, the epididymis, ductus deferens, and ejaculatory duct. Remnants of the duct persist in the female and are referred to as Gartner's duct cysts.

175. **(A, B, C, E)** Only the distal one third of the vagina is formed from the urogenital sinus. The proximal vagina is formed by fusion of the müllerian ducts. This explains why, in cases of müllerian agenesis, patients have a rudimentary vagina.

176. **(A, B, C, D)** The various types of uterine duplication and vaginal malformation that occur with improper fusion include uterus didelphys, which is a double uterus with a double vagina, bicornuate uterus with a fusion defect isolated to the uterine fundus but no vagina, unicornuate uterus with a rudimentary horn, and a longitudinal septum where a caudal fusion problem exists but uterine fusion is adequate.

177–181. **(177-A, 178-E, 179-C, 180-D, 181-B)** The zygote is the cell resulting from the union of the sperm and ovum (egg) or the fertilized ovum. The blastocele is the name applied to the 12 to 16 blastomeres composing the ball of cells from the division of the zygote. The embryonic period begins at the third week of development. During this time most of the major structures are formed, and the greatest risk from teratogens exists. The fetal period begins in the ninth developmental week and extends to birth. The ninth week to birth is more remarkable for rapid growth than for major developmental change. This is a period of growth and maturation of the existing structures. Trophoblastic invasion is the process by which the embryo implants into the uterine lining at the blastocyst stage. The blastocele is the fluid-filled cavity that forms immediately prior to blastocyst formation.

182–186. **(182-B, 183-C, 184-D, 185-B, 186-A)** A transverse vaginal septum and an imperforate hymen imply that canalization of the vaginal plate at its junction with the sinusal (müllerian) tubercle did not proceed completely. A longitudinal septum implies that the caudal fusion of the müllerian ducts did not result in complete canalization of the uterovaginal primordium. When the vagina is absent, in most cases it will be due to aplasia of the müllerian ducts. When the urogenital sinus persists, it causes any number of anomalies, most representing either no opening for the anus or an aberrant opening.

CHAPTER 4

Genetics and Teratology
Questions

DIRECTIONS (Questions 187 through 214): Each of the numbered items or incomplete statements in this section is followed by answers or by completions of the statement. Select the ONE lettered answer or completion that is BEST in each case.

187. The number of chromosomes in the human somatic cell is

    (A) 24
    (B) 44
    (C) 46
    (D) 48
    (E) 23

188. Alleles are

    (A) alternate forms of a gene occupying the same locus on homologous chromosomes
    (B) abnormal chromosomes
    (C) paired chromosomes
    (D) genes changed by mutation
    (E) none of the above

189. Which of the following best describes the composition of nucleic acids, such as DNA and RNA?

    (A) a five-carbon sugar, a nitrogen-containing base, and a phosphate
    (B) two purine bases and two pyrimidine bases
    (C) a double helix composed of interlocking codons
    (D) a combination of polypeptide proteins and protein isomers
    (E) a base, a phosphate, and a sugar

190. Gene transcription refers to the process whereby

    (A) messenger RNA (mRNA) is spliced to the double-stranded DNA and carried outside the cell to centers for protein synthesis
    (B) mRNA is used to make new DNA
    (C) nuclear DNA is used to make mRNA in the cell nucleus
    (D) cytosomes divide to form a new strand of DNA with identical messages
    (E) ribosomes synthesize new nuclear proteins

191. Translation is the process whereby

    (A) the strands of the DNA–mRNA unwind and break so that the interspersed fragments can replicate to form a new protein messenger
    (B) adenosine triphosphate is converted to a second messenger in order to allow hormonal input in the synthesis of DNA
    (C) phosphodiesterase bonds release energy that allows the DNA–RNA complex to split and form daughter strands
    (D) cytosolic codons and anti-codons are "read" for base link matching
    (E) mRNA, with the help of transfer RNA (tRNA), synthesizes protein in the cytoplasm of the cell, specifically at the site of the ribosomal RNA

192. A restriction endonuclease is

(A) the cell product responsible for most chromosomal mutations

(B) an artificial product that allows cells to reproduce rapidly and uncontrollably for research purposes

(C) the cell product that prohibits cross-species fertilization

(D) a product of bacteria that cuts DNA into specifically sequenced fragments

(E) a theoretical means of cutting out abnormal sequences on genes of diseased individuals

193. Which of the following, if any, is the usual pattern of inheritance for a rare autosomal dominant gene?

(A) TT × TT

(B) tt × tt

(C) TT × tt

(D) TT × Tt

(E) none of the above

194. Which of the following, if any, is the usual pattern of inheritance for a rare autosomal recessive trait?

(A) AA × aa

(B) Aa × aa

(C) Aa × Aa

(D) aa × aa

(E) none of the above

195. Because a male has only one X chromosome, he would be called which of the following in regard to any X-linked gene?

(A) codominant

(B) heterozygous

(C) hemizygous

(D) homozygous

(E) intermediate

196. A female who possesses an X-linked trait may do so because either she inherited a recessive gene from both her mother and father or

(A) she inherited a recessive gene from one of her parents and may express the recessive characteristic as a function of the Lyon hypothesis

(B) she has undergone spontaneous mutation from an environmental source

(C) she is really a testicular feminization patient

(D) she lacks the genetic expressor gene for dominance

197. The Hardy–Weinberg law in genetics

(A) explains the inactivation of one X chromosome

(B) expresses the frequency relationship between heterozygotes and homozygotes in a stable population

(C) predicts the penetration of recessive genes

(D) expresses a prediction of the spontaneous mutation rate

(E) none of the above

198. Expressivity in genetics refers to the

(A) percentage of individuals who have a gene in which there is an effect

(B) percentage of individuals in a population who have a gene

(C) phenotypic variation among the individuals who have a gene

(D) change in the form of a gene with chromosomal aging

(E) shape and number of chromosomes

199. Penetrance in genetics refers to the

(A) percentage of individuals who have a gene in which there is an effect

(B) percentage of individuals in a population who have a gene

(C) phenotypic variation among the individuals who have a gene

(D) change in the form of a gene with chromosomal aging

(E) shape and number of chromosomes

200. You are seeing a patient who has been exposed to a medication. You look it up in the register of pregnancy medications. It is listed as Category C. The patient asks you what this means. Your best response is

(A) the drug has been evaluated in well-controlled human studies and no fetal risk has been shown

(B) animal studies have not shown any fetal risk, or suggested some risk not confirmed in humans, or there are not adequate studies in women

(C) animal studies have shown adverse effects, but there are no adequately controlled studies in humans

(D) there are some fetal risks, but benefits may outweigh risks under certain circumstances; thus, patients should be warned

(E) fetal abnormalities have occurred in animal and human studies, the risk is greater than the benefit, and the drug is contraindicated in pregnancy

201. Approximately what percentage of spontaneous first-trimester abortions show chromosomal abnormalities?

(A) 1%

(B) 10%

(C) 25%

(D) 50%

(E) 75%

202. Live births of infants would demonstrate approximately what percentage of chromosomal abnormalities?

(A) less than 1%

(B) 1 to 5%

(C) approximately 10%

(D) 15 to 20%

(E) 40 to 50%

203. The most common chromosomal abnormality in abortuses is

(A) trisomy

(B) 45,XO

(C) triploidy

(D) unbalanced translocation

Questions 204 and 205

A 19-year-old woman comes to your office with a complaint of never having had menses. Physical examination shows that she is 1.37 m tall and weighs 94 pounds. She lacks breast and pubic hair development. There is webbing of her neck and cubitus valgus.

204. The simplest, yet most useful, initial test to begin her evaluation would be

(A) serum estrogen level

(B) prolactin

(C) thyroid index

(D) serum follicle-stimulating hormone (FSH) and luteinizing hormone (LH)

(E) a cardiogram

205. Given the description of this patient, her most likely diagnosis is

(A) testicular feminization

(B) Klinefelter syndrome

(C) Turner syndrome

(D) congenital adrenal hyperplasia

(E) normal but delayed development

206. Patients with a 45,XO karyotype are invariably of short stature because the locus responsible for short stature is located on the missing

(A) long arm of X

(B) short arm of X

(C) centromere of the O chromosome

(D) long arm of chromosome 45

(E) short arm of chromosome 45

207. What percentage of ovarian dysgenesis patients are chromatin positive?

(A) 0%

(B) less than 1%

(C) about 10%

(D) 40%

(E) 95%

208. Aneuploidy is a characteristic of

(A) cystic fibrosis
(B) Down syndrome
(C) testicular feminization
(D) Lesch–Nyhan syndrome

209. Enzymatic diseases (or inborn errors of metabolism) that are diagnosable in utero are generally

(A) not genetic diseases
(B) autosomal dominants
(C) autosomal recessives
(D) sex-linked
(E) polygenic in origin

210. A woman with blood type O gave birth to an AB infant. This could be explained by which of the following?

(A) Lyon's hypothesis
(B) chimerism
(C) Bombay phenotype
(D) laboratory error
(E) X-linked inheritance

211. The Barr body is

(A) the condensed, nonfunctioning X chromosome
(B) the darkest, widest band found on chromosomes
(C) an extra lobe on the female polymorphonuclear leukocytes
(D) found only in the female
(E) the largest chromosome in the female genotype

212. Tests that may increase the ability to diagnose inherited diseases prenatally include

(A) ultrasound
(B) direct fetal blood sampling
(C) x-ray
(D) gene-specific probes
(E) all of the above

213. A couple presents to your office during the ninth week of pregnancy. Their previous child was diagnosed with trisomy 18. They are extremely anxious and would like prenatal diagnosis as early as possible. Which of the following statements about chorionic villus sampling (CVS) is/are correct?

(A) CVS may be performed between 9 and 12 weeks' gestation.
(B) CVS done in the 9- to 10-week range has a very small association (less than 1:1000) with limb malformations.
(C) CVS can provide complete chromosomal analysis.
(D) CVS is performed either transvaginally or transabdominally.
(E) all of the above

214. A mother with blood group AB has an AB child. Which of the following are possible paternal genotypes?

(A) AA
(B) BB
(C) BO
(D) AO
(E) all of the above

DIRECTIONS (Questions 215 through 223): Each of the numbered items or incomplete statements in this section is followed by answers or by completions of the statement. Select the answers or completions that may apply.

215. Which three of the following genetic types will differentiate into a male?

(A) XY
(B) XXY
(C) XYY
(D) YO
(E) XX

216. Which four of the following are suppositions of the Lyon hypothesis?

(A) In the somatic cells of females, only one X chromosome is active. The second X is condensed and inactive and known as the sex chromatin.

(B) Inactivation of the X occurs early in embryonic life.

(C) The inactive X can be either the paternal or maternal X in different cells of the same individual.

(D) Once the X is inactivated by the cell, all the clonal descendants of that cell will inactivate the same X.

(E) X inactivation occurs at the time the second polar body is extruded from the cell.

217. Which of the following are indications for chromsomal evaluation with prenatal diagnosis?

(A) maternal age 35 or greater

(B) previous chromosomally abnormal child

(C) family history of open neural tube defect

(D) abnormal serum marker

(E) possible female carrier of X-linked disease

218. Which four of the following are characteristic of a teratogen?

(A) a chemical that causes gross malformations

(B) any agent that can produce a malformation or raise the incidence of a given malformation

(C) a naturally occurring substance that can cause malformation during the intrauterine period of life

(D) a mutation in maternal or paternal DNA that will affect the phenotype of the offspring

(E) a nonembryocidal mutagen

219. Alterations in the biological process of development may be due to which two of the following?

(A) heredity

(B) drugs

(C) x-rays

(D) infection

220. Which two of the following describe couples who suffer recurrent miscarriage?

(A) They are no more likely than any other couple to have chromosomal anomalies.

(B) They may be affected by thrombophilias.

(C) They may have up to a 25% rate of chromosomal anomalies.

(D) They are more likely to live under high-voltage electric power lines.

(E) They are found to have unsuspected consanguinity in 4 to 8% of cases.

221. A pregnant woman presents to your clinic with a history of a previous child who was diagnosed with phenylketonuria (PKU) as a neonate. Her partner is not the father of the first child. The mother remembers that she had to have a special diet when she was a child. Which three of the following statements are correct?

(A) PKU is an autosomal recessive disease.

(B) Because this is a new father, the pregnancy cannot result in an affected child although the child may be a carrier.

(C) If ph is the PKU gene and the father's genotype is PhPh, the fetus cannot have the disease.

(D) The fetus may be affected in utero if the mother has PKU.

(E) Unless the first baby's father can be tested, the neonate cannot be adequately tested.

222. Which two of the following statements are true?

(A) Any sex-linked recessive disease normally occurring in males can also occur in 45,XO females.

(B) In patients with Klinefelter syndrome, cells have two Y chromosomes.

(C) 45,XO gestations cannot be identified through routine maternal blood screening; amniocentesis or CVS is necessary to diagnose this lesion.

(D) Pituitary gonadotropins are elevated in pregnant women whose offspring have gonadal dysgenesis.

223. Anomalies from polygenic/multifactorial inheritance include which four of the following?

(A) cleft lip
(B) tetralogy of Fallot
(C) pyloric stenosis
(D) achondroplasia
(E) clubfoot (talipes equinovarus)

DIRECTIONS (Questions 224 through 279): Each set of questions in this section consists of a list of lettered options followed by several numbered items. For each numbered item, select the ONE lettered option that is most closely associated with it. Each lettered option may be selected once, more than once, or not at all.

Questions 224 through 234

(A) mitosis
(B) interphase
(C) meiosis
(D) centromere
(E) chromatid
(F) open square
(G) darkened square
(H) diamond shape
(I) a single line
(J) proband
(K) phenotype
(L) codominance
(M) chiasmata
(N) recessive
(O) linkage

224. Cell division in which cells containing a haploid number of chromosomes are produced

225. A period of time when a cell is active but the chromosomes are not recognizable

226. A normal male

227. The propositus

228. Unspecified sex

229. Nonrelated mating

230. A recognizable expresson of genetic information

231. Joining points of paired chromosomes

232. A situation in which each of a pair of genes has equal expression

233. Refers to close proximity of gene loci

234. Division of a cell in which DNA is doubled and two diploid cells result

Questions 235 through 242

(A) mosaicism
(B) polyploidy
(C) aneuploidy
(D) deletion
(E) translocation
(F) isochromosome
(G) inversion
(H) insertion
(I) nondisjunction

235. More than one cell line present in the same individual

236. $2n + 1$ or $2n - 1$

237. $4n$

238. May be either reciprocal or Robertsonian

239. Results when a chromosome divides by horizontal rather than longitudinal split at the centromere

240. May be either paracentric or pericentric

241. May result in a ring chromosome

242. The most common cause of chromosomal abnormalities

Questions 243 through 247

    (A) 47,XY 21+

    (B) 45,XY 46,XY

    (C) 46XY, t (Bp–;Dq+)

    (D) 45,XX, D–, G–, t(Dq Gq)+

    (E) none of the above

243. A balanced translocation between the long arm of a B group and the short arm of a D group chromosome

244. Down syndrome

245. A balanced translocation

246. A translocation resulting in the loss of genetic material

247. An isochromosome

Questions 248 through 253

Match the chromosomal complement with the phenotype.

    (A) 45,XO

    (B) 46,XY

    (C) 47,XXY

    (D) 46,XX, (D/G)

    (E) 46,XX, 5p–

    (F) 46,XX/XY

248. Tall stature, eunuchoidism, sometimes gynecomastia

249. Edema of the hands and feet in a newborn

250. Epicanthic folds, hypertelorism, mental deficiency, single palmar crease

251. Large breasts, scanty axillary hair, absent uterus

252. Microcephaly, severe mental retardation

253. True hermaphrodite

Questions 254 through 261

    (A) autosomal dominant

    (B) autosomal recessive

    (C) X-linked

    (D) polygenic or multifactorial

    (E) not a genetic disease

254. Diabetes mellitus

255. Sickle cell anemia

256. Hemophilia

257. Thalidomide baby

258. Transmitted through the daughter to half of the grandsons

259. Most such diseases have a carrier rate in the general population of less than 1%

260. Congenital adrenal hyperplasia (CAH)

261. Neurofibromatosis

Questions 262 through 264

Match the treatment with the genetic disease.

    (A) restriction of any substance that the patient is incapable of metabolizing

    (B) replacement of a product that the patient cannot synthesize

    (C) superphysiologic replacement of a vitamin

    (D) enzyme replacement

    (E) avoidance of precipitating agents

262. Congenital adrenal hyperplasia (CAH)

263. Treatment of glucose-6-phosphate dehydrogenase (G6PD) deficiency

264. Treatment of PKU

Questions 265 through 270

Match the item with its associated description.

  (A) carcinoma of the lung
  (B) Burkitt's lymphoma
  (C) chronic myelogenous leukemia (CML)
  (D) c-myc
  (E) retinoblastoma

265. Associated with a reciprocal translocation between chromosome 22q and 9q

266. Reciprocal translocation between chromosomes 8 and 14,t (8q;14)

267. Deletion in chromosome 13

268. Loss of a suppressor gene, either TP53 or WT1

269. The Y chromosome may be lost in males

270. May be activated by retroviruses (RNA virus) or mutational events

Questions 271 through 273

  (A) seminoma
  (B) first-degree relative with the disease
  (C) Lynch type II family
  (D) autosomal dominant in selected families

271. Doubles the risk of breast cancer in the proband

272. Ovarian cancer

273. Ovarian, endometrial, and nonpolypoid colorectal cancer

Questions 274 through 279

Match the maternal drug exposure with a potential neonatal effect.

  (A) no effect
  (B) cardiac lesions
  (C) craniofacial lesions
  (D) limb anomalies
  (E) renal lesions
  (F) hypospadias

274. Lithium

275. Warfarin (Coumadin)

276. Carbamazepine (Tegretol)

277. Alcohol

278. Acyclovir

279. Metronidazole

Answers and Explanations

187. (C) There are 23 pairs of chromosomes in the normal human cell. Twenty-two are alike in males and females and are called autosomes. The remaining pair are sex chromosomes, the X and the Y, and determine genetic sex. In Figure 4–1, a 47,XX + 21 chromosome complement is illustrated.

188. (A) Alleles influence the phenotype of the individual, depending on whether they are dominant or recessive. They are genes in the same location on a pair of homologous chromosomes. When both alleles are the same, the individual is said to be a homozygote; when they are different, a heterozygote. Needless to say, alleles affect a similar function.

189. (A) The nucleic acids, DNA and RNA, are composed of three kinds of structures: a five-carbon sugar (either deoxyribose or ribose), a nitrogen-containing base, and a phosphate. The bases are either a purine or a pyrimidine. In DNA the purines are either adenine or guanine, and the pyrimidines are either thymine or cytosine. In RNA, uracil replaces thymine as one of the pyrimidines. The chains themselves are double helices. A codon is simply the triplet code of adjacent bases that specifies an amino acid building block in the genetic code.

190. (C) Transcription of DNA takes place in the cell nucleus. The DNA makes a complementary mRNA strand. The mRNA then passes into the cytoplasm of the cell for translation and the building of cell protein.

191. (E) Translation in the cytoplasm occurs when mRNA is translated into protein, using tRNA to bring complementary amino acids from the cytoplasm to their position along the mRNA template. Amino acids will be added in order beginning at the 5′ and progressing to the 3′ end of the chain. The ribosomes (ribosomal RNA) are the site of protein synthesis in this process.

192. (D) A restriction endonuclease is a bacterial product that can cleave sequences of DNA at specific sites for analysis. It is a nucleic acid-cleaving enzyme that is very widely used to analyze the genome. It is also being used to insert new sequences into genomes (e.g., the *Escherichia coli* that can produce human insulin). It may one day produce a cure for many genetic diseases. This serves as the basis for recombinant DNA research.

193. (E) Dominant traits are represented as capital letters, recessive as lowercase letters. Dominant traits are expressed when they are present on only one chromosome of a pair. If a trait is dominant and rare, few people will have it, and it is usually inherited from one parent only (i.e., Tt × tt). T is dominant; t is recessive. One in four offspring is affected. In autosomal dominant inheritance, the trait should appear with equal frequency in both sexes, at least one parent should possess the trait, and most affected persons will be heterozygous for the trait.

194. (C) If the trait is rare, only a few people have it; if it is recessive, it will not be manifest unless both genes for it are present. Therefore, to get aa, two asymptomatic carriers (het-

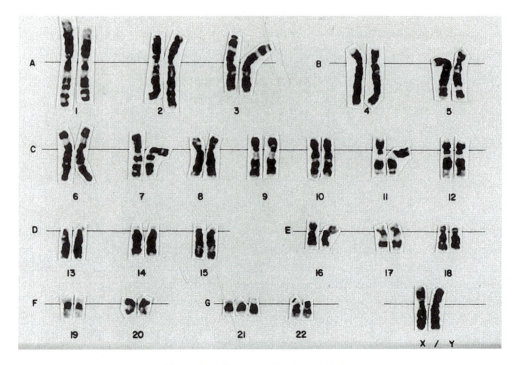

Figure 4–1. Abnormal female karyotype.
(Reproduced, with permission, from Cunningham FG et al.: *Williams Obstetrics*, 21st ed. New York: McGraw-Hill, 2001.)

erozygotes) must be crossed. Even then, only one in four offspring would be affected. Again, the characteristic should occur equally in both sexes. Both parents must be carriers. If both parents have the phenotypic trait, all offspring must have it.

195. **(C)** The female, having two X chromosomes, can be either heterozygous or homozygous for an X-linked gene. The male with only one X will express all the characteristics of the lone X, hence the term hemizygous, rather than heterozygous. In this form of inheritance (X-linked or sex-linked), the condition occurs more commonly in males. If both parents do not possess the trait and an affected male is born, the mother is a carrier. If the father is affected and an affected male is born, the mother is a heterozygote. While a characteristic linked to a Y chromosome is possible, there seem to be none of real clinical significance.

196. **(A)** All females are mosaics (have more than one cell line) for the X chromosome. It is believed that this occurs because as an embryo,

every female cell selects one X to be expressed and the other to become inactive. The selection is more or less random. By chance, a genotypical heterozygote could express a recessive trait phenotypically. The inactive material of each X appears in the cell as a clump of chromatin called the Barr body.

197. **(B)** The Hardy–Weinberg law defines a predictable relationship between heterozygote and homozygote possessors of dominant and recessive pairs of genes found at the same locus. It explains why, given random mating, recessive individuals do not become extinct. It works only in populations with random mating.

198. **(C)** Expressivity means the gene has a different effect or appearance in different kindreds. Sometimes the gene may be expressed in mild, moderate, or severe forms. It is an example of how the entire genome must be taken into account when considering the effect of some genes.

199. **(A)** Penetrance is the percentage of persons having the gene in whom there is an effect. For example, if not all the people who have a certain gene have the corresponding phenotype, the gene has reduced penetrance.

200. **(C)** Teratogenicity drug labeling is required by the Food and Drug Administration (FDA). The FDA has established five categories of drugs based on their potential for causing birth defects. The categories are A through D, which correspond directly to distractors A through D in this question. The fifth category is X and corresponds to distractor E.

201. **(D)** The 50% number represents testable products of conception in the first trimester. Second trimester losses are significantly less.

202. **(A)** Elective abortions and term births have approximately the same incidence of chromosomal abnormalities: 1/200 (less than 1%). Spontaneous abortions may have 50 to 75 times the incidence, according to some studies.

203. **(A)** Of abortuses that are abnormal, nearly one half are trisomic. One third of the trisomies are trisomy 16, which does not occur in the liveborn since all such fetuses die. Next is 45,XO, which occurs in about roughly 20% of chromosomally abnormal abortuses.

204. **(D)** An evaluation of serum gonadotropins would demonstrate ovarian failure, one of the hallmarks of this syndrome. Karyotyping is not always necessary.

205. **(C)** The initial three anomalies described by Turner were short stature, cubitus valgus, and webbing of the neck. Lymphedema of the hands and feet is a sign often present at the birth of these infants and may be the first diagnostic sign. Clogging of lymphatics causes webbing of the fetal neck with the resultant skin bridges and edema of the extremities. Coarctation of the aorta and absence of a kidney may also be present. Normal fertility is not possible since the gonads are dysfunctional (gonadal dysgenesis).

Only two thirds of the patients, however, have the classic 45,XO chromosomal complement. The syndrome is synonymous with the term of gonadal dysgenesis. Patients with pure gonadal dysgenesis lack the associated physical findings of Turner syndrome.

206. **(B)** Patients who lack an X (such as XO) or have Xp (short arm of X) missing will be short. X inactivation (Lyons) appears to be incomplete. More specifically, those missing the distal-most portion of the short arm of X are of short stature.

207. **(D)** More than one third of the patients with gonadal dysgenesis are chromatin positive. They are not all XO Turner's. Some of the chromatin-positive patients are mosaics or have structural defects of the X chromosomes, such as isochromosomes, and there are some who are 46,XX.

208. **(B)** Aneuploidy is characterized by any number of chromosomes that is not an exact multiple of the haploid number. Down syndrome has 47 chromosomes (2n + 1); the extra being a trisomy of chromosome 21. It is commonly associated with advanced maternal age and thought to be caused most often by maternal chromosomal nondisjunction. About 4% of Down patients are euploidy.

209. **(C)** Many of these enzyme defects lend themselves to biochemical determinations, either on the amniotic fluid itself or on cells cultured from it. Unfortunately, in most instances you must know prospectively which defect to screen. They cannot all be routinely screened. PKU, galactosemia, Tay–Sachs disease, Hurler syndrome, Sanfilippo A, and Sanfilippo B all fit this category.

210. **(C)** The Bombay phenotype is very rare and has inactive alleles for H antigen. If no H is formed, neither A nor B antigen can be formed, and the patient's blood will be type O even if the A or B gene is present. Laboratory error is always possible, but given the caution with which blood typing is done, it is unlikely.

211. **(A)** The Barr body is the inactivated X chromosome and is also known as the sex chromatin. The number of Barr bodies is generally one less than the number of X chromosomes. It tells nothing about the number of Y chromosomes. It equals the total number of X chromosomes minus one.

212. **(E)** Ultrasound is performed in over one half of pregnancies in the United States. It is useful in finding many structural defects. X-ray can be useful in some of the same situations. Direct fetal blood sampling has some promising indications. DNA analysis with gene-specific probes is available for several prenatal conditions. Screening with maternal serum alpha-fetoprotein, estriol, human chorionic gonadotropins, and inhibin are also used. Even fetal cells obtained from maternal blood can be used.

213. **(E)** Chorionic villus sampling, also known as chorionic villus biopsy, has been performed in the United States for the past 15 to 20 years. It is associated with a 1 per 200 pregnancy loss rate. One complication is the very small risk of less than one per thousand limb malformations when CVS is performed at 9 to 10 weeks. Thus, many centers will perform CVS only around 10½ to 11½ weeks. CVS is performed by placing a small catheter or needle into the placenta (not into the chorionic membranes or into the amniotic fluid) and removing a small bit of villus through suction aspiration. The chorionic villus is then dissected, and cells are harvested for chromosomal analysis. The analysis made from CVS can essentially give the same information as the chromosomal analysis from amniocentesis.

214. **(E)** All of the options are possible, as is AB. The father could not be type O, unless of the very rare Bombay phenotype.

215. **(A, B, C)** The crucial factor in male development is the presence of a Y chromosome. Even in the presence of multiple Xs, a male will develop. In a YO genotype, there will be no offspring. It is incompatible with life.

216. **(A, B, C, D)** In somatic cells of human (and all mammal) females, only one X chromosome is active. The second X becomes condensed and inactive and known as the sex chromatin or Barr body. Inactivation of the X occurs early in embryonic life, but scientists are not certain when. The inactive X can be either the paternal or maternal X in different cells of the same individual. Once the cell has inactivated an X, all the clones of that cell will inactivate the same X.

217. **(A, B, D, E)** Since development by Liley in 1962, amniocentesis and CVS for prenatal diagnosis and therapy have become very common. There are now several hundred diagnosable diseases. Structural lesions are usually diagnosed by ultrasound.

218. **(A, B, C, E)** A teratogen is any agent that can produce a malformation or raise the incidence of a malformation in a given population. In identifying a teratogen, four factors must be considered: (1) The time of exposure to the teratogen. The affected organ should be rapidly growing to be affected. (2) The amount of exposure. Has there been a large enough dose and a long enough time to show an effect? (3) Are there known anomalies associated with the agent, and are those the anomalies present? (4) Are there known anomalies present in other family members not exposed to the agent? A mutation is genetic, not a teratogen.

219. **(A, B, C, D)** Not all chromosomal abnormalities are hereditary. Couples who have a child with a nonhereditary defect have a very low risk of a similar defect occurring in a subsequent pregnancy. Proven causes of chromosomal abnormalities in vivo are few but do exist. Irradiation, viruses, some bacteria, gases, and chemical agents have all been associated with anomalies.

220. **(B, C)** Couples suffering recurrent miscarriage (three or more early pregnancy losses) make up about 1/200 couples. A chromosomal abnormality is reported in 10 to 25% of these couples. The most types of anomaly are related to chromosomal nondisjunction. Two to 3% demonstrate balanced translocations. Thrombophilia diseases may be associated with this condition as well.

221. **(A, C, D)** PKU is an autosomal recessive disease in which an affected individual lacks the enzyme phenylalanine hydroxylase. When excessive amounts of phenylalanine accumulate, mental retardation usually occurs. The disease may be treated with a low phenylalanine diet in childhood. If a woman with PKU becomes pregnant and is not on a special diet, the maternal phenylalanine levels may cause fetal abnormalities, growth retardation, and microcephaly. Thus, her fetus may be affected even though the fetus does not have the disease. Because individuals who carry one gene are asymptomatic, the father of this pregnancy may be a carrier and still have an affected infant. Additionally, testing the previous child's father has no bearing on this pregnancy.

222. **(A, C)** If the X chromosome with the recessive gene is the only X chromosome present, the female can certainly have an X-linked disease. Gonadal dysgenesis results in increased gonadotropins only in the affected offspring, not in the mother. Pregnant women have very low gonadotropin production. There is no blood test that is routinely done to detect 45,XO patients in utero, and amniocentesis is necessary.

223. **(A, B, C, E)** Polygenic/multifactorial inheritance is involved in many abnormalities. These inheritance patterns present with a greater than expected recurrence rate than that seen at random, usually 2 to 5%. Many structural abnormalities, including cleft lip and palate, tetralogy of Fallot, pyloric stenosis, and clubfoot, are examples of such inheritance. Achondroplasia is an autosomal dominant inheritance.

224. **(C)** Germ cells (gametes) undergo this type of division only once in a lifetime to produce gametes with a haploid number of chromosomes. Reduction to the haploid number occurs in the first meiotic division.

25. **(B)** Interphase is a period of time during a cell's division when the chromosomes are active but not individually recognizable. Interphase is a relatively long period in the mitotic cycle; DNA replication takes place in this phase.

226. **(F)** The symbol for a normal male is an open square.

227. **(J)** The propositus (proband) is the individual who brought the family to the geneticist's attention. He is designated by an arrow. If the propositus were female, the symbol would be a blackened circle with an arrow pointing to it.

228. **(H)** When the sex is not known for assignment, a diamond figure is used rather than a circle or square.

229. **(I)** The male and female symbol joined by one line signifies a nonrelated marriage. If joined by a double line, the symbols refer to a consanguineous marriage.

230. **(K)** Phenotype refers to how the individual can be recognized, while genotype refers to genetic constituency.

231. **(D)** A centromere is a constant feature of every chromosome. Some are in the middle (metacentric), some acrocentric (near one end), and some submetacentric (off-center). It appears as a small, clear structure microscopically.

232. **(L)** An example would be the AB blood group, in which both A and B antigens are recognized.

233. **(O)** Linked genes (i.e., lying close together) that are crossing over are apt to cross over together. Therefore, the phenotypic patterns produced by the two remain together also.

234. **(A)** Mitosis results in the doubling of the genetic material.

235. **(A)** Chromosomal abnormalities may be numerical or structural and may involve auto-

somes, sex chromosomes, or both simultaneously. The abnormality may be present in all
body cells or only some of the cells, producing what is called mosaicism (or more than
one cell line).

236–237. (236-C, 237-B) Each species has a characteristic number of chromosomes (ploidy). In
man, this 2n number is 46. Any multiple of
the haploid number (1n) is called euploid.
Polyploid means any exact multiple greater
than 2n (3n, 4n, etc.). Aneuploid means any
number of chromosomes that is not an exact
multiple of 1n.

238. (E) Translocations consist of two chromosomes breaking and exchanging material between them. They may be of two types, either
reciprocal (the exchange of chromatin between two nonhomologous chromosomes) or
Robertsonian (fusion of two chromosomes at
the centromere with loss of their heterochro-
matic short arms).

239. (F) A chromosome divides such that the two
arms separate, rather than the two chromatids. This is an isochromosome. The most
common isochromosome involves the long
arm of the X, i(Xq). Fifteen to 20% of Turner
syndrome patients have this karyotype.

240. (G) Breakage and rearrangement of a chromosome such that a fragment ends up rotated 180 degrees. If the rearrangement takes
place in a single arm, the inversion is called
paracentric. If it involves the region of the
centromere, it is called pericentric.

241. (D) A ring chromosome is a type of deletion
chromosome in which two broken ends are
reunited to form a ring-shaped chromosome.
As long as the ring chromosome retains a
centromere, it is capable of division.

242. (I) Nondisjunction is the failure of paired
chromosomes to separate in anaphase. It is
the most common cause of an error in chromosome number.

243. (E) The short arm is designated by p and the
long arm by q. Remember that p stands for

petite. (The conventions were developed in
France.) (See Figure 4–2.)

244. (A) Trisomy 21 is revealed. The patient is a
male with 47 chromosomes, three of which
are number 21.

245. (C) The 46 reveals that the proper number of
chromosomes is present, and the semicolon
between the involved chromosomes desig-
nates a balanced translocation without loss of
genetic material.

246. (D) The long arms of a D and a G chromosome have united to form a single chromosome, and the short arms have been lost.

247. (E) Isochromosomes are identified by a lowercase i after the chromosome involved.

248. (C) Klinefelter syndrome can also be found
with 48,XXXY. This patient would have two
Barr bodies per cell, yet still be male.

249. (A) Early diagnosis is important, as other developmental defects such as coarctation of
the aorta and renal abnormalities are also associated. Any child born with lymphedema
of the extremities should be thoroughly investigated for possible Turner syndrome.

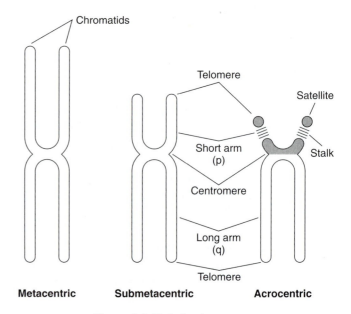

Figure 4–2. Part of a chromosome.

250. **(D)** Translocation can cause Down syndrome with 46 chromosomes present. The occurrence of this entity does not increase with age and is rarely transmitted by the male. The current terminology for this condition would be t(14q 21q)–.

251. **(B)** Testicular feminization patients have a normal male chromosome pattern and target organs that are insensitive to testosterone. They generally are of a normal female phenotype but with the potential for gonadal malignancy.

252. **(E)** Cry of the cat, or cri du chat, syndrome is due to deletion of the short arm of chromosome 5. It can also occur because of a parental translocation. It, however, is the most common human chromosomal syndrome caused by deletion.

253. **(F)** In the true hermaphrodite, both testicular and ovarian tissue (ovotestes) must be present. The external genitalia may resemble either a male or female, depending on the ratio of estrogens and androgens present. Some are XX, some XY, while others are chimeras (XX/XY).

254. **(D)** Diabetes mellitus is another entity that has no single known genetic defect and no definite age of onset. It does exhibit characteristics indicating multifactorial genetic inheritance with associated human lymphocyte antigen (HLA) types.

255. **(B)** Sickle cell anemia is caused by an abnormal hemoglobin resulting from a change in the amino acid sequence of the globin chain. The abnormality is the result of a single amino acid in the six position on the 146 amino acid chain being substituted.

256. **(C)** Hemophilia is due to a defect in the production of antihemophilic globulin. Fortunately, it is rare, occurring in about 1 in 10,000 male births. One third of all cases arise from new mutations in lethal X-linked diseases but are much less common in nonlethal diseases such as hemophilia.

257. **(E)** Thalidomide is a drug that causes defects when the fetus is exposed to it between the 28th and the 42nd day of gestation. Congenital anomalies of phocomelia and hearing defects are produced, but they are not genetic. It is one of the few known cause–effect teratogens and one of the most severe teratogens known in humans.

258. **(C)** This sequence is characteristic of X-linked recessive inheritance. In X-linked dominant inheritance, an affected male transmits the disease to all of his daughters and none of his sons. This is a rare situation.

259. **(B)** Dominant inheritance diseases do not have a carrier state, and sex-linked recessives occur only in males. The incidence may be as low as one in a thousand.

260. **(B)** This disease is usually discussed under the heading of intersex or ambiguous genitalia. Its genetic etiology may be overlooked. It can be lethal within the first few days of life or produce adrenal insufficiency and short stature in other cases. It is the most common cause of female pseudohermaphroditism, causing virilization of female infants. It is the most common cause of ambiguous genitalia in the newborn. These patients have normal XX chromosomes but lack an enzyme needed for normal steroid metabolism. They are deficient in 21, 17, or 11 hydroxylase enzymes. The site of the block determines the manifestations of the disease.

261. **(A)** The defect resulting in neurofibromatosis (von Recklinghausen disease) is autosomal dominant. It is one of the genetic diseases that increases (shows evidence of greater mutation) with increasing paternal age. It shows a very high mutation rate in man and also shows extremely variable patterns of inheritance. Duchenne's muscular dystrophy has similar patterns of transmission.

262. **(B)** CAH is an autosomal recessive disease that can be treated by replacing cortisol or an equivalent, which then by feedback inhibi-

tion decreases the excess production of androgens. Some forms require vigorous sodium replacement to save the adrenal insufficient infant.

263. (E) Hemolysis will develop only when the patient is exposed to certain drugs such as primaquine. If the genetic defect is known, such drugs can be avoided.

264. (A) These patients cannot convert phenylalanine to tyrosine. By restricting phenylalanine, the sequelae of this defect can be decreased. Even with a special diet, problems cannot be avoided completely. Diet is especially important when the patient is pregnant.

265. (C) This is seen in about 95% of adults with CML and a much smaller portion of patients with other types of leukemia. The deleted chromosome 22 is called the Philadelphia chromosome.

266. (B) This is seen in Burkitt's lymphoma and B-cell acute lymphocytic leukemia.

267. (E) Retinoblastoma often has a deletion in chromosome 13 in bond 13g 14. Most cases are due to somatic mutation but about 40% are hereditary.

268. (A) Sporadic carcinoma of the lung is associated with loss of tumor-suppressor genes TP53 and W1.

269. (C) This distinctive, nonrandom chromosomal defect may be acquired during the development of a malignancy. In CML, a second Philadelphia chromosome and an additional chromosome 8, or isochromosome of the long arm of 17, may be found in terminal patients. The Y chromosome may be lost in males.

270. (D) Oncogenes are present in all cells and, in their natural state, are in charge of orderly division. They consist of more than 50 functionally heterogeneous genes that are important in the transformation of cells to the malignant state. They may be activated by retroviruses (RNA virus) or mutational events. Names for the genes are acronyms for their origins (c-myc was found in B-cell avian myelocytoma).

271. (B) The risk of breast cancer in a woman doubles when a first-degree relative has the disease.

272. (D) Cancer of the breast, endometrium, and ovary all seem to have genetically inherited risk. Ovarian cancer may even be an autosomal dominant trait in some families, but in most cases there is probably no familial relationship. The highest risk-associated ovarian cancer appears to be the papillary serous cystadenocarcinoma. It probably represents only 3% of all cases of ovarian cancer. Women with two first-degree relatives with ovarian cancer may have a 50% chance of getting the disease, but with one probably a 2 to 3% risk (about double that of the general population)—certainly not the 25% reported in some places.

273. (C) The Lynch type II family has a genetic transmission of ovarian, endometrial, and nonpolypoid colorectal cancer. It appears to be passed as an autosomal dominant with variable penetrance.

274. (B) Lithium has been associated in some reports with Ebstein's anomaly, an abnormality of the tricuspid valve.

275. (C) Warfarin crosses the placenta and has been associated with several lesions, including nasal hypoplasia and other craniofacial anomalies.

276. (C) Carbamazepine, which is commonly used as an anticonvulsant, has been associated with several lesions including craniofacial anomalies.

277. (C) Fetal alcohol syndrome is a group of anomalies including minor facial anomalies and mental retardation.

278–279. (278-A, 279-A) Acyclovir and metronidazole are not associated with anomalies in the neonate.

Physiology of Reproduction
Questions

280. Gonadotropin-releasing hormone (GnRH) stimulates the release of

    (A) adrenocorticotropic hormone (ACTH)
    (B) growth hormone (GH)
    (C) luteinizing hormone (LH)
    (D) opiate peptide
    (E) thyroid-stimulating hormone (TSH)

281. Which of the following substances stimulates GnRH secretion?

    (A) beta-endorphin
    (B) dopamine
    (C) dynorphin
    (D) norepinephrine
    (E) serotonin

282. GnRH-associated peptide (GAP) is a/an

    (A) stimulator of gonadotropins and an inhibitor of prolactin
    (B) inhibitor of gonadotropins and a stimulator of prolactin
    (C) stimulator of gonadotropins and a stimulator of prolactin
    (D) inhibitor of gonadotropins and an inhibitor of prolactin
    (E) stimulator of gonadotropins and has no effect on prolactin

283. Tyrosine is an essential amino acid for the biosynthesis of

    (A) dopamine
    (B) dynorphin
    (C) GnRH
    (D) prostaglandins
    (E) vasopressin

284. X-rays on a 35-year-old after a motor vehicle accident reveal a basilar skull fracture and raise a concern about an interruption of the hypophyseal portal circulation. This would cause a decline in circulating

    (A) arginine vasopressin
    (B) dopamine
    (C) gonadotropins
    (D) oxytocin
    (E) prolactin

285. A patient presents with amenorrhea and galactorrhea. Her prolactin levels are elevated. She is not and never has been pregnant. In addition to evaluating her for a prolactinoma, one also needs to evaluate for other causes that would increase prolactin such as elevated

    (A) corticotropin-releasing hormone
    (B) dopamine
    (C) gamma-aminobutyric acid (GABA)
    (D) histamine type II receptor activation
    (E) thyrotropin-releasing hormone (TRH)

286. Since the workup of an elevated prolactin level can be expensive, it is appropriate to draw prolactin levels when the lowest values are to be expected. Prolactin levels

(A) decrease shortly after sleep
(B) increase after ingesting high-carbohydrate meals
(C) increase during stress
(D) decrease during surgery
(E) decrease after exercise

287. During which of the following conditions would the serum prolactin level be greatest?

(A) menopause
(B) ovulation
(C) parturition
(D) sleep

288. Which of the following statements regarding GnRH-stimulated LH secretion is accurate?

(A) It is enhanced by gonadotrope exposure to progesterone.
(B) It is increased by gonadotrope exposure to testosterone.
(C) It is enhanced by gonadotrope exposure to estrogen.
(D) It is enhanced by gonadotrope exposure to continuous GnRH.
(E) It is associated with steady LH release.

289. Low-density lipoprotein (LDL) cholesterol serves as the principal substrate for steroidogenesis. Which of the following statements regarding circulating LDL is correct?

(A) LDL is formed after addition of triglyceride to very low-density lipoprotein (VLDL).
(B) LDL levels are negatively correlated with cardiovascular disease.
(C) LDL is the major carrier of cholesterol in the plasma.
(D) LDL enters the cells by passive diffusion.
(E) LDL facilitates the transport of polar lipids in the blood plasma.

290. Steroid hormones are classified as

(A) amino acids
(B) phospholipids
(C) lipids
(D) glycoprotein
(E) none of the above

291. The progressive sequence (with steps omitted) in the metabolism of steroid hormones is

(A) cholesterol–estradiol–testosterone–pregnenolone
(B) cholesterol–pregnenolone–cortisol–estradiol
(C) cholesterol–pregnenolone–estrone–androstenedione
(D) cholesterol–androstenedione–pregnenolone–estrone
(E) cholesterol–pregnenolone–androstenedione–estrone

292. Adrenal corticoids belong to which of the following groups?

(A) aldehydes
(B) androstanes
(C) cholesterols
(D) estranes
(E) pregnanes

293. The three principal estrogens in women in decreasing order of potency are

(A) estradiol, estriol, estrone
(B) estradiol, estrone, estriol
(C) estriol, estradiol, estrone
(D) estriol, estrone, estradiol
(E) estrone, estriol, estradiol

294. Which of the following sequences best describes estrogen action?

(A) cell membrane diffusion; steroid receptor–DNA complex formation; transcription; translation
(B) cell membrane receptor activation; steroid receptor–DNA complex formation; transcription; translation

(C) cell membrane diffusion; steroid receptor–DNA complex formation; translation; transcription

(D) cell membrane diffusion; adenylate cyclase activation; cyclic adenosine monophosphate (cAMP) production; protein phosphorylation

(E) cell membrane receptor activation; adenylate cyclase activation; cyclic AMP production; protein phosphorylation

295. Which of the following compounds was used in the 1950s to 1960s in an attempt to hormonally support a pregnancy and avoid a miscarriage? Instead, it caused vaginal adenosis in female offspring.

(A) dehydroepiandrosterone

(B) diethylstilbestrol (DES)

(C) estradiol

(D) estrone

(E) testosterone

296. Addition of an ethinyl group at the 17C position of estradiol was critical in the development of the oral contraceptive pill because it

(A) decreases biological activity

(B) increases androgenic activity

(C) increases hepatic degradation

(D) increases sex hormone–binding globulin affinity

(E) maintains biological activity after oral absorption

297. A 50-year-old menopausal patient wishes to stay on her oral contraceptive pill. Her health care provider tries to explain that this provides more estrogen than she needs postmenopausally. What dose of ethinyl estradiol is roughly biologically equivalent to the typical postmenopausal dose of 0.625 mg of conjugated estrogens?

(A) 0.005 to 0.010 mg

(B) 0.05 to 10 mg

(C) 0.50 to 1.0 mg

(D) 5.0 to 10.0 mg

(E) 50.0 to 100.0 mg

298. The three principal androgens in decreasing order of potency are

(A) androstenedione, testosterone, dihydrotestosterone

(B) dihydrotestosterone, androstenedione, testosterone

(C) dihydrotestosterone, testosterone, androstenedione

(D) testosterone, androstenedione, dihydrotestosterone

(E) testosterone, dihydrotestosterone, androstenedione

299. A patient with polycystic ovarian syndrome will often have an increase in insulin resistance. This will result in an increase in

(A) follicle-stimulating hormone (FSH)

(B) free estrogen level

(C) free testosterone level

(D) hepatic production of sex hormone–binding globulin

300. The chemical name of the compound shown in Figure 5–1 is

(A) 5-cholesten-3 b-ol

(B) 17b-hydroxy-4-androstene-3-one

(C) 3b-hydroxy-5-pregnane-20-one

(D) 4-androstene-3, 17-dione

(E) none of the above

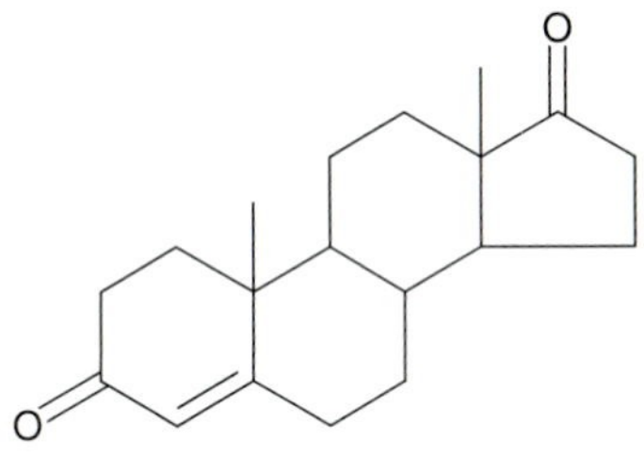

Figure 5–1.

301. Which of the following substances is the precursor to prostaglandins (PGs)?

(A) arachidonic acid

(B) isobutyric acid

(C) isoleucine

(D) linoleic acid

(E) phospholipase A

302. Given that prostaglandins appear to be involved in preterm labor, which of the following medications might provide some help in stopping preterm labor?

(A) ACTH

(B) indomethacin

(C) progesterone

(D) prolactin-inhibiting factor (PIF)

(E) thyroid hormone

303. During human development the Rathke's pouch differentiates into the

(A) anterior pituitary

(B) arcuate nucleus

(C) medial basal hypothalamus

(D) median eminence

(E) posterior pituitary

304. Normal fetal gonadotropins are necessary to control and coordinate the phenotypic sexual differentiation of the fetus during intrauterine development. Which of the following statements best describes circulating gonadotropin levels in the human fetus?

(A) They are low during the first trimester, rise to maximal levels during the second trimester, and return to low levels by term.

(B) They are low during the first trimester, rise to maximal levels during the second trimester, and remain elevated to term.

(C) They are low during the first trimester, remain low during the second trimester, and rise to maximal levels by term.

(D) They are high during the first trimester, decrease to undetectable levels during the second trimester, and remain low to term.

(E) They are low throughout intrauterine life.

305. Which of the following embryonic tissues contributes to the adult fallopian tube?

(A) coelomic epithelium

(B) mesenchyme

(C) mesonephric duct

(D) paramesonephric duct

(E) urogenital ridge

306. Which of the following statements best describes the role of testosterone in developing a phenotypic male fetus?

(A) Testosterone causes elongation of the genital tubercle into the phallus.

(B) Testosterone is mainly responsible for corpus spongiosum development.

(C) Testosterone is mainly responsible for paramesonephric duct development.

(D) Testosterone secretion is stimulated by maternal circulating gonadotropins.

(E) Testosterone secretion is stimulated by human chorionic gonadotropin (hCG).

307. The most common ovarian lesion associated with excessive estrogen stimulation in infants is a

(A) granulosa cell tumor

(B) leiomyoma

(C) serous cystadenoma

(D) single large follicular cyst

(E) theca cell tumor

308. Initiation of puberty results from

(A) diminished hypothalamic sensitivity to sex steroid negative feedback

(B) diminished "intrinsic" central nervous system (CNS) inhibition

(C) both

(D) neither

Questions 309 through 313

A mother and her 16-year-old daughter present to your office because the daughter has not yet menstruated. They are very concerned that something is wrong. By applying principles of puberty to this patient, it is possible to determine if the teen is simply undergoing a slightly delayed puberty versus potentially manifesting a significant problem.

309. The normal sequence of pubertal changes in the female is

    (A) maximal growth velocity, menarche, thelarche

    (B) maximal growth velocity, thelarche, menarche

    (C) menarche, maximal growth velocity, thelarche

    (D) thelarche, maximal growth velocity, menarche

    (E) thelarche, menarche, maximal growth velocity

310. Menarche usually occurs between the ages of

    (A) 8 and 10 years

    (B) 11 and 13 years

    (C) 14 and 16 years

    (D) 17 and 18 years

311. Which of the following pubertal events is not mediated by gonadal estrogen production and therefore would occur even in the absence of estrogen production?

    (A) breast development

    (B) menstruation

    (C) pubic hair growth

    (D) skeletal growth

    (E) vaginal cornification

312. The sequence of pubertal changes should occur over a period of

    (A) 0.5 years

    (B) 1.5 years

    (C) 4.5 years

    (D) 7.5 years

    (E) 9.5 years

313. Which of the following causes of delayed puberty accompanies elevated circulating gonadotropin levels?

    (A) chronic illness

    (B) gonadal dysgenesis

    (C) hypothalamic tumors

    (D) Kallmann's syndrome

    (E) malnutrition

314. A 7-year-old girl is brought in for evaluation. On examination, she has well-developed pubic hair and breasts. She is at 99% of height for her age. Her mother recently noted some blood stains on her underwear. Which of the following conditions is most likely the cause of these findings?

    (A) estrogen-producing ovarian cyst

    (B) hepatoma

    (C) hypothalamic tumor

    (D) sex steroid-containing medication

    (E) thecal/Leydig cell tumor

315. A 6-year-old girl experiences irregular vaginal bleeding. She is taller than her peers and has early breast development. Serum gonadotropin levels are low and remain unchanged after intravenous administration of GnRH. The most likely diagnosis is a/an

    (A) corpus luteum cyst

    (B) endometrioma

    (C) epoophoron

    (D) fibroma

    (E) granulosa cell tumor

316. The inhibitory action of sex steroids on GnRH secretion is primarily mediated by

    (A) dopamine

    (B) melatonin

    (C) norepinephrine

    (D) opioid peptides

    (E) serotonin

317. Which of the following statements best describes the role of FSH in menstruation?

    (A) FSH stimulates follicular growth only in the early preantral stage.
    (B) FSH increases its own receptor number on theca cells.
    (C) FSH induces theca cell aromatase.
    (D) FSH stimulates granulosa cell androgen production.
    (E) FSH induces granulosa cell LH receptors within the dominant follicle.

318. The midcycle LH surge

    (A) enhances thecal cell androgen production
    (B) luteinizes granulosa cells
    (C) initiates resumption of meiosis
    (D) facilitates oocyte expulsion
    (E) all of the above

319. Which statement best describes estrogen-positive feedback on LH release?

    (A) It is affected by the level of circulating estrogen.
    (B) It is enhanced by testosterone.
    (C) It is increased by opioid peptides.
    (D) It is unaffected by progesterone.
    (E) It is unaffected by the duration of estrogen stimulation.

320. Which of the following gametes is released from the graafian follicle during ovulation?

    (A) primary oocyte
    (B) primary oocyte and first polar body
    (C) secondary oocyte
    (D) secondary oocyte and first polar body
    (E) secondary oocyte and second polar body

321. Which of the following hormone(s) is/are produced by the corpus luteum?

    (A) progesterone only
    (B) progesterone and estrogen only
    (C) progesterone, estrogen, and inhibin only
    (D) progesterone, estrogen, inhibin, and relaxin only
    (E) progesterone, estrogen, inhibin, relaxin, and contractin

322. During an evaluation for infertility, a woman may have an endometrial biopsy to evaluate the quality of her ovulation since the development of the corpus luteum is most closely associated with the

    (A) fertilization of an ovum
    (B) follicular phase of the endometrium
    (C) proliferative phase of the endometrium
    (D) secretory phase of the endometrium
    (E) shedding phase of the endometrium (menstruation)

323. The postcoital test used in an infertility evaluation assesses the cervical mucus for ferning. The presence of ferning depends on which of the following hormones?

    (A) estrogen
    (B) estrogen and progesterone
    (C) hCG
    (D) LH
    (E) progesterone

324. Spinnbarkeit describes the

    (A) amount of cervical mucus
    (B) clarity of cervical mucus
    (C) elasticity of cervical mucus
    (D) ferning of cervical mucus
    (E) viscosity of cervical mucus

Questions 325 through 327

A 47-year-old patient presents wondering if her problems with mood swings, insomnia, and vaginal dryness represent menopause. She had a hysterectomy 10 years ago for abnormal uterine bleeding, but the ovaries were not removed. Since she cannot afford hormonal testing, a maturation index is done on her Pap smear.

325. Ideally, cytologic cells for evaluation of hormonal status should be obtained from the

    (A) ectocervix
    (B) endocervix
    (C) labia minora
    (D) lateral vaginal wall
    (E) posterior vaginal fornix

326. Ninety percent of the cells found on her Pap smear have thick, rounded cytoplasm and plump, round, vesicular nuclei with an intact chromatin pattern. The maturation index (MI) would most likely be

    (A) 90/0/10
    (B) 90/10/0
    (C) 10/0/90
    (D) 10/90/0
    (E) 0/90/10

327. Based on this result, one would anticipate that if hormonal levels were obtained they would show

    (A) elevated estrogen levels
    (B) elevated progesterone levels
    (C) low estrogen levels
    (D) normal FSH levels
    (E) normal progesterone levels

328. Which of the following target tissue effects is mediated by progesterone?

    (A) mammary ductal development
    (B) proliferative endometrium
    (C) shortened GnRH pulse interval
    (D) thermogenic effect
    (E) thin, stretchy cervical mucus

329. A patient presented to the emergency department with an infected incomplete abortion. During the dilatation and curettage (D&C) excessive bleeding developed that required vigorous curetting to control. She returns to the physician 6 months later complaining that she has not had a menstrual cycle since. She has all the symptoms of getting ready to start a period but never sees any bleeding. This history implies that what layer of endometrium is damaged?

    (A) basal zone
    (B) compact zone
    (C) functional zone
    (D) spongy zone
    (E) none of the above

330. Menstrual flow is associated with the

    (A) prolonged maintenance of estrogen
    (B) prolonged maintenance of progesterone
    (C) withdrawal of FSH
    (D) withdrawal of LH
    (E) withdrawal of progesterone

331. The amount of blood lost during an average normal menses is about

    (A) 10 to 25 mL
    (B) 25 to 75 mL
    (C) 80 to 120 mL
    (D) 125 to 175 mL
    (E) 180 to 220 mL

332. Menstrual blood is usually nonclotting because of

    (A) heparin
    (B) "organ hemophilia"
    (C) prior clotting and liquefaction
    (D) toxins that inhibit clotting
    (E) none of the above

333. The normal vaginal pH during the menstrual cycle is

    (A) 3 to 4.5
    (B) 4.5 to 5.5
    (C) 5.5 to 6.5
    (D) 6.5 to 7.5
    (E) 7.5 to 8.5

334. Even after menopause most women have circulating estrogen. In high enough levels, this can promote the development of endometrial cancer. It mainly originates from the aromatization of

(A) androstenedione to estrone by ovarian granulosa cells

(B) androstenedione to estrone by ovarian thecal cells

(C) androstenedione to estrone by adipose tissue

(D) testosterone to estradiol by adipose tissue

(E) estradiol to estrone by adipose tissue

335. A 50-year-old woman presents to her health care provider complaining of hot flushes. Hot flushes are often the symptom in a perimenopausal woman that causes her to seek medical assistance. Hot flushes entail

(A) peripheral redistribution of blood flow leading to sweating and elevated heart rate

(B) peripheral vasodilatation reflecting an increase in core body temperature

(C) subjective symptoms always accompanying objective signs of vasomotor instability

(D) peripheral vasodilatation resulting from a direct LH action on sympathetic neurons

(E) an average duration of about 30 minutes

336. Prior to initiating estrogen replacement therapy (ERT), the patient is counseled regarding the long-term risks of estrogen deficiency associated with menopause. These are osteoporosis and cardiovascular disease. With osteoporosis the accelerated bone loss occurs 1 to 8 years after menopause

(A) causes an elevation in circulating parathyroid hormone levels

(B) causes increased urinary loss of phosphorus and hydroxyproline

(C) does not influence trabecular bone

(D) primarily affects cortical bone

337. Cardioprotective actions of estrogen may include

(A) depression of high-density lipoprotein (HDL) levels

(B) dilatation of coronary vessels

(C) elevation of LDL levels

(D) production of thromboxane

(E) widening of pulse pressure

338. This postmenopausal patient is interested in hormone replacement therapy (HRT) with progesterone but is concerned about its dangers. Which of the following statements should be included in your discussion regarding the risks of HRT with combined therapy relative to no HRT?

(A) Just as oral contraceptives may increase blood coagulability, HRT will also, due to higher doses.

(B) HRT may increase the risk of cholelithiasis.

(C) HRT may increase the risk of endometrial carcinoma.

(D) HRT is likely to greatly increase the risk of breast carcinoma.

(E) HRT may increase the risk of renal dysfunction.

DIRECTIONS (Questions 339 through 364): Each group of items in this section consists of lettered headings followed by a set of numbered words or phrases. For each numbered word or phrase, select the ONE lettered heading that is most closely associated with it. Each lettered heading may be selected once, more than once, or not at all.

Questions 339 and 340

(A) increased prolactin

(B) increased arginine vasopressin (AVP)

(C) decreased oxytocin

(D) decreased prolactin

339. Destruction of the supraoptic and paraventricular hypothalamic nuclei would result in _____.

340. Destruction of the dopamine tuberoinfundibular tract would result in _____.

Questions 341 through 347

   (A) androstenedione

   (B) dihydrotestosterone (DHT)

   (C) dehydroepiandrosterone sulfate (DHEAS)

   (D) estradiol

   (E) estrone

   (F) hCG

   (G) pregnenolone

   (H) testosterone

   (I) 17-hydroxyprogesterone

341. The lack of 5-alpha-reductase will result in the birth of an infant that looks female (phenotype) but is genetically male due to an inability to make _____.

342. Developing hirsutism in a 24-year-old woman prompts one to suspect an adult-onset 21-hydroxylase deficiency. The principal marker for such an enzyme deficiency is _____.

343. Principal androgen of adrenal origin.

344. Principal estrogen formed in a postmenopausal woman in peripheral tissue (e.g., adipose and muscle).

345. Hormone that can be used to simulate an LH surge and promote ovulation in an artifically stimulated cycle because it cross-reacts antigenically with LH.

346. Precursor for all hormonally active steroids.

347. Steroid hormone synthesized without 17-hydroxylase.

Questions 348 through 352

To understand the abnormalities of menstruation or ovulatory problems, one must understand the role of each of the involved hormones during the normal ovulatory menstrual cycle.

   (A) androstenedione

   (B) arachidonic acid

   (C) cholesterol

   (D) DHEAS

   (E) estradiol

   (F) inhibin

   (G) progesterone

348. Secretory endometrium

349. Breast duct development

350. Substrate for aromatase

351. Thermogenic hormone

352. Proliferative endometrium

Questions 353 through 356

Refer to Figure 5–2 for Questions 353 through 356.

353. FSH

354. LH

355. Estradiol

356. Progesterone

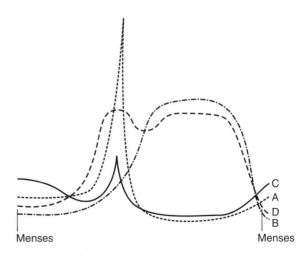

Figure 5–2.

Questions 357 through 359

    (A) high circulating estradiol

    (B) high circulating estrone

    (C) high circulating FSH

    (D) high circulating progesterone

    (E) high circulating testosterone

357. Castrated young adult female

358. Obesity

359. Dominant follicle

Questions 360 through 364

Women go through very distinctive stages relative to their reproductively related hormonal balance. A knowledge of these changes allows the provider to anticipate the physical manifestations of these changes. When do the following hormonal changes occur?

    (A) childbearing

    (B) fetal life

    (C) infancy

    (D) perimenopause

    (E) peripuberty

360. Rising serum DHEAS levels

361. Rising serum estrogen levels

362. Decreasing serum estrogen levels

363. Low serum DHEAS levels

364. Low serum estrogen levels

Answers and Explanations

280. **(C)** Anterior pituitary hormones are regulated by hypothalamic hormones, which reach the pituitary via the portal hypophyseal vessels. The six hypothalamic hormones are: (1) thyrotropin-releasing hormone (TRH), which stimulates TSH; (2) gonadotropin-releasing hormone (GnRH), which stimulates follicle-stimulating hormone (FSH) and LH; (3) corticotropin-releasing hormone (CRH), which stimulates ACTH; (4) somatostatin inhibits GH; (5) growth hormone-releasing hormone (GRH), which stimulates GH; and (6) prolactin inhibitory factor (PIF), which inhibits prolactin (PRL).

281. **(D)** Dopamine administration in vivo inhibits GnRH secretion. Serotonin and opiate peptides (produced under stressful conditions) also appear to inhibit GnRH release. Norepinephrine is produced in the mesencephalon and in the lower brain stem and stimulates GnRH secretion.

282. **(A)** The precursor protein for GnRH contains a 56-amino acid sequence called GnRH-associated peptide (GAP). GAP is a potent stimulator of gonadotropins and an inhibitor of prolactin. In mice, absence of gonadal function (hypogonadism) accompanies partial deletion of the gene responsible for the common precursor of GnRH and GAP.

283. **(A)** Tyrosine is an essential amino acid for the biosynthesis of all catecholamines, including dopamine. Tyrosine is converted to L-dihydroxyphenylalanine (DOPA) by the rate-limiting enzyme tyrosine hydroxylase.

DOPA is rapidly decarboxylated to dopamine by L-amino acid decarboxylase. Dopamine is the precursor of norepinephrine.

284. **(C)** Interruption of the hypophyseal portal circulation inhibits GnRH and dopamine delivery to the anterior pituitary, causing a decline in circulating gonadotropin values and an increase in circulating prolactin levels. AVP and oxytocin secretion from the posterior pituitary into the circulation is unaffected by interruption of the portal hypophyseal vessels (see Figure 5–3).

285. **(E)** Prolactin secretion is dominated by the inhibitory action of hypothalamic dopamine. Other mechanisms of prolactin inhibition are GABA and histamine type II receptor activation. TRH is a potent stimulator of prolactin and may induce galactorrhea under conditions of primary hypothyroidism, which should be checked for by measuring TSH.

286. **(C)** Circulating prolactin levels exhibit a diurnal variation with highest values occurring during sleep. High-protein meals (presumably mediated by ingestion of neurotransmitters) also cause a large increment in serum prolactin levels, while carbohydrate meals have no such effect. Several stressful stimuli, including surgery, exercise, and hypoglycemia, cause an elevation in prolactin secretion.

287. **(C)** Although prolactin is elevated throughout pregnancy, it rises sharply during labor and delivery, reaching levels of 200 ng/mL. It also increases with sleep, but not as much as

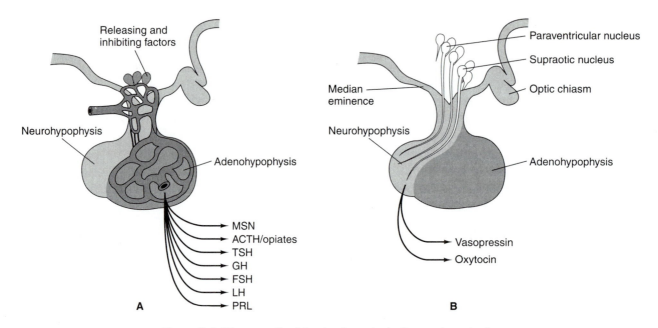

Figure 5–3. Diagrammatic of A. adenohypophysis, B. neurohypophysis.

during labor. Breast-feeding in the immediate postpartum period (< 7 days) may promote the release of prolactin enough to have serum levels that exceed 200 ng/mL. However, with established lactation the levels are much lower. Menopause and ovulation are not associated with increased prolactin.

288. **(C)** Pituitary cells that secrete LH and FSH are called gonadotropes. GnRH action on LH secretion is enhanced by gonadotrope exposure to estrogen and diminished by gonadotrope exposure to testosterone. Pulsatile GnRH reduces a similar LH release pattern and stimulates LH synthesis, causing a greater amount of LH release during subsequent GnRH stimulation. The GnRH stimulation test used to diagnose the etiology of sexual precocity is based on this phenomenon. In contrast, exposure of gonadotropes to continuous GnRH reduces pituitary desensitization to GnRH, resulting in a decrease in LH release during subsequent continuous GnRH stimulation.

289. **(C)** Cholesterol is the basic substrate for steroid-producing cells. LDL contains two thirds of plasma cholesterol and serves to

transport nonpolar lipids in the blood plasma. LDL is formed by removal of triglyceride from very low-density lipoprotein (VLDL). Circulating LDL levels are positively correlated with cardiovascular disease, while circulating HDLs are inversely associated with atherosclerosis. Cellular entry of LDL is mediated by specific cell membrane receptors; sex steroids readily enter cells by rapid diffusion.

290. **(C)** Steroids are relatively insoluble in water but are soluble in alcohol and ether, as are lipids. With the common precursor of steroids being cholesterol, the lipid character of these molecules would be expected.

291. **(E)** Steroid metabolism begins with cholesterol, which contains 27 carbons (C27), and proceeds from C21 compounds (pregnanes) through C19 compounds (androstanes) to C18 compounds (estranes). During this sequence of enzymatic events, the number of carbon atoms in the steroid molecule is reduced but never increased (see Figure 5–4).

292. **(E)** Twenty-one-carbon steroid compounds (which include the corticoids) are known as

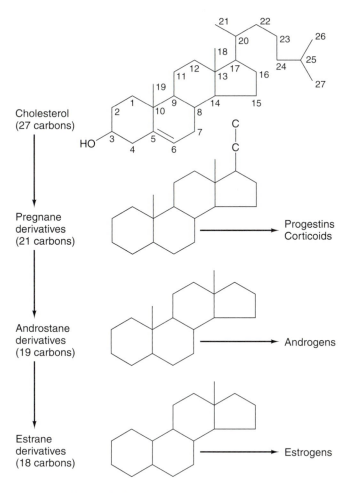

Figure 5–4. Pathway of steroid metabolism.

pregnanes; pregnanes are precursors of androstanes and estranes.

293. **(B)** Estrogens are derived from androgens by aromatization, a process creating a phenol configuration of the A ring. There are three main estrogens—estradiol (E2), estrone (E1), and estriol (E3)—and their potency, in decreasing order, is E2, E1 (0.1 that of E2), and E3 (0.01 that of E2) (see Figure 5–5).

294. **(A)** The action of steroids on their target cells involves cellular entry by diffusion, binding to intracellular receptor, formation of steroid receptor–DNA complex, transcription, and translation. In contrast, hypothalamic-releasing hormones and pituitary glycoproteins bind with cell membrane receptors and mediate their action through a variety of second messengers, including cAMP and calcium-dependent mechanisms.

295. **(B)** Although DES is the only one of these compounds without a steroid configuration, it is strongly estrogenic. Before its ban as an anti-abortifacient in 1971, the use of DES for miscarriage prevention was associated with müllerian tract abnormalities and clear cell adenocarcinoma of the vagina in offspring exposed in utero. The most frequent müllerian tract abnormality was a T-shaped uterus, with a small uterine cavity, accompanied by structural abnormalities of the cervix.

296. **(E)** The major breakthrough in steroid contraception occurred in 1938, when it was discovered that addition of an ethinyl group at the 17C position made estradiol active because of its reduced rate of hepatic degradation after oral ingestion.

297. **(A)** Ethinyl estradiol is a potent estrogen and is prescribed in microgram doses (1 µg =

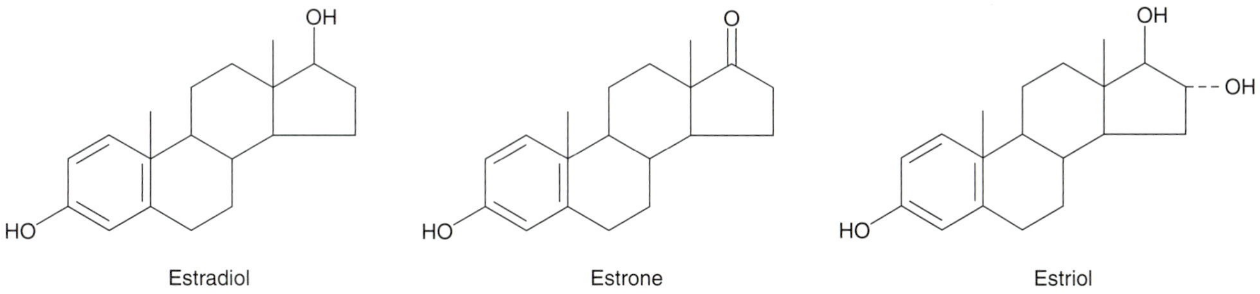

Estradiol

Estrone

Estriol

Figure 5–5. Classification of estrogens.

0.001 mg). The 0.625-mg dose of conjugated estrogens is roughly equivalent to 5 to 10 μg (i.e., 0.005 to 0.010 mg) ethinyl estradiol. Therefore, the most commonly used dosage of estrogen required for menopausal hormone replacement (0.625 mg conjugated estrogens) is less than that found in oral contraceptives, which contain approximately 30 μg of ethinyl estradiol.

298. **(C)** Androgens are steroids that stimulate the development of male secondary sex characteristics. Androgenic potency, in decreasing order, is dihydrotestosterone, testosterone, and androstenedione.

299. **(C)** The metabolic clearance rate (MCR) is defined as the volume of blood that is cleared of a substance per unit time. The circulating level of a substance is determined by its blood production rate (PR) divided by its MCR. With increased insulin resistance, insulin levels rise and inhibit hepatic production of sex hormone-binding globulin (SHBG). As most circulating testosterone is bound to SHBG, a decrease in SHBG will increase the amount of free testosterone and decrease the amount of free estrogen. The free testosterone and levels of estrone from peripheral conversion of androstenedione will keep FSH levels low.

300. **(D)** An understanding of steroid nomenclature is required to comprehend the steroid literature. The common name for 4-androstene-3, 17-dione is androstenedione.

301. **(A)** Arachidonic acid is found in several tissues, including fetal membranes and decidua. The liberation of intracellular arachidonic acid is followed by enzymatic oxidation via cyclooxygenase to form prostaglandins.

302. **(B)** Indomethacin is an inhibitor of prostaglandin synthesis and is used as a tocolytic. Inhibitors of PG synthesis may be prescribed for pain relief during menstruation (dysmenorrhea) since prostaglandins also play a role in dysmenorrhea.

303. **(A)** The primitive neural tube gives rise to the diencephalon, which differentiates into the hypothalamus, median eminence, and posterior pituitary by 9 to 11 weeks' gestation. The anterior pituitary appears as an evagination of Rathke's pouch arising from a diverticulum of the stomadeum. The fetal hypothalamus secretes neurohormones into the portal circulation by 16 weeks' gestation.

304. **(A)** The hypothalamus does not develop until 9 to 11 weeks' gestation so that circulating fetal gonadotropin levels are low during the first trimester. By midgestation, the hypothalamo-pituitary unit is functional, producing adult levels of circulating gonadotropins. This elevation in circulating gonadotropins is maximal during the second trimester and appears to play a role in gametogenesis. Fetal plasma gonadotropin levels decline as gestation continues, so that circulating fetal FSH and LH are undetectable at term. This phenomenon reflects the earliest manifestation of sex steroid negative feedback on the fetal hypothalamus.

305. **(D)** The medial aspect of the urogenital ridges forms the genital ridges, which give rise to the gonads. During the fifth gestational week, primordial germ cells originate in the yolk sac endoderm and migrate from the dorsal mesentery to reach the urogenital ridges. With their arrival, the coelomic epithelium covering the urogenital ridges divides into finger-like projections and carries germ cells into the underlying mesenchyme of the gonad as primitive sex cords. The paramesonephric (müllerian) duct develops into the fallopian tube and uterus. The mesonephric duct develops into the wolffian duct and the epididymis.

306. **(E)** Fetal Leydig cells are the source of testosterone, which is produced in response to circulating hCG and fetal LH. Testosterone induces the mesonephric system (male internal genitalia) to undergo male sexual differentiation. Dihydrotestosterone (DHT) is responsible for formation of the external genitalia, including the prostate and Cowper's glands (from the urogenital sinus). DHT causes elongation of the genital tubercle into the phallus, forward migration of the urethral folds to create the penile shaft (corpus spongiosum), and caudal migration of the genital swellings to form the scrotum.

307. **(D)** With removal of the placenta at birth, the decline in circulating sex steroid levels causes loss of sex steroid negative feedback to the neonatal hypothalamus. A transient elevation in circulating gonadotropin levels temporarily stimulates gonadal steroidogenesis and disappears by age 6 months in males and 1 to 2 years in females. During this time, circulating gonadotropins in infants may transiently induce formation of ovarian cysts, which results in estrogen stimulation of breast tissue.

308. **(C)** The hypothalamo-pituitary system governing gonadotropin secretion is called the gonadostat. During childhood (ages 4 to 10 years), the gonadostat is 6 to 15 times more sensitive to sex steroid negative feedback than in adulthood. In addition, the gonadostat is inhibited by "intrinsic" central nervous system (CNS) signals. Both mechanisms operate together to profoundly inhibit the childhood gonadostat, resulting in low circulating levels of gonadotropins and sex steroids. During puberty (8 to 13 years in females; 9 to 14 years in males), a decrease in the exquisite sensitivity of the childhood gonadostat to sex steroids, combined with the loss of "intrinsic" CNS inhibition, initiates nocturnal pulsatile GnRH secretion. This pattern of GnRH release is characteristic of pubertal onset and does not occur before or after puberty. Circulating gonadotropin levels increase nocturnally in cadence with hypothalamic GnRH release and stimulate gonadal steroidogenesis (gonadarche). An elevation in circulating sex steroid levels is initially sleep entrained but later persists throughout the day as maturation of the hypothalamo-pituitary unit leads to an adult pattern of pulsatile GnRH release.

309. **(D)** Sex steroid production during puberty stimulates development of secondary sex characteristics, growth of long bones (e.g., growth spurt), and changes in bone composition (maturation). The normal sequence of pubertal changes in the female is thelarche, maximal growth velocity, and menarche.

310. **(B)** The age at which menstruation begins has steadily decreased in the United States. The normal age range in which the first menstruation occurs is from 10 to 16 years, with an average of 12.8 years.

311. **(C)** During puberty, an increase in circulating gonadotropin levels stimulates gonadal steroidogenesis. The production of sex steroids induces secondary sex characteristics, endometrial proliferation (leading to menstruation), vaginal cornification, and growth of long bones. Between ages 6 and 9 years, an increase in adrenal function (adrenarche) is accompanied by an elevation in circulating DHEA and DHEAS levels, which induce pubic and axillary hair growth (pubarche).

312. **(C)** Puberty is one step in the continuum of development and bridges the period of transition between the juvenile state and adulthood. You should know the normal sequence of pubertal changes and that they should all occur within a 4- to 5-year time span. Beyond this time, evaluation may be indicated.

313. **(B)** Puberty is delayed when secondary sex development fails to occur by age 13 years in females or 14 years in males. Low circulating sex steroid levels delay epiphyseal closure, leading to prolonged growth of extremities. Delayed puberty results from either absence of gonadal or hypothalamo-pituitary function. Absence of gonadal function due to defective gonadal development (gonadal dysgenesis) leads to a rise in circulating gonadotropin levels (hypergonadotropic hypogonadism) because negative feedback restraint is removed from the hypothalamus and pituitary. Absence of pulsatile GnRH due to hypothalamic suppression causes a decline in circulating gonadotropin levels (hypogonadotropic hypogonadism). Suppression of hypothalamic GnRH may reflect the presence of CNS tumors and diseases, malnutrition, chronic illness, or stress. Kallmann's syndrome refers to GnRH deficiency, combined with anosmia due to olfactory bulb agenesis. This syndrome may be due to a defect in migration of GnRH-containing neurons from the nasal placode to the hypothalamus.

314. **(C)** Precocious puberty refers to the onset of puberty prior to age 8 years in females or 9 years in males. Premature onset of pubertal changes may reflect either (1) early activation of the gonadostat (true precocious puberty), or (2) exposure of target tissues to sex steroids without activation of the gonadostat (pseudo-precocious puberty). True precocious puberty occurs more commonly in females than males and leads to full reproductive function (e.g., ovulation or spermatogenesis). Ten percent of females with true precocious puberty have an underlying CNS abnormality (e.g., tumors, obstructions to cerebral spinal fluid outflow, granulomatous and infectious diseases, neurofibromatosis, head trauma). Ninety percent of females have the idiopathic (constitutional) form of this disorder, in which no abnormality is detected.

315. **(E)** The response of circulating gonadotropins to exogenous GnRH differentiates children with true sexual precocity (exhibiting an adult-pattern rise) from those with pseudo-precocious puberty (exhibiting an attenuated, prepubertal rise). Pseudoprecocious puberty, as evidenced in this patient, is responsible for 20 to 30% of sexual precocity and does not lead to fertility. It can be due to estrogen-secreting neoplasms of the adrenal and ovary (e.g., gonadoblastoma, teratoma, granulosa cell tumor, cystadenoma), benign ovarian follicular cysts, and sex steroid–containing creams and medications. Although its mechanism is unclear, hypothyroidism also is associated with pseudo-precocious puberty and regresses with thyroid hormone replacement.

316. **(D)** Opioid peptides are a group of peptides that bind to opiate receptors and demonstrate analgesic activity (like morphine). Opioid peptides inhibit gonadotropin secretion by suppressing hypothalamic GnRH release. The effect of opioid peptides on hypothalamic GnRH release is responsible for the low frequency of pulsatile LH secretion during the luteal phase. Melatonin, produced by the pineal gland (in response to environmental light and endogenous rhythm-generating mechanisms), suppresses GnRH release but has little apparent significance in humans. Norepinephrine stimulates GnRH release.

317. **(E)** FSH regulates ovarian steroidogenesis and stimulates folliculogenesis beyond the early preantral stage. The central principle of gonadotropin-dependent ovarian steroidogenesis is the "two cell theory" of estrogen synthesis. This theory proposes that a developing follicle requires both granulosa cells and surrounding stromal cells (theca interna) for estrogen synthesis. Granulosa cells possess FSH receptors, and respond to FSH by synthesizing aromatase and increasing FSH receptor sites. Thecal cells contain LH receptors and produce androgens in the presence of LH. Under these conditions, granulosa cells are able to convert androgens, produced locally by thecal cells, to estrogens and are the major source of circulating E2.

318. **(E)** The midcycle LH surge is the ovulatory signal, triggering ovulation about 36 hours later. The elevated circulating LH levels at midcycle promote androgen production by thecal cells, resulting in 15% and 20% increases in plasma androstenedione and testosterone levels. This transient rise in androgens assures sufficient substrate for estrogen production, induces atresia of nondominant follicles, and may enhance libido. As ovulation approaches, granulosa cells of the graafian follicle respond to LH by producing a yellow pigment (luteinization) and synthesizing progesterone. Finally, the LH surge overcomes oocyte maturation inhibitory factor (OMIF), causing the primary oocyte to complete its first meiotic division.

319. **(A)** Exposure of the hypothalamus and pituitary to a threshold E2 level (> 200 pg/mL) for a critical interval (approximately 50 hours) induces a surge of circulating LH. This transient phenomenon is referred to as estrogen-positive feedback. As ovulation approaches, luteinized granulosa cells synthesize progesterone, which facilitates the E2-induced LH surge. Conversely, testosterone inhibits LH release by decreasing gonadotrope sensitivity to GnRH. Opioidergic mechanisms decrease LH secretion by diminishing the release of hypothalamic GnRH.

320. **(D)** The LH surge causes the primary oocyte to complete its first meiotic division, forming a secondary oocyte and first polar body. Each cell contains 23 double-structured chromosomes (haploid) with every chromosome consisting of two chromatids.

321. **(D)** The three principal hormones synthesized by the corpus luteum are progesterone, estrogen, and inhibin. These hormones are produced in greatest quantity 7 to 10 days after ovulation. The corpus luteum also secretes relaxin, which rises in concentration 10 to 12 days after ovulation. There is no hormone called contractin.

322. **(D)** The development of secretory endometrium by progesterone action on an estrogen-primed endometrium is an indirect method of assessing whether ovulation has occurred. The changes are so characteristic that the histologic pattern can determine the postovulatory age of the endometrial tissue. This histologic analysis is called *endometrial dating.*

323. **(A)** Although the amounts vary with the menstrual cycle, 90% of cervical mucus consists of water and sodium chloride (NaCl). In the early follicular phase, a scant amount of cervical mucus containing leukocytes acts as a barrier to sperm and bacteria. During the late follicular phase a rise in circulating estrogen levels alters vascular epithelial permeability and increases the water content of cervical secretions. The sodium chloride content of the mucus allows it to form a palm-leaf

crystallization pattern upon drying, a phenomenon referred to as *ferning.* Ferning is maximal when circulating estrogen levels are highest and is prevented by progesterone.

324. **(C)** Spinnbarkeit describes the elasticity of cervical mucus. High circulating estrogen levels cause the mucus to become profuse, thin, acellular, and clear, resulting in a high degree of stretchability (8 to 10 cm) when pulled from the cervix or stretched between a slide and a coverslip. Ferning will also occur at this time. These properties of estrogen-stimulated mucus promote formation of glycoprotein channels favoring sperm penetration. A high degree of spinnbarkeit in cervical mucus that ferns is clinically useful to time the postcoital test.

325. **(D)** Cells from the cervix or external genitalia do not yield accurate endocrinologic data and should not be used for this purpose. Cells obtained from the lateral vaginal wall yield an excellent maturation index.

326–327. **(326-B, 327-C)** The vaginal maturation index uses the relation between parabasal, intermediate, and superficial cells to describe sex steroid action. The cells described are parabasal cells and are characteristically thick and contain much cytoplasm. They are predominant in states characterized by lack of estrogen and progesterone. This could represent hypothalamic–pituitary suppression due to stress but given her age is most likely due to ovarian failure and menopause. If FSH levels were obtained, they would be elevated. The least expensive way to confirm the diagnosis is to provide conjugated estrogen and see if the symptoms resolve.

328. **(D)** Progesterone produced during the luteal phase inhibits GnRH pulsatility and shifts core body temperature upward 0.6 to 1.0°F. Progesterone also produces secretory endometrium; induces thick, opaque cervical mucus (preventing passage of sperm and bacteria); and stimulates mammary alveolar development. Estrogen causes endometrial proliferation.

329. **(A)** The compact and spongy zones, collectively called the functional zone, are shed at menstruation. Endometrial shedding is facilitated by two different types of arteries: the spiral arteries of the functional zone (which spasm from progesterone withdrawal) and the permanent arterioles of the basalis.

330. **(E)** Menstruation implies the sloughing of an estrogen- and progesterone-primed endometrium in response to the withdrawal of progesterone. Progesterone withdrawal induces spasm of the spiral arteries, leading to vascular collapse, endometrial necrosis, and sloughing.

331. **(B)** Blood loss in a normal period ranges from 25 to 75 mL. Consistent losses of blood greater than 80 mL can cause iron deficiency anemia unless supplemental iron is given.

332. **(C)** The endometrium contains a potent thromboplastin that initiates clotting. Activation of plasminogen causes lysis of blood clots. If menstrual bleeding is excessive, some clotting will remain, although the "coagulum" usually represents a collection of mucoid material and red cells rather than a true clot.

333. **(A)** The pH of the vagina is alkaline prepubertally, but becomes acidic after menarche. An acidic vaginal milieu promotes the growth of normal vaginal flora and decreases the ability of abnormal flora to flourish. The level of acidity (pH) is an important factor in the diagnosis and treatment of a number of causes of vaginitis.

334. **(C)** The major circulating estrogen in postmenopausal women is estrone. Almost all of the estrone produced in postmenopausal women is derived from the peripheral conversion of androstenedione by fat, muscle, and other peripheral tissues.

335. **(A)** The physiological changes accompanying the hot flush include peripheral vasodilation, sweating, elevated heart rate, and increased oxygen consumption. These events promote heat loss via redistribution of blood flow to the periphery, and reflect a change in the set point of the hypothalamic thermoregulatory center. Peripheral blood flow increases approximately 1.5 minutes before and continues for several minutes beyond the subjective symptoms of the hot flush. Perspiration begins 2 to 3 minutes later and is followed by an increase in peripheral temperature, occurring several minutes after the initial rise in peripheral blood flow. At this time, core body temperature drops 0.2°C, and chills begin.

336. **(B)** Osteoporosis results when there is an imbalance between bone resorption and formation, with a chronic negative calcium balance causing mobilization of calcium from trabecular bone. Estrogen deficiency is a significant factor in the development of osteoporosis and has been associated with a transient increase in serum calcium, a compensatory decrease in serum parathyroid hormone levels, hypercalciuria (indicating negative calcium balance), and increased urinary loss of phosphorus and hydroxyproline. The rate of trabecular bone loss is 4 to 8% annually in the 5 to 8 years following menopause, and women lose 35% of their cortical bone and 50% of their trabecular bone through life. The bone loss can be slowed by estrogen replacement therapy even if it is begun many years after menopause.

337. **(B)** Postmenopausal women are at greater risk of cardiovascular disease (CVD) than age-matched premenopausal women. Evidence that estrogen exerts a cardioprotective effect comes from studies showing greater mortality rates in men than in premenopausal women and an increased heart attack rate in women after menopause. Bilateral oophorectomy in premenopausal women also increases the frequency of heart disease. Oral administration of estrogen increases serum HDL concentrations, and decreases serum LDL and total cholesterol levels. However, the lipid hypothesis accounts for only 25 to 50% of the beneficial effect of estrogen on CVD, and other estrogen actions on car-

diovascular function must be operative, such as coronary vessel vasodilatation, arterial prostacyclin production (thereby decreasing platelet aggregation), and blood pressure reduction.

338. **(B)** The amounts of estrogen used for postmenopausal HRT are less than those found in oral contraceptives. Thus, they may theoretically still slightly increase the risk of thromboembolic disease but far less so than oral contraceptive pills. However, the administration of estrogen by the transdermal patch, thereby avoiding the first pass through the liver, appears to have no effect on clotting factors. The use of exogenous estrogen unopposed by progesterone is associated with an increase in the incidence of endometrial carcinoma (four- to eightfold), but with the addition of progesterone the risk is less than half of the risk of using no replacement therapy at all. ERT may increase the risk of breast carcinoma, particularly after long-term therapy (> 9 years), but most studies do not demonstrate this increased risk. Estrogen therapy also increases the risk of cholelithiasis. It does not increase the risk of renal dysfunction.

339–340. **(339-C, 340-A)** Neurosecretory cells within the supraoptic and paraventricular hypothalamic nuclei produce AVP and oxytocin and transport them via transport proteins (neurophysins) to the posterior pituitary. Destruction of the supraoptic and paraventricular hypothalamic nuclei causes a decline in circulating AVP and diabetes insipidus, a condition in which large urinary losses occur from inadequate renal tubular resorption of water. Dopamine is transported to the median eminence by the dopamine tuberoinfundibular tract. Interruption of this tract diminishes dopamine delivery to the anterior pituitary, resulting in an increase in circulating prolactin levels.

341. **(B)** DHT is the principal androgen formed in target tissues containing 5-alpha-reductase. This enzyme converts circulating testosterone to a more potent androgen, DHT.

342. **(I)** The 21-hydroxylase enzyme is required to convert 17-hydroxyprogesterone (17-OHP) to 11-desoxycortisol. Its absence is associated with a marked elevation in circulating 17-OHP levels. A deficiency of 21-hydroxylase is the cause of the most common form of congenital adrenal hyperplasia.

343. **(C)** DHEAS is produced almost entirely by the adrenal gland. The adrenal and ovary generally contribute about 50% each to androstenedione production. In females, approximately 50% of testosterone arises from peripheral conversion of androstenedione, while the adrenal and ovary contribute equal amounts (25%) to circulating testosterone levels. Any rapid or sudden development of hirsutism in a woman requires the determination of the source of the androgen.

344. **(E)** Estrone is the principal estrogen formed in peripheral tissue (e.g., adipose and muscle). In obese women with chronic anovulation, circulating estrone levels may be elevated.

345. **(F)** The strong antigenic similarity between LH and hCG is useful in clinical practice. Administration of hCG in the presence of a dominant follicle will induce ovulation by mimicking an LH surge.

346. **(G)** Pregnenolone is the steroid precursor for all hormonally active steroids.

347. **(G)** Pregnenolone does not require 17-hydroxylase for its synthesis. Without 17-hydroxylase, sex steroid production decreases, while circulating gonadotropin levels increase.

348. **(G)** Progesterone action on the endometrium increases glandular epithelial secretion, stimulates glycogen accumulation in stromal cell cytoplasm (decidualization), and promotes stromal vascularity (spiral arterioles) and edema. These changes vary daily throughout the luteal phase and are the basis of the histological analysis referred to as *endometrial dating*.

349. **(E)** Estradiol induces mammary duct development, while progesterone induces mammary alveolar development.

350. **(A)** Theca interna cells of the ovary supply androstenedione to granulosa cells for aromatization to estrone.

351. **(G)** Progesterone is thermogenic, causing a rise in basal body temperatures during the luteal phase of the menstrual cycle. A biphasic temperature usually confirms an ovulatory cycle, and persistence of the temperature elevation suggests pregnancy.

352. **(E)** Estrogen stimulates the endometrium to proliferate during the follicular phase of the menstrual cycle. The endometrium increases in thickness during folliculogenesis, at which time mitotic figures are abundant throughout the glands and stroma.

353. **(C)** The small FSH midcycle peak is induced by the preovulatory rise in serum progesterone. Midcycle FSH production serves to free the oocyte from its follicular attachments (via hyaluronic acid), aid in follicular rupture (via plasminogen activator), and ensure sufficient LH receptor number for adequate luteal function. There is a rise of FSH at the very end and at the beginning of each cycle in response to the low estrogen levels. This recruits the next set of follicles.

354. **(A)** The LH surge is initiated by the positive feedback effect of unopposed estrogen. For purposes of ovulation induction, the LH surge can be mimicked by exogenous hCG administration.

355. **(D)** Circulating estradiol levels rise steadily during the follicular phase and have negative feedback on FSH release.

356. **(B)** Notice that circulating levels of progesterone (ng/mL) during the luteal phase are greater than those of estradiol (pg/mL). Progesterone withdrawal during luteolysis induces normal menses.

357. **(C)** With castration, loss of negative gonadal feedback (e.g., estrogen, progesterone, and inhibin) on FSH secretion causes a profound increase in circulating FSH levels.

358. **(B)** Peripheral aromatization of androstenedione to estrone accounts for the high circulating estrone levels associated with obesity. Since anovulation is common under these conditions, circulating estradiol levels remain in the early follicular range.

359. **(A)** Circulating estradiol is derived mostly from the dominant follicle and increases steadily in concentration to over 200 pg/mL by the late follicular phase.

360. **(E)** A portion of the adrenal cortex, called the zona reticularis, increases in size during the peripubertal period (ages 6 to 9 years). This increase in adrenal function (adrenarche) is accompanied by an elevation in circulating DHEA and DHEAS levels, which induce pubic and axillary hair growth (pubarche).

361. **(E)** Approximately 2 years after adrenarche (8 to 13 years in females; 9 to 14 years in males), a decrease in the exquisite sensitivity of the childhood gonadostat to sex steroids, combined with the loss of "intrinsic" CNS inhibition, initiates nocturnal pulsatile GnRH secretion. An elevation in circulating estrogen levels in females and androgen levels in males is initially sleep entrained but later persists throughout the day.

362. **(D)** Ovarian function is altered by the depletion of oocytes and surrounding granulosa cells that occurs throughout life. With ovarian senescence, a decline in circulating estradiol levels due to loss of granulosa cells induces amenorrhea after a final episode of uterine bleeding (menopause).

363. **(C)** Low serum DHEAS levels occur during infancy and rise during adrenarche (ages 6 to 9 years). Serum DHEAS levels remain at this level throughout reproductive life and menopause and eventually decline in the elderly.

364. **(C)** During infancy, the hypothalamo-pituitary unit is inhibited by exquisite sensitivity to steroid-negative feedback and by "intrinsic" CNS signals. Both mechanisms operate together to lower circulating levels of gonadotropins and sex steroids during infancy and childhood.

CHAPTER 6

Maternal Physiology During Pregnancy
Questions

365. Cessation of menses is regarded as a presumptive sign of pregnancy in a menstrual-age female. In what percentage of cases does macroscopic vaginal bleeding occur during an otherwise normal pregnancy that does not abort?

    (A) never
    (B) approximately 1%
    (C) approximately 10%
    (D) approximately 20%
    (E) approximately 50%

366. Most state-of-the art serum pregnancy tests have a sensitivity for detection of β-hCG of 25 mLU/mL. Such tests would diagnose pregnancy as early as

    (A) 5 days after conception
    (B) 24 hours after implantation
    (C) the day of the expected (missed) period
    (D) 5 weeks' gestation

367. Changes of the vagina that occur during pregnancy include

    (A) decreased secretions
    (B) decreased vascularity
    (C) hypertrophy of the smooth muscle
    (D) vaginal cells appear similar microscopically to those in the follicular phase of the cycle
    (E) decrease in the thickness of the vaginal mucosa

368. Changes that occur in the cervix during pregnancy include

    (A) progressive hypertrophy and enlargement of the entire cervix
    (B) retraction of the squamocolumnar junction into the cervical canal
    (C) generalized erythema
    (D) normal small amounts of bleeding
    (E) softening

369. Which of the following cervical changes may be found more frequently in the pregnant than in the nonpregnant state?

    (A) atypical glandular hyperplasia
    (B) dysplasia
    (C) metaplasia
    (D) neoplasia
    (E) vaginal adenosis

370. The increase in total body water in pregnancy

    (A) begins at 8 to 10 weeks' gestation
    (B) occurs in response to an increase in plasma osmolality
    (C) is associated with elevated plasma levels of antidiuretic hormone (ADH)
    (D) is in part due to the decreased clearance of ADH
    (E) all of the above
    (F) none of the above

371. At the fifth lunar month, the uterus in a normal pregnancy is

(A) not palpable abdominally
(B) palpable just over the symphysis pubis
(C) palpable at the level of the umbilicus
(D) palpable midway between the umbilicus and the sternum
(E) palpable at the level of the xiphoid

372. A soft, blowing sound that is synchronous with the maternal pulse and heard over the uterus is

(A) borborygmus
(B) uterine souffle
(C) funic souffle
(D) fetal movement
(E) maternal femoral vessel bruit

373. The hemostatic mechanism most important in combating postpartum hemorrhage is

(A) increased blood clotting factors in pregnancy
(B) intramyometrial vascular coagulation due to vasoconstriction
(C) contraction of interlacing uterine muscle bundles
(D) markedly decreased blood pressure in the uterine venules
(E) fibronolysis inhibition

374. The uterine muscle mass enlarges during pregnancy because of

(A) atypical hyperplasia
(B) anaplasia
(C) hypertrophy and hyperplasia
(D) involution
(E) none of the above; the total muscle mass actually does not change

375. During early pregnancy a pelvic examination may reveal that one adnexa is slightly enlarged. This is most likely due to

(A) a parovarian cyst
(B) fallopian tube hypertrophy
(C) an ovarian neoplasm
(D) a follicular cyst
(E) a corpus luteum cyst

376. During pregnancy there is a decrease in the size of

(A) uterine muscle cells
(B) uterine fibrous and elastic tissue
(C) uterine blood vessels
(D) Frankenhauser's ganglion
(E) the maternal ovarian follicles

377. Progesterone production increases during pregnancy. By the third trimester, what is the approximate rate of production per day?

(A) 50 µg
(B) 350 µg
(C) 50 mg
(D) 100 mg
(E) 250 mg

378. Pregnancy is rare

(A) after one episode of pelvic inflammatory disease (PID)
(B) before the age of 18
(C) in physically active women
(D) after the age of 50
(E) in women who have used an intrauterine device (IUD)

379. Maternal mortality is lowest in mothers between ages

(A) 10 and 20
(B) 20 and 30
(C) 30 and 40
(D) 40 and 50
(E) 50 and 60

380. During normal pregnancy, a weight gain is anticipated. For a normal-weight woman, the recommended weight gain is approximately

(A) 5 to 10 lb
(B) 10 to 15 lb
(C) 15 to 20 lb
(D) 25 to 35 lb
(E) 30 to 40 lb

381. A characteristic posture of pregnancy is

    (A) hyperextension
    (B) kyphosis
    (C) scoliosis
    (D) lordosis
    (E) none of the above

382. The skin changes common to both liver disease and normal pregnancy include

    (A) striae and chloasma
    (B) spider angiomata and palmar erythema
    (C hyperpigmentation and spider angiomata
    (D) linea nigra and chloasma
    (E) striae and linea nigra

383. Which of the following would normally be expected to increase during pregnancy?

    (A) plasma creatinine
    (B) thyroxine-binding globulin (TBG)
    (C) hematocrit
    (D) aspartate aminotransferase (AST)
    (E) alanine aminotransferase (ALT)

384. During normal pregnancy, which of the following physiologic effects occur?

    (A) increased serum beta globulins (transport proteins) and decreased triglycerides
    (B) increased serum corticosteroid-binding globulin and free cortisol
    (C) increased levels of immunoglobulins A, G, and M
    (D) increased thyroid-binding globulin and iodide levels
    (E) decreased serum ionized calcium levels and parathyroid hormone (PTH)

385. Epulis of pregnancy is a/an

    (A) enlarged hemorrhoid
    (B) circumscribed vascular swelling of the gums
    (C) spider hemangioma found on palms and soles

    (D) syndrome of nausea and vomiting
    (E) placental vascular shunt

386. Changes in the gastrointestinal (GI) tract during pregnancy include

    (A) compression and downward displacement of the appendix by the uterus
    (B) increased intestinal tone and mobility
    (C) physical elevation of the stomach
    (D) more rapid gastric emptying
    (E) increased intestinal absorption helping to ensure weight gain

387. Changes in hepatic and gallbladder function during pregnancy include

    (A) decreased serum albumin/globulin (A/G) ratio and decreased bromosulfophthalein (BSP) secretion
    (B) increased alkaline phosphatase (ALP) and lactate dehydrogenase (LDH)
    (C) decreased biliary cholesterol saturation and rate of gallbladder emptying
    (D) increased AST and ALT
    (E) decreased fibrinogen and ceruloplasmin

388. Changes in the urinary tract during normal pregnancy include a/an

    (A) increase in glomerular filtration rate (GFR)
    (B) decrease in renal plasma flow (RPF)
    (C) marked increase in both GFR and RPF when the patient is supine
    (D) increase in the amount of dead space in the urinary tract
    (E) increase in blood urea nitrogen (BUN) and creatinine

389. If an intravenous pyelogram (IVP) were performed in the third trimester of a normal pregnancy, you would be likely to find

(A) the kidneys appearing smaller than normal because of diaphragmatic compression

(B) obstruction of the right ureter secondary to the dextrorotation of the uterus

(C) sediment in the renal collecting system due to the stasis effect of progesterone

(D) vesicoureteral reflux secondary to stretching of the trigone by the enlarging uterus

(E) ureteral dilation, probably secondary to progesterone effect and compression of the lower urinary tract by the uterus

390. The increase in red blood cells (RBCs) during pregnancy

(A) causes the hematocrit to rise

(B) is due to the prolonged life span of the erythrocytes

(C) is due to increased production of erythrocytes

(D) results despite decreased levels of erythropoiesis in maternal plasma

391. Iron metabolism in women is characterized by

(A) greater iron stores than men

(B) greater iron absorption during pregnancy

(C) decreased iron absorption from the GI tract during pregnancy

(D) greater iron requirements in early pregnancy than in late pregnancy

(E) decreased absorption of iron in the presence of ascorbic acid

392. Iron supplementation is recommended in pregnancy in order to

(A) prevent iron deficiency in the fetus

(B) raise the maternal hemoglobin concentration

(C) maintain the maternal hemoglobin concentration

(D) prevent iron deficiency in the mother

(E) prevent postpartum hemorrhage

393. Which of the following maternal measurements or findings is first decreased by the iron requirements of pregnancy?

(A) red cell size

(B) bone marrow iron

(C) serum iron-binding capacity

(D) hemoglobin

(E) jejunal absorption of iron

394. Maternal blood volume in a normal pregnancy

(A) remains stable

(B) decreases 10%

(C) increases 10%

(D) decreases up to 40%

(E) increases up to 40%

395. The increase in blood volume in normal pregnancy is made up of

(A) plasma only

(B) erythrocytes only

(C) more plasma than erythrocytes

(D) more erythrocytes than plasma

(E) neither plasma nor erythrocytes

396. Women who become hypertensive during late pregnancy have a decreased resistance to which of the following in early pregnancy?

(A) epinephrine

(B) angiotensin I

(C) prostaglandin F_2-alpha

(D) prostaglandin E_2

(E) angiotensin II

397. The cardiovascular system undergoes great change during pregnancy. During this time

(A) the heart enlarges greatly, as can be demonstrated by standard chest x-rays

(B) apical systolic murmurs are heard in approximately half of pregnant patients

(C) cardiac output is decreased by lying in the lateral position

(D) the stroke volume decreases

(E) arrhythmias are common

398. Which of the following is probably responsible for physiologic hyperventilation during pregnancy?

(A) large fluctuations in plasma bicarbonate

(B) increased estrogen production

(C) increased progesterone production

(D) decreased functional residual volume

(E) decreased plasma P_{O_2}

399. Which of the following statements regarding immunity in pregnancy is TRUE?

(A) Humoral immunity against measles, herpes simplex, and influenza A decreases in pregnancy.

(B) Alpha-interferon is abundant in maternal tissues.

(C) Polymorphonuclear leukocyte chemotaxis and adherence increases from the second trimester onward in a normal pregnancy.

(D) The leukocytosis of pregnancy is one manifestation of the maternal hyperimmune state.

(E) all of the above

400. Regarding C-reactive protein in pregnancy, which of the following statements is TRUE?

(A) C-reactive protein is elevated in most pregnancies, especially during labor.

(B) Gestational age greatly affects C-reactive protein values.

(C) In pregnancy, C-reactive protein loses its usefulness as a harbinger of infection.

(D) A C-reactive protein of twice its normal value would be a good predictor of infection in pregnancy.

401. Pregnancy induces which of the following changes in adrenal hormones?

(A) increases only bound cortisol

(B) increases only free cortisol

(C) decreases aldosterone

(D) increases aldosterone

402. Antibodies to human chorionic gonadotropin (hCG) will cross-react most commonly with

(A) follicle-stimulating hormone (FSH)

(B) adrenocorticotropic hormone (ACTH)

(C) thyroid-stimulating hormone (TSH)

(D) melanocyte-stimulating hormone (MSH)

(E) luteinizing hormone (LH)

403. During pregnancy, maternal estrogen increases markedly. Most of this estrogen is produced by the

(A) ovaries

(B) adrenals

(C) fetus

(D) placenta

(E) uterus

404. Which of the following cardiorespiratory changes is abnormal during pregnancy?

(A) systolic murmur

(B) increased cardiac output

(C) increased pulmonary vascular markings

(D) alterations in electrical axis

(E) resting pulse rate of 100 beats per minute

405. An ocular change associated with normal pregnancy is

(A) decreased corneal thickness

(B) visual field defects

(C) decreased intraocular pressure

(D) increased retinal thickness

(E) increased corneal permeability

406. Cardiac output is highest

(A) in the first trimester

(B) in the second trimester

(C) in the third trimester

(D) during labor

(E) immediately postpartum (10 to 30 minutes)

(F) at 1 hour after delivery

407. A 29-year-old primigravida at 36 weeks' gestation complains of dizziness and nausea when reclining to read in bed before retiring at night. Suspecting that her symptoms are the result of normal physiologic changes of pregnancy, you recommend

(A) elevation of both her feet while lying in bed

(B) a small late night snack

(C) improved room lighting

(D) rolling toward the right or left hip while reading

(E) a mild exercise before retiring to bed

Questions 408 and 409

A 24-year-old nurse at 32 weeks' gestation complains of shortness of breath during her pregnancy, especially with physical exertion. She has no prior medical history. Her respiratory rate is 16; her lungs are clear to auscultation; and your office oxygen saturation monitor reveals her oxygen saturation to be 98% on room air.

408. You reassure her that this sensation is normal and explain that

(A) small amniotic fluid emboli are shed throughout pregnancy

(B) maximal breathing capacity is not altered by pregnancy

(C) airway conductance is decreased during pregnancy

(D) pulmonary resistance increases during pregnancy

409. She urges you to perform pulmonary function tests. Assuming that your medical judgment is correct, these tests should show a/an

(A) diminished vital capacity

(B) increased tidal volume

(C) increased functional residual capacity

(D) increased residual volume

(E) unchanged expiratory reserve volume

DIRECTIONS (Questions 410 through 423): Each of the numbered items or incomplete statements in this section is followed by answers or by completions of the statement. Select the answers or completions that may apply.

410. Which four of the following are presumptive signs/symptoms of pregnancy?

(A) cessation of menses

(B) development of hirsutism

(C) quickening

(D) nausea and vomiting

(E) swelling of the hands and face

(F) breast changes

(G) darkening of the skin on the palms of the hands

411. During pregnancy, several ovarian changes can occur that are normal but can be disturbing if not understood. These changes include which three of the following?

(A) luteoma of pregnancy

(B) follicular cyst

(C) decidual reaction on the ovarian surface

(D) corpus luteum cyst

(E) dermoid cysts

412. Physiologic findings usually associated with previous parity include which three of the following?

(A) earlier engagement of the fetal head in subsequent pregnancy

(B) gaping vulva

(C) narrow vagina

(D) healed lacerations of the cervical os represented by cervical deformities or nabothian cysts

(E) significant cervical effacement in the second trimester of pregnancy

413. The improvement in peptic ulcer disease generally seen during pregnancy may be related to which three of the following?

(A) increase in gastric mucous secretion

(B) more rapid gastric emptying

(C) increased tone of the stomach

(D) protective affect of prostaglandins on gastric mucosa

(E) effect of progesterone on gastrointestinal motility

414. Which three of the following proteins produced by the liver are elevated during pregnancy?

(A) fibrinogen

(B) albumin

(C) ceruloplasmin

(D) sex hormone-binding globulin (SHBG)

(E) prothrombin (factor II)

415. The supine position is important during late pregnancy because it may cause which three of the following?

(A) an elevation of uterine artery pressure compared with brachial artery pressure

(B) complete occlusion of the inferior vena cava

(C) a significant reduction in maternal ventilatory capacity

(D) hypotension and syncope

(E) a significant reduction in renal blood flow and glomerular filtration

416. Which three of the following physiologic changes accompany pregnancy?

(A) an increase in cardiac output

(B) an increase in blood volume

(C) a decrease in peripheral vascular resistance

(D) an increase in functional residual volume

(E) a decrease in renal perfusion

417. Many physiologic changes of pregnancy mimic disease states. Which six of the following normal physiologic changes commonly occurring during pregnancy can also be present during disease?

(A) peripheral edema

(B) spider angiomata

(C) hyperventilation

(D) palmar erythema

(E) systolic murmur

(F) increase in serum creatinine

(G) reduction in peripheral vascular resistance

(H) elevation in blood pressure

(I) decreased serum cholesterol concentration

418. Which six of the following hormones increase during pregnancy?

(A) prolactin

(B) FSH

(C) insulin

(D) calcitonin

(E) thyroid-releasing hormone (TRH)

(F) testosterone

(G) vasopressin

(H) aldosterone

(I) progesterone

419. A 25-year-old G3P2 in her sixth week of pregnancy by last menstrual period (LMP) calculation has an endovaginal ultrasound examination because of vaginal bleeding. The ultrasound confirms an intrauterine pregnancy with fetal cardiac activity present and fetal pole length consistent with 6 weeks' gestation. Scan of the adnexae reveals a 3-cm simple cyst on the left ovary. Which two of the following statements are true?

(A) This patient likely has both an intrauterine pregnancy and an ectopic pregnancy.

(B) This patient should be told she will probably miscarry.

(C) The ovarian cyst should not be removed.

(D) First trimester vaginal bleeding is not uncommon.

(E) This patient has a blighted ovum.

420. Which three of the following factors contribute to the increase in cardiac output in late pregnancy?

(A) increase in heart rate

(B) increase in ejection fraction

(C) decrease in systemic vascular resistance

(D) increase in blood volume

(E) increase in left ventricular stroke work index

Questions 421 and 422

A healthy 30-year-old primigravida presents at 34 weeks' gestation. She reports that she has been experiencing abdominal discomfort that increases after eating, especially when in the recumbent position. A series of tests is performed. She has normal vital signs, an unremarkable examination, a fundal height of 33 cm, and a negative urinalysis.

421. Which one of the following tests represent abnormal values?

(A) a white blood count (WBC) of 11,000/mL

(B) a hemoglobin of 9.0 g/dL

(C) an alkaline phosphatase double that of the reference range

(D) serum albumin of 3.0 g/dL

(E) AST of 25 U/L

422. You recommend which three of the following?

(A) frequent small meals

(B) antacid preparations such as aluminum or magnesium hydroxide

(C) an abdominal ultrasound

(D) iron supplementation

(E) postpartum cholecystectomy

423. Positive signs of pregnancy should include which three of the following?

(A) enlargement of the uterus

(B) changes in the cervix

(C) positive hormonal pregnancy test

(D) ballottement of the fetus

(E) fetal heart tones

(F) imaging the fetal body

(G) palpating fetal motion

Answers and Explanations

365. **(D)** Although any painless vaginal bleeding during early pregnancy has to be regarded as a threatened abortion and investigated and followed, many of these women do not abort and deliver perfectly normal children. In some studies, multiparas were found to have a much higher incidence of bleeding than primigravidas.

366. **(C)** Circulating β-hCG in early pregnancy at a level of 25 mLU/mL is detected in most women by 12 to 13 days after the LH peak. Therefore, the test should be positive by the date of the expected menses.

367. **(C)** In keeping with the other general changes during pregnancy, there is increased secretion, vascularity, and thickness of mucosa. The vaginal cells will look like those of the luteal phase with progesterone influence. Secretions will be copious.

368. **(E)** The cervix softens and displays a characteristic bluish appearance. Endocervical cells hypertrophy (but not squamous cells) and appear everted. Other than for passage of the blood-streaked cervical mucus (called bloody show) near the onset of labor, the cervix does not normally bleed at any time during pregnancy. The red columnar epithelium on the cervical portio is often erroneously called an erosion. Erosion refers to an area where the epithelium has been denuded, which is not the case with a cervical ectropion. Increased blood flow causes cyanosis, not erythema.

369. **(C)** The cervix can be histologically evaluated for malignant change during pregnancy as well as during the nonpregnant state. Pap smears and colposcopy are both reliable. Dysplasia is probably best not treated until the postpartum period.

370. **(F)** Plasma volume expansion begins shortly after conception. Serum sodium level and osmolality decrease during a normal pregnancy. The threshold for thirst and antidiuretic hormone is lowered. The metabolic clearance rate of antidiuretic hormone is increased, yet plasma levels of this hormone are similar to nonpregnant levels, resulting from increased production.

371. **(C)** This measurement is only a rough guide to the duration of gestation. It may be increased by twins, myomas, and hydramnios and decreased by oligohydramnios, intrauterine growth retardation, fetal death, and so on. Considerable individual variation is also common. One study found up to 3 cm difference, depending on whether the fundal height was measured with the gravida's bladder full or empty (see Figure 6–1).

372. **(B)** The funic or umbilical cord souffle is timed with the fetal pulse, while the femoral vessels are rarely heard over the uterus. When the uterus is small, however, maternal vessels are easily heard. A rapid maternal pulse may therefore be mistaken for the fetal heart tones.

373. **(C)** If uterine atony exists, the muscle does not provide the pressure on the endometrial vessels needed to occlude them. Methods such as massage and oxytocin administration

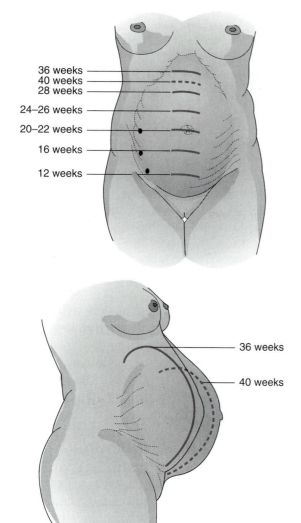

Figure 6–1. Fundal height in pregnancy. (Reproduced, with permission, from DeCherney AH, Nathan L. *Current Obstetric and Gynecologic Diagnosis and Treatment*, 9th ed. New York: McGraw-Hill, 2003).

will usually cause sufficient uterine contraction to inhibit such bleeding. Methergine and prostaglandins (PGs) are also used as therapeutic agents.

374. (C) Involution occurs postpartum, when the uterus decreases from about 1,000 g to about 60 g. During pregnancy, both the appearance of new cells and the enlargement of old cells contribute to the growth.

375. (E) The corpus luteum normally decreases in its function after 4 weeks of gestation. In

midgestation, it is no longer needed to maintain the hormonal milieu of pregnancy (the placenta does). Often, a positive pregnancy test and an adnexal mass signal normal pregnancy but can be present with an ectopic pregnancy as well. Ultrasound can be very helpful in differentiating the two.

376. (E) All components of the uterus enlarge to accommodate the fetus. The uterine wall is thicker and stronger, and the muscle cells can exert greater force as their longer fibers contract. If the uterus is overdistended (twins, polyhydramnios), poor contractility is often found. Though the ovary may enlarge, there are few if any developing follicles.

377. (E) Progesterone is present in milligram amounts both during pregnancy and during the luteal phase of the cycle. Estrogens are present in microgram amounts. Similar ratios exist in combination birth control pills.

378. (D) Though the reasons are unclear, the average age of menarche is getting earlier, and the average age of menopause is getting later. Therefore, the number of years a woman is capable of bearing children is increasing. However, fertility declines markedly toward the end of the reproductive years. Approximately 13% of women experience tubal infertility after one episode of pelvic inflammatory disease.

379. (B) Mothers between 20 and 30 years of age have the fewest deaths, according to vital statistics. Babies born to mothers in this age range do best also. Age and parity both correlate directly with maternal mortality after the age of 30.

380. (D) In 1990 the Institute of Medicine summarized studies and published guidelines for weight gain during pregnancy, which the American College of Obstetrics and Gynecology supports. It recommended a weight gain of 25 to 35 lb for normal-weight women. The weight gain is accounted for by adding up the components that contribute to it, such as the fetus, placenta, increased blood volume, increased maternal fat stores, and so on. More and more evidence is accumulating to show that low weight gain when associated with inadequate diet is detrimental to the pregnancy. Women who are morbidly obese can gain less weight, but dieting to lose weight during pregnancy is never recommended.

381. **(D)** The change in center of gravity caused by the enlarging uterus predisposes to a lordotic position and puts strain on paraspinal muscles and pelvic joints. Backache is a common complaint during pregnancy. Less commonly, the neck flexion and depressed shoulder girdle may cause median and ulnar nerve traction. Treatment is generally not effective and those complaints regress only after delivery.

382. **(B)** Hyperpigmentation in pregnancy includes the transformation of the linea alba to the linea nigra and the development of the "mask of pregnancy" or chloasma. Striae result from stretching of the skin under hormonal influences. The vascular changes occurring during states of high estrogen are common to both liver disease and normal pregnancy. These include the development of spider angiomata and palmar erythema.

383. **(B)** The mother and a rapidly growing infant use an increased amount of oxygen, resulting in an increased basal metabolic rate (BMR). When combined with elevated binding protein secondary to estrogen effect, one can be misled to diagnose hyperthyroidism when, in fact, these are normal pregnancy changes. Even mild hyperthyroidism probably does not merit treatment during pregnancy. AST and ALT are not elevated in normal pregnancy but may be elevated in patients with severe preeclampsia.

384. **(B)** Serum beta globulins increase in pregnancy, including corticosteroid-binding globulin and thyroid-binding globulin. Triglyceride levels rise two- to threefold. The elevation in free cortisol seen after the first trimester is related in part to an increase in corticotropin-releasing hormone (CRH) dur-

ing pregnancy. Due to increased renal loss, serum iodide levels fall. Serum ioinized calcium levels are unchanged during pregnancy, and PTH levels remain in the low-normal range. While antibody-mediated immunity is enhanced in pregnancy, the levels of immunoglobulins A, G, and M all decrease.

385. **(B)** This rather unusual lesion tends to regress spontaneously with delivery. There is no link to dental caries or permanent changes. Gums may bleed more easily in pregnancy.

386. **(C)** With prolonged gastric emptying time and an elevated stomach and progesterone acting to relax the sphincter mechanism of the stomach, the reflux of gastric contents into the esophagus becomes more frequent. These physiologic events are translated into the physical symptom of heartburn, about which many patients complain. Appendicitis can be more difficult to diagnose because of the abnormal position of the appendix. It is elevated toward the right upper quadrant of the abdomen. The stomach is elevated and also somewhat compressed. Intestinal tone and mobility are slowed by progesterone effect. Intestinal absorbency remains the same, and for weight gain to take place, the gravida must increase caloric intake.

387. **(A)** Serum albumin levels fall in pregnancy but many proteins increase. ALP is increased in pregnancy, although most of the increase is the heat-stable isoenzyme produced by the placenta. The gallbladder empties more slowly, fasting and residual volumes are greater, and biliary cholesterol saturation is increased—all contributing to a greater propensity for gallstone formation in pregnancy.

388. **(A)** Renal function is generally enhanced during pregnancy but is also dependent on position during pregnancy. This is largely due to the marked hemodynamic changes that occur in the upright and supine position. There is also marked dilation (2×) of the urinary tract, which is probably due to the effect of progesterone on smooth muscle. BUN and creatinine are markedly decreased during pregnancy.

389. (E) The kidneys hypertrophy slightly in pregnancy. The effect of progesterone is dilatory on the collecting system. It does not dilate the ureterovesical junction and does not normally cause reflux. In rare cases the enlarging uterus will cause ureteral obstruction, but this is not true in the great majority of pregnancies.

390. (C) Increased levels of erythropoietin are found, which apparently stimulate increased RBC production. Reticulocyte count is slightly elevated. However, there is a greater increase in plasma, so the hematocrit tends to drop slightly. Adequate iron supplementation will attenuate this drop.

391. (B) Women generally do have lower iron stores than men and need supplemental iron, especially in the latter half of pregnancy. Under conditions of increased iron needs, such as pregnancy, the fraction of iron absorbed is increased. With good dietary supplementation, depletion of maternal iron stores can be avoided. The presence of vitamin C enhances the absorption of oral iron supplements, and that is why there are compounds that combine the two.

392. (D) Because iron is actively transported to the fetus by the placenta against a high concentration gradient, fetal hemoglobin levels do not correlate with maternal levels. Further, the physiologic anemia of pregnancy occurs in both supplemented and nonsupplemented pregnant women because the increase in plasma volume exceeds the increase in RBC mass. Iron supplementation is to prevent iron deficiency in the mother. It has been estimated that women who are iron sufficient at the beginning of pregnancy and who are not iron supplemented need about 2 years after delivery to replenish their iron stores from dietary sources.

393. (B) Bone marrow iron will be depleted before the RBCs or binding is affected. Iron ab-

sorption would increase as the patient became anemic. Oral iron can be used to prevent depletion of bone marrow stores.

394. (E) This increase can occur even in the presence of a hydatidiform mole. It is a safeguard against blood loss at delivery and helps meet the demands of an increased intravascular space. There is great individual variability, with some increases near zero and others almost double.

395. (C) The erythrocytes increase approximately 33%, while total blood volume increases approximately 40 to 45%. This helps explain "physiologic" anemia. Again, adequate iron stores and intake will prevent iron depletion.

396. (E) Being refractory to the pressor response to angiotensin II during pregnancy may be mediated by PGs. Therefore, administration of PG synthetase inhibitors may cause a loss of resistance to angiotensin II, resulting in hypertension. This has not been the case, however, in patients taking PG inhibitors on a regular basis.

397. (B) The heart appears to enlarge on x-ray, but this is a function of position change. An electrocardiogram also reveals a left-axis shift. Systolic murmurs are common and often benign, but diastolic murmurs are pathologic. Because of the normal changes due to pregnancy, it can be very difficult to diagnose cardiac disease during gestation. Arrhythmia is not normal in pregnancy.

398. (C) Progesterone affects both the respiratory center and the smooth muscles of the bronchi. The smooth muscles generally are relaxed by progesterone, leading to decreased GI (gastrointestinal) motility and ureteral dilation, as well as bronchodilation. Tidal volume, minute volume, and oxygen uptake all increase (see Figure 6–2).

399. (A) While the fetus produces alpha-interferon, the gravida's tissues contain almost none. Humoral immunity seems to be less in pregnancy, and the leukocytosis of pregnancy

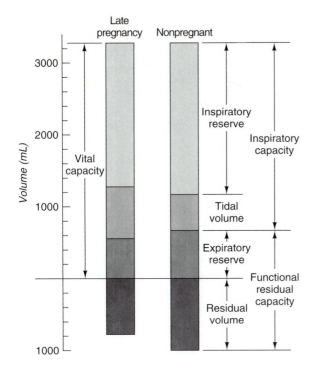

Figure 6–2. Lung volumes in pregnancy.
(Reproduced, with permission, from DeCherney AH, Nathan L. *Current Obstetric and Gynecologic Diagnosis and Treatment*, 9th ed. New York: McGraw-Hill, 2003.)

is probably secondary to demargination of WBCs, not to immunity.

400. **(A)** C-reactive protein is an acute-phase serum reactive protein that rises rapidly to 1,000 times its usual value in response to infection or trauma in tissue. It is mildly elevated in normal pregnancy but may increase greatly in labor.

401. **(D)** Estrogen elevates the concentration of the protein that binds cortisol (transcortin) and, therefore, there is a large increase in bound cortisol. However, there is an increase in unbound cortisol as well. Aldosterone levels are increased, possibly in response to progesterone. Aldosterone may protect against the natriuretic effect of progesterone.

402. **(E)** The molecules of LH and hCG are structurally very similar. In fact, hCG has been used clinically as an injection to stimulate the LH surge and trigger ovulation. It is the al-

pha chain of these protein hormones that is most similar; therefore, the pregnancy tests that are immunologically specific for the molecule (including the beta chain) will not cross-react.

403. **(D)** Estriol is formed in large amounts by the placenta from maternal and fetal precursors. It is used as an indicator of fetal well-being. Its production relies on interaction of fetus with the placenta and excretion into the maternal serum and urine. Problems with any of these decreases estriol in maternal serum.

404. **(E)** The resting pulse rate increases about 10 to 15 beats per minute so it is not generally more than 85 bpm. Systolic murmurs, increased cardiac output, increased pulmonic markings on x-ray, and a slight change in the cardiac electrical axis all occur normally.

405. **(C)** Intraocular pressure typically falls by about 10% during pregnancy, resulting in an improvement for some women with preexisting glaucoma.

406. **(E)** Cardiac output increases by 30 to 50% in pregnancy. Additionally, it further increases as labor progresses to as much as 50% above baseline term pregnancy values. It reaches its maximum in the immediate postpartum period (10 to 30 minutes after delivery) with a further increase of 10 to 20%. At 1 hour postpartum, cardiac output returns to prelabor baseline values.

407. **(D)** In the supine position, the compression of the inferior vena cava in late pregnancy markedly diminishes venous return, stroke volume, and cardiac output. Symptoms of supine hypotension include dizziness, lightheadedness, nausea, and even syncope. The lateral recumbent position increases cardiac output 10 to 30% over the supine position.

408. **(B)** Vital capacity and maximal breathing capacity remain the same in normal pregnancy. The loss in lung volume due to elevation of the diaphragm is taken from the functional residual capacity and, therefore, does not affect the vital capacity. Pulmonary resistance decreases, making air conduction easier.

409. (B) In pregnancy there is a 30 to 40% increase in tidal volume, which occurs at the expense of expiratory reserve volume (ERV). Due to the elevation of the diaphragm, the residual volume (RV) is decreased approximately 20%. The functional residual capacity (FRC), comprised of the ERV and RV, is therefore also decreased. The vital capacity is unchanged and large airway function is unimpaired.

410. (A, C, D, F) The recognition that many of the most common signs looked for during examinations to confirm pregnancy are only presumptive is extremely important. All of these signs can be due to many conditions other than pregnancy. Finding them in an amenorrheic woman should immediately make one consider the possibility of pregnancy. Rarely, luteomas of pregnancy can cause maternal virilization. Dependent edema, while not a sign of pregnancy, is physiologic in pregnancy. But swelling of the hands and face may be a sign of preeclampsia.

411. (A, C, D) Decidual reaction results in elevated red patches on the ovarian surface that are friable. They should not be mistaken for adhesions or malignancy. The corpus luteum produces progesterone, which sustains the pregnancy in the early weeks of gestation. Luteomas are solid ovarian tumors occurring during pregnancy as a result of an exaggeration of the luteinization reaction of the ovary. They normally regress after delivery. Follicular cysts appear prior to ovulation and not during pregnancy when a woman is not cycling. Dermoid cysts or mature teratomas are among the most common ovarian neoplasms. They are comprised of mature cells, usually from all three germ layers. They are not associated with pregnancy and are found bilaterally in 10 to 15% of cases.

412. (B, D, E) The cervix is often damaged during delivery, resulting in scarring or deformity. The nabothian cyst is basically a gland that is

covered over during healing. In second or later pregnancies, the fetal head usually engages later than in first pregnancies. Vaginal and vulvar widening and relaxation to some degree occurs after all vaginal deliveries. None of these signs of prior parity is absolute. Other possible signs include striae, laxity of the abdominal wall, and sagging of the breasts.

413. (A, D, E) Both the tone and motility of the stomach are decreased during pregnancy, probably because of the smooth muscle-relaxing effects of progesterone. Additionally, pregnancy is associated with a normal increase in gastric mucous and PG production, which have a protective effect on the gastric mucosa. Gastric acid secretion is reduced below nonpregnant values in the first and second trimesters.

414. (A, C, D) During pregnancy, the serum concentrations of many proteins produced by the liver increase in response to estrogen. Fibrinogen levels rise 50% by the end of the second trimester, but prothrombin levels remain unchanged during pregnancy. The levels of ceruloplasmin and the binding proteins for corticosteroids, sex steroids, thyroid hormone, and vitamin D are also increased. Serum albumin levels fall progressively during pregnancy and at term are 30% lower than nonpregnant values.

415. (B, D, E) Because the blood return to the heart is compromised by vena cava occlusion, cardiac output falls, thereby reducing tissue perfusion. Ventilation does not change significantly. The lateral recumbent position will generally restore normal blood flow and normalize blood pressure.

416. (A, B, C) The RV decreases to compensate for the elevated diaphragm. Cardiac output, renal perfusion, and blood volume all increase. Peripheral resistance and blood pressure decrease during normal pregnancy.

417. (A, B, C, D, E, G) Peripheral edema is a common finding in later pregnancy, occurring as a result of the increased venous pressure in the legs, obstruction of lymphatic flow, and reduced plasma colloid osmotic pressure. Both spider angiomata and palmar erythema, the result of elevated estrogen levels, are normal and regress after pregnancy. Hyperventilation of pregnancy, mediated through progesterone, occurs by an increase in tidal volume and not respiratory rate. Systolic ejection murmurs result from increased flow across the aortic and pulmonic valves. Glomerular filtration rate increases; therefore, creatinine declines. Blood pressure declines as a result of decreased peripheral vascular resistance, which likely occurs from the smooth muscle–relaxing effects of progesterone. Cholesterol levels are twice the normal values by the end of pregnancy.

418. **(A, C, D, F, H, I)** There is a marked increase in prolactin, which is highest prior to delivery. Prolactin is necessary for lactation. Insulin levels are increased and demonstrate an exaggerated response to glucose. Calcitonin acts to increase skeletal calcification during times of calcium stress such as pregnancy and lactation. Levels are elevated during these periods. Aldosterone is elevated in pregnancy, seemingly mediated by elevated progesterone. Plasma progesterone levels as well as estradiol and estriol increase throughout pregnancy. Androgens such as testosterone and androstenedione increase in pregnancy and are converted to estradiol in the placenta. TRH and vasopressin levels are not elevated in pregnancy. Inhibin, produced by the placenta, results in a lowered FSH acting to inhibit ovulation.

419. **(C, D)** Any woman in early pregnancy with unexplained vaginal bleeding should be evaluated for the possibility of an ectopic pregnancy. The risk of heterotopic pregnancy, that is, simultaneous intrauterine and ectopic pregnancy, is rare. Therefore, in general, confirming the presence of an intrauterine pregnancy by ultrasound effectively rules out ectopic pregnancy. First-trimester vaginal bleeding occurs in approximately 20% of intrauterine pregnancies that do

not abort, and it is reported to be more common among multiparous women. A "blighted ovum" is defined as a gestational sac of 2.5 cm or more in which no fetus can be identified on ultrasound. Such pregnancies are not viable. The corpus luteum of pregnancy produces progesterone to sustain pregnancy in the early weeks of pregnancy. Surgical removal before 7 weeks' gestation results in a rapid decline of maternal serum progesterone and ensuing spontaneous abortion.

420. **(A, C, D)** Cardiac output is the product of stroke volume and heart rate. Heart rate increases by approximately 15 to 20 beats per minute above the pre-pregnancy rate, and stroke volume increases, largely as a result of increased blood volume. Under the influence of the smooth muscle–relaxing effects of elevated progesterone, systemic vascular resistance decreases. Normal pregnancy is not associated with a hyperdynamic left ventricular function, however.

421. **(B)** Blood volume increases 40 to 45% in pregnancy, but plasma volume increases by 50%, whereas erythrocyte production increases by only 30%. Because of the greater increase in plasma, a physiologic anemia of pregnancy occurs and hematocrit reaches a nadir at 30 to 34 weeks' gestation. The fifth percentile of hemoglobin concentration for normal iron-supplemented women at 32 weeks' gestation is 11.0 g/dL. The Centers for Disease Control and Prevention defined anemia as less than 11 g/dL in the first and third trimesters and less than 10.5 g/dL in the second trimester. The woman in question has likely depleted her iron stores. All other laboratory values presented are normal for pregnancy. This woman's symptoms are those of heartburn (pyrosis), common in pregnancy, caused by reflux of gastric contents into the lower esophagus. The physical findings are normal.

422. **(A, B, D)** The recommendation for ameliorating the symptoms of heartburn are frequent small meals and antacid preparations.

In addition, because of her anemia, iron supplementation should be encouraged.

423. **(E, F, G)** The first four choices are all probable or presumptive signs of pregnancy. The main purpose for knowing the positive signs is not to become too dogmatic about the diagnosis of pregnancy without them. There are three positive signs which are completely reliable: (1) identification of a beating fetal heart (auscultation or ultrasound), (2) perception of fetal movement by the examiner (not just ballottement of an object), and (3) ultrasound and/or radiography.

CHAPTER 7

Placental, Fetal, and Newborn Physiology
Questions

DIRECTIONS (Questions 424 through 467): Each of the numbered items or incomplete statements in this section is followed by answers or by completions of the statement. Select the ONE lettered answer or completion that is BEST in each case.

424. Because the human placenta has the syncytiocytrophoblast directly bathed by maternal blood, it is called

    (A) allantoic
    (B) choroidal
    (C) hemochorial
    (D) of endodermal origin
    (E) an example of countercurrent flow

425. The placental cotyledons are formed primarily by

    (A) mesenchymal differentiation secondary to unknown factors
    (B) arterial pressure on the chorionic plate and decidua
    (C) fetal angiogenesis
    (D) maternal angiogenesis
    (E) folding of the yolk sac

426. The fetus is totally dependent on the placenta for transporting nutrients and elimination of wastes. The effectiveness of the placenta as an organ of transfer for any substance is determined by a number of variables. These include

    (A) rate of maternal blood flow
    (B) metabolism of the substance by the placenta
    (C) concentration of the substance in fetal and maternal blood
    (D) rate of fetal blood flow
    (E) all of the above

427. Because the fetus is growing rapidly its need for nutrients and energy exceeds the mother's on a gram-for-gram basis. Often, the placental transport will achieve a fetal concentration greater than maternal, but occasionally the converse occurs. Which of the following has a lower concentration in the fetus than in the mother?

    (A) vitamins
    (B) phosphate
    (C) amino acids
    (D) oxygen

428. The placenta is supplied by two umbilical arteries that carry deoxygenated fetal blood. This blood flows into intravillous capillaries and back to the fetus in the single umbilical vein. The maternal blood flows from

    (A) arteries to placental capillaries to veins
    (B) veins to placental capillaries to arteries
    (C) intravillous space to arteries to veins
    (D) veins to intravillous spaces to arteries
    (E) arteries to intravillous spaces to veins

429. The placenta

(A) maintains absolute separation between the maternal and fetal circulations

(B) allows total mixing of the maternal and fetal blood

(C) allows maternal blood to enter the fetal circulation but not vice versa

(D) allows only large molecules to pass

(E) allows mainly small molecules and a few blood cells to pass

430. Which of the following statements regarding the placenta is true?

(A) In the placenta, fetal blood is in lacunae that bathe maternal capillaries.

(B) The placenta fulfills some of the functions of lung, kidney, and intestine for the fetus.

(C) Infectious organisms cannot cross the placenta from mother to fetus.

(D) The placenta produces only human chorionic gonadotropin (hCG).

431. A chronic hypertensive patient presents with complaints of decreased fetal movement. Her prenatal care has been sporadic but it appears she is at 37 weeks' gestation with an estimated fetal weight of 2,200 g. Concerns are raised regarding placental reserves for oxygenating the fetus. This can be most directly assessed by

(A) maternal estriol production

(B) oxytocin challenge testing

(C) a fetal ultrasound growth curve

(D) lecithin/sphingomyelin (L/S) ratio

(E) maternal alpha-fetoprotein

432. Labor is induced at 38 weeks due to severe oligohydramnios. The infant is born with a congenital absence of the left hand. This is likely due to

(A) maternal trauma

(B) amniotic bands

(C) chorioangioma

(D) true knots in the umbilical cord

(E) genetic abnormalities

Questions 433 and 434

A patient presents at 28 weeks' gestation for prenatal care. Her last pregnancy was complicated by no prenatal care and delivery of a term infant with minimal hydrops and eventual jaundice due to Rh sensitization to D. The father of that pregnancy also fathered this pregnancy. He is homozygous for D. The amniotic fluid obtained from amniocentesis at 28 weeks shows an optical density (OD) at 450 millimicrons of 0.29, placing it in zone 3 of the Liley curve. The fetus appears normal on ultrasound.

433. At this time, which of the following should be done?

(A) no further study

(B) repeat titer in 4 weeks

(C) amniocentesis in 1 to 2 weeks

(D) intrauterine transfusion

(E) immediate delivery

434. At 30 weeks' gestation, the amniocentesis reveals a delta OD at 450 millimicrons of 0.24. The infant continues to look normal on ultrasound. Which of the following should be done?

(A) no further study

(B) repeat titer in 4 weeks

(C) amniocentesis in 1 week

(D) intrauterine transfusion

(E) immediate delivery

435. A poorly controlled class D diabetic patient desired a repeat cesarean section. An amniocentesis to verify pulmonary maturity was done prior to scheduled surgery at 37 weeks' gestation. The lecithin/sphingomyelin (L/S) ratio was 2:1 and phosphotidyl glycerol was absent. An infant was delivered who developed infant respiratory distress syndrome (IRDS). The most likely reason was

(A) fetal lung maturation may be delayed in maternal diabetes

(B) the L/S test was done on fetal urine

(C) maternal blood was present in the specimen

(D) a foam test was not done

(E) diabetic patients do not produce lecithin

436. Although the parents want to know the total length of the infant, the more accurate measurement is the crown–rump length. The average fetus at term is approximately how long from crown to rump?

(A) 36 cm

(B) 40 cm

(C) 50 cm

(D) 66 cm

(E) 80 cm

437. A patient presents to labor and delivery complaining of regular uterine contractions. Upon reviewing her gestational dating criteria, the following is determined:

Last menstrual period (LMP) places her at 36 weeks estimated gestational age (EGA).

Ultrasound done at 10 weeks places her at 38 weeks.

Ultrasound done at presentation places her at 35 weeks.

Clinical size at presentation places her at 34 weeks.

You determine that she is

(A) 34 weeks EGA

(B) 35 weeks EGA

(C) 36 weeks EGA

(D) 38 weeks EGA

438. The fetal head is usually the largest part of the infant. Depending on the positioning of the head as it enters the pelvis, labor will progress normally or experience a dystocia due to cephalopelvic disproportion. The smallest circumference of the normal fetal head corresponds to the plane of the

(A) suboccipitobregmatic diameter

(B) occipitofrontal diameter

(C) occipitomental diameter

(D) bitemporal diameter

(E) biparietal diameter

439. During the last month of normal pregnancy, the fetus grows at a rate of approximately

(A) 100 g/week

(B) 250 g/week

(C) 500 g/week

(D) 1,000 g/week

440. Fetal nutrition is dependent on

(A) maternal nutrient stores

(B) maternal diet

(C) placental exchange

(D) maternal metabolism

(E) all of the above

441. A patient is found to be blood type A negative during her first pregnancy. She receives antenatal RhoGAM at 28 weeks. At 32 weeks she develops severe preeclampsia and is induced, resulting in an uncomplicated vaginal delivery. The infant does well and is found to be A positive. The mother is found to have anti-D immunoglobulin at a titer of 1:1. The patient should receive

(A) no RhoGAM since she is sensitized

(B) mini RhoGAM dose

(C) 1 dose of RhoGAM

(D) 2 doses of RhoGAM

442. A patient has an emergent cesarean section for an abruption. Due to a large anterior placenta, the placenta was entered during the surgery. The mother is Rh negative. The infant appears anemic and is Rh positive. To determine the amount of Rhogam that needs to be given, an estimate of the amount of fetal red blood cells (RBCs) in the maternal circulation is necessary. Fetal RBCs can be distinguished from maternal RBCs by their

(A) shape

(B) resistance to acid elution

(C) lack of Rh factor

(D) lower amounts of hemoglobin

443. It is found that approximately 40 cc of fetal blood has gotten into the maternal circulation. The patient should receive

(A) no RhoGAM since she is already becoming sensitized

(B) one ampule of RhoGAM

(C) two ampules of RhoGAM

(D) 15 cc RhoGAM

(E) 30 cc RhoGAM

444. The oxygen dissociation curve of fetal blood lies to the left of the curve of maternal blood. This implies that

(A) at any given O_2 tension and pH, fetal hemoglobin (Hb F) binds less O_2 than adult hemoglobin (Hb A)

(B) the fetus needs a greater O_2 tension than the mother

(C) there is more Hb F than Hb A

(D) O_2 should transfer easily to the fetus

Questions 445 through 448

In utero the fetus exists in a "water"-filled environment. All oxygen is derived from the placenta. The fetal lungs are filled with amniotic fluid. Given the lower oxygen tension of the fetal blood, the circulation through the heart and lungs is altered to allow optimal oxygen delivery to the most critical structures. Yet this unique circulation must convert in minutes upon delivery to a typical adult circulatory flow.

445. Oxygenated blood from the umbilical vein enters the fetal circulation via the

(A) portal sinus and ductus venosus

(B) the inferior vena cava

(C) intrahepatic artery

(D) the lesser hepatic veins

(E) ductus arteriosus

446. In the fetus the most well-oxygenated blood is allowed into the systemic circulation by the

(A) foramen ovale

(B) ductus arteriosus

(C) right ventricle

(D) ligamentum teres

(E) ligamentum venosum

447. In the fetal circulation the highest oxygen content occurs in the

(A) superior vena cava

(B) aorta

(C) ductus arteriosus

(D) umbilical arteries

(E) ductus venosus

448. In systemic circulation of the fetus the highest oxygen content occurs in the

(A) ascending aorta

(B) descending aorta

(C) ductus arteriosus

(D) umbilical vein

(E) left ventricle

449. Hematopoiesis takes place in the early embryo within the _____. It then takes place in the _____ and finally in the _____. In chronological order these hematopoietic organs are

(A) yolk sac, fetal liver, fetal bone marrow

(B) yolk sac, fetal kidney, fetal bone marrow

(C) placenta, fetal liver, fetal bone marrow

(D) placenta, fetal kidney, fetal bone marrow

(E) maternal circulation, placenta, fetal liver

450. Fetal coagulation at birth

(A) is generally the same as the adult

(B) shows significantly less clotting capabilities than in the adult

(C) demonstrates a hypercoagulable state

(D) differs significantly between male and female fetuses

(E) depends solely on platelet activity until well into the first week of life when clotting factors are activated

451. The fetus can produce immune antibodies. In the fetal blood at birth (compared to maternal blood) there is/are generally

(A) more immunoglobulin G (IgG)
(B) similar IgG levels
(C) more immunoglobulin M (IgM)
(D) more immunoglobulin A (IgA)
(E) similar IgM levels

452. Characteristics of the fetal respiratory system includes

(A) no evidence of respiratory movement until 8 months' gestation
(B) slow aspiration of amniotic fluid
(C) normal maturation sufficient to support long-term extrauterine existence by the end of the fifth lunar month
(D) high level of surfactant by term

453. Lung surfactant is critical to pulmonary functioning by keeping surface tension in the alveoli low and thereby decreasing the occurrence of atelectasis and atrioventricular (AV) shunting. Surfactant is formed in the

(A) type I pneumocytes of the lung alveoli
(B) type II pneumocytes of the lung alveoli
(C) epithelium of the respiratory bronchi
(D) hilum of the lung
(E) placental syncytiocytotrophoblast

454. The presence of which of the following substances is most reassuring that fetal lungs will be mature?

(A) phosphatidylinositol
(B) phosphatidylethanolamine
(C) phosphatidylglycerol
(D) phosphatidylcholine
(E) phosphatidylinositol deacylase

455. Fetal breathing movements can be an indicator of fetal well-being in utero and should occur about

(A) every 30 to 60 seconds
(B) every 30 to 60 minutes
(C) every 24 hours
(D) 5 times per week
(E) every 1 to 2 weeks

456. Characteristics of the fetal digestive tract include

(A) swallowing of amniotic fluid by 16 weeks' gestation
(B) lack of hydrochloric acid until after delivery
(C) production of meconium only in the eighth month of gestation
(D) esophageal atresia until the seventh lunar month
(E) peristalsis starting at approximately 20 weeks' gestation

457. The presence of meconium-stained amniotic fluid is felt to be indicative of possible fetal stress. It is thought that the release of meconium by the fetus may be caused by

(A) the release of cholecystokinin (pancreozymin) in response to fetal hypoxia
(B) a fetal gut reflex secondary to ischemia
(C) the release of arginine vasopressin by the fetal pituitary secondary to hypoxia
(D) intermittent fetal bowel obstruction
(E) excessive levels of endogenous oxytocin

458. A fetus has an infection that is causing acute hemolysis. At birth, the infant is not jaundiced though the liver is enlarged. The lack of fetal jaundice is because

(A) the fetus has a great capacity for conjugating bilirubin
(B) the liver has high levels of uridine diphosphoglucose dehydrogenase
(C) the liver plays no part in fetal blood production
(D) the fetus produces biliverdin
(E) unconjugated bilirubin is cleared by the maternal liver

459. The serum insulin and glucose levels in the *newborn* infant of a poorly controlled diabetic mother in comparison to the newborn infant of a euglycemic mother are generally

	Insulin	Glucose
(A)	higher	lower
(B)	same	same
(C)	lower	lower
(D)	higher	higher
(E)	lower	higher

460. The fetal kidneys

(A) are first capable of producing highly concentrated urine at 3 months

(B) are first capable of producing highly concentrated urine at 6 months

(C) produce only nomotonic urine

(D) if absent are associated with pulmonary hypoplasia

(E) are not affected by urinary tract obstruction in utero

461. Fetal neurologic injury or developmental abnormalities may have many symptoms, including

(A) failure to nurse

(B) seizures

(C) apathy

(D) weak cry

(E) all of the above

462. Which of the following statements is true regarding fetal endocrine systems?

(A) The adrenal is relatively larger than it is in adults.

(B) Inadequate fetal thyroid hormone is compensated for by maternal thyroid hormone.

(C) The testes are incapable of secreting androgens at birth.

(D) A fetus does not produce growth hormone.

(E) all of the above

463. Which of the following statements regarding the fetal pituitary is true?

(A) The anterior pituitary function is dependent on function of the remaining central nervous system (CNS).

(B) Arginine vasopressin is demonstrable only late in the third trimester of pregnancy.

(C) There is a well-developed intermediate lobe of the pituitary in the human fetus.

(D) Fetal pituitary extract has been shown to alleviate nearly all signs of parkinsonism when injected into adults with that disease.

(E) The pituitary thyroid axis begins to function in the fetus just before birth.

464. The interaction between maternal and fetal physiology relative to thyroid function is complex. Which of the following is an accurate description of this interaction?

(A) Maternal thyrotropin easily crosses the placenta.

(B) The placenta serves as a barrier to maternal iodine crossing to the fetus.

(C) The athyroid fetus is growth retarded at birth.

(D) The fetal thyroid concentrates iodide.

(E) Maternal thyroid hormones (T_4 and T_3) readily cross the placenta.

465. A term infant is born with normal external female genitalia. Which of the following is not possible?

(A) There are ovaries.

(B) There are no functioning gonads.

(C) There is androgen insensitivity.

(D) There is inadequate androgen production.

(E) There is functional dihydrotestosterone (DHT).

466. A fetus has genotype 46,XY. Early in embryogenesis the right testis does not form (dysgenesis). What will be the resulting developments?

(A) female phenotype
(B) development of the right paramesonephric duct
(C) development of the right mesonephric duct
(D) development of a right ovary

467. A female fetus has partial fusion of the two müllerian ducts and complete failure of septal resorption. The resulting uterine anomaly is called

(A) müllerian agenesis
(B) vaginal septum
(C) unicornuate uterus
(D) didelphys uterus
(E) septate uterus

DIRECTIONS (Questions 468 through 471): Each group of items in this section consists of lettered headings followed by a set of numbered words or phrases. For each numbered word or phrase, select the ONE lettered heading that is most closely associated with it. Each lettered heading may be selected once, more than once, or not at all.

Questions 468 through 471

Match the appropriate gestational age with the intrauterine onset of the corresponding behavior.

(A) 10 weeks
(B) 14 to 16 weeks
(C) 24 to 26 weeks
(D) 28 weeks

468. Local stimuli evoke squinting, opening the mouth, and flexion of the toes.

469. Swallowing and respiratory movements occur.

470. Fetus hears some sounds.

471. Fetus is responsive to taste.

Answers and Explanations

424. **(C)** In primates, the allantoic sac fuses with the chorion, forming the chorioallantoic placenta. Fetal trophoblast invades the myometrium, and a decidual plate is formed. In humans, maternal blood comes in direct contact with the fetal trophoblast as the placental villi are suspended in lacuni of maternal blood in the placental bed. Therefore, the human placenta is described as a hemochorial placenta.

425. **(B)** About 6 weeks after conception the trophoblast has 12 to 15 major arteries invading deeply into the myometrium and 20 or more lesser arteries. The pressure generated by these major vessels forces the chorionic plate away from the decidua and forms 12 to 20 cotyledons. Fetal angiogenesis is partly contributory to cotyledon formation as well.

426. **(E)** There are at least ten variables that determine the course of placental transfer. Other variables include placental surface area, physical properties of the intervening tissue, gradients of the substance on each side of the placenta, and the amount of active transport. The placenta is a respiratory and excretory organ for the fetus.

427. **(D)** Although much of placental transport is passive, a large number of necessary metabolic products are actively transported against a concentration gradient. This accounts for many instances of nutritional sparing of the fetus even though maternal nutrition is poor. Fetal P_{O_2}, however, is significantly less than maternal.

428. **(E)** Oxygenated maternal arterial blood flows into the intravillous spaces, exchanging oxygen with the fetal blood across the placental tissues. It is then collected in maternal veins and reenters the maternal vascular system. The fetal and maternal vascular systems do not normally mix maternal and fetal blood.

429. **(E)** The placenta allows a few maternal and a few fetal cells to cross. There may be as much as 0.1 to 3.0 mL of fetal blood in the maternal circulation normally. However, there is not free passage. The systems should be separate and to the degree to which they are not, maternal sensitization may occur.

430. **(B)** Small amounts of fetal and maternal blood do cross the placental barrier, but they do not mix freely. Spirochetes (e.g., *Treponema pallidum*) can cross the placenta and have been known to do so. The placenta is a respiratory and excretory organ for the fetus and is capable of producing several hormones, including hCG and human placental lactogen (HPL).

431. **(B)** The stress test consists of stimulating the pregnant uterus until three contractions occur every 10 minutes and observing monitored fetal heart rate for abnormal decelerations that would indicate marginal placental reserve. It is the only immediate and direct measure of placental respiratory function. Estriol can be delayed as can a fall-off in fetal growth. L/S ratio is a test for lung maturity of the fetus, not the placental reserve. Maternal serum alpha-fetoprotein (MSAFP) is a prenatal screen for neural tube defects. Although asymmetric intrauterine growth retardation can result from a decreased reserve and be detected by ultrasound, this is not an immediate assessment of status.

432. **(B)** Amniotic bands can cause severe fetal deformities and even amputations by constricting fetal parts. They are thought to result when small areas of amnion tear and form tough bands from the resultant scarring with healing. The phenomenon is also associated with oligohydramnios. Placental abnormalities have also been noted with a full-blown amniotic band syndrome.

433. **(C)** At this level the infant is affected but not in danger. The amniocentesis should be repeated in 1 to 2 weeks. The fetal cardiovascular reserve (level of hemoglobin from the effects of fetal hemolytic anemia) is still adequate given normal ultrasound despite the finding of zone 3 (see Figure 7–1). Direct fetal umbilical blood sampling can also be used, but has a fetal loss rate of 0.5 to 2.0% and other morbidities of up to 5%.

434. **(C)** The slightest decrease in delta OD 450 is encouraging, and one can hope that these values will parallel the zone 3 line (see Figure 7–1) and that the infant can be delivered at 38 weeks. However, weekly amniocentesis should be done to follow the patient. The status may be tenuous at best.

435. **(A)** In diabetics the lecithin/sphingomyelin (L/S) ratio alone may not be adequate to predict the onset of infant respiratory distress syndrome (IRDS). Hence the recommendation to assess for the presence of PG as a better indicator of lung maturity. Fetal urine would not have a high L/S ratio. Maternal

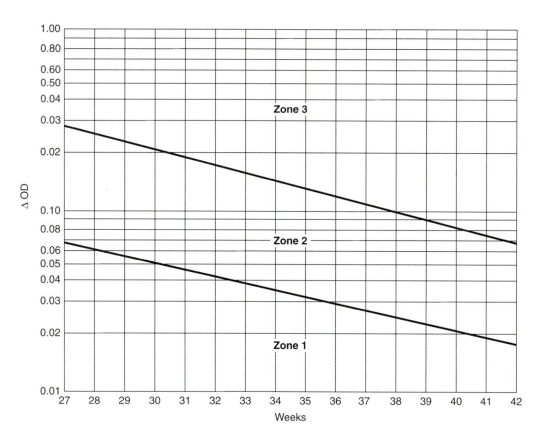

Figure 7–1. The Liley graph (curve).
(Reproduced, with permission, from Cunningham FG et al. *Williams Obstetrics,* 21st ed. New York: McGraw-Hill, 2001.)

blood would lower the L/S ratio in most cases, as it has an L/S ratio of about 1.4. Fetal lung biochemical measurements are less reliable predictors of fetal lung maturity in poorly controlled pregnant diabetic patients.

436. **(A)** Fifty centimeters, or 20 inches, is an average crown-to-heel length, and that is the standard way to assess newborn length. Crown-to-rump lengths were found to be more accurate in predicting growth in utero. Average sitting height is 36 cm, or 14 in. With the difficulty involved in measurement of the newborn, many nursery height measurements are less than completely accurate. Haase suggested this approximation. During the last half of gestation, the fetus's length can be approximated by taking the number of lunar months (4 weeks per lunar month) times five. In this circumstance, the LMP may not be totally accurate. Although a foot length may be useful, most of the data available refer to crown–rump lengths. Fetal weight is not useful for determining gestational age and should be used only as a last resort. Abdominal circumference is too dependent on nutritional status and possible associated anomalies to be of much use.

437. **(D)** Dating a pregnancy is critical to determining the best management. Traditionally the first day of the last menstrual period is used. However, with the advent of ultrasound, which allows measurement of the fetus, dating has become more accurate. The first ultrasound done during a pregnancy should be compared to the dating from the LMP. If dating based on the LMP is within the error of the ultrasound, LMP dating is used. The error of the ultrasound is roughly +1 week for the first trimester, +2 weeks for the second trimester, and +3 weeks for the third trimester. Since the initial ultrasound was done in the first trimester and was 2 weeks different from the LMP, the ultrasound dating is used. Later ultrasounds are not used to change the due date but can be used for estimating the fetal growth rate. Given that the ultrasound and clinical sizing is smaller than the EGA of 38 weeks deter-

mined by the initial ultrasound, concerns of growth restrictions or a constitutionally small fetus can be raised.

438. **(A)** A vertex presentation offers the smallest circumference of the fetal head to the pelvic passage. The circumference at this point is about 32 cm. At the greatest point of the circumference (the occipitofrontal diameter), it is about 34 cm. In addition to the circumference, the ability of the fetus to negotiate the pelvic curve is very dependent on the position of the presenting vertex with a well-flexed head in the OA position.

439. **(B)** A good rule of thumb is that the fetus gains one-half pound a week during the last few weeks of gestation. Of course, if placental insufficiency exists, such weight gain does not occur. In uncontrolled diabetes mellitus, classes A, B, and C, growth during this period is accelerated. More severe forms of diabetes (e.g., F, R, or H) may have small-vessel disease with resulting placental insufficiency.

440. **(E)** More and more evidence is accumulating that the fetus does not get everything it needs from the mother unless the mother is and has been well nourished and in good health. The fetus will, however, serve as a sink for glucose and iron. Active transport will also supply fetal nutrients, even against an unfavorable gradient.

441. **(C)** RhoGAM consists of anti-D immunoglobin. Since she received RhoGAM only a month earlier, there would still be some detected during the "RhoGAM" workup postpartum. She should still receive one ampule of RhoGAM unless testing determines a large fetal–maternal bleed, which is not likely in an uncomplicated vaginal delivery.

442. **(B)** Small numbers of fetal red cells can be detected in the maternal circulation by the Kleihauer–Betke test, which uses the fetal cells resistant to acid elution for identification. Fetal red cells can exist and function at lower pH values than adult red blood cells (RBCs). Fetal RBCs have less than two thirds

the life span of adult RBCs. Fetal RBCs may also be nucleated. The nucleation helps identify fetal RBCs on a smear. This nucleation disappears early in normal pregnancy. Fetal cells then closely resemble reticulocytes.

443. **(C)** An ampule of RhoGAM neutralizes approximately the equivalent of 30 cc of fetal blood. Since the estimate is 40 cc, she should receive 2 ampules.

444. **(D)** The pH of the fetus is slightly lower than the maternal pH. The difference in O_2 affinity is very small in vivo. The fetus lives at a lower O_2 concentration with an oxygen-loving hemoglobin (Hb F). There is still, however, more Hb A than Hb F.

445. **(A)** The umbilical vein comes directly from the placenta and distributes highly oxygenated blood to the liver, the portal system, and the inferior vena cava. The umbilical vein enters the fetus and divides immediately into the portal sinus (carrying blood to the hepatic veins) and the ductus venosus (carrying blood to the vena cava). The ductus arteriosus connects the fetal pulmonary vasculature with the fetal aorta (see Figure 7–2).

446. **(A)** The foramen ovale lets oxygenated blood into the left side of the heart. The ligaments mentioned are found after birth and represent occluded vessels from the fetal circulation. Before birth, however, they serve as the shunting mechanism that makes fetal oxygenation possible.

447. **(E)** The fetal venous blood from the placenta has the highest oxygen content. This is true because fetal venous blood in the ductus venosus has most recently received oxygenation. Pulmonary fetal oxygenation does not occur until the infant's first breath.

448. **(D)** The umbilical vein always has the highest oxygen concentration. The next highest oxygen concentration in the systemic circulation is in the ascending aorta prior to the insertion of the ductus arteriosis. The arteries supplying the fetal brain branch off that part of the as-

cending aorta, allowing the blood with the highest systemic oxygen levels to be preferentially shunted to the brain. The umbilical vein is not part of the systemic circulation.

449. **(A)** Hematopoiesis in the early embryo takes place first in the yolk sac, then the liver, and finally the bone marrow. The spleen and lymph nodes also make a minor contribution. While kidney function is needed for normal erythropoiesis in the adult, it is not needed in the fetus. No fetal blood comes from a maternal source or from placenta.

450. **(B)** Fetal and early neonatal blood clotting may be compromised because the fetus is low in factors II, VII, IX, X, XI, XII, and XIII and fibrinogen. Newborn infants are given vitamin K to stimulate the lipid-soluble coagulation factors.

451. **(B)** IgG crosses the placenta easily from 16 weeks' gestation onward. At birth, fetal and maternal IgG levels are equal since most of the IgG present is from maternal diffusion. IgM cannot cross, and a normal fetus (noninfected) produces very little IgM. IgA is not produced and later will be absorbed through the fetal gut from the colostrum in small to moderate amounts. The fetus normally has lower levels of IgM and IgA than the mother. In contrast to what occurs in adults, however, the IgM response is the primary immunologic reaction of the fetus for up to 4 weeks postexposure.

452. **(D)** Surfactant, which decreases surface tension of the alveoli, is not present in high amounts until near term. Fetal breathing of amniotic fluid is present early on in pregnancy and may be an indicator of fetal well-being. Amniotic fluid is the medium allowing for prebirth lung expansion. In fact, preterm rupture of membranes at an early gestational age (< 25 weeks) with resultant oligohydramnios interferes with the normal breathing process and hence pulmonary development. If severely affected, the fetus can have pulmonary hypoplasia with increased risk of neonatal death.

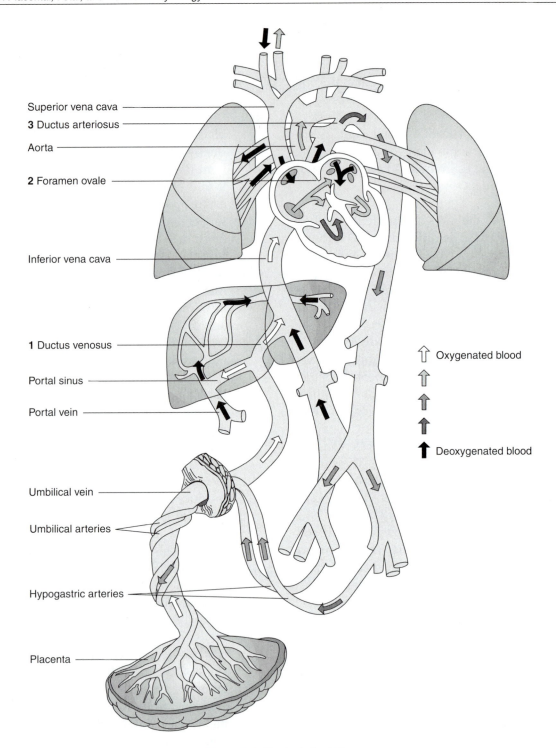

Figure 7–2. The fetal circulation.
(Reproduced, with permission, from Cunningham FG et al. *Williams Obstetrics,* 21st ed. New York: McGraw-Hill, 2001.)

453. **(B)** There are more than 40 cell types in the fetal lung. Surfactant is specific to the type II pneumocytes of the alveoli. Surfactant is produced in the lamellar bodies of these cells. The presence of air-to-tissue interface as the infant takes its first breath allows the surfactant to "uncoil" from the lamellar bodies and line the alveolus, thus preventing alveolar collapse. It is the capacity for the lungs to produce surfactant and not the actual laying down of it in utero that establishes lung maturity before birth.

454. **(C)** The first four are all components of mature surfactant. Fifty percent of surfactant is composed of phosphatidylcholine, but the presence of phosphatidylglycerol seems to play the crucial role in prevention of infant respiratory distress. Its presence is nearly a guarantee of fetal lung maturity.

455. **(B)** Fetal breathing movements can be seen episodically in the normal human fetus. They occur about every 30 to 60 minutes. Asphyxia appears to reduce the frequency of fetal breathing movements.

456. **(A)** The fetus has peristalsis by 11 weeks' gestation and swallows amniotic fluid from 16 weeks onward. Esophageal atresia should not be present since the consequent inability to effectively swallow will cause the development of hydramnios. Gastric acid and meconium continue to be produced from early on, although an extremely preterm infant may have transient deficiencies of digestive enzymes.

457. **(C)** Hypoxia is implicated in the passage of meconium from the large bowel in utero. The mechanism may result from the fetal pituitary release of arginine vasopressin stimulating the smooth muscle of the colon to contract (just as it will in adults).

458. **(E)** Because of a relative lack of enzymes, the liver conjugates bilirubin poorly. Some is excreted into the bowel where it is oxidized to biliverdin and colors the meconium. However, the unconjugated bilirubin is transported across the placenta and cleared by the maternal liver. This prevents fetal jaundice. Neonatal jaundice will appear hours to days after birth due to the poor ability of the newborn liver to conjugate bilirubin and excrete it through the intestines. The fetal liver is active in blood production early in pregnancy, hence the liver enlargement in this case. Uri-

dine diphosphoglucose dehydrogenase plays only a minor role in intermediary metabolism. Fetal levels of glycogen are two to three times that of adult levels.

459. **(A)** Insulin levels are elevated in the infants of diabetic mothers. In fact, high insulin levels may cause a precipitous drop in newborn serum glucose, causing the baby to be metabolically unstable. This is why all babies of diabetic mothers and macrosomic infants (potentially undiagnosed diabetic mothers) are screened quickly after birth and for the first few hours for hypoglycemia.

460. **(D)** The number and function of glomeruli can be used as a rough index of fetal maturity. Creatinine concentration in the amniotic fluid mirrors renal function. Maximum fetal urine production is about 650 mL/day of hypotonic solution. Fetal urine production is often decreased in infants with growth retardation. Intrauterine obstruction of the fetal urinary tract can cause severe damage to the fetal kidneys. Absence of fetal kidneys will result in severe oligohydramnios and pulmonary hypoplasia and is incompatible with life. Many of these infants have a specific syndrome called Potter syndrome.

461. **(E)** Other signs are difficult breathing, cyanosis, and vomiting. Since there are few fetal activities that are more than vegetative, these are the functions affected. Neurologic examination may also reveal abnormalities.

462. **(A)** Basically, a fetus is capable of manufacturing most of the hormones found in an adult. Fetal endocrine organs function to regulate thyroxine, insulin, and some adrenal hormones. They are necessary for normal fetal development. Fetal adrenals are very enlarged, which makes them vulnerable to injury during a difficult delivery, especially a breech presentation.

463. **(C)** The control of fetal anterior pituitary secretion is independent of maturation of the CNS. Vasopressin is produced from the first trimester onward by the fetus. The interme-

diate lobe of the pituitary is well developed in the fetus and produces melanocyte-stimulating hormone and beta-endorphin. Fetal pituitary extract may someday play a key role in the treatment of parkinsonism but does not at present. The pituitary thyroid axis functions from the first trimester onward.

464.   **(D)** Generally, the placenta serves as a barrier to maternal thyrotropin and thyroid hormones. The fetus concentrates iodide very effectively, hence the need to avoid radioactive iodine and high iodide-containing medications. There is limited action of the thyroid hormone during fetal life. The athyroid fetus will appear normally grown at birth. This is why all newborns are screened in the first week of life for thyroid function.

465.   **(E)** Functional androgens with active androgen receptors are required for the phenotypic male development. In the presence of inactive androgens (androgen insensitivity syndrome), no gonads (gonadal dysgenesis), inadequate androgen production, or normally functioning ovaries, the infant phenotype will be female even though the chromosomes may be 46,XY.

466.   **(B)** The müllerian inhibiting substance (MIS) is active only in the immediate area. Thus, the lack of a testis on the right will mean there is no MIS, the müllerian ducts (paramesonephric) will develop, and the wolffian duct will regress. Because DHT is present from the left testis, the external genitalia will be male. Thus, the newborn will have a male phenotype. Since there was gonadal dysgenesis, there will not be a right ovary.

467.   **(D)** The formation of a normal internal female reproductive system requires the fusion of the two müllerian tubes and then reabsorption of the resulting septum to a single uterine cavity and cervix. Vaginal agenesis is a failure of the müllerian ducts to elongate to the level of the urogenital sinus. A vaginal septum is formed when there is a septal reabsorption defect. A septate uterus has successful müllerian fusion but incomplete reabsorption of the septum. A unicornuate uterus results when there is agenesis of one müllerian duct. A uterine didelphys results when there is partial fusion and complete septal resorption defect. This results in two uterine cavities and two cervices.

468–471.   **(468-A, 469-B, 470-C, 471-D)** At 10 weeks, local stimuli evoke squinting, opening the mouth, finger closure, and flexion of the toes. By 16 weeks, the fetus can swallow and has spontaneous respiration. At 24 weeks or later, sucking begins as does the perception of some sound. By 28 weeks' gestation, the fetus responds to the maternal ingestion of some substances, indicating the presence of taste.

CHAPTER 8

Prenatal Care
Questions

DIRECTIONS (Questions 472 through 514): Each of the numbered items or incomplete statements in this section is followed by answers or by completions of the statement. Select the ONE lettered answer or completion that is BEST in each case.

472. Worldwide, the most common problem during pregnancy is

    (A) diabetes
    (B) toxemia
    (C) heart disease
    (D) urinary tract infection (UTI)
    (E) iron-deficiency anemia

473. In the United States, the leading causes of maternal mortality include

    (A) infection, cardiomyopathy, and stroke
    (B) motor vehicle accidents, homicide, and suicide
    (C) embolism, hypertension, and ectopic pregnancy
    (D) complications related to abortion and anesthesia
    (E) human immunodeficiency virus (HIV) and infections related to immunodeficiency

474. The expected date of delivery of a human pregnancy can most correctly be calculated by

    (A) adding 254 to the date of the start of the last menstrual period (LMP)
    (B) counting 10 lunar months from the time of ovulation

    (C) counting 40 weeks from the first day of the LMP
    (D) counting 280 days from the last day of the LMP
    (E) adding 256 to the date of the elevated urinary luteinizing hormone (LH) when detected by home testing

475. The LMP was June 30. The expected date of confinement (EDC) is approximately

    (A) March 23
    (B) April 7
    (C) March 28
    (D) April 23
    (E) March 7

476. Pregnancy may occur during a period of amenorrhea such as during lactation or following discontinuance of hormonal methods of contraception. In such a situation, determination of the most accurate estimated date of delivery can then be made by

    (A) eliciting when breast tenderness or morning sickness began
    (B) assessing uterine size by physical exam
    (C) counting 280 days from the first positive serum pregnancy test
    (D) asking the patient when she first felt pregnant
    (E) obtaining fetal biometry by ultrasound prior to 20 weeks' gestation

477. A 24-year-old patient who has signs and symptoms of renal lithiasis is to have an intravenous pyelogram (IVP) as part of a urologic investigation. Before proceeding with the study, a determination should be made if she

(A) is using contraception
(B) is in the follicular phase of a menstrual cycle
(C) is sexually active
(D) has a history of children with birth defects
(E) may be pregnant

478. A 20-year-old primigravida who is 24 weeks' pregnant expresses concern about the normality of her fetus after learning that a close friend has just delivered an infant with hydrocephalus. Details about hydrocephalus that should be included in her counseling include the fact that it

(A) occurs spontaneously in 1 in 500 pregnancies
(B) has a multifactorial etiology
(C) is usually an isolated defect
(D) can be cured by intrauterine placement of shunts
(E) can be identified as early as 10 weeks' gestation

479. Fundal height, part of the obstetric examination, is taken from the top of the symphysis pubis to the top of the fundus. It is measured

(A) by calipers, approximating the week of gestation
(B) in inches, approximating the lunar month of gestation
(C) in centimeters and divided by 3.5, approximating the lunar months of gestation
(D) in centimeters, approximating the weeks of gestation between 18 and 34 weeks
(E) by calipers in centimeters, prognosticating the fetal weight

480. Using your knowledge of normal maternal physiology, which of the following would you employ if a patient at 38 weeks became faint while lying supine on your examination table?

(A) smelling salts
(B) turning the patient on her side
(C) oxygen by face mask
(D) intravenous (IV) drugs to increase blood pressure
(E) IV saline solution

481. A woman in early pregnancy is worried because of several small, raised nodules on the areola of both breasts. There are no other findings. Your immediate management should be

(A) reassurance after thorough examination
(B) needle aspiration of the nodules
(C) excisional biopsies of the lesions
(D) mammography
(E) testing for herpes simplex virus II antibodies

482. Immunologic tests for pregnancy can detect human chorionic gonadotropin (hCG) in the urine in which of the following concentrations?

(A) 2 IU/L
(B) 20 IU/L
(C) 100 IU/L
(D) 200 IU/L
(E) 1,000 IU/L

483. Pap smears taken from the uterine cervix during a normal pregnancy

(A) should be part of routine obstetric care
(B) are indicated only in patients with clinically assessed risks
(C) are difficult to interpret because of gestational changes
(D) are a cost-effective replacement for cultures for sexually transmitted diseases (STDs)
(E) are likely to induce uterine irritability

484. A 39-year-old woman (gravida 3, para 1, abortus 1, living children 2) is seen for prenatal care at 14 weeks' gestation. Her history is unremarkable, and her entire family is in good health. Physical examination is within normal limits and confirms a 14-week gestation. Suggested laboratory studies need not include

(A) hematocrit
(B) determination of fetal karyotype
(C) rubella titer
(D) Pap smear
(E) pregnancy test

485. In assessing risk factors in pregnancy, which of the following would create the most concern?

(A) maternal age of 39
(B) maternal age of 17, with menarche at age 13
(C) past history of four normal deliveries
(D) history of ovarian dermoid cyst removed 4 years ago
(E) a clinically measured pelvic diagonal conjugate of 12 cm

486. A pregnant woman at 4 weeks' gestation had an upper gastrointestinal (GI) series and is worried about possible fetal effects from radiation. You inform her that the risk for mental retardation to the fetus is greatest during the

(A) implantation stage from 0 to 7 days
(B) 1st to 8th week of gestation
(C) 8th through 15th week of gestation
(D) 15th through 25th week of gestation
(E) last trimester

487. Advising a 34-year-old woman at 12 weeks' gestation about the risk of chromosomal defects in the fetus, you can correctly state that

(A) there is little worry regarding Down syndrome before the age of 35
(B) paternal age is very important in the etiology of Down syndrome

(C) maternal serum alpha-fetoprotein (MSAFP) is a very specific test for Down syndrome
(D) screening for Down syndrome can be improved by checking amniotic fluid and acetylcholinesterase level
(E) efficacy of screening for Down syndrome is improved by adding estriol and hCG concentration to the MSAFP

488. Counseling of a pregnant patient during early prenatal care should include advice and education on which of the following?

(A) smoking
(B) alcohol abuse
(C) drug abuse
(D) avoiding infection
(E) all of the above

489. Of the following, the most worrisome sign or symptom of potentially serious pathology in late pregnancy is

(A) swollen ankles
(B) constipation
(C) visual changes
(D) nocturia
(E) heartburn

490. During late pregnancy, which of the following implies urinary tract disease?

(A) decreased serum creatinine
(B) failure to excrete a concentrated urine after 18 hours without fluids
(C) glucosuria
(D) dilation of the ureters
(E) decreased creatinine clearance

491. Compared with single pregnancies, multiple pregnancies have a higher rate of which of the following?

(A) abortion
(B) abnormal presentations
(C) prolapsed cords
(D) vasa previa
(E) all of the above

492. Which of the following is a true statement regarding HIV testing in pregnancy?

(A) It should not be offered to patients in low-risk populations.

(B) Universal screening is required by law.

(C) It is performed routinely without patient consent in federal facilities serving high-risk populations.

(D) Testing is done only at the request of the patient.

(E) Universal screening with patient notification is recommended.

493. Routine screening procedures at her first prenatal care visit for a 35-year-old primigravida with an estimated gestational age (EGA) of 8 weeks should include

(A) MSAFP

(B) 1-hour glucose challenge

(C) family history

(D) *Toxoplasma* titer

(E) ultrasound

494. Which of the following fetal findings is LEAST often associated with other congenital anomalies?

(A) omphalocele

(B) gastroschisis

(C) diaphragmatic hernia

(D) duodenal atresia

(E) posturethral value

495. Which of the following factors is NOT measured as part of a biophysical profile (BPP)?

(A) amniotic fluid volume

(B) a contraction stress test (CST)

(C) a nonstress test (NST)

(D) fetal breathing motion

(E) fetal limb movements

496. Positive sign(s) of pregnancy include

(A) amenorrhea, morning sickness, and breast tenderness

(B) bluish or purplish discoloration of the uterine cervix

(C) softening of the lower uterine segment

(D) a positive pregnancy test

(E) ultrasound demonstration of an intrauterine sac

497. A pregnant woman not previously known to be diabetic who is at 26 weeks' gestation had a routine 50-g glucose tolerance test (GTT) with a 1-hour blood glucose value of 144 mg/dL. A follow-up 100-g, 3-hour oral GTT revealed plasma values of fasting blood sugar of 102; 1 hour, 180; 2 hours, 162; and 3 hours, 144. You should

(A) begin diet and insulin therapy

(B) repeat the GTT in early or mid third trimester

(C) start oral hypoglycemic agents in the diet

(D) perform an immediate CST

(E) follow the patient as a normal gestation

498. The best method to safely and reliably diagnose twins is

(A) ultrasonography

(B) Leopold's maneuvers

(C) auscultation

(D) x-rays

(E) computed tomography (CT) scan

499. Ultrasound is used to determine

(A) estimation of fetal weight

(B) presence of multiple pregnancies

(C) whether abdominal masses are cystic or solid

(D) placental position

(E) all of the above

500. Using the NST tracing in Figure 8–1, which of the following is TRUE?

(A) The tracing does not meet the criteria for reactivity.

(B) A fetus with this pattern is at risk for fetal death in utero within the next week.

(C) The pattern demonstrates short-term but not long-term variability.

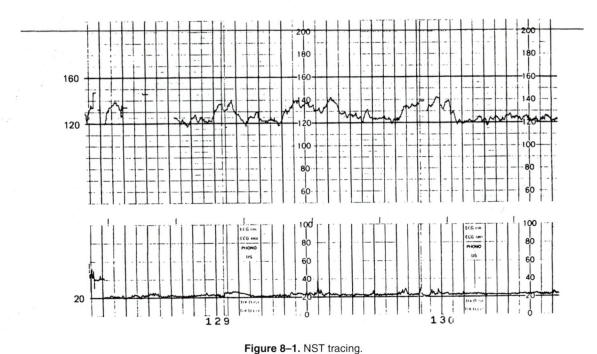

Figure 8–1. NST tracing.
(Reproduced, with permission, from DeCherney AH, Nathan L. *Current Obstetric and Gynecologic Diagnosis and Treatment,* 9th ed. New York: McGraw-Hill, 2003.)

(D) The pattern is common during the sleep cycle of the fetus.

(E) A tracing from the same fetus taken later may demonstrate no accelerations.

501. CSTs and NSTs are used for evaluation of fetal well-being. Which of the following is a TRUE statement?

(A) NST is contraindicated in situations in which labor is contraindicated.

(B) A positive nonreactive CST contraindicates labor.

(C) A positive CST is an excellent predictor of fetal well-being.

(D) A CST is falsely negative less frequently than an NST is falsely reactive.

502. The side effects of oral iron that often cause patients to complain seem to be related most to the

(A) amount of iron ingested

(B) amount of iron needed

(C) amount of iron absorbed

(D) degree of anemia

(E) prior presence of duodenal ulcers

503. Of the following evaluations done during routine prenatal care in a normal pregnancy, the most important in the initial clinic visit is

(A) routine measurement of the fundus

(B) determination of the gestational age

(C) determination of maternal blood pressure

(D) maternal urinalysis

(E) maternal weight

504. There is good evidence that a woman who gave birth to an infant with a neural tube defect (NTD) can substantially reduce the risk of recurrence by taking periconceptional folic acid supplementation. The recommended amount for such a woman would be

(A) 0.4 mg

(B) 0.8 mg

(C) 1.0 mg

(D) 4 mg

(E) 8 mg

505. Which of the following medications, when given before and during pregnancy, may help to prevent NTDs?

   (A) pyridoxine (vitamin B$_6$)
   (B) iron
   (C) folic acid
   (D) zinc
   (E) manganese

506. Which of the following is the greatest cause of pregnancy wastage?

   (A) contraception
   (B) stillbirths
   (C) neonatal mortality
   (D) fetal deaths in utero
   (E) abortion

507. If a patient gains weight rapidly during pregnancy, you should first

   (A) give the patient diuretics
   (B) determine whether the weight gain is from edema or fat
   (C) markedly restrict her diet
   (D) encourage vigorous exercise
   (E) place her on bed rest

508. An 18-year-old single, sedentary, obese female (gravida 1, para 0) is first seen by you for prenatal care at 16 weeks' gestation. Her history is unremarkable, and she claims to be in good health. Her dietary history includes high carbohydrate intake with no fresh vegetables. Physical examination is within normal limits except that she is somewhat pale. Suggested nutritional counseling should include

   (A) a strict diet to maintain her current weight
   (B) 25 to 30 g of protein in the diet every day
   (C) intake of 1,200 calories a day
   (D) folic acid supplementation
   (E) at least 1 hour of vigorous aerobic exercise daily

509. Often, an increase in vaginal discharge may be noted during pregnancy. It may be

   (A) bacterial vaginosis
   (B) *Trichomonas* vaginitis
   (C) *Candida* vaginitis
   (D) physiologic
   (E) all of the above

510. A 19-year-old primigravida with unsure LMP presents to initiate prenatal care. You attempt to estimate gestational age. The uterine fundus is palpable at the level of the pubic symphysis, and fetal heart tones are audible by electronic Doppler. Based on this information, the gestational age is approximately

   (A) 8 weeks
   (B) 12 weeks
   (C) 16 weeks
   (D) 20 weeks
   (E) 24 weeks

511. A 28-year-old gravida 3, para 1, abortus 1 at 30 weeks' gestation reports some recent intermittent contractions. Which of the following correlates with the greatest risk for preterm labor?

   (A) patient is a smoker (1/2 pack per day)
   (B) prior 32-week delivery
   (C) history of colposcopy
   (D) history of *Chlamydia trachomatis*
   (E) prior 8-week spontaneous abortion

512. A 32-year-old gravida 2, para 1 initiates care at 10 weeks' gestation. Which of the following is most worrisome for poor obstetric outcome?

   (A) trace proteinuria on urine dipstick
   (B) blood pressure of 144/92
   (C) inaudible fetal heart tone by electronic Doppler
   (D) maternal height of 4 ft 10 in
   (E) the presence of curdlike discharge consistent with *Candida* on speculum examination

513. Ultrasound is most accurate in dating a pregnancy

    (A) between 2 and 4 weeks after LMP

    (B) between 7 and 9 weeks after LMP

    (C) between 12 and 14 weeks after LMP

    (D) between 19 and 21 weeks after LMP

    (E) between 30 and 32 weeks after LMP

514. Ultrasound is most useful in evaluating fetal anatomy

    (A) between 2 and 4 weeks after LMP

    (B) between 7 and 9 weeks after LMP

    (C) between 12 and 14 weeks after LMP

    (D) between 19 and 21 weeks after LMP

    (E) between 30 and 32 weeks after LMP

DIRECTIONS (Questions 515 through 519): Each of the numbered items or incomplete statements in this section is followed by answers or by completions of the statement. Select the answers or completions that may apply.

515. Nutrients required in increased amounts during pregnancy include which three of the following?

    (A) iron

    (B) iodine

    (C) vitamin A

    (D) calcium

    (E) sodium

516. Compared with singleton pregnancies, twin pregnancies have a higher risk of which five of the following conditions?

    (A) shoulder dystocia

    (B) pregnancy-induced hypertension

    (C) cesarean delivery

    (D) postterm delivery

    (E) perinatal death

    (F) placenta previa

    (G) congenital anomalies

517. A 25-year-old primigravida presents at 30 weeks' gestation complaining of intermittent "menstrual-like cramps" persisting for 4 hours. Which two of the following steps would be most useful in determining whether she is in preterm labor?

    (A) NST

    (B) complete blood count (CBC)

    (C) serial cervical examination

    (D) biophysical profile

    (E) measurement of amniotic fluid volume

518. Periconceptional dietary adjustments have been shown to have a profound impact on which two of the following diseases or malformations?

    (A) Tay–Sachs

    (B) NTDs

    (C) clubfoot (talipes equinovarus)

    (D) diabetes mellitus

    (E) cystic fibrosis

519. Which two of the following should be prescribed for the average pregnant woman?

    (A) an increase of no more than 15 to 20 lb in pregnancy

    (B) iron supplementation

    (C) continuation of moderate exercise

    (D) Jacuzzi hot tub baths for relaxation

    (E) vinegar–water douches in the third trimester

DIRECTIONS (Questions 520 through 540): Each group of items in this section consists of lettered headings followed by a set of numbered words or phrases. For each numbered word or phrase, select the ONE lettered heading that is most closely associated with it. Each lettered heading may be selected once, more than once, or not at all.

Questions 520 through 523

A pregnant woman asks when during gestation the developing conceptus is at greatest risk of a teratogenic insult. You explain the different stages of development. Match the stage of development with the name of that particular stage.

(A) zygote
(B) embryo
(C) fetus
(D) infant

520. Liveborn individual from birth to 1 year

521. The diploid cell resulting from the union of a sperm and an egg

522. The conceptus from the time of formation of the inner-cell mass to the eighth week of development

523. The conceptus from the eighth week of gestation to delivery

Questions 524 through 527

During prenatal care, history often determines the need for screening of uncommon abnormalities. Match the laboratory measure with the abnormality for which it serves as a screening test.

(A) acetylcholinesterase
(B) electrophoresis
(C) hexosaminidase A
(D) Delta F 508
(E) glycosylated hemoglobin

524. Tay–Sachs

525. Thalassemia

526. Cystic fibrosis

527. NTD

Questions 528 through 532

During prenatal evaluation, ultrasound has become a frequent procedure. Match the specific ultrasound findings with the commonly associated abnormality.

(A) interventricular defect
(B) NTD
(C) duodenal atresia
(D) Potter syndrome
(E) thalassemia

528. Absent kidneys

529. Banana sign

530. Lemon sign

531. Double bubble sign

532. Hydrops fetalis

Questions 533 through 540

(A) craniofacial abnormalities
(B) Ebstein's anomaly
(C) spina bifida
(D) scalp defects
(E) abortion
(F) stillbirth
(G) none of the above

533. Fluoxetine

534. Podophyllin resin

535. Ofloxacin

536. Captopril

537. Valproic acid

538. Isotretinoin

539. Methimazole

540. Misoprostol

Answers and Explanations

472. (E) In the United States, the average woman has iron stores of less than 1 g. This amount is needed for the increased maternal blood volume and fetal growth during pregnancy. Poorly nourished women have an even greater deficiency. Supplemental iron should be given during and for several months after pregnancy.

473. (C) Maternal death is the demise of any woman from any pregnancy-related cause while pregnant or within 42 days after termination of pregnancy. A direct maternal death is the result of obstetric complications of pregnancy, labor, or the puerperium. An indirect maternal death is not directly due to obstetric causes but may be aggravated by the physiologic changes of pregnancy. Studies vary in reporting the most frequent causes of maternal death, but collectively embolism, hypertension, and ectopic pregnancy represent nearly 50% of direct maternal deaths. Maternal mortality, along with other statistics of pregnancy outcome, is a measure of the effectiveness of obstetrical care.

474. (C) In calculating the expected date of confinement (EDC) by using the LMP, one must take into account the duration of the patient's normal cycle. If it is longer than 28 days, the EDC will be further from the LMP than calculated by Nägele's rule. From the LMP, gestation is 280 days; from conception, it is 266 days.

475. (B) Nägele's rule allows rapid estimation of the expected date of delivery. From the LMP, add 7 days, subtract 3 months, and add 1 year. It works for the patient with regular monthly cycles and good dating.

476. (E) A certain, documented LMP in a woman with normal, regular menstrual cycles is an excellent means to determine gestational age and estimated date of delivery. Without this, we must rely on other clinical information to date the pregnancy. The most accurate means is an early ultrasound, preferably in the first trimester (crown–rump length), or, at the latest, biometry done before 20 weeks' gestation. Assessment of uterine size—if done in the first trimester by an experienced obstetrical clinician—can also provide an accurate estimate, but objective early ultrasound measurements are preferable.

477. (E) One should always determine whether the patient is pregnant before ordering diagnostic x-rays on any menstrual-age woman. While mutagenic radiation is unlikely from low doses, cumulative effects may be more damaging.

478. (B) Hydrocephalus occurs in approximately 1/2,000 births and may be due to neoplasm infections (such as toxoplasmosis) or genetic inheritance, frequently by the mechanisms of aqueductal stenosis. It is usually found in conjunction with other neurologic or systemic anomalies. Ultrasound has greatly facilitated our ability to diagnose hydrocephalus in utero by using either the absolute size of greater than 10 mm of the lateral ventricular atrium, or a ratio of greater than 50% of the lateral ventricular width to the hemispheric width of the brain.

Although surgery has been tried, results have been discouraging.

479. **(D)** Measurement of fundal height is a routine component of prenatal care. The repetitive, consistent measurements may allow the obstetrician to detect failure of the fetus to grow. Precise knowledge of the age of the fetus is essential for appropriate obstetric management.

480. **(B)** The supine hypotensive syndrome can be corrected by moving the gravid uterus off the vena cava and aorta either by lateral pressure or by turning the patient. Administration of fluids or pressors is usually unnecessary.

481. **(A)** Montgomery nodules are hypertrophied sebaceous glands and occur normally during pregnancy. No further evaluation is necessary. A mass in the breast parenchyma would dictate treatment in the pregnant or nonpregnant state.

482. **(B)** The lower range of detectable hCG has dropped dramatically in recent years. Because of this sensitivity, one can use pregnancy tests to detect low hCG levels. More sensitive tests have greatly improved the ability to diagnose pregnancy. The tests are now inexpensive, specific, sensitive, and highly accurate.

483. **(A)** Every pregnant patient, regardless of her age, should have a Pap smear as part of a routine workup. Routine health care screening must be done during pregnancy.

484. **(E)** Hematocrit is necessary to rule out anemia, as is urinalysis to rule out urinary tract infection or renal disease. Amniocentesis should be recommended at this time because of the probability of chromosomal aberrations when a mother is her age. The incidence of aberration in a patient of this age is 2%. A pregnancy test is not indicated to determine pregnancy when it is clinically apparent.

485. **(A)** Older women have an increased risk during pregnancy for chromosomal abnor-malities, mostly due to nondisjunction. They also have an increased number of abnormalities associated with advancing age, such as hypertension. Extremely young women are also at a greater risk for problems during pregnancy. This is particularly true under the age of 16 and particularly if menarche occurs less than 2 years before the pregnancy. Normal deliveries are not a problem, but a history of prior abnormal deliveries, such as preterm delivery and cesarean section, are concerning. The presence of an ovarian cyst that is treated adequately is of little concern regarding current pregnancy risk. The diagonal conjugate of 12 cm is normal.

486. **(C)** Data derived from the survivors of the atomic bomb place the greatest risk for mental retardation from radiation when the fetus is exposed at 8 to 15 weeks' gestation and virtually no risk with small (i.e., < 5 rads) doses before 8 or after 25 weeks' gestation.

487. **(E)** Although the risk of Down syndrome increases with maternal age, most Down infants are born to women under age 35, because there are a greater number of pregnancies in this age group. Therefore, a good test to detect it is important. Paternal age does not have much effect on the incidence of Down syndrome, although it is important in autosomal dominant genetic disease. MSAFP is a reasonably good test for NTDs when elevated, and a low serum value of AFP is useful, particularly when combined with maternal age to detect Down syndrome. Still, most women who have a low MSAFP will not have children with Down syndrome. The efficacy of screening can be improved by adding estriol and hCG, in which case the hCG tends to be higher and the estriol tends to be lower than normal in mothers with Down syndrome fetuses. This is the so-called triple screen and is performed between 16 and 20 weeks' gestation. Amniotic fluid acetylcholinesterase is valuable for detecting NTDs but not for Down syndrome. Screening for Down syndrome can be performed in first trimester, when indicated, by chorionic villous sampling. In certain centers, first-

trimester detection of Down syndrome by ultrasound is being investigated.

488. **(E)** Information should be obtained on smoking, alcohol and drug abuse, and behavior that increases the risk of infection. Information given about these risks by the caregiver during pregnancy has a powerful effect on the actions of the pregnant woman. Smoking has been shown to decrease birth weight, probably due to multiple causes such as vasoconstriction, carbon monoxide, and decreased nutrition; alcohol abuse can lead to fetal alcohol syndrome with mental retardation or more subtle fetal alcohol effects with mild retardation and milder forms of other abnormalities. Drug abuse is of concern because of the effect of the specific drug and also the impurities and dilutents that are taken with them. Cocaine is a highly potent vasoconstrictor, leading to marked increase in blood pressure in both the mother and fetus, and has been associated with numerous congenital anomalies and premature delivery. Heroin and methadone have severe withdrawal symptoms in neonates, and also the methods by which drugs are obtained often exposes patients to STDs. Certain known teratogenic infections can be controlled by immunization, but use of live viral vaccines, such as rubella and measles and mumps, is contraindicated during pregnancy. If adequate antibody resistance is not present, avoidance of high-risk groups is the only protection. Patients should also avoid cat feces and eating undercooked meat because of the risk of toxoplasmosis. Prescribed drugs, which also must be considered as possible items of abuse, should not necessarily be discontinued during pregnancy. For example, the advisability of continuing psychiatric drugs for seizure disorders may depend on whether the benefits outweigh the risks and should be dealt with on an individual basis.

489. **(C)** Cerebral visual disturbances such as scotomata can occur in preeclamptic patients, and such women require further evaluation. The other listed choices are common nuisances related to the physiologic changes of pregnancy.

490. **(E)** Because of increased glomerular filtration rate (GFR), serum creatinine is usually low during pregnancy and creatinine clearance is increased. The increased GFR is also responsible for glucosuria in gravidas with normal glucose levels. The kidneys often excrete excess extracellular fluid after a period of recumbency, so the urine may not be concentrated after decreased oral intake of fluid, and urine is often the least concentrated in the morning. There is usually normal dilation of the collecting system on IVP during pregnancy.

491. **(E)** Pregnancy-induced hypertension and the aggravation of hypertension is more common in multiple gestations. The percentage of male fetuses in the human species *decreases* as the number of fetuses per pregnancy increases. The combination of hydramnios and breech presentation provides a good setup for cord prolapse. Because of separate placentas with interconnecting blood vessels, vasa previa becomes a greater possibility as well.

492. **(E)** Universal HIV testing with patient notification was recommended by the Institute of Medicine in an effort to reduce the rate of perinatal HIV transmission in the United States. In 1999, both the American College of Obstetricians and Gynecologists and the American Academy of Pediatrics supported the recommendation. The use of patient notification allows the woman to decline to be tested.

493. **(C)** Women over the age of 35 should be offered amniocentesis or MSAFP if they decline amniocentesis. However, these tests are done between 15 and 20 weeks' gestation. If serum alpha-fetoprotein is elevated, there is an increased possibility of open spinal cord abnormalities. If low, there is an increase in the likelihood of a trisomy. A 1-hour glucose challenge test is done routinely in the second trimester to predict gestational diabetes in otherwise asymptomatic women. A family

history to evaluate familial retardation or birth defects, as well as different ethnic origins, is important for screening purposes and needs to be done at the first visit to guide subsequent recommendations. A *Toxoplasma* titer is not beneficial as the incidence in the United States is very low, and the treatment is not good. It may be done in selected cases in a preconceptual testing program but as yet is not routine in the United States. Ultrasound at 8 weeks' gestation may be used to date a pregnancy if LMP is uncertain, but it need not be performed routinely.

494. **(E)** Omphalocele, diaphragmatic hernia, and duodenal atresia are associated approximately 50% of the time with other congenital anomalies. Gastroschisis, a defect in the anterior abdominal wall, is associated with other anomalies approximately 30% of the time. Other stenotic areas of the GI tract do not usually indicate chromosomal abnormalities. Posterior urethral valves may cause significant dilation of the urinary collecting system. It is amenable to surgical correction, because if one can stop the renal damage, the outcome is quite good.

495. **(B)** The biophysical profile (BPP) measures (1) amniotic fluid volume (requiring a fluid pocket of 12 cm), (2) the results of the NST, (3) an episode of fetal breathing that lasts at least 30 seconds, (4) three discrete limb movements of the fetus, and (5) at least one episode of extension with return to flexion by a fetal limb or trunk. Each of these factors is given two points. A normal score is 8 or 10, indicating fetal well-being. The advantage is that the BPP involves no fetal risk. It does require some expertise in ultrasound evaluation. Progressive perinatal mortality rate correlates with decreasing BPP score.

496. **(E)** Often, determination of pregnancy is a critical part of patient management. Traditionally, texts classify the findings associated with pregnancy according to whether they are presumptive, probable, or positive. Presumptive manifestations include amenorrhea, morning sickness, breast tenderness,

urinary frequency, and others. There is a likelihood that these symptoms may be present in the absence of pregnancy. Probable manifestations of pregnancy include various physical findings such as discoloration of the cervix (Chadwick's sign), softening of the lower uterine segment (Hegar's sign), abdominal enlargement, uterine enlargement, and others. These too may not be associated with a pregnancy. A positive pregnancy test may be associated with a pregnancy but also with certain endocrine neoplasms. Positive manifestations and the ones most reliable in diagnosing a pregnancy include the detection of fetal heart tones, palpation of a fetus, and diagnostic imaging techniques, the most practical and commonly used one being ultrasound. Ultrasound scanning either transabdominally or endovaginally may provide one of the earliest positive signs of pregnancy, being useful by the fifth or sixth week of gestation. A fetal sac, fetal pole, or cardiac movement can usually be seen by 5 or 6 weeks.

497. **(B)** Many authorities advise universal screening of pregnant women with a GTT because at least one third of women with gestational diabetes will be missed when only women who have risk factors for diabetes are screened. Many physicians would check the GTT again in the early to mid third trimester as the increased placental lactogen and the stresses of the pregnancy can cause a significant change and the GTT was so close to being abnormal. The screening test in this patient is positive, and therefore a 3-hour test is indicated. The diagnosis of gestational diabetes is made when two of the four values exceed normal criteria. Since perinatal mortality is not changed in patients diagnosed with gestational diabetes, it would appear that the value of diagnosing the condition has to do with the development of overt diabetes in more than half the women in the ensuing 20 years. There is also mounting evidence of long-range complications that include obesity and diabetes in the offspring of patients diagnosed as having gestational diabetes. The test is negative now, there is no

need to begin insulin, and oral hypoglycemics are contraindicated in pregnancy. A CST, without other concerns, is not necessary.

498. **(A)** Leopold's maneuvers are used to assess fetal lie, presentation, and engagement by palpation of the gravid abdomen. They are not intended as a means to diagnose twins. Auscultation of two fetal heart beats may help in diagnosing twins, but the diagnosis may be uncertain and is generally confirmed by ultrasound. The three radiologic methods listed can all diagnose twins, but the use of ultrasound can reliably make the diagnosis early and safely in pregnancy.

499. **(E)** Thus far, no fetal or maternal damage caused by ultrasound has been reported. For dating pregnancy, determining placental location, and finding anomalies, older, less sophisticated techniques cannot compete with it.

500. **(E)** Fetal heart rate tracings are a common method for assessing fetal well-being. Nonstress testing is done by recording fetal heart rates during a 20-minute period. The test requires at least two accelerations of the fetal heart rate of at least 15 beats and lasting for at least 15 seconds. A reactive tracing demonstrates both short-term (instantaneous change in heart rate from one heartbeat to the next), and long-term (changes occurring in the course of 1 minute in a cycle of three to five waves per minute) variability. With a reactive NST, the probability of fetal demise is less than 3 per 1,000 within the next week. Reactivity, such as seen in the tracing in Figure 8–1, is unlikely during a fetal sleep cycle. If a reactive pattern is not seen within the first 20 minutes, attempts to stimulate the fetus may be done because a nonreactive pattern is often due to a sleep cycle and will become reactive within the following 20 minutes.

501. **(D)** An advantage of the NST is that it can be done in situations in which labor itself might be contraindicated (such as prior classical cesarean section), because it does not involve the risk of uterine stimulation. Frequently, a fetus that has had a nonreactive positive CST will tolerate labor. Labor may be initiated with close fetal monitoring, particularly if the cervix is favorable. CST is a better predictor of fetal demise within a week of test than is NST. One per thousand infants die in the week following a negative CST versus 3/1,000 dying within a week of a normal NST.

502. **(C)** As iron is absorbed primarily in the proximal jejunum, iron preparations that do not release their elemental iron during the time they are in transit through the proximal jejunum do not provide much iron for absorption. Some preparations may not have as many side effects because they do not provide much usable iron. Constipation may be the most common complaint during iron supplementation.

503. **(B)** The early determination of the gestational age allows informed decision making if any pregnancy complication demands treatment that depends on knowledge of the gestational age. Although it is true that all of the evaluations listed are important, the accurate assessment and recording of gestational age is generally deemed most important in otherwise clinically normal pregnancies.

504. **(D)** In a randomized prospective trial of women with a previously affected child, the recurrence risk of NTDs was lowered by 72% in women taking 4 mg of folic acid daily. For women without a previously affected child, the recommended amount is 0.8 mg daily immediately prior to conception and during the early weeks of neural tube closure.

505. **(C)** The use of 4 mg of folic acid per day for 1 month before and during the first 3 months of gestation has been shown to reduce the recurrence risk of NTDs among women with previously affected children. Currently, the

Centers for Disease Control and Prevention recommends this level of folic acid supplementation for women with such history. Also recommended is that all fertile women of childbearing age consume at least 0.4 mg of folic acid daily.

506. **(E)** Contraception that prevents pregnancy is not pregnancy wastage. Abortion, which is the termination of pregnancy before the period of viability, exceeds all other causes of loss of pregnancy. Over 1 million voluntary abortions are performed yearly in the United States, accounting for the loss of 25% of all pregnancies.

507. **(B)** Diuretics are rarely indicated in pregnancy. A well-balanced, protein-rich diet with adequate rest in a lateral recumbent position is better treatment for edema than diuretics. Rapid weight gain secondary to fluid retention may be a sign of impending preeclampsia.

508. **(D)** Overweight women should limit weight gain to 15 to 25 lb in pregnancy. Most weight gain occurs in the second half of pregnancy. Folic acid requirements are increased during pregnancy, and an individual with this dietary history is apt to be severely deficient in folic acid as well as having deficiencies of iron, protein, and many other nutrients. She needs 70 g of protein a day, plus other nutrients. Her diet should be supplemented in any area of deficiency: calories, constituents, or minerals. While aerobic exercise is recommended and would be of benefit to her, it is inadvisable to initiate a vigorous program in a previously sedentary woman during pregnancy.

509. **(E)** The endocervical crypts enlarge during pregnancy and form increased mucus. Pregnancy does not confer any protection against the common causes of vaginitis, which should be evaluated. Treatment should be given as necessary. The presence of a sexually transmitted vaginal infection during pregnancy requires an inquiry into sexual activity and possible risk-taking behaviors. Bacterial vaginosis has been associated with preterm delivery in some populations. The diagnosis is made by microscopic examination of vaginal discharge for clue cells and the lack of lactobacilli, determination of vaginal pH, and "whiff test." Treatment with either clindamycin in early pregnancy or metronidazole later is recommended.

510. **(B)** Fetal heart tones can be documented by 12 weeks' gestation by Doppler devices. Before 12 to 14 weeks' gestation, uterine size can give a fairly accurate estimate of gestational age. At about 12 weeks' gestation the uterus has reached the pubic symphysis.

511. **(B)** Prior preterm delivery is the single most significant risk factor associated with preterm birth. Preterm birth is also associated with smoking, but the association is not as strong. Other risk factors include maternal genital tract infection, reduced cervical competence, low socioeconomic status, and uterine malformations. Colposcopy alone would not increase a woman's risk for cervical incompetence, but depending on the amount of tissue removed, cervical conization may. First-trimester spontaneous abortion is common, and it is not associated with preterm delivery in subsequent pregnancies.

512. **(B)** Minimal protein loss of 100 to 300 mg/24 hours is normal in nonpregnant women and in pregnancy. Fetal heart tones are not consistently audible by Doppler until about 12 weeks' gestation. Candidiasis, a common cause of vaginitis, is common in pregnancy and can safely be treated with topical agents. Short stature in itself does not portend a poor prognosis for pregnancy. Gravidas with chronic hypertension (BP > 140/90 before 20 weeks' gestation), however, are more likely to develop superimposed preeclampsia, one of the leading causes of maternal morbidity and mortality.

513. **(B)** Ultrasound measurement of crown-to-rump length in the first trimester will provide accurate estimation of gestational age to within a few days. Because of variation in

growth among fetuses, ultrasound is much less accurate for dating pregnancies beyond the second trimester. In women with normal cycles, conception should occur approximately 2 weeks after LMP. At 4 weeks, the conceptus is implanting within the uterus and is not yet visible by ultrasound.

514. **(D)** The best time to thoroughly evaluate fetal anatomy is between 16 and 20 weeks' gestation. Often, a complete evaluation of the fetal heart is more easily accomplished a few weeks later in gestation.

515. **(A, B, D)** Dietary allowances for most substances increase during pregnancy, and a nutritious diet is of prime importance to the pregnant woman. Vitamin A, however, is not required in greater amounts in pregnancy since it is felt to be stored adequately. Extra sodium is not needed.

516. **(B, C, E, F, G)** Twin pregnancies are high-risk pregnancies, accounting for a disproportionately large share of adverse pregnancy outcomes. Twin (and higher-order) pregnancies carry a higher risk of preterm delivery, low birthweight, and perinatal death. Possibly because the placenta is quite large in multiple gestations, placenta previa is more common than in single pregnancies. Congenital anomalies are more common, as is pregnancy-induced hypertension.

517. **(A, C)** The diagnosis of preterm labor is made by the combination of persistent uterine contractions in the face of cervical change—dilation and/or effacement—by digital examination. Therefore, either palpation of regular contractions or observing them on the tocodynamometer during an NST, and a cervical examination are required to establish the diagnosis. It is noted, however, that the accuracy of this diagnosis is poor, with a large number of false-positive diagnoses.

518. **(B, D)** There is evidence that periconceptional folic acid supplementation decreases the risk of recurrence of NTDs. Periconceptional glycemic control in diabetic women

has been shown to decrease the risk of congenital malformations in their offspring.

519. **(B, C)** For the average woman, a weight gain of 25 to 35 lb is optimal in pregnancy. Moderate exercise should be encouraged in the normal pregnancy, but fatigue should be avoided. Iron supplementation is recommended to improve iron stores. Jacuzzi hot tub baths are advised against, particularly in the first trimester because of the potential teratogenic effect of increased maternal core temperature. Douching is not recommended for the pregnant or nonpregnant woman.

520–523. **(520-D, 521-A, 522-B, 523-C)** The sperm and egg join to form a zygote, which then divides to form blastomeres. These first make up a morula and then a blastocyst with a central cavity. The blastocyst will implant in the uterus 5 to 7 days after ovulation. The inner cell mass (embryonic cell mass) from which an embryo develops is next to form, and all major organ systems will develop in the next 7 weeks. This is the time of greatest teratogenic risk, except for radiation, which is more dangerous to the brain at 8 to 15 weeks, when it can cause microcephaly and mental retardation. The fetal period begins at 8 weeks after conception or 10 weeks after the onset of the LMP. It consists of the maturation and growth of structure formed when an embryo. An infant is defined as an individual from the time of live birth to 1 year.

524–527. **(524-C, 525-B, 526-D, 527-A)** Tay–Sachs is a recessive disorder resulting from a deficiency in hexosaminidase A. It can be detected by measuring the amount of hexosaminidase A activity in blood. The carrier state is quite common in Ashkenazi Jews. Thalassemia is due to a genetic lack causing the defect in alpha or beta globulin chains. In both cases, different types of hemoglobin exist, which can be determined by electrophoresis, which should be done in the case of microcytic anemias with high iron levels. Cystic fibrosis is the most common autosomal recessive disorder in the Caucasian population. It is caused by several different mutations, the most common of which is called Delta F 508, which alone accounts for 75% of the mutations occurring in Caucasians. Several other common mutations are checked for, and these, along with the Delta F 508, will cause approximately 85% of the carrier individuals. The NTDs can be detected by acetylcholinesterase in the amniotic fluid. This test is particularly valuable in patients whose amniotic fluid alpha-fetoprotein level is elevated due to fetal blood contamination in the amniotic fluid. Glycosylated hemoglobin allows an assessment of blood glucose control over a long period of time.

528–532. (528-D, 529-B, 530-B, 531-C, 532-E) Bilateral renal agenesis will result in severe oligohydramnios because of no urine production. The infant develops pulmonary hypoplasia and atypical facies and has frequent cardiac anomalies. This is Potter syndrome. The banana sign is found frequently in infants with open spina bifida. It is due to a flattening of the cerebral hemispheres with an obliteration of the cisterna magna, which results in a centrally curved banana-like appearance on ultrasound. The lemon sign is also associated with NTDs and may occur with spina bifida. It is a scalloping of the frontal bones to give a lemon-shaped appearance of the head and usually disappears after 24 weeks. One should be suspicious of an open spina bifida if there is a small head, lemon and banana signs, enlarged ventricles, and absence or obliteration of the cisterna magna. The double bubble sign is found with duodenal atresia. Homozygous alpha-thalassemia results in the formation of tetramers of beta chains known as Bart's hemoglobin. This hemoglobinopathy can result in hydrops fetalis.

533. (G) For any drug to be prescribed during pregnancy, its benefits must outweigh its risks. According to the Food and Drug Administration classification, fluoxetine is Category B; that is, animal studies show no fetal risks, but human studies have not been done. While not teratogenic, several neonatal effects have been reported, including difficulty in environmental adaptation.

534. (F) Podophyllin resin, a common treatment for condyloma acuminata, has been associated with stillbirth. It causes local vascular spasm, ischemia, and necrosis of tissue. During pregnancy the lesions are profuse and vascular, predisposing to systemic absorption. This is a Category X drug.

535. (G) Ofloxacin is a Category C; that is, there are no adequate studies either animal or human, or there are adverse effects in animals but no data on humans. This drug is especialy useful in treating urinary tract infections. Use in immature animals has been associated with an arthropathy. The use of quinolones is not recommended in children and adolescents.

536. (G) Captopril is an angiotensin-converting enzyme (ACE) inhibitor. ACE inhibitors are Category C/D. Category D means that fetal risk has been identified, but use in pregnancy may be indicated if benefits outweigh the risks. Its use in pregnancy has been associated with severe oligohydramnios, pulmonary hypoplasia, and neonatal anemia. In general, there is reduction in uteroplacental perfusion, which can be fatal. Patients who use this drug and then become pregnant must seek alternative antihypertensive medications.

537. (C) Valproic acid, a drug used in the treatment of seizure disorders, has been associated with a 1 to 2% risk of spina bifida. It is Category C/D.

538. (A) Isotretinoin (Accutane) is a vitamin A isomer marketed for treatment of severe cystic acne. It is a Category X drug. Use of this drug in pregnancy poses a significant risk of both structural anomalies and mental retardation. Malformed infants have a characteristic pattern of craniofacial, cardiac, thymic, and central nervous system (CNS) anomalies.

539. (D) Methimazole is used for treatment of hyperthyroidism. A small number of cases of unusual scalp defects, aplasia cutis, have occurred in infants born to mothers taking the

drug. Like propylthiouracil, it is a Category D drug.

540. **(E)** Misoprostol is a synthetic prostaglandin E_1 that induces uterine contractions. In obstetrics, it is effective in ripening the cervix for labor induction. In the first trimester, it is used in conjunction with mifepristone or methotrexate to produce a medical abortion.

CHAPTER 9
Diseases Complicating Pregnancy
Questions

DIRECTIONS (Questions 541 through 628): Each of the numbered items or incomplete statements in this section is followed by answers or by completions of the statement. Select the ONE lettered answer or completion that is BEST in each case.

541. After convulsions are controlled in an eclamptic patient, the therapy should be aimed at

(A) reducing edema with diuretics
(B) giving hypotensive agents until the blood pressure is 110/70
(C) giving 3 g of magnesium sulfate every 3 hours
(D) obtaining a term infant
(E) keeping the patient free of convulsions, coma, and acidosis

542. The most common warning sign of pre-eclampsia is

(A) proteinuria
(B) headache
(C) edema
(D) increased blood pressure
(E) epigastric pain

543. Of the following, the most common cause of death from eclampsia is

(A) infection
(B) uremia
(C) congestive heart failure
(D) fever
(E) cerebral hemorrhage

544. Severely preeclamptic patients have a decrease in

(A) response to pressor amines
(B) plasma volume
(C) total body sodium
(D) uric acid
(E) serum liver functions

545. The renal lesion most associated with eclampsia is

(A) glomerular endothelial swelling
(B) pyelonephritis
(C) hydroureter
(D) cortical necrosis
(E) acute tubular necrosis

546. You are seeing a 19-year-old woman (gravida 1, para 0) in the third trimester of pregnancy in the emergency room. While being examined, she has a convulsion. You should

(A) obtain neurologic consultation
(B) perform an emergency cesarean delivery
(C) give intravenous (IV) phenytoin
(D) protect the patient from self-harm
(E) obtain a chest film

547. Which of the following is characteristic of magnesium sulfate ($MgSO_4$) used in the treatment of toxemia?

(A) excreted via the kidney
(B) smooth-muscle constrictor
(C) narrow margin of safety
(D) central nervous system (CNS) stimulant
(E) does not cross the placenta

548. In eclampsia there are several unfavorable prognostic signs. They include

(A) absence of edema
(B) 2+ proteinuria
(C) urine output greater than 100 cc/hr
(D) more than one but less than three convulsions
(E) swelling of the tongue

549. In preeclampsia, lesions may be found in the

(A) brain
(B) kidney
(C) heart
(D) lungs
(E) all of the above

550. Eye findings observed in preeclampsia include

(A) exudates and hemorrhage
(B) loss of corneal curvature
(C) retinal edema
(D) arteriolar dilation
(E) macular degeneration

551. A 24-year-old gravida 1, para 0 at 37 weeks' gestation was noted to have a 6-lb weight gain and an increase in blood pressure from 100/60 to 130/80 in the past week. She also has 1+ proteinuria. The examination was repeated 6 hours later and the same results were obtained. The best diagnosis is

(A) normal pregnancy
(B) preeclampsia
(C) eclampsia
(D) pregnancy-induced hypertension
(E) transient hypertension of pregnancy

552. The perinatal mortality rate in eclampsia is about

(A) 1%
(B) 5%
(C) 15%
(D) 30%
(E) 45%

553. The treatment for preeclampsia is

(A) magnesium sulfate
(B) delivery
(C) an antihypertensive drug
(D) renal dialysis
(E) bed rest

554. According to the New York Heart Association classification, a patient with cardiac disease and slight limitation of physical activity would be

(A) class 0
(B) class I
(C) class II
(D) class III
(E) class IV

555. Which of the following accounts for most heart disease in pregnancy?

(A) rheumatic fever
(B) previous myocardial infarction
(C) hypertension
(D) thyroid disease
(E) congenital heart disease (CHD)

556. Which of the following congenital heart defects is the most common?

(A) ventricular septal defect (VSD)
(B) patent ductus arteriosus
(C) pulmonary stenosis
(D) atrial septal defect (ASD)
(E) aortic stenosis

557. The diagnosis of valvular heart disease in pregnancy may be made when there is

(A) a history of rheumatic fever
(B) arrhythmia
(C) a diastolic murmur
(D) a soft systolic murmur along the left sternal border (LSB)
(E) an S_4

558. Occasionally, a patient with a cardiac valvar prosthesis will become pregnant. During the pregnancy, she should be

(A) evaluated for valve replacement due to cardiac enlargement

(B) anticoagulated with dicumarol

(C) anticoagulated with dextran

(D) anticoagulated with heparin

(E) kept on low-dose oral antibiotics

559. If heart disease is severe enough to cause cyanosis and polycythemia of greater than 65%, the fetal outcome of pregnancy is usually

(A) not affected

(B) marked prematurity

(C) intrauterine growth retardation

(D) abortion or fetal death

(E) postmaturity

560. A pregnant patient has a history of insulin-dependent diabetes for 14 years. In the absence of other findings, which would be the diabetic class according to White's classification?

(A) A

(B) B

(C) C

(D) D

(E) E

561. If the patient in question 560 were found to have diabetic nephropathy, she would be a class

(A) C

(B) D

(C) E

(D) F

(E) R

562. A 33-year-old Type 1 diabetic patient (gravida 1, para 9) is scheduled for induction of labor at 37 weeks' gestation. Her insulin dosage should be

(A) maintained at her preinduction level

(B) increased by 10 to 15%

(C) decreased by half

(D) put on a sliding scale with q3–4h blood glucose measurements

(E) put on an IV insulin infusion

563. Which of the following histories might lead you to suspect the existence of diabetes in a patient now pregnant for the third time?

(A) Spontaneous rupture of the membranes occurred during the second trimester in both preceding pregnancies.

(B) Jaundice appeared in the last trimester of her second pregnancy.

(C) Both preceding infants were premature.

(D) Unexplained intrauterine death occurred at 38 weeks' gestation in her last pregnancy.

(E) Abruptio placentae occurred in the second pregnancy.

564. Generally, anemia can best be defined as

(A) lack of iron stores

(B) a genetic defect

(C) deficiency of folic acid

(D) a hemoglobin below 11 g/dL

(E) low blood volume

565. The most common type of anemia in pregnancy is due to

(A) iron deficiency

(B) sickle cell disease

(C) folate deficiency

(D) hemolytic disease

(E) vitamin B_{12} deficiency

566. Folic acid deficiency results in

(A) microcytic anemia

(B) megaloblastic anemia

(C) aplastic anemia

(D) glucose-6-phosphate dehydrogenase (G6PD) deficiency

(E) white blood cell (WBC) stippling

567. Microcytic hypochromic anemia may be due to

(A) folate deficiency

(B) vitamin B_{12} deficiency

(C) thalassemia

(D) vitamin B_6 deficiency

(E) acute blood loss

568. Sickle cell disease is found in approximately what percentage of African-Americans?

(A) less than 1%

(B) 5%

(C) 10%

(D) 25%

(E) 50%

569. If one parent has sickle cell disease and the other has the trait, what proportion of their children will have the disease?

(A) 0%

(B) 25%

(C) 50%

(D) 75%

(E) 100%

570. G6PD homozygous deficiency is present in what percentage of African-American women?

(A) less than 1%

(B) 2%

(C) 5%

(D) 10%

(E) 33%

Questions 571 and 572

A 22-year-old patient presents with a hematocrit of 31% at 28 weeks' gestation. Her mean corpuscular volume (MCV) is 105, her mean corpuscular hemoglobin (MCH) is 33, and her mean corpuscular hemoglobin concentration (MCHC) is 36. Serum iron is 100 mg/dL. There is no evidence of abnormal bleeding.

571. The most appropriate diagnosis is

(A) normocytic, normochromic anemia

(B) normal

(C) macrocytic anemia

(D) microcytic anemia

(E) hemolysis

572. The most likely cause of the anemia in the patient in question 571 is

(A) gastrointestinal (GI) bleeding

(B) G6PD deficiency

(C) iron deficiency

(D) folic acid deficiency

(E) pernicious anemia

573. You are seeing a 28-year-old woman (gravida 3, para 2) with suspected urinary tract infection (UTI). To obtain a urine specimen, you should order

(A) clean-void midstream urine

(B) catheterization

(C) suprapubic tap

(D) 24-hour urine

(E) first morning void

574. A pregnant patient at 16 weeks' gestation has normal blood pressure, proteinuria (4 g/day), serum albumin of 2.0 g/dL, creatinine 0.8 mg/dL, and peripheral edema. Which of the following diagnoses is most appropriate?

(A) glomerulonephritis

(B) pregnancy-induced hypertension

(C) nephrotic syndrome

(D) polycystic kidney disease

(E) chronic renal failure

575. A pyelogram taken during the eighth month of gestation would normally reveal

(A) a nonfunctioning right kidney

(B) the same findings as those of a normal, nonpregnant woman

(C) hydroureter bilaterally

(D) occlusion of the ureters bilaterally

(E) nephroptosis

576. Proper treatment for the hydroureter of pregnancy is

(A) bladder catheterization

(B) ureteral catheterization

(C) bed rest

(D) increased fluid intake

(E) no treatment

Questions 577 and 578

A 21-year-old patient, gravida 1, is seen for the first time when 16 weeks' pregnant. History and examination are entirely normal except for a large solid mass in the posterior pelvis. It is slightly lobulated, immobile, and smooth and cannot be completely palpated. There is some question as to whether or not it will obstruct labor.

577. Which of the following procedures should be carried out?

(A) "one shot" intravenous pyelogram (IVP)

(B) barium enema

(C) exploratory laparotomy

(D) abortion

(E) ultrasound

578. Of the following, the most likely possibility is

(A) anterior meningomyelocele

(B) pelvic kidney

(C) carcinoma of the bowel

(D) sacculated uterus

(E) idiopathic retroperitoneal fibrosis

Questions 579 and 580

A 34-year-old gravida 3, para 2 at 35 weeks' gestation complains of sharp, excruciating pain in the right flank radiating into her groin. No chills or fever have been noted. The pain resolved shortly after the patient was seen. Urinary analysis reveals numerous red blood cells (RBCs), some WBCs, and no bacteria. WBC and hematocrit are normal.

579. Of the following options, the most likely diagnosis is

(A) appendicitis

(B) pyelonephritis

(C) round ligament pain

(D) ureteral lithiasis

(E) Meckel's diverticulum

580. Which of the following laboratory tests should be performed?

(A) serum iron

(B) serum glutamic oxaloacetic transaminase (SGOT)

(C) tine test

(D) bilirubin

(E) serum calcium

581. Ureteral stones during pregnancy are rare. Which of the following is true?

(A) They are more likely to produce pain during pregnancy than in the nonpregnant state.

(B) They are usually discovered during workup for vague abdominal pain.

(C) They are associated with hyperparathyroidism.

(D) They are frequently a cause of acute obstruction.

(E) A prophylactic ureteral filter may need to be placed.

582. A 14-year-old girl is seen for her first prenatal visit at 34 weeks' gestation by menstrual history. On examination her BP is 135/85 and her fundus measures 33 cm. Her urine dipstick is 1+ positive for protein. The most likely diagnosis is

(A) hypertensive disease with superimposed preeclampsia

(B) mild eclampsia

(C) third-trimester pregnancy

(D) preeclampsia

(E) chronic hypertension

583. If the patient has hyperparathyroidism, the infant may be at increased risk for postpartum

(A) hyaline membrane disease
(B) tetany
(C) coma
(D) hyperglycemia
(E) malabsorption syndrome

584. A healthy mother delivers a term infant with microcephaly. The mother's urine was found to contain cells with inclusion bodies. The most likely diagnosis is

(A) chromosomal abnormality
(B) cytomegalovirus disease
(C) syphilis
(D) poliomyelitis
(E) granuloma inguinale

585. A patient is seen in the early third trimester of pregnancy with acute onset of chills and fever, nausea, and backache. Her temperature is 102° F. The urinary sediment reveals many bacteria and WBCs. Which of the following is the most likely diagnosis?

(A) acute appendicitis
(B) ruptured uterus
(C) pyelonephritis
(D) abruptio placentae
(E) labor

586. Toxoplasmosis is transmitted to the infant by

(A) ascending passage of a virus
(B) delivery through the infected tissue
(C) transplacental passage of the protozoa
(D) sexual intercourse by the mother during pregnancy
(E) hematogenesis spread of the bacteria

587. A disease that may be reactivated during pregnancy after being dormant for years is

(A) infectious hepatitis
(B) syphilis
(C) tuberculosis (TB)

(D) poliomyelitis
(E) Huntington's chorea

588. The most common reportable bacterial sexually transmitted disease (STD) in women is

(A) gonorrhea
(B) syphilis
(C) chlamydia
(D) herpes
(E) chancroid

589. An asymptomatic pregnant woman consults you because she has been sexually exposed to a man with gonorrhea. You should

(A) reassure her and await symptoms
(B) culture her endocervix and treat on the basis of a positive culture
(C) treat when she is past 12 weeks' (the first trimester) pregnant
(D) treat her with 2.4 million units of oral penicillin over 10 days
(E) treat her with ceftriaxone 250 mg IM

590. The major complication of maternal gonorrhea in the third trimester is

(A) gonorrheal ophthalmia of the newborn
(B) gonococcal arthritis
(C) miscarriage in subsequent pregnancies
(D) infection of the patient's sexual partner
(E) tubo-ovarian abscess

Questions 591 through 593

A 24-year-old married white woman was exposed to rubella at 7 to 8 weeks' gestation. Several days later she developed a red macular rash and had a rubella antibody titer of 1:160 when seen by you at 11 weeks' gestation.

591. What is the approximate risk of the fetus having serious congenital abnormalities?

(A) 0%
(B) 1 to 24%
(C) 25 to 50%
(D) 50 to 75%
(E) 100%

592. Which of the following may be anticipated in an infant born to this mother?

   (A) rhagades
   (B) hepatosplenomegaly
   (C) trisomy 21
   (D) Hutchinson's incisors
   (E) cri du chat syndrome

593. The mother refused therapeutic abortion and under caudal anesthesia delivered a fetus with a marked purpuric rash. This was most likely due to

   (A) the classic skin lesions of rubella in the newborn
   (B) marked thrombocytopenia
   (C) placental heparinase
   (D) an allergic reaction to the anesthetic agent
   (E) a cause unrelated to the rubella

Questions 594 through 598

A 24-year-old patient now 17 weeks' pregnant is found to have a positive VDRL (Venereal Disease Research Laboratory) of 1:16 titer. She gives no past history of syphilis. A fluorescent treponemal antibody test (FTA) is drawn but will require 1 to 2 weeks to be returned. Cerebrospinal fluid (CSF) tests are negative. The patient denies allergies.

594. Serologic tests for syphilis will usually first be positive in which of the following periods of time after contact with the disease?

   (A) 1 to 2 days
   (B) 6 to 8 hours
   (C) 18 to 20 days
   (D) 4 to 6 weeks
   (E) 4 to 6 months

595. Of the following, the most appropriate course of action is to

   (A) wait until the FTA results are known
   (B) treat with 4.8 million units of procaine penicillin
   (C) treat with 2.4 million units of benzathine penicillin IM
   (D) treat with 3.5 g of ampicillin PO
   (E) redraw the VDRL

596. After adequate treatment, the maternal VDRL titer slowly decreases but is still positive. At the time of delivery, the fetus appears normal but the cord VDRL is also positive. Which of the following is the most likely explanation?

   (A) The baby has a biologic false positive.
   (B) The baby has congenital syphilis.
   (C) The baby has levels of maternal antibody.
   (D) The baby has been treated but its antibody level is still elevated.
   (E) The mother was treated but the baby was not and has reinfected the mother.

597. To distinguish whether or not the infant is infected, you should

   (A) do skin biopsies
   (B) do serial VDRLs
   (C) do serial Frei tests
   (D) perform darkfield examinations
   (E) do an x-ray of long bones

598. Which of the following is recommended as treatment for early syphilis diagnosed by a positive VDRL, and FTA-ABS during pregnancy?

   (A) 4.8 million units procaine penicillin IM stat
   (B) 4.8 million units procaine penicillin IM stat with probenecid
   (C) 2.4 million units benzathine penicillin IM stat
   (D) 1.2 million units procaine penicillin IM stat
   (E) 600,000 units benzathine penicillin IM

599. Which of the following is most likely to be born to a woman with Graves' disease that is currently under control?

(A) hypothyroid infant

(B) mongoloid infant

(C) hyperthyroid infant

(D) infertile infant

(E) infant with ambiguous genitalia

Questions 600 and 601

An agitated patient is seen during the first trimester of pregnancy with an enlarged thyroid, a BP of 110/70, a resting pulse of 110, and an increased RBC uptake of triiodothyronine T_3.

600. You should

(A) measure thyroid-stimulating hormone (TSH)

(B) obtain an iodine 131 (I^{131}) uptake by the thyroid

(C) obtain a basal metabolic rate (BMR)

(D) evaluate free thyroxine (T_4)

(E) evaluate thyroid-binding globulin

601. Among other tests, the free thyroxine is elevated. Your initial treatment should be

(A) treat with I^{131}

(B) give propylthiouracil (PTU)

(C) give PTU and propranalol

(D) give PTU and low-dose thyroid hormone

(E) advise subtotal thyroidectomy in the second trimester

602. A 35-year-old patient at 31 weeks' gestation complains of a firm lump in her left breast. On examination, a $2 \times 3 \times 3$-cm firm nodule surrounded by some erythema is discovered in the upper outer quadrant. There is no skin retraction, and the nodule is somewhat mobile. The most appropriate plan of management is

(A) to reassure the patient, see her regularly, and evaluate the mass at 6 weeks' postpartum

(B) mastectomy

(C) hot packs on the breast and antibiotics for mastitis

(D) mammogram

(E) biopsy

603. The combined incidence of carcinoma (both invasive and in situ) of the cervix in pregnancy is

(A) less than 0.5%

(B) 1%

(C) 2 to 3%

(D) 5 to 6%

(E) 8 to 10%

604. During pregnancy, Pap smears are

(A) contraindicated in the third trimester

(B) consistently overread and to be judged with caution

(C) normally return as atypical or ASCUS

(D) of poor diagnostic importance

(E) part of the normal workup

605. A pregnancy luteoma is generally

(A) easily differentiated from a hilus cell tumor

(B) not a part of the corpus luteum of pregnancy

(C) made up of small basophilic cells

(D) cystic

(E) malignant

606. A patient 8 weeks' pregnant is found to have Stage III carcinoma of the cervix. In regard to the malignancy, the best treatment would be to

(A) deliver by cesarean section at 34 weeks and irradiate

(B) deliver vaginally at term and irradiate

(C) perform hysterotomy now and irradiate

(D) perform radical hysterectomy and pelvic lymphadenectomy now

(E) irradiate now

607. Which of the following diseases in pregnancy has the highest maternal mortality rate when it occurs?

(A) diabetes insipidus

(B) gestational diabetes

(C) pheochromocytoma

(D) syphilis

(E) obesity

Questions 608 through 610

A 17-year-old single female (gravida 1, para 0), last menstrual period (LMP) 32 weeks ago, menstrual formula (MF) 12/28/4–5, with occasional cramps and no history of contraception, comes for her first OB clinic visit and routine care.

History: The patient admits to a 40-lb weight gain during pregnancy with ankle swelling for the past 4 weeks. Rings on her fingers are tight. Otherwise, she feels well. She has been staying with a cousin who is on welfare. She has had no prior prenatal care and no iron or vitamin supplementation.

Past history: Noncontributory except for appendectomy, age 14. Generally in good health.

Social history: High school dropout; parents divorced.

Family history: No history of renal disease, diabetes, cancer, hypertension, congenital anomalies, or twins.

Physical findings: BP 135/85; P 84; T 37; R 20. HEENT: Fundi not examined.

Neck: Thyroid 1–1½ times enlarged; chest: clear; breasts: full, slightly tender; heart: grade 11/VI, systolic murmur at LSB.

Abdomen: Uterus measures 42 cm, fetal heart tones (FHTs) 136 and 156 taken simultaneously; extremities: 2+ edema, 3+ reflexes. Brief ultrasound confirms twins in breech, breech presentation.

Pelvis: Normal measurements; cervix: one-half effaced, soft, and not dilated. Station +1. The above findings were all confirmed 6 hours later.

Laboratory tests: UA: color cloudy yellow; specific gravity 1.013; protein 2+; RBCs rare; WBC 2 to 5; bac. 0; WBC: 9,800; Rh, VDRL, rubella titer, and Pap smear were obtained but not yet returned.

608. Which of the following complications would you expect to be found with increased frequency in a patient such as this?

(A) abruption

(B) accreta

(C) acute fatty necrosis of the liver

(D) abortion

(E) Crohn's disease

609. Given the history, you would expect which of the following laboratory findings?

(A) chest x-ray to show decreased pulmonary vascular markings

(B) urine to show infection

(C) creatinine clearance to be increased above normal pregnancy levels

(D) serum uric acid to be increased

(E) a decreased hematocrit

610. Procedure(s) that may be helpful to clarify the diagnosis at this time include

(A) arteriograms

(B) dilation and curettage (D&C)

(C) x-ray with instillation of radiopaque material in the uterine cavity

(D) complete ultrasound examination

(E) serum quantitative pregnancy test

611. A missed abortion is the death of the fetus

(A) that the patient does not realize has occurred

(B) in which the products of conception are retained after the embryo or fetus has died

(C) in which the products of conception are partially expelled

(D) in which the products of conception cause bleeding and there is an open cervical os

(E) in which the products of conception are no longer recognizable

612. An unconscious obstetric patient is admitted to the emergency room in the eighth month of pregnancy with a BP of 60/20 and a pulse of 120. If there has been no vaginal bleeding, which diagnosis may be excluded?

(A) abruptio placentae

(B) placenta previa

(C) premature rupture of membranes with septic shock

(D) eclampsia

(E) amniotic fluid embolism

613. A 23-year-old patient, amenorrheic for 16 weeks, had vaginal spotting. She was found to have a uterus enlarged to 20 weeks' size and no FHTs audible with the Doppler or fetoscope. Human chorionic gonadotropin (hCG) serum levels were approximately 150 IU/mL. Which of the following tests is most appropriate at this time?

(A) human chorionic somatomammotropin (hCS)

(B) pelvic ultrasound

(C) serial hCGs

(D) Apt test on vaginal blood

(E) serial clotting function studies

614. Signs and symptoms that should alert you to the possibility of gestational trophoblastic disease include

(A) persistent titer of hCG after pregnancy

(B) hematuria

(C) weight loss

(D) persistent postpartum anovulation

(E) nocturnal fever

615. Gestational trophoblastic disease may occur

(A) after abortion

(B) spontaneously

(C) after hydatidiform mole

(D) after normal pregnancy

(E) all of the above

Questions 616 through 618

A 28-year-old woman noted loss of fetal motion at 36 weeks' gestation by dates. FHTs were not heard at 40 weeks by dates, when the patient was next seen. The uterus measured 30 cm from symphysis to fundus.

616. Amniocentesis would be likely to reveal

(A) a lithopedion

(B) Spaulding's sign

(C) thick, dark brown fluid

(D) fetal distress

(E) air

617. A valuable test to perform at this time would be

(A) maternal serum estriol

(B) clotting screen

(C) lecithin sphingomyelin (L/S) ratio

(D) karyotype of amniotic cells

(E) amniotic fluid creatinine

618. The most well-recognized maternal complication that may occur in this case is

(A) uterine rupture

(B) coagulation defect

(C) amniotic fluid embolus

(D) thrombophlebitis

(E) all of the above

619. If you found that a 25-year-old patient with amenorrhea of 18 weeks' duration had an elevated serum hCG, which of the following would be the most likely diagnosis?

(A) pregnancy

(B) hydatidiform mole

(C) choriocarcinoma

(D) endometriosis

(E) primary ovarian cancer

620. Massive hydramnios (> 3,000 mL) is associated with congenital malformation in what percentage of cases?

(A) less than 1%

(B) 5 to 10%

(C) 20 to 30%

(D) 50 to 60%

(E) 90 to 100%

621. Complications associated with hydramnios include

(A) maternal high blood pressure

(B) fetal urinary tract anomalies

(C) maternal diabetes

(D) postmature pregnancy

(E) all of the above

622. Hydramnios is characterized by

(A) a volume greater than 2,000 mL

(B) no increase in perinatal morbidity

(C) a lack of symptoms, depending on rapidity of onset

(D) marked increase in intrauterine pressure

(E) an increase in endometritis

Questions 623 and 624

A 23-year-old gravida 1 at about 12 weeks' gestation develops persistent nausea and vomiting that progresses from an occasional episode to a constant retching. She has no fever or diarrhea but loses 5 lb in 1 week and appears dehydrated.

623. Your diagnosis is

(A) anorexia nervosa

(B) morning sickness

(C) ptyalism

(D) hyperemesis gravidarum

(E) gastroenteritis

624. Among those listed below, the best therapy for this patient is

(A) phenothiazines

(B) hypnosis

(C) intravenous hydration

(D) psychiatric referral

(E) outpatient antiemetic therapy

625. A patient at 34 weeks' gestation develops marked pruritus and mildly elevated liver function tests. Among the diagnostic possibilities is

(A) pancreatitis

(B) hyperthyroidism

(C) diabetes insipidus

(D) cholestasis of pregnancy

(E) progesterone allergy

626. Under which of the following conditions are the pruritus and jaundice likely to recur?

(A) menopause

(B) after discontinuation of breast feeding

(C) poor diet

(D) another pregnancy

(E) with the use of antihypertensive medication

627. Which of the following histologic findings is present in cholestatic hepatosis?

(A) necrosis

(B) inflammation

(C) centrolobular bile staining

(D) extrahepatic cholestasis

(E) glomeruloendotheliosis

628. You are seeing a 25-year-old woman (gravida 1, para 0) with sickle cell disease at 12 weeks' gestation for her first prenatal visit. Suggestions for her care should include which of the following?

(A) folic acid

(B) transfusions of fresh hemoglobin for hematocrit less than 25%

(C) antibiotic prophylaxis to prevent urinary tract infection

(D) oral iron in double the usual dosage (650 mg tid)

(E) delivery at 36 weeks after documentation of fetal lung maturity

629. Magnesium sulfate is used in the treatment of eclampsia. Magnesium sulfate has which two of the following characteristics?

   (A) is metabolized by the liver
   (B) has vitamin K as an antidote
   (C) can cause convulsions if given in excess
   (D) can be given IM or IV
   (E) may cause respiratory arrest

630. Which four of the following cardiovascular conditions results in cyanosis?

   (A) VSD
   (B) patent ductus arteriosus
   (C) tetralogy of Fallot
   (D) Ebstein's anomaly
   (E) Marfan syndrome

631. Hypertensive patients are at increased risk during pregnancy. Changes that increase their risk include which three of the following?

   (A) poor renal function
   (B) cardiac hypertrophy
   (C) advanced retinal changes
   (D) short stature
   (E) low weight gain

632. Which two of the following items in a pregnant patient's history suggest the possibility of the patient's having diabetes?

   (A) jaundice in previous children
   (B) past history of twins
   (C) previous 9½-lb infant
   (D) diabetic husband
   (E) unexplained stillbirth

633. During pregnancy, blood tests for diabetes are more apt to be abnormal than in the nonpregnant state. This is due in part to which two of the following?

   (A) decreased insulin production
   (B) increased food absorption from the gastrointestinal (GI) tract
   (C) increased placental lactogen
   (D) estrogen increase
   (E) hemoconcentration

634. Signs of folic acid deficiency include which three of the following?

   (A) hypersegmentation of neutrophils
   (B) perioral blisters
   (C) thrombocytopenia
   (D) microcytes
   (E) anemia

635. Hemolytic anemia may be due to which of the following?

   (A) *Clostridium* exotoxin
   (B) medications
   (C) G6PD deficiency
   (D) preeclampsia
   (E) group B streptococcus colonization

636. Hemoglobin C trait has which two of the following characteristics?

   (A) an occurrence of the gene in about 1 in 50 of the black population in the United States
   (B) generally causes a severe anemia in the homozygous condition
   (C) when combined with hemoglobin S trait, it may cause significant problems in pregnancy
   (D) combination with hemoglobin S trait in the nonpregnant state results in greater morbidity than sickle cell disease
   (E) a diagnosis of exclusion

637. Which three of the following are associated with an increased risk of spontaneous embolism?

   (A) increased antithrombin III
   (B) decreased protein C
   (C) increased protein S

(D) Factor V Leiden

(E) lupus anticoagulant

638. Consumptive coagulopathy is a known complication of which of the following?

(A) abruptio placentae

(B) fetal death in utero

(C) acute cystitis

(D) amniotic fluid embolus

(E) postdates (> 42 weeks' gestation)

639. Anti-D immune globulin should be given for which three of the following situations?

(A) after an abortion occurring beyond 6 weeks' gestation in an Rh-negative female

(B) to an Rh-negative mother who has an Rh-positive baby

(C) to an Rh-negative female infant with an Rh-positive mother

(D) postpartum to Rh-positive females with Rh-negative husbands

(E) after a motor vehicle accident to an Rh-negative mother

640. The treatments of choice for folic acid deficiency anemia include which three of the following?

(A) folic acid

(B) iron

(C) vitamin B_{12}

(D) nutritional counseling

(E) vitamin K

641. A 24-year-old woman (gravida 3, para 0, abortus 2) comes to you for prenatal care. Her sister had a clot on the pill and was found to have Factor V Leiden. You tell her which three of the following?

(A) She has a 50% chance of having the disease.

(B) She may need low-dose aspirin during this pregnancy.

(C) She may need heparin during this pregnancy.

(D) You need to order Factor V levels.

(E) You need to order activated protein C resistance.

642. Predisposing factors in the development of pyelonephritis during pregnancy include which three of the following?

(A) asymptomatic bacteriuria

(B) high levels of progesterone

(C) small maternal stature (< 5 ft 2 in)

(D) increased blood flow

(E) expanding uterus

643. Lesions of the vulva that may be seen during pregnancy include which four of the following?

(A) varicosities

(B) condyloma acuminata

(C) condyloma lata

(D) Montgomery tubercles

(E) Bartholin gland cysts

Questions 644 and 645

A 44-year-old married white woman (gravida 4, para 3, abortus 0) has had amenorrhea for 4 months. She comes to you because of vaginal spotting over 4 days.

644. You should do which four of the following?

(A) obtain more history

(B) prescribe 10 mg of progesterone for 10 days

(C) perform a physical examination

(D) perform an ultrasound

(E) obtain laboratory tests

Further history reveals that the patient is married, sexually active, and her youngest child is 17 years old. She has been healthy with no history of high blood pressure. She would like to have a normal child. Examination is within normal limits except for a blood pressure of 140/90, slight bleeding from the cervix, and a uterus consistent with a 14- to 16-week gestation. No FHTs are heard with either the fetoscope or Doppler. Urine pregnancy test is positive.

645. Of the following diagnoses, in your differential you should include which four of the following?

(A) intrauterine gestation
(B) missed abortion
(C) hydatidiform mole
(D) uterine myomas
(E) ovarian cancer

646. A woman with class II cardiac disease is pregnant. Care should include which three of the following?

(A) adequate bed rest
(B) limiting weight gain to 20 to 25 lb
(C) avoidance of hypotension
(D) vaginal delivery if possible
(E) deliver with pulmonary maturity

647. Asthma is a chronic respiratory disease. In pregnancy it is associated with which three of the following?

(A) higher incidence of respiratory infection
(B) prematurity
(C) postdates
(D) higher incidence of preeclampsia
(E) chorioamnionitis

648. Dangers associated with acute pyelonephritis of pregnancy include which three of the following?

(A) gram-negative sepsis
(B) hepatitis
(C) tubo-ovarian abscess
(D) respiratory distress syndrome
(E) premature labor

649. A 34-year-old woman with long-standing systemic lupus erythematosus (SLE) is pregnant for the first time. You are seeing her at 10 weeks' gestation. Special testing will be required for her during pregnancy because of marginal renal function secondary to the severity of her disease. Which three of the following tests are indicated?

(A) serum blood urea nitrogen (BUN)
(B) serum calcium and phosphorus
(C) serum creatinine
(D) serum C3 and C4 levels
(E) C-reactive protein

650. A patient with cholestasis of pregnancy develops a slight hyperbilirubinemia and slight elevation of SGOT. Relief of the pruritus may be obtained by which two of the following?

(A) delivery
(B) bland diet
(C) oral H_2 blockers
(D) cholestyramine
(E) mild diuretic therapy

651. Which two of the following often are true regarding obstetric patients with nonendocrine obesity?

(A) They do not need vitamin supplements.
(B) They have adequate stores of body iron.
(C) They are malnourished.
(D) They need nutritional counseling.
(E) They are accepting of their weight.

652. The three most common causes of maternal mortality are

(A) hemorrhage
(B) congenital cardiac disease
(C) infection
(D) hypertension
(E) pulmonary embolism

653. The two most common causes of nonmaternal mortality are

(A) domestic violence
(B) amniotic fluid emboli
(C) motor vehicle accidents
(D) heart disease
(E) asthma

654. On her first prenatal visit, a 17-year-old single woman (gravida 1, para 0), 32 weeks by good dates, is found to have vital signs as follows: blood pressure 135/85, pulse 84, temperature 98.6° F, respiration 20. She also has ankle and hand edema and a uterine fundus measuring 42 cm with breech concordant twins on ultrasound. She has normal pelvic measurements and the cervix is closed and soft, with the presenting part at station −1. Her urinalysis revealed no WBCs or bacteria with 2+ protein. Her hematocrit is 38, and her white count is 9,800. The care of this patient over the first 6 to 8 hours should include which two of the following?

(A) evaluation of urine output and level of proteinuria
(B) hospitalization with bed rest and frequent vital signs
(C) oxytocin induction of labor
(D) antihypertensive drugs
(E) cesarean section because of the twins

DIRECTIONS (Questions 655 through 688): Each set of items in this section consists of a list of lettered headings followed by several numbered words or phrases. For each numbered word or phrase, select the ONE lettered option that is most closely associated with it. Each lettered option may be selected once, more than once, or not at all.

Questions 655 through 658

Match the following medications' effects during pregnancy with the appropriate medication.

(A) tetracycline
(B) nitrofurantoin
(C) sulfas
(D) streptomycin
(E) chloramphenicol

655. Is excreted after binding, utilizing glucuronyl transferase

656. May cause aplastic anemia in the neonate

657. Ototoxic

658. Discolors decidual teeth

Questions 659 through 661

(A) radiologic examinations
(B) ultrasonographic examinations
(C) both
(D) neither

659. Utilize ionizing radiation

660. Allow visualization of the chorionic plate

661. Are 100% accurate

Questions 662 through 666

Match the following causes of bleeding with the time of pregnancy during which they most commonly occur.

(A) first trimester
(B) second trimester
(C) third trimester
(D) immediately postpartum
(E) at any time during gestation

662. Spontaneous abortion

663. Carcinoma of the cervix

664. Placenta previa

665. Uterine atony

666. Hydatidiform mole

Questions 667 through 671

(A) mild preeclampsia
(B) severe preeclampsia
(C) chronic hypertensive disease
(D) eclampsia
(E) none of the above

667. A 30-year-old woman at 16 weeks' gestation with a BP of 144/95, no edema, no proteinuria, FHT 140

668. A 19-year-old woman at 36 weeks' gestation with a BP of 150/100, 2+ edema, and 2+ proteinuria with no other symptoms

669. A 21-year-old woman in early labor at 39 weeks' gestation who has just convulsed

670. A 16-year-old woman at 37 weeks' gestation with a BP of 145/105, 2+ proteinuria, and pulmonary edema

671. A 35-year-old woman (gravida 5, para 4), now at 32 weeks' gestation with a BP of 180/120, no proteinuria or edema, but retinal exudates and hemorrhage, as well as a history of hypertension for 8 years

Questions 672 through 678

(A) lymphogranuloma venereum
(B) chancroid
(C) granuloma inguinale
(D) *Neisseria*
(E) syphilis

672. Condylomata

673. Cutaneous induration and vulvar elephantiasis

674. Rectal strictures

675. *Haemophilus ducreyi*

676. Donovan bodies

677. Chlamydial disease

678. Monoarticular arthritis

Questions 679 through 684

Pregnant women may be affected by the same diseases that affect nonpregnant women. Match the following disease entities with the most applicable statement.

(A) SLE
(B) carcinoma of the breast
(C) herpes gestationis
(D) melanoma
(E) influenza

679. Is occasionally associated with nephritis and hypertension

680. May cross the placenta to cause fetal malignancy

681. May be mistaken for toxemia

682. A rare skin disorder characterized by erythema, vesicles, bullae, and pruritus

683. Appears to affect pregnant women much more severely than nonpregnant women

684. May be exacerbated in the postpartum period

Questions 685 through 688

(A) *Listeria monocytogenes*
(B) multiple sclerosis
(C) hiatal hernia
(D) polyostotic fibrous dysplasia (McCune–Albright syndrome)
(E) influenza

685. Associated with the occurrence of pregnancy in early childhood

686. Associated with fetal demise

687. Is often worse postpartum than antepartum

688. May be causally related to heartburn in pregnancy

DIRECTIONS (Questions 689 through 693): Each group of items in this section consists of lettered headings followed by a set of numbered words or phrases. For each numbered word or phrase, select

(A) if the item is associated with (A) only,
(B) if the item is associated with (B) only,
(C) if the item is associated with both (A) and (B),
(D) if the item is associated with neither (A) nor (B).

Questions 689 and 690

(A) type I pregnant diabetic women
(B) pregnant women with gestational diabetes

(C) both

(D) neither

689. Have an above-average incidence of hydramnios

690. Have an above-average incidence of fetal malformations

Questions 691 through 693

(A) hyperthyroidism

(B) pregnancy

(C) both

(D) neither

691. Diffuse enlargement of the thyroid gland

692. Persistent tachycardia

693. Decreased red cell uptake of triiodothyronine

Answers and Explanations

541. (E) Diuretics are contraindicated in eclampsia, and a rapid decrease in blood pressure may not allow adequate tissue perfusion. Magnesium sulfate should be titrated to keep reflexes 1+. As soon as the patient is stabilized, delivery should be attempted.

542. (D) Although all of the signs listed can occur in preeclampsia, the most common one is an acute elevation of the blood pressure. Five percent of pregnancies will be complicated by preeclampsia.

543. (E) Prevention of eclampsia is one of the concerns in the treatment of preeclampsia. Both the fetal and maternal mortality rate rise if the disease becomes so complicated by convulsions. There may be a severe compromise of cardiac function, gastric content aspiration, and pulmonary edema. Of the choices listed, the most frequent cause of death is cerebral hemorrhage.

544. (B) Severely preeclamptic or eclamptic patients have marked hemoconcentration due to a decrease in plasma volume. The hematocrit is uniformly high. Albumin is low in spite of the hemoconcentration. The plasma volume may decrease by as much as 30%.

545. (A) This lesion is transient and will usually regress rapidly after delivery. This is often associated with subendothelial deposition of proteinaceous material. The process has been called *glomerular capillary endotheliosis*.

546. (D) In such an emergency situation, the immediate concern is to protect the patient from self-inflicted injury and to stop the convulsion. Morphine, magnesium sulfate, barbiturates, and diazepam have all been used acutely to decrease convulsions and relax the patient. Care must be exercised not to depress respiration.

547. (A) Magnesium sulfate ($MgSO_4$) is excreted by the kidney. Therefore, if kidney function is decreased, the amount of $MgSO_4$ given must also be decreased. Because of its smooth muscle–relaxing properties, blood vessels relax slightly and blood supply to the uterus may be increased. This agent is thought to have a wide margin of safety.

548. (A) Prolonged coma, rapid pulse, more than 10 convulsions, and high proteinuria are other poor diagnostic signs. Given these problems, maternal and fetal mortality are high.

549. (E) Eclampsia associated with vasoconstriction causes a widespread arteriolitis and thereby affects many body organs. Bleeding at these affected sites can cause serious and permanent damage secondary to infarct.

550. (C) Exudates and hemorrhages are usually found in chronic hypertensive states and not in preeclampsia. The arteriolar spasm is representative of the generalized vasospasm that occurs in preeclampsia. Retinal hemorrhage or detachment may occur. It is usually unilateral and seldom causes total visual loss.

551. (B) Criteria for mild preeclampsia are met— namely, a rise in systolic BP of 30 mm Hg and in diastolic of more than 15 mm Hg, along with proteinuria. These signs and symptoms were observed on two occasions 6 hours apart. The patient should be treated in the appropriate manner.

552. **(C)** In preeclampsia, the perinatal death rate varies from 5 to 20%, depending on severity. Maternal mortality is near zero, but if eclampsia occurs, maternal mortality is about 5%.

553. **(B)** Once delivery is accomplished, most patients show marked improvement within 48 hours. Magnesium sulfate may be used for seizure prevention. Antihypertensive medication also helps prevent complications. Only delivery is a cure.

554. **(C)** The classification according to the degree to which activity is limited by the heart disease appears to be a very practical one. There is no class 0. Most patients with class I or II can go through a pregnancy; however, they must be monitored closely throughout, as heart failure can occur.

555. **(E)** As the incidence of rheumatic fever decreased, CHD gained in importance. More of the congenital defects are repaired and rheumatic fever decreased secondary to good antibiotic therapy. CHD has now become the most common heart defect.

556. **(A)** Combined data show that VSD is much more common than the other forms of congenital heart defects. The physiologic effects of VSD are related to its size. Large unrepaired defects result in pulmonary hypertension and risk of bacterial endocarditis.

557. **(C)** Other signs of valvular disease are a harsh, loud systolic murmur and evidence of true cardiac enlargement. As pregnancy causes some change in cardiac contour and sounds, one must be careful the changes noticed are not physiologic only. A diastolic murmur is always abnormal. Echocardiography can detect early abnormalities.

558. **(B)** Anticoagulation is recommended to prevent embolic phenomena. Heparin and low-molecular-weight heparin do not cross the placenta and will not harm the fetus, but dicumarol does cross the placenta and may cause fetal bleeding and other abnormalities. However, heparin is not as protective as dicumarol for the mother and has been associated with an increased risk of maternal mortality. Dextran is difficult to administer. Patients with three artificial heart valves have had successful pregnancies. Antibiotics are necessary at the time of operative procedures.

559. **(D)** Such patients should not become pregnant if possible. Their own life expectancy is markedly diminished. Maternal concerns must be considered first in such situations. The fetus will almost always be lost.

560. **(C)** In general, the more severe the diabetes, the greater the risk to the mother and the infant. This is the purpose of White's classification. It is very useful in predicting maternal and fetal outcome in a general manner but is less useful for the individual patient.

561. **(D)** If the renal disease is severe, patients are quite unlikely to become pregnant. If they do, the chance of perinatal death is markedly increased, and delivery is usually indicated several weeks before term. Hypertension is very common and usually severe.

562. **(E)** Induction of labor usually is intense and long in a primiparous woman. Insulin infusion is most commonly the optimal form of management for these patients.

563. **(D)** Alertness to several clinical and historical signs may allow one to diagnose diabetes early in pregnancy and by proper care decrease the fetal mortality associated with the disease. However, approximately one half of the pregnant patients with gestational diabetes will be missed if only high-risk factors are used for diagnosis.

564. **(D)** Anemia is a common finding in pregnancy. A fairly standard definition of anemia is

important. In pregnancy, a hemoglobin below 10 g/dL is considered to reflect an anemic state. The anemia may be partly "physiologic," but it should and can be treated in most cases.

565. **(A)** Many women have small iron stores secondary to blood loss during menses, childbirth, and inadequate intake. Their intake should be increased to make up for the lack of bone marrow iron. The poor tolerance to iron and poor intestinal absorption also add to the problem.

566. **(B)** The anemia occurs as a late manifestation of folic acid deficiency. If iron is also low, the megaloblastic character of the folate deficiency may be masked.

567. **(C)** Thalassemia is a disease of defective production of either the alpha or beta globin that make up the hemoglobin molecule. Deficient production may lead to microcytic anemia. Acute blood loss does not manifest as a change in the red cell indices.

568. **(A)** Sickle cell disease is found in less than 1 in 500 African-Americans. Sickle cell *trait* is found in approximately 8% of African-Americans.

569. **(C)** Sickle cell disease is autosomal recessive. Thus, the children must have both copies of the abnormal gene to have the disease. Each child will receive an abnormal gene from one parent and have a 50% chance of receiving an abnormal gene from the parent who has sickle cell trait.

570. **(B)** G6PD deficiency is a disease found in 2% of African-American women. The enzyme deficiency may lead to anemia when a woman is exposed to certain drugs.

571. **(C)** The MCV is greater than normal with a lower than normal hematocrit.

572. **(D)** Folic acid deficiency is the most common cause in a young person of macrocytic anemia. B_{12} deficiency also may cause macrocytic anemia but is more rare in this age group.

573. **(A)** A clean-void urine specimen is best for routine cultures, provided meticulous care is taken during collection. Other methods that avoid contamination of the specimen—namely, catheterization and suprapubic aspiration—may be used, but both invade the bladder, and catheterization is known to predispose to UTIs.

574. **(C)** The combination of proteinuria, hypoalbuminemia, and hyperlipidemia characterize the nephrotic syndrome, which may be due to many causes. Generally, women with nephrosis who do not have renal insufficiency or hypertension have a successful pregnancy; however, if either of these appear, prognosis becomes increasingly poor.

575. **(C)** X-rays of the lower abdomen should not be done routinely during pregnancy because of the radiation exposure to both mother and fetus. However, one should be aware of the physiologic hydroureters present during pregnancy. This finding may be misinterpreted as obstruction.

576. **(E)** As this is a normal physiologic finding, it does not require any treatment. Total obstruction is unlikely. Stenting is unnecessary.

577. **(E)** Pelvic kidney must always be considered in the presence of a large, firm, posterior pelvic mass. In pregnancy, ultrasound is an even better study than an IVP, which gives a low dose of radiation.

578. **(B)** A single pelvic kidney is susceptible to trauma at the time of delivery and to infection during pregnancy. However, if it is functioning properly, there is no need to terminate the pregnancy. Transplant patients deliver vaginally with few problems.

579. **(D)** Stones can be passed during pregnancy. The possibility of long-standing renal calculi must be kept in mind, in which case low-grade chronic infection is likely to be present. Symptomatic treatment is provided with surgical removal, if necessary.

580. (E) Hyperparathyroidism during pregnancy is a rare disease, usually caused by an adenoma or hyperplasia of the parathyroids. However, the presence of renal stones in young women should make one think of this disease. Other tests, such as urine cultures and serum calcium and phosphorus, should also be done. The urine can be strained for other stones.

581. (C) Because of the rarity (< 0.01%) of ureteral stones in the normal age group of pregnant women and the large ureters secondary to pregnancy hormones, one should look for predisposing factors such as hyperparathyroidism if renal stones are discovered. The diagnosis, evaluation, and therapy are similar as in the nonpregnant patient, except lithotripsy is contraindicated. Pain caused is usually excruciating. There is no such thing as a ureteral filter.

582. (D) Eclampsia requires the presence of convulsions and/or coma. Preeclampsia is the only diagnosis that can be substantiated. The blood pressure in a young pregnant girl would normally be low, and therefore the 135/85 BP may well represent an increase of 30 mm Hg systolic or 15 mm Hg diastolic.

583. (B) During intrauterine life, the infant of a hyperparathyroid mother is exposed to high serum calcium levels, which may result in tetany when no longer present. Such symptoms in the newborn may be the first indication of the maternal disease.

584. (B) Fortunately, cytomegalic disease is almost never recurrent and often does not affect the infant even if the asymptomatic mother excretes the virus. Up to 1% of all newborns excrete the virus at birth. Only 5 to 10% of these infants are symptomatic.

585. (C) Generally, the signs and symptoms of pyelonephritis are clear-cut. Women with prior asymptomatic bacteriuria are at greater risk of developing pyelonephritis than women without bacteriuria. Up to 2% of pregnancies are complicated by pyelonephritis.

586. (C) The mother may contract the protozoa from exposure to cat feces or by eating undercooked meat. Most women are asymptomatic. Many of the newborns will be infected. Fetal infection with toxoplasmosis may be devastating.

587. (C) While it was once thought that pregnancy did cause exacerbations of TB, there is no proof of this. However, there is an increasing incidence of TB with high-risk behavior such as IV drug use and HIV, resulting in crowding. TB in pregnancy must be treated just as in the nonpregnant patient.

588. (C) All of the STDs listed occur in pregnancy and should be thought of in high-risk women. Herpes, HIV (human immunodeficiency virus), and human papillomavirus are three viral conditions that are also common in pregnancy. With maternal chlamydia, there is an increased incidence of conjunctivitis and pneumonia in the newborn, and there might be late postpartum endometritis in the mother. Chancroid is a rare disease in the United States, although it is becoming more common. The causative agent is *Haemophilus ducreyi,* which causes painful, soft, genital ulcers and is associated with painful inguinal nodes.

589. (E) Because of the large number of asymptomatic carriers of gonorrhea (both male and female), the decreasing sensitivity of the organism, and the inability to culture the gonococci adequately from the female, this patient should be treated with ceftriaxone 250 mg IM if she is not allergic. She should be recultured in 2 weeks. Her partner should also be treated. She should also be evaluated and/or treated for chlamydia, as the probability of simultaneous exposure is high.

590. (A) Most pregnant patients should have a gonococcal culture taken. Any disease so discovered should be treated promptly. Prevention is the best means to avoid poor neonatal outcome. Given the seriousness of gonococcal ophthalmia, all newborns receive prophylactic eye drops.

591. (C) During the second month of pregnancy, maternal rubella results in an 80% fetal infection, with a 25 to 50% incidence of major abnormalities. With rubella, during the first month, the incidence of anomalies is even higher. The anomalies can be and usually are multiple.

592. (B) Several major anomalies are also known to occur following rubella. These include eye and heart lesions, intrauterine growth retardation, and chromosomal abnormalities. Most common is congenital hearing loss.

593. (B) Purpura is a recognized abnormality occurring in infants with congenital rubella. It is due to thrombocytopenia. Anemia is also possible.

594. (D) Obtaining a VDRL only at the time of contact or within a few days may lead one to a sense of false security. However, the serologic tests for syphilis will almost always be positive within 4 to 6 weeks postexposure.

595. (C) If syphillis in pregnancy can be treated early, it is less likely to cross the placenta and infect the fetus. Treatment beyond 18 weeks often leaves the fetus with serious sequelae. A titer of 1:16 is unlikely to be a biologic false positive. Any patient with a positive test for syphilis should be screened for HIV.

596. (C) There is a slim chance that the mother was reinfected, but it is far more likely that the baby has maternal antibody. The VDRL should become negative without therapy.

597. (B) If the baby has the disease, the VDRL titer will increase. If the infant simply has passive maternal antibody, the titer will disappear within 3 months. Positive IgM levels provide a useful, though not specific, indication of infection. If there is any doubt, it is better to treat the infant. Darkfield examinations will help if lesions are present, but otherwise there is no place from which to obtain specimens.

598. (C) Short-acting penicillin may cure incubating syphilis but is not adequate for the established disease. Late syphilis requires higher doses. If duration is greater than 1 year or if neurosyphilis is suspected, spinal fluid must be obtained for analysis.

599. (C) Long-acting thyroid stimulators can cross the placenta and affect the fetus for some time after delivery. The fetus may require symptomatic therapy or even antithyroid medication.

600. (D) BMR, protein-bound iodine (PBI), and binding globulin will all be elevated during pregnancy. I^{131} uptake determination is contraindicated during pregnancy. The T_3 uptake is normally decreased in pregnancy because the increased serum-binding globulin competes with the RBCs added for the test for uptake of labeled T_3. To diagnose hyperthyroidism, measurements of unbound or free T_4 can be done. PBI, BMR, and assays other than TSH, T_4, and T_3 resin (or RBC) uptake are seldom done.

601. (B) I^{131} treatment is contraindicated in pregnancy, and thyroidectomy may not be necessary. Some arguments exist as to the best medical regimen. However, initial treatment is thyroid suppression with PTU.

602. (E) Carcinoma of the breast can arise at any time, and nodules should be worked up in spite of pregnancy. Mistaking a cancer for a mastitis is not unusual. Delay in evaluation or treatment only decreases the chance of long-term survival.

603. (A) The absolute figure is not as important as the knowledge that a significant number of women will have cancer of the cervix during pregnancy and that pregnancy may be the only time when they will see a physician for a checkup. An abnormal Pap smear must always be investigated, even during pregnancy. Therapy may be tempered to some extent in pregnancy. The primary concern is optimal outcome for mother and fetus.

604. **(E)** Many women see a physician for the first time in years when they are pregnant. Pap smears should be done routinely. Pregnancy does not alter cytologic findings significantly enough to alter the reading of Pap smears in pregnancy.

605. **(B)** This tumor probably arises from the stromal theca cells, which become luteinized, large, and eosinophilic. Hilar cells are probably homologues of the testicular Leydig cells and may resemble hyperplastic theca lutein cells. Luteoma should regress following delivery.

606. **(E)** In general, the best results are achieved if one disregards the pregnancy and treats the cancer. Irradiation will soon result in abortion. Radical surgery has no place in Stage III disease, and hysterotomy is not necessary so early in gestation. The patient, of course, may desire another course of action after all the possibilities have been explained.

607. **(C)** Fortunately, pheochromocytoma is extremely rare. Diabetes insipidus is also rare but does not seem to give rise to problems during pregnancy if enough antidiuretic hormone (ADH) is given. Syphilis, obesity, and gestational diabetes seldom are causes of maternal mortality.

608. **(A)** Hypertension predisposes to abruptio placentae, and many infants have died in utero because of abruptio. Therefore, after the patient is stabilized, delivery should be accomplished if the twins are mature, especially if the patient is severely toxemic. If the fetuses are not mature, delivery may be temporized with the patient in the hospital.

609. **(D)** Increased uric acid levels are probably from microangiopathic cell destruction and endothelial damage.

610. **(D)** A D&C at this time would be unsafe in an intrauterine gestation and would destroy the fetus. Although both arteriogram and an x-ray after dye installation would clarify the diagnosis, they are expensive and more dangerous than ultrasound, which at this stage of gestation can identify IUG, mole, and/or fibroid.

611. **(B)** The uterus enlarges until the embryo dies, and then it decreases in size. The pregnancy test also reverts to negative. This term applies to in utero embryonic or fetal loss without expelled products. Ultrasound has made the diagnosis easier and earlier.

612. **(B)** Septic shock, as well as coma, postictal state, or pulmonary hypertension, could cause such symptoms. The absence of vaginal bleeding virtually rules out placenta previa as a diagnosis for a state of shock. Abruptio placentae can have hidden bleeding. Eclampsia usually has associated hypertension. Amniotic embolism usually occurs during labor.

613. **(B)** If the patient had a hydatidiform mole, which is certainly a strong possibility from the history, you would anticipate a very low level of hCS. Serial hCG would be elevated well beyond normal levels. Ultrasound will show classic signs of molar tissue and is the test of choice. The Apt test is to detect fetal hemoglobin, of which there is none in complete molar pregnancies. Serial clotting function will not help in the immediate diagnosis.

614. **(A)** Gestational trophoblastic disease such as choriocarcinoma may follow hydatidiform mole, normal pregnancy, or abortion, and a common sign is persistent positive hCG.

615. **(E)** Those occurring after gestation seem to be related to poor nutrition and an advanced maternal age. Spontaneous occurrence is extemely rare. Asian patients are at the highest risk.

616. **(C)** Fetal death is quite likely under the circumstances. The cause of death remains unclear, as is often the case. The dark fluid may be due to meconium or bleeding.

617. (B) In the presence of long-standing fetal death, tests to determine fetal viability are fruitless. The mother, however, may develop a consumptive coagulopathy. This is rare before 1 month after fetal death.

618. (B) A dead fetus that is retained in utero beyond 5 weeks is likely to cause hypofibrinogenemia; therefore, maternal clotting ability should be evaluated. This should be done at least weekly. Delivery is indicated.

619. (A) The situation is classic for pregnancy. Serum hCG could also be elevated with hydatidiform mole or with choriocarcinoma, but these are much less likely. Amenorrhea means pregnancy until proven otherwise.

620. (C) Defects that inhibit fetal swallowing appear to be most common. The importance of recognizing the association of poor fetal outcome with severe degrees of hydramnios is greater than the importance of knowing the absolute percentages. Most fetuses will not have anomalies, and the cause of hydramnios is usually not found. Amniotic fluid index, calculated by adding the vertical depth of the largest pocket of amniotic fluid in each of four quadrants, has been used as a measure.

621. (C) The distention of the uterus will tend to cause preterm labor. Fetal urinary tract anomalies are associated with a decreased volume of amniotic fluid because urine makes up a lot of the amniotic fluid. Hypertension is generally not related to hydramnios, although often it is related to oligohydramnios. Diabetes in the mother will cause an osmotic diuresis in the infant, resulting in increased fluid, and neurologic deficits may compromise swallowing; both can increase amniotic fluid.

622. (A) The pressure within the amnion is not elevated in the majority of cases but may be increased in the presence of uterine contractions. Hydramnios implies greater than 2,000 mL of fluid, with severe hydramnios being more than 3,000 mL. Hydramnios is associated with a variety of fetal abnormalities. The uterus is often overdistended and may contract very poorly.

623. (D) The duration and intensity place this episode beyond the realm of usual nausea and vomiting of pregnancy. Ptyalism is excessive salivation. Flu is possible but less likely without associated intestinal symptoms.

624. (C) If the patient is acutely dehydrated and unable to retain ingested food, she should be admitted and treated with fluids and electrolytes. Often, hydration with a dilute glucose solution will relieve the vomiting.

625. (D) Cholestatic hepatosis or cholestasis of pregnancy is characterized by mild icterus and pruritus. This entity may be associated with adverse fetal outcome.

626. (D) High estrogen levels appear to be etiologically implicated in the syndrome of cholestatic hepatosis. Why they predispose to cholestasis is unclear. This may also recur with the use of birth control pills.

627. (C) The hyperbilirubinemia is mainly due to conjugated bilirubin. Obstruction is intrahepatic. No long-term sequelae are evident. Delivery results in complete recovery. Glomeruloendotheliosis is a finding in preeclampsia.

628. (A) Sickle cell anemia is not managed with iron supplementation because the patient has high iron stores. Transfusions are with the packed cells, not with hemoglobin.

629. (D, E) Urine output is extremely important, as this is the only route of excretion of MgSO4, which causes marked muscle and central nervous system (CNS) depression in overdose and can be counteracted by calcium. Respiratory arrest is perhaps the most dangerous side effect. The compound, however, has a wide margin of safety.

630. (A, B, C, D) In Ebstein's anomaly, there is downward displacement of an abnormal tricuspid valve into the right ventricle. Cyanosis is due to right-to-left shunting through the foramen ovale. Tetralogy of Fallot is a combination of VSD, right ventricular hypertrophy, and an overriding aorta with cyanosis. Cyanosis gets worse during pregnancy when peripheral resistance decreases and the shunt increases. Patent ductus arteriosus (PDA) also allows right-to-left shunting when systemic pressure falls. VSD will allow right-to-left shunting when pulmonary hypertension develops. Marfan syndrome is an inherited weakness of connective tissue that commonly leads to aortic dilation and dissecting aneurysm.

631. **(A, B, C)** A history of preeclampsia is a grave omen. More than half of the hypertensive patients will have a recurrence. Nonhypertensive patients are unlikely to have preeclampsia in subsequent pregnancies.

632. **(C, E)** Unexplained stillbirths should always make one think of maternal diabetes, as should urinary glucose, family history of diabetes, and excessively large babies such as 9½ lb. However, with improved control of glucose before and during pregnancy, the perinatal mortality of diabetic patients now approaches that of nondiabetics.

633. **(C, D)** Human placental lactogen and estrogen both act to inhibit insulin activity.

634. **(A, C, E)** Folic acid deficiency leads to a megaloblastic or "large" cell anemia. In late stages, platelet deficiency may occur.

635. **(A, B, C, D)** Intravascular hemolysis may be precipitated by inherited causes, medication exposures, and acquired diseases.

636. **(A, C)** Homozygous C-C disease is usually a benign condition with a mild anemia. Hemoglobin S-C is problematic in pregnancy.

637. **(B, D, E)** Decreased antithrombin III or protein S (not increased levels) leads to higher risk of embolism.

638. **(A, B, D)** The release of placental thromboplastin into the maternal circulation may lead to the coagulopathy.

639. **(A, B, E)** Anti-D immune globulin is given after an event such as trauma, amniocentesis, or delivery, which may lead to exposure of maternal Rh-negative blood to the Rh antigen.

640. **(A, B, D)** Folic acid may be given orally, and dietary supplements should be encouraged as well.

641. **(A, C, E)** Factor V Leiden is an abnormal Factor V that cannot bind with protein C, and thus cannot be inhibited. In thrombogenic conditions such as pregnancy, this may lead to thrombosis.

642. **(A, B, E)** Dilation of the renal collecting system results from the effect of progesterone on smooth muscle. It may also predispose to pyelonephritis because of the stasis and predisposition to reflux. Use of any instrumentation would also predispose to infection. The presence of infection is a risk factor. Increased uterine size contributes to ureteral obstruction.

643. **(A, B, C, E)** Montgomery tubercles are found in the areola of the breast. Venereal warts and the lesions of secondary syphilis can be confused with them, but the treatment is quite different. Varicosities are common secondary to increased valvar blood flow and dependent stasis. They demand no treatment.

644. **(A, C, D, E)** Perform an accurate history and physical before diagnosis or treatment. Each should give a fair indication and together should enable a diagnosis to be made. If there are questions, pregnancy tests or ultrasound may be needed.

645. **(A, B, C, D)** The normal-sized uterus does not rule out hydatidiform mole, as approximately one half of these patients have small or normal uteri. The high blood pressure may be an early sign of toxemia, which may occur

prior to 24 weeks' gestation if there is a hydatidiform mole. Normal pregnancy is possible, as is a missed abortion. A fibroid can enlarge a pregnant uterus. Ovarian cancer should not enlarge the uterus.

646. (A, C, D) Patients should be closely monitored to detect the early signs of congestive heart failure (CHF). Decreasing vital capacity is an early sign of CHF. If CHF occurs, rapid medical treatment with digitalis, oxygen, diuretics, and so on is indicated. A functional class II patient, if followed properly, should have an excellent outcome.

647. (A, B, D) Sometimes minor health problems play a more significant role when a patient is pregnant. Severe asthma is associated with an increase in maternal morbidity and mortality. Asthma is not a risk factor for tuberculosis. There is a higher rate of prematurity.

648. (A, D, E) Pyelonephritis may cause preterm labor and, if untreated, leads to sepsis. There is also an association with respiratory distress syndrome.

649. (A, C, D) Most often in pregnancies complicated by SLE, the worst complications will be renal. Declining function with exacerbation or onset of hypertensive disease are the manifestations. Renal function must be monitored throughout pregnancy. While BUN and creatinine levels are specifically used to monitor current renal function, sharply declining C3 and C4 levels are predictors of exacerbations of this disease. Many authorities recommend monthly monitoring of these serum complement levels.

650. (A, D) The signs and symptoms of obstetric hepatosis disappear after delivery. Antihistamines and cholestyramine have been reported to be helpful.

651. (C, D) The concept that obese people have good dietary habits is false. They usually lack proteins, vitamins, and minerals, although they often have a high caloric intake. Most obesity is of a nonendocrine type.

652. (A, D, E) The three most common causes of maternal mortality are hemorrhage, hypertension, and pulmonary embolism. Anesthesia, heart disease, collagen diseases, and asthma are also causes of maternal death, but they are not among the top three as recorded in current maternal death statistics. Maternal mortality is steadily declining, and causes are changing in relative incidence.

653. (A, C) Nonmaternal deaths are due to factors that have nothing to do with the pregnancy, such as gunshot wounds or motor vehicle accidents.

654. (A, B) The patient should be stabilized before any attempt at induction. One must be sure that the fetuses are mature. If the mother and fetuses are not in danger, there is no great urgency for delivery. Antihypertensives are not used at this level of blood pressure.

655. (C) Sulfas compete with bilirubin for an excretory pathway. This may result in increased bilirubin in the fetus and may require therapy.

656. (E) Aplastic anemia from chloramphenicol is a rare occurrence and one that can be avoided. Usually, many other effective drugs are available that do not have so serious a side effect. However, it remains the first choice for treatment of typhoid fever.

657. (D) Streptomycin is not a drug of choice for the usual infections, as the range of bacterial coverage is not great and there is risk of toxicity. Many broad-spectrum aminoglycosides are now available that can be used in place of streptomycin.

658. (A) High concentrations of tetracycline will develop in patients with decreased renal function, as excretion will be impaired. Therefore, dosage should be decreased if renal function is impaired. It can cause staining of deciduous teeth and has been associated with acute fatty liver.

659. (A) Irradiation is far less with radioisotope procedures than with soft-tissue x-ray. Both maternal and fetal radiation must be considered, including thyroid uptake of I^{131}. Any procedures involving radiation have teratogenic and mutagenic potential.

660. **(B)** The echo pattern of various structures is fairly typical. The chorionic plate appears as a white line. Other structures appear as shades of gray.

661. **(D)** Accuracy in diagnosing abnormalities of pregnancy, placental implantation, or pelvic masses increases with experience in the technique. Both methods have failure rates in the 5 to 15% range. Because of its dynamic quality and lack of ionizing radiation, sonographic examination is preferred.

662. **(A)** Abortion, by definition, has to occur early in gestation. If the fetus weighs over 500 g, its expulsion from the uterus is technically a premature or immature delivery. Gestational age must be less than 20 weeks for a pregnancy loss to be considered an abortion.

663. **(E)** Cervical carcinoma can occur and bleed at any stage of gestation. Routine Pap smears should be taken in all pregnancies and suspicious cervical lesions biopsied. The treatment is altered only slightly by pregnancy.

664. **(C)** Although bleeding from placenta previa can occur prior to the third trimester, it is much more common after the 28th week. It is a tenuous and dangerous situation, often requiring extended hospitalization.

665. **(D)** A flaccid uterus postpartum prevents the constriction of the myometrial blood vessels by contraction of the interlacing fibers of the myometrium. Bleeding can be severe. Oxytocin, methergine, and massage have all been used with success in controlling atony.

666. **(B)** Other causes of bleeding in the second trimester, especially abortion, are more common. However, a hydatidiform mole is most likely to bleed during the second trimester. It can also be associated with hypertension and a large-for-dates uterus.

667. **(C)** In this instance, the BP elevation was discovered before 20 weeks' gestation, and there was no evidence of hydatidiform mole. Therefore, the most likely diagnosis is chronic hypertensive disease. Preeclampsia is usually a disease of the third trimester.

668. **(A)** This patient does not have any of the signs or symptoms required to make the diagnosis of severe preeclampsia. These signs are somewhat arbitrary and constitute a continuum.

669. **(D)** The presence of convulsions or coma, or both, in late pregnancy must be considered eclampsia until proved otherwise. Epilepsy, brain tumors, or hepatic disease may be at fault, but the most likely diagnosis is eclampsia. Primary seizure disorders may present in pregnancy, but pregnancy-related seizures are more likely.

670. **(B)** The presence of pulmonary edema or cyanosis is sufficient to make the diagnosis of severe preeclampsia. Pulmonary complications are one of the major causes of death from preeclampsia. It is treated best by delivery and supportive measures.

671. **(C)** The long history of increased BP with the retinal changes make the most likely diagnosis chronic hypertensive disease. However, this patient must be observed closely for superimposed toxemia.

672. **(E)** Secondary luetic lesions are known as condyloma lata and are to be distinguished from condyloma acuminata. Serology differentiates them.

673. **(A)** Culture and/or a complement fixation test are also diagnostic. The differential diagnosis includes syphilis, chancroid, and tuberculosis. Biopsy may be needed to make the correct diagnosis.

674. **(A)** These debilitating sequelae are more common in women than in men. (Men tend to have more inguinal buboes.) Vaginal deliv-

ery is sometimes contraindicated in the presence of severe perineal fibrosis.

675. **(B)** The soft chancre and inguinal adenopathy are self-limiting but very painful. Treatment with the sulfas is usually adequate. Culture of aspirated pus from buboes is best for diagnosis. Biopsy can also be used to help differentiate this lesion.

676. **(C)** These microbacilli are seen in stained, large, mononuclear cells found in the diseased tissue. Granuloma inguinale can cause severe vulvar deformity. Fistulous tracts may form as a result of these lesions.

677. **(A)** The marked rectal stricture that lymphogranuloma venereum can cause must again be emphasized. Colostomy may be indicated. The disease may require surgery to eradicate it.

678. **(D)** Asymptomatic and, therefore, untreated or inadequately treated gonorrhea should always be suspected when a patient presents with monoarticular arthritis.

679. **(A)** SLE is a diagnosis that must be kept in mind when patients present with proteinuria and increased blood pressure. However, preeclampsia is much more common and does not have antinuclear and anti-DNA antibodies. Preeclampsia is not associated with arthritis.

680. **(D)** Fortunately, malignant melanoma is rare but is one of the few tumors known to cross the placenta and metastasize in the fetus.

681. **(A)** Lupus flares may often mimic symptoms of preeclampsia.

682. **(C)** This disease tends to recur in subsequent pregnancies and is associated with an increased rate of preterm birth. Steroids and local therapy are the most common treatment.

683. **(E)** Pneumonia, as a complication of epidemic influenza, is very serious in the pregnant woman. Children, pregnant women, and the aged appear to be at the greatest risk from this disease. Vaccination for influenza during pregnancy is safe and recommended.

684. **(A)** Many autoimmune diseases become more severe, or "flare" after delivery.

685. **(D)** Polyostotic fibrous dysplasia causes bony sclerosis and is associated with the development of precocious puberty, which in turn allows pregnancy to occur at an early age.

686. **(A)** *Listeria* have been found in abortuses, although the exact association with abortion in humans is unclear. It can cause fetal infection, with a high fetal mortality rate.

687. **(B)** For unknown reasons, perhaps due to a depressed immune response with a rebound during postpartum, multiple sclerosis often flares postpartum.

688. **(C)** Hiatal hernia is quite common during pregnancy, perhaps from reflux of gastric acid into the esophagus, causing the symptom of heartburn. This is common because of increased intra-abdominal pressure. Antacids are the best treatment. The symptom of heartburn can be mistaken for the epigastric pain of preeclampsia and vice versa.

689. **(C)** The mildly diabetic woman also tends to have large babies. The combination of hydramnios and large infants predisposes to maternal discomfort, increased postpartum bleeding, and difficult delivery. Injuries to the infant are also more common with macrosomia.

690. **(A)** Early (prepregnancy) control of glucose may decrease the overall incidence of anomalies. Abortion is increased in patients with poorly controlled diabetes. Tight glucose control from conception provides the greatest aid toward a good outcome.

691. **(C)** The thyroid increases 50% in size during pregnancy. Its increase should be diffuse and not nodular. Pregnancy does not predispose to hyperthyroidism.

692. **(A)** In hyperthyroidism, the rapid pulse is often present even during sleep, and this is a good clinical diagnostic feature to discriminate between hyperthyroidism and pregnancy. The tachycardia of pregnancy is usually milder than in the hyperthyroid patient.

693. **(B)** Many tests are changed by pregnancy to mimic the hyperthyroid state. Care must be taken not to diagnose hyperthyroidism erroneously and thus institute a plan of management detrimental to both mother and fetus.

CHAPTER 10

Normal Labor and Delivery
Questions

DIRECTIONS (Questions 694 through 742): Each of the numbered items or incomplete statements in this section is followed by answers or by completions of the statement. Select the ONE lettered answer or completion that is BEST in each case.

694. At term, the ligaments of the pelvis change. This can result in

    (A) increasing rigidity of the pelvis
    (B) degeneration of pelvic ground substance
    (C) decreasing width of the symphysis pubis
    (D) enlargement of the pelvic cavity
    (E) posterior rotation of the levator muscles

695. During clinical pelvimetry, which of the following is routinely measured?

    (A) true conjugate
    (B) transverse diameter of the inlet
    (C) shape of the pubic arch
    (D) flare of the iliac crests
    (E) elasticity of the levator muscles

696. The birth canal is made up of a number of tissue layers. The proper order of these layers as the fetus passes through them is

    (A) levator ani, deep transverse perineal muscles, peritoneum, bulbocavernosus, skin
    (B) peritoneum, levator ani, bulbocavernosus, deep transverse perineal muscles, skin
    (C) peritoneum, deep transverse perineal muscles, levator ani, bulbocavernosus, skin

    (D) peritoneum, levator ani, deep transverse perineal muscles, bulbocavernosus, skin
    (E) peritoneum, bulbocavernosus, levator ani, deep transverse perineal muscles, skin

697. During the delivery, the fetal head follows the pelvic axis. This axis is best described as

    (A) a straight line
    (B) a curved line, first directed anteriorly and then caudad
    (C) a curved line, first directed posteriorly and caudad
    (D) a curved line, first directed posteriorly and cephalad
    (E) none of the above

698. The interspinous diameter of a normal pelvis should be at least

    (A) 5 cm
    (B) 8 cm
    (C) 10 cm
    (D) 11 cm
    (E) 12 cm

699. The greatest diameter of the normal fetal head is the

    (A) occipitofrontal
    (B) occipitomental
    (C) subocciput bregmatic
    (D) bitemporal
    (E) biparietal

700. The diagram in Figure 10–1 depicts which position of the fetus in the female pelvis?

(A) right occipitoposterior (ROP)
(B) left mentotransverse (LMT)
(C) left occipitoanterior (LOA)
(D) left sacrotransverse (LST)
(E) left occiput transverse (LOT)

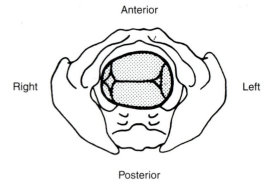

Anterior

Right   Left

Posterior

Figure 10–1.

701. The pudendal nerve can be easily blocked by local anesthetics. The neurologic effect of the pudendal nerve is

(A) motor to levator ani muscle
(B) motor to obturator internus muscle
(C) sensory to the uterus
(D) motor to the bladder
(E) sensory to the perineum

702. A pudendal anesthetic blocks which of the following nerves?

(A) autonomic motor pathways
(B) autonomic sensory pathways
(C) T11, 12
(D) L2,3,4
(E) S2,3,4

703. Caudal anesthesia is given in the

(A) subarachnoid space
(B) subdural space
(C) peridural space

(D) presacral space
(E) peripheral nerve terminal

704. Epidural anesthesia is placed in the same space as the

(A) spinal block
(B) local
(C) pudendal
(D) paracervical
(E) caudal

705. Which of the following methods may provide adequate pain relief in labor?

(A) general anesthesia
(B) paracervical and pudendal blocks
(C) caudal block
(D) psychological methods
(E) all of the above

706. Which of the following anesthetic techniques will produce the greatest uterine relaxation?

(A) spinal block
(B) caudal
(C) nitrous oxide
(D) halothane
(E) paracervical

707. The major problem with the administration of barbiturates during labor is

(A) sudden fetal death
(B) fetal depression after birth
(C) lack of maternal cooperation during the birth process because of narcosis
(D) the likelihood of maternal aspiration causing pneumonitis
(E) their effect is not better than placebo

708. The average blood loss during normal deliveries when measured appears to be about

(A) 700 mL
(B) 500 mL
(C) 250 mL
(D) 100 mL
(E) 50 mL

709. The physiologic retraction ring occurs at the

(A) internal os
(B) external os
(C) level of the round ligament insertion
(D) junction of the upper and lower uterine segments
(E) vulva

710. If the large fontanel is the presenting part, the presentation is

(A) vertex
(B) sinciput
(C) breech
(D) face
(E) brow

711. Methods of determining fetal presentation and position include

(A) Cullen's sign
(B) Leopold's maneuvers
(C) Mauriceau–Smellie–Veit maneuver
(D) careful history taking
(E) all of the above

712. The designation SRT refers to what fetal position?

(A) vertex presentation
(B) brow presentation
(C) face presentation
(D) breech presentation
(E) transverse lie

713. In a cephalic presentation, the position is determined by the relationship of what fetal part to the mother's pelvis?

(A) mentum
(B) sacrum
(C) acromion
(D) occiput
(E) sinciput

714. The relation of the fetal parts to one another determines the

(A) presentation of the fetus
(B) lie of the fetus
(C) attitude of the fetus
(D) position of the fetus
(E) none of the above

715. The relationship of the long axis of the fetus to the long axis of the mother is called the

(A) lie
(B) presentation
(C) position
(D) attitude
(E) none of the above

716. Average durations of labor in primigravidas are best expressed by which of the following?

(A) first stage, 750 minutes; second stage, 80 minutes; third stage, 30 minutes
(B) first stage, 80 minutes; second stage, 20 minutes; third stage, 5 minutes
(C) first stage, 120 minutes; second stage, 80 minutes; third stage, 5 minutes
(D) first stage, 80 minutes; second stage, 20 minutes; third stage, 20 minutes
(E) first stage, 750 minutes; second stage, 80 minutes; third stage, 5 minutes

717. A Montevideo unit is the

(A) number of contractions in 10 minutes
(B) number of contractions per minute times their intensity
(C) intensity of any 10 contractions times the time it took for them to occur
(D) number of contractions over 50 mm Hg in 10 minutes
(E) number of contractions in 10 minutes times their average intensity

718. In the normal labor, the pressure produced by uterine contractions is greatest at which of the following times?

(A) latent phase
(B) active phase
(C) second stage
(D) third stage
(E) when Braxton Hicks sign is evident

719. Which of the following, when released from lysosomes, may initiate labor?

(A) arachidonic acid
(B) phosphatidylinositol
(C) phospholipase A
(D) thromboxane
(E) phosphatidylglycerol

720. Mechanical stretching of the cervix produces increased uterine activity. This has been called the

(A) Moro reflex
(B) Ferguson reflex
(C) Valsalva maneuver
(D) Hoffmann's reflex
(E) Hering–Breuer reflex

721. The process by which mature products of conception are expelled by the mother is called

(A) parturition
(B) childbirth
(C) labor and delivery
(D) accouchement
(E) all of the above

722. Forces acting to aid delivery include

(A) birth canal friction
(B) maternal intra-abdominal pressure during the first stage of labor
(C) cervical resistance
(D) uterine contractions
(E) epidural anesthesia

723. Choose the option in which the cardinal movements of labor are arranged in the proper order. Disregard any omissions of certain movements.

(A) descent, internal rotation, engagement, explusion
(B) engagement, external rotation, descent, extension
(C) engagement, extension, flexion, internal rotation

(D) engagement, extension, descent, flexion, expulsion
(E) engagement, flexion, extension, external rotation

724. Engagement strictly defined is

(A) when the presenting part goes through the pelvic inlet
(B) when the presenting part is level with the ischial spines
(C) when the greatest biparietal diameter of the fetal head passes the pelvic inlet
(D) when the greatest biparietal diameter of the head is level with the ischial spines
(E) none of the above

725. In a vertex presentation, if the sagittal suture is transverse or oblique but closer to the symphysis than the promontory, a specific condition exists. It is called

(A) posterior asynclitism
(B) internal rotation
(C) anterior asynclitism
(D) extension
(E) restitution

726. "Bloody show" is

(A) a result of placenta previa
(B) not seen in breech presentations
(C) a consequence of effacement and dilatation of the cervix
(D) a sign of impending obstetrical hemorrhage
(E) all of the above

727. Molding of the fetal head

(A) usually causes brain damage
(B) becomes progressively easier as gestational age increases
(C) increases the difficulty of delivery
(D) does not have time to occur during breech delivery
(E) does not happen when the maternal pelvis is adequate

728. Crowning is best defined as

(A) when the greatest diameter of the fetal head comes through the vulva

(B) when the presenting part reaches the pelvic floor

(C) when the perineum bulges in front of the fetal head

(D) when the fetal head is first visible through the vulva

(E) when the head is delivered

729. During the delivery of a breech, the infant has been spontaneously expelled to the umbilicus, and the legs are delivered. The next step is

(A) application of forceps

(B) the Mauriceau–Smellie–Veit maneuver

(C) to apply gentle traction until the tip of the scapula is seen

(D) to deliver the anterior arm

(E) to rotate the fetus to a chest-up position

730. Placental separation is facilitated by

(A) deep placental growth into the myometrium

(B) presence of a layer of decidua

(C) decreased uterine muscle contractibility

(D) the changing configuration of the uterus after fetal delivery

(E) all of the above

731. The three signs of placenta separation after delivery include

(A) a gush of blood, a change in uterine shape from discoid to globular, and lengthening of the umbilical cord

(B) descent of the fundus, a gush of blood, and lengthening of the umbilical cord

(C) a darkening of the perineum, a change in uterine shape from discoid to globular, and a gush of blood

(D) a gush of blood, vaginal retraction, and lengthening of the umbilical cord

(E) descent of the fundus, vaginal retraction, and lengthening of the umbilical cord

732. Eight minutes after a normal delivery under pudendal anesthesia, the patient has not completed the third stage of labor. The uterus is discoid and firm; no bleeding is evident. You should

(A) pull vigorously on the cord

(B) perform Crede's maneuver

(C) invert the uterus

(D) manually remove the placenta

(E) gently massage the uterus and wait

733. The tissues incised at the time of routine episiotomy include skin, subcutaneous tissue, and vaginal mucosa, as well as

(A) the rectovaginal septum, intercolumnar fascia of superior fascia of the pelvic diaphragm, and the lowermost fibers of the puborectalis portion of the levator ani muscles

(B) the urogenital sinus, the pelvic diaphragm, and the lowermost fibers of the puborectalis portion of the levator ani muscles

(C) the urogenital diaphragm, intercolumnar fascia of superior fascia of the pelvic diaphragm, and the lowermost fibers of the puborectalis portion of the levator ani muscles

(D) the urogenital septum, intercolumnar fascia of superior fascia of the pelvic diaphragm, and the lowermost fibers of the coccygeus and levator ani muscles

(E) the urogenital septum, superior fascia of the pelvic diaphragm, bulbocavernosus muscle, and the lowermost fibers of the puborectalis portion of the levator ani muscles

734. Which of the following is a characteristic of oxytocin?

(A) half-life of about 8 minutes

(B) prolonged effect

(C) immediate hypertensive effect if given intravenously

(D) inactivated by oxytocinase

(E) inhibited by nonsteroidal anti-inflammatory agents

735. Natural childbirth means

(A) elective induction of labor

(B) continuous conduction analgesia in labor

(C) many things to different people, many being misinterpreted

(D) painless delivery

(E) no physician in attendance

Questions 736 and 737

A 21-year-old primigravida at 39 weeks' gestation presents to labor and delivery with complaints of uterine contractions since 5 A.M. that day. She was seen for a routine clinic visit at 3 P.M. and her cervix was found to be 2 cm dilated, 50% effaced, midposition, and moderate in consistency, with the fetal vertex at 0 station. Reexamination on labor and delivery at 7 P.M. shows no significant cervical change. Fetal heart tones are reassuring.

736. This gravida's Bishop score is

(A) 8, cervix unripe

(B) 4, cervix unripe

(C) 2, cervix ripening

(D) 6, cervix ripening

(E) 9, cervix ripe

737. The optimal obstetrical management at that time would be

(A) labor augmentation with a high dose of oxytocin

(B) performance of primary cesarean section for prolonged labor with presumed cephalopelvic disproportion

(C) reassurance and rest, offering narcotics to aid relaxation and sleep

(D) artificial rupture of the membranes

Questions 738 through 740

A 32-year-old woman (gravida 3, para 1, abortus 1) at term is admitted in labor with an initial cervical examination of 6-cm dilatation, complete effacement, and the vertex at −1 station. Estimated fetal weight is 8 lbs, and her first pregnancy resulted in an uncomplicated vaginal delivery of an 8-lb infant. After 2 hours there is no cervical change. An intrauterine pressure catheter is placed. This shows three contractions in a 10-minute period, each with a strength of 40 mm Hg.

738. This degree of uterine activity in Montevideo units is

(A) considered adequate, 400 Montevideo units

(B) considered inadequate, 120 Montevideo units

(C) considered inadequate, 400 Montevideo units

(D) considered adequate, 240 Montevideo units

(E) considered inadequate, 240 Montevideo units

739. This abnormality of labor is termed

(A) prolonged latent phase

(B) active phase arrest

(C) failure of descent

(D) arrest of latent phase

(E) protraction of descent

740. The best course of action at this time is to

(A) wait 2 more hours and repeat the cervical examination

(B) start oxytocin augmentation

(C) perform a cesarean section

(D) discharge the patient, instructing her to return when contractions become stronger

Questions 741 and 742

A 29-year-old woman (gravida 2, para 1) has a rapid labor. Within minutes of her admission, she is found to be completely dilated, with the vertex at 0 station, and she begins pushing. You are called by her nurse to evaluate her. Contractions are regular, every 2 to 3 minutes, and palpated to be strong. Fetal heart tones are approximately 70 beats per minute. Cervical examination reveals the vertex to be ROP at 0 station with no caput appreciated. Thick meconium is noted.

741. Initially, you

   (A) instruct the patient to ambulate
   (B) turn the patient on her side and administer oxygen by face mask
   (C) begin amnioinfusion and increase IV fluids
   (D) await vaginal delivery

742. Your efforts yield no change in the above parameters. Next, you

   (A) take steps to perform an emergency cesarean section
   (B) continue your initial course of action
   (C) request forceps to perform an assisted vaginal delivery promptly
   (D) ask the anesthesiologist to administer halothane for uterine relaxation

DIRECTIONS (Questions 743 through 752): Each of the numbered items or incomplete statements in this section is followed by answers or by completions of the statement. Select the answers or completions that may apply.

743. The use of midline episiotomy has been shown to do which two of the following?

   (A) prevent urinary stress incontinence after delivery
   (B) expedite delivery when the fetal head is crowning
   (C) decrease maternal blood loss
   (D) increase the incidence of third- and fourth-degree lacerations
   (E) prevent rectal incontinence after delivery

744. Three actions of oxytocin include

   (A) antidiuretic activity
   (B) production of transient hypertension
   (C) increase in uterine muscle contractibility
   (D) nausea and vomiting
   (E) activation of myoepithelial cells of the breast

745. Characteristics of uterine muscle cells during normal labor include which four of the following statements?

   (A) Intermittent contractions are the rule in early labor.
   (B) The entire uterus contracts simultaneously.
   (C) Muscle cells generate adenosine triphosphate (ATP).
   (D) They demonstrate a contractile sensitivity to oxytocin.
   (E) Muscle cells return to the original length after contraction.
   (F) Muscle does not regain full strength between contractions.

746. Which four of the following are characteristics of normal labor?

   (A) progressive cervical dilation
   (B) low-grade fever (100.5°F)
   (C) increasing intensity of contractions
   (D) lack of fetal movement
   (E) uterine relaxation between contractions
   (F) moderate bleeding
   (G) pain associated with contractions

747. Which two of the following statements regarding postpartum hemorrhage are TRUE?

   (A) It is prevented primarily by the increased concentration of clotting factors in maternal blood.
   (B) Grand multiparity is a risk factor.
   (C) Women with severe preeclampsia are more tolerant of heavy blood loss.
   (D) Changes in pulse and blood pressure are good early indicators of excessive blood loss.
   (E) Uterine atony and retained placenta are the most frequent causes.

748. Indications for induction of labor include which four of the following?

(A) prolonged pregnancy

(B) severe preeclampsia

(C) intrauterine growth retardation

(D) grand multiparity, posterior cervix

(E) prolonged rupture of membranes without labor

(F) placenta previa

749. Which three of the following are principles in the active management of labor?

(A) early amniotomy

(B) frequent pelvic examination

(C) encouragement of ambulation

(D) relatively high concentration of oxytocin for labor augmentation

(E) hospital admission during latent-phase labor

(F) expected cervical dilatation of 3 cm per hour

750. Psychoprophylaxis in childbirth means which three of the following?

(A) facilitating pregnancy by common sense

(B) using slow, deep breathing and shallow, quick breathing to take away some of the associated pain

(C) using comfort aids such as massage, positioning, or objects that help the patient concentrate on things other than pain

(D) in most cases, specialized predelivery classes and preparation in techniques

(E) routinely using pharmacologic agents during delivery

Questions 751 and 752

A 19-year-old primigravida at term presents to labor and delivery reporting irregular contractions and rupture of membranes 21 hours prior to arrival. She has not received prenatal care but reports that her pregnancy was uncomplicated. She is afebrile, and electronic fetal monitoring is reactive with occasional mild variable decelerations.

751. Which three methods, when all are positive, confirm rupture of membranes?

(A) nitrazine test

(B) vaginal pooling

(C) pelvic exam

(D) ferning

(E) Coombs' test

752. Cervical exam reveals a dilatation of 3 cm, 50% effacement, −1 station, vertex presentation. The best course of action at this time is to

(A) perform an immediate low transverse cesarean section

(B) start IV antibiotics for group B streptococcal prophylaxis

(C) begin an amnioinfusion

(D) conduct a contraction stress test

(E) ambulate the patient

DIRECTIONS (Questions 753 through 767): Each group of items in this section consists of lettered headings followed by a set of numbered words or phrases. For each numbered word or phrase, match the ONE lettered heading that is most closely associated with it. Each lettered heading may be selected once, more than once, or not at all.

Questions 753 through 758

(A) diagonal conjugate

(B) midplane

(C) inlet

(D) true conjugate or conjugate vera

(E) outlet

753. In most women, the plane of least pelvic dimension

754. Is at the level of the ischial spines

755. The distance from the top of the symphysis to the sacral promontory

756. The upper boundary of the true pelvis

757. Distance from the lower margin of the symphysis to the sacral promontory

758. Made up of two triangles

Questions 759 through 762

    (A) first stage of labor
    (B) second stage of labor
    (C) third stage of labor
    (D) effacement
    (E) lightening

759. Dropping of the fetal head into the pelvis

760. Ends with complete dilation of the cervix

761. Begins with the delivery of the baby

762. Ends with the delivery of the baby

Questions 763 through 767

    (A) McRoberts maneuver
    (B) Mauriceau–Smellie–Veit maneuver
    (C) external cephalic version
    (D) Ritgen maneuver
    (E) Leopold's maneuvers

763. At 39 weeks' gestation, a woman is admitted to labor and delivery. Her cervix is long and closed. The fetus is found to be a vertex presentation.

764. Gentle constant pressure is applied to squeeze the vertex out of the fundal area and into the lower uterine segment.

765. The vertex delivers, but gentle downward traction fails to effect delivery of the anterior shoulder.

766. Traction is maintained on the shoulders and not on the mandible.

767. A rapid labor with a vertex presentation has taken place, and the infant is crowning.

Answers and Explanations

694. **(D)** The change is one of relaxation of the ligaments, allowing more mobility and on occasion some instability. Whether or not these changes truly add to pelvic size has not been determined, but they seem to allow passage more easily, perhaps by accommodation.

695. **(C)** Clinical pelvimetry cannot directly measure the midplane of the pelvis, but its capacity can be estimated by the evaluation of the sacrosciatic notch, the ischial spines, and the concavity of the sacrum. Parallel pelvic sidewalls and a wide pubic arch are crucial to the outlet evaluation.

696. **(D)** One should know the layers of tissue making up the deep and superficial pelvic floor. The anatomy here becomes most important when a postdelivery bleeding source must be identified. Knowledge of basic anatomy is very important to stopping bleeding.

697. **(C)** A common misconception is that the fetal head follows a straight line through the pelvis. On the contrary, it describes nearly a 90-degree angle following the pelvic axis. The pelvic axis (curve of Carus) reflects a line in the center of the pelvic inlet (directing it posterior into the sacrum), then caudally toward the center of the outlet (extending the head). The classic mechanisms of labor can be better understood through a knowledge of the pelvic axis.

698. **(C)** The interspinous diameter is the lateral distance between the ischial spines. The ischial spines should not be too prominent on pelvic examination. The distance is generally considered to be the smallest pelvic diameter and the "obstetric limit" in preventing or allowing delivery.

699. **(B)** The occipitomental diameter is about 13.5 cm. A brow presentation tries to force the greatest diameter of the head through the pelvis. The greatest circumference is the occipitofrontal (see Figure 10–2).

700. **(E)** In vertex presentations, the relation of the occiput to the maternal pelvis determines the position. The position of the occiput can be detected by finding the posterior fontanel. As it is on the left lateral side of the mother and the sagittal suture is transverse, the position is left occiput transverse (LOT).

701. **(E)** The pudendal block is often used for delivery or minor surgery on the vulva. The pudendal nerve can be blocked either transvaginally or percutaneously through the buttock. The latter route may be used in the presence of a Bartholin's abscess without causing the pain of vaginal manipulation.

702. **(E)** The pudendal nerve is blocked near the ischial spines. This block will not interfere with uterine contractions and will provide anesthesia to the perineum. Because there is considerable overlap of innervation, midline infiltration anterior to the rectum is needed to provide the best block.

703. **(C)** A real danger with caudal anesthesia is penetration of the dura and arachnoid and instillation of a large dose of anesthetic agent in the subarachnoid space, causing a high

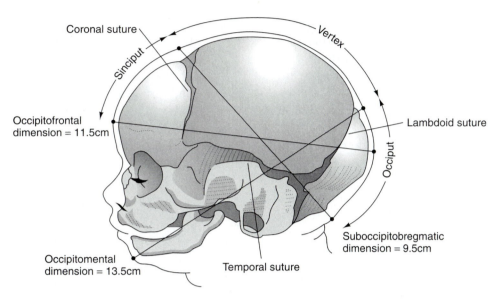

Figure 10–2.

spinal block. This can result in respiratory paralysis, hypotension, and even central nervous system (CNS) reactions. Ventilation and vascular support may be necessary.

704. **(E)** Both the caudal and epidural blocks are given in the extradural space (also called peridural). The difference is in the site of needle insertion. Also different is the level to which the anesthetic agent is allowed to migrate. The caudal is the lower block.

705. **(E)** What constitutes adequate pain relief depends on the patient's perception; the physician does well to remember that such adequacy can be had with many methods, depending on the patient. The physician's prime concern is to provide adequate pain relief safely. In experienced hands, any of these methods may be used to those ends.

706. **(D)** Ether also produces great uterine relaxation but is seldom used in modern obstetric units. The regional techniques may decrease uterine contractions but will not result in the profound uterine relaxation caused by halothane. Halothane should be used only when profound uterine relaxation is desired. Atony is seldom desired unless a fetus is "trapped."

707. **(B)** Fetal depression is the best reason to minimize the use of barbiturates in labor. For example, after a dose of thiopental is given, it will reach the fetal circulation in 2 to 3 minutes. A dose of 250 mg will have little effect on an otherwise healthy infant, but it does have some effect. All the other distractors have been claimed. Remember, a barbiturate alone is a poor substitute for a true analgesic agent. It seldom is given in large enough doses to truly sedate or narcotize the mother, but when given with narcotics, it certainly can. Anesthetic and analgesic effects on the fetus are a never-ending source of controversy. There is no clear-cut "best" anesthetic or analgesic regimen for delivery. Judgment should be used, subject to local availability.

708. **(B)** This value is greater than that generally estimated by the obstetrician. In fact, the classic definition of postpartum hemorrhage is more than 500 mL at delivery and in the ensuing 24 hours—obviously a gross mistake. If the maternal reserves are good, however, there will be little change in the postpartum hematocrit unless the blood loss is substantially more than 500 mL. Blood loss is often difficult to measure without completely weighing sponges, drapes, and towels.

709. **(D)** A distinct boundary exists between the thin lower segment and the thicker upper uterine segment. It can easily be identified at the time of cesarean section if labor has progressed for some time. Retraction rings generally occur only when labor has been obstructed for quite some time. This ring can obstruct labor at times (pathologic retraction ring or Bandl's ring).

710. **(B)** The diameter of the head presented to the pelvis may be larger or smaller, depending on the presentation. Therefore, the possibility of vaginal delivery may depend on the proper presentation of the fetus to the pelvis. The sinciput diameter is generally larger than the occiput presentation.

711. **(B)** Methods include examination, x-ray, and sonography. Leopold's maneuvers and vaginal examination are readily performed and require no special equipment. Together, they will yield the proper diagnosis in most cases.

712. **(D)** SRT stands for sacrum right transverse and, therefore, signifies a breech presentation. Know the difference between position, presentation, and lie. Each must be determined on examination.

713. **(D)** The most common presentation is cephalic. Position is the relationship between the denominator of the fetus (occiput in cephalic presentations) and the planes of the birth canal.

714. **(C)** Generally, the fetus assumes an attitude with the arms and legs crossed in front of the body and the back curved in a convex manner. The head is generally flexed for best delivery. The cord usually occupies the space between the extremities.

715. **(A)** A common error is to refer to the position as the lie. A transverse position of the fetal head in labor carries a far different connotation than a transverse lie in labor. The lie is usually directly in line with the maternal longitudinal axis. It may also be oblique or transverse.

716. **(E)** Fourteen-hour labors are average, but there is a great deal of variation. However, marked prolongation of any stage merits reevaluation to determine the reason. Warning signs must be observed to prevent catastrophe. Labor curves can give an excellent indication as to diagnosis of abnormalities and prediction of when delivery will occur.

717. **(E)** By considering both frequency and intensity during a time period, an evaluation of contractile forces can be made. Quality of the contractions must also be known. Palpation or external monitoring cannot be used. Internal monitors must be used to accurately determine the pressure measurement.

718. **(D)** Pressures produced by the uterine fundus around the placenta have been measured at 300 mm Hg. Such pressure is enough to stop uterine bleeding and is a physiologic protective mechanism.

719. **(C)** A theory to explain the initiation of labor is that lysosomes containing phospholipase A become unstable at term due to decreased progesterone. The phospholipase A is released and causes release of arachidonic acid from phosphatidylglycerol found in the fetal membranes. The arachidonic acid then forms prostaglandins that initiate myometrial contractions. This is one of several theories regarding the initiation of labor. None have been shown to be completely satisfactory in explaining the phenomenon.

720. **(B)** The name of the phenomenon is not as important as the recognition that it exists. The mechanism is unknown, but it can be blocked by spinal anesthesia. Inflation of a Foley bulb through the cervical os is an acceptable means of labor induction.

721. **(E)** These are all synonymous terms referring to the series of events culminating in delivery, which is the actual birth of the infant. Labor should be thought of as a continuum of events and not as a single episode. The pas-

senger, passageway, and powers of labor all come into play.

722. **(D)** Although all the options are involved in labor, only the uterine contractions and voluntary effort contribute toward delivery, while the resistance offered by the birth canal and cervix inhibit delivery and must be overcome for parturition to occur. Forced dilation of external fundal pressure has been used but probably does more harm than good.

723. **(E)** These movements are best understood in the context of pelvic and cranial anatomy and the forces of labor. Some of these movements may occur simultaneously, but some must precede others. To understand labor as a mechanical process, extensive knowledge of the anatomy of passenger and passageway is necessary.

724. **(C)** When engagement has occurred, the inlet is adequate for that particular head. The midplane or outlet may not be. Also, the attainment of zero station by the head does not automatically imply engagement, although the head usually is engaged. If molding has changed the normal skull measurements, the presenting part may be at zero station before the greatest biparietal diameter of the head passes the pelvic inlet.

725. **(C)** This condition usually corrects itself as the head seeks the largest area in the pelvis. Posterior asynclitism means the sagittal suture is closer to the sacrum. This may occur as the head seeks more room.

726. **(C)** *Bloody show* is a term used to describe the blood-tinged mucus that often precedes labor by a few hours to days. It is not pathologic and bleeding is not profuse. It occurs as a result of tearing of small veins in the cervix secondary to cervical effacement and dilatation in preparation for labor.

727. **(D)** During a breech delivery, the fetal head must traverse the pelvis in a short time because the oxygen supply to the fetus is occluded. This time span of less than 8 minutes

is not adequate to allow significant molding, thus substantially increasing the risk of breech deliveries. Some authorities feel that forceps-assisted delivery of the head should be routine.

728. **(A)** This is a time of great stretch on the perineum, when perineal tears often occur. Crowning should indicate that delivery is imminent.

729. **(C)** In an assisted breech delivery, the fetus should not be disturbed until the breech is delivered. Gentle traction should be applied to keep the back up after delivery to the lower tip of the scapula. Delivery of the posterior arm should follow easily. In many instances, the breech will be allowed to deliver spontaneously to the level of the scapula; then assistance is provided.

730. **(D)** Placental accretion markedly inhibits placental separation. If the uterus does not contract well postpartum, it may not exert sufficient force to shear the placenta from the decidua of the uterus. This will keep the uterus from contracting to close uterine sinusoids, resulting in heavy bleeding. The change in uterine configuration occurs during and after delivery.

731. **(A)** Uterine contractions normally cease for a short time immediately after delivery and then continue whether or not the placenta has separated. These uterine contractions are instrumental in causing placental separation by cleavage through the decidual plane of attachment. Traction does not aid in normal placental separation.

732. **(E)** The lack of bleeding and shape of the uterus are clues that the placenta has not yet separated. The firm uterus makes retroplacental bleeding unlikely. Gentle massage to stimulate uterine contractions will probably result in placental separation, after which expulsion will occur rapidly. Pulling on the cord may avulse it from the placenta or even invert the uterus.

733. (A) The structures involved are the skin and subcutaneous tissue, vaginal mucosa, the rectovaginal septum, intercolumnar fascia of superior fascia of the pelvic diaphragm, and the lowermost fibers of the puborectalis portion of the levator ani muscles (if the episiotomy is made deeply enough). Each episiotomy can be tailored to needs at the time.

734. (D) Because of a rapid onset of action and a rapid metabolism, oxytocin should be closely monitored during its administration. Its IV use can cause transient hypotension that may be especially dangerous in patients with heart disease. The half-life of oxytocin is about 3 minutes. Why oxytocin does not always work to induce contractions is unknown.

735. (C) Natural childbirth has come to mean different things to different people, and there are some erroneous concepts. It does not mean no physician, no drugs, or no pain. It is the desire to make labor and delivery easier by reducing pain and fear through education and understanding of the birth process, and cooperation between caregiver and patient.

736. (D) The Bishop score was originally developed to evaluate patients prior to induction of labor. It predicts the ease of inducibility based on cervical dilatation, effacement, consistency, position, and station of the vertex. Scores of 0 to 3 are assigned for each parameter, with higher total scores predicting a more favorable prognosis for induction. This patient's score is 6, indicating that the cervix is becoming ripe.

737. (C) This woman is in the latent phase of labor, which is the period between regular contractions and the onset of more rapid cervical dilatation (active phase). Latent phase is considered prolonged when it lasts longer than 20 hours in the nullipara and more than 14 hours in the parous woman. This primigravida has had 14 hours of latent-phase labor, which is not considered prolonged. Most authorities recommend therapeutic rest, if any action is to be taken.

738. (B) The Montevideo unit is used to define uterine activity. By definition, it is the product of the intensity of uterine contraction, which is the increased uterine pressure above baseline tone, multiplied by the contraction frequency in 10 minutes. In this case, the value is 120 (or 40 mm Hg × 3). When inadequate progress in active labor occurs in the face of uterine activity less than 200 Montevideo units, then augmentation is indicated provided no contraindications exist.

739. (B) This gravida is in the active phase of labor, when there is an increased rate of cervical dilatation. This occurs by 4-cm dilation for most women. No cervical change after 2 hours is defined as an active-phase arrest.

740. (B) An appropriate step in the evaluation of abnormal labor patterns is the determination of the adequacy of uterine contractions, which can be done accurately with the use of an intrauterine pressure catheter. Since this patient's uterine activity is suboptimal, augmentation with oxytocin is indicated.

741. (B) Intrapartum fetal heart rate monitoring is routinely used to assess fetal well-being in labor. A rate below 100 or above 160 bpm is generally regarded as evidence of distress. The association of thick meconium with abnormal heart rate is even more predictive of distress. Therefore, rapid intervention is imperative. Supplemental oxygen can be helpful, as can maternal position change to potentially alleviate cord compression.

742. (A) In the face of prolonged sudden deceleration nonresponsive to corrective measures, an immediate cesarean section is indicated if vaginal delivery is not imminent. With the vertex at 0 station and ROP position, an operative vaginal delivery is contraindicated.

743. (B, D) Routine episiotomy is performed less frequently in recent years. It can be useful to expedite deliveries in the setting of fetal heart rate abnormalities or to enable appropriate maneuvers in relieving a shoulder dystocia. There is no evidence that episiotomy reduces the likelihood of pelvic relaxation later in life. Furthermore, recent studies have demonstrated an increased likelihood of third- or fourth-degree lacerations after cutting an episiotomy.

744. **(A, C, E)** One must be aware of the antidiuretic effect of oxytocin, especially when it is given diluted in large volumes of D_5W for a long period of time. Water intoxication can be iatrogenically produced. It can rapidly induce hypotension. It also contracts smooth muscles in both the uterus and the breast.

745. **(A, C, D, F)** The ability of uterine muscle to retract allows a progressive diminution of the intrauterine cavity size, which gradually expels the fetus through the thinned-out lower segment and vagina. The upper segment contracts while the lower segment and cervix thins out and dilates to result in expulsion of the fetus. Uterine muscle is unique in function.

746. **(A, C, E, G)** A cervical dilation should not only be progressive but should be constantly accelerating. Frank bleeding during labor is a warning sign and should not be regarded as normal. Low-grade fever could be a sign of developing chorioamnionitis. Fetal movement may not be appreciated as much during the throes of labor pain, but it should still be present as a sign of well-being. Uterine relaxation is necessary to ensure normal placental blood flow.

747. **(B, E)** Uterine bleeding is minimized postpartum by contraction of the myometrium and not by an increase in clotting factors. Women of high parity are at risk for uterine atony. Gravidas with severe preeclampsia are volume contracted and are less tolerant of excessive blood loss. Significant changes in pulse and blood pressure generally do not occur until large amounts of blood have been lost. Atony and retained placenta, followed closely by genital tract lacerations, are the most common causes of postpartum hemorrhage.

748. **(A, B, C, E)** Indications for induction of labor include prolonged pregnancy, diabetes mellitus, Rh isoimmunization, preeclampsia, premature or prolonged rupture of membranes, chronic hypertension, placental insufficiency, and suspected intrauterine growth retardation. Ideally, the fetus should be mature and the cervix should be favorable or "ripe": anterior, well effaced (50% or more), and dilated 1 to 2 cm. The head should also be well down in the pelvis. There are, unfortunately, no guarantees of delivery based on cervical assessment alone. Contraindications to induction include cephalopelvic disproportion, placenta previa, transverse lie, breech presentations, multiple gestation, and grand multiparity.

749. **(A, B, D)** "Active management of labor" refers to methods used to minimize the rate of cesarean section. The principles were developed at the National Maternity Hospital in Dublin, where the rate of primary cesarean delivery was 5 to 6% from its introduction in 1968 through 1980. It involves strict criteria for admission in labor, early amniotomy, frequent examinations to check for progress in labor, and administration of relatively high doses of oxytocin for cervical dilatation rates less than 1 cm/hr.

750. **(B, C, D)** Psychoprophylaxis relies on individual instructions of both partners in the birthing process, again to allay fears and provide alternatives for pain management. It may consist of any of a number of methods—all designed to educate the family-to-be.

751. **(A, B, D)** Speculum exam revealing vaginal pooling, demonstrating an alkaline pH on nitrazine paper and ferning on microscopic exam after drying on a slide confirm rupture of membranes. Pelvic exam may suggest this as well because, as the cervix dilates, palpation of amniotic membranes covering the presenting part (or an absence of the membranes) is usually possible. Coombs' test is a serologic test evaluating maternal sensitization to fetal red blood cells.

752. (B) This patient has premature rupture of membranes. Using the risk-based approach, she should receive group B streptococcal (GBS) prophylaxis, since rupture of membranes is greater than 18 hours. Other criteria for administering antibiotics would be maternal fever greater than or equal to 100.4°F or a history of a previous birth of an infant with GBS disease. To minimize infectious complications for both the patient and her infant, she should be delivered promptly, but labor augmentation rather than cesarean section is indicated.

753. (B) As the fetus has to negotiate the entire pelvis, the smallest portion of the pelvic passage assumes considerable significance. This is where arrest usually occurs. It is also the place where instrument delivery is most dangerous.

754. (B) The midplane cannot be measured directly but can be estimated by clinical pelvimetry. The interspinous diameter should not be less than 10 cm. The intertuberous diameter is an indirect indicator of this measurement.

755. (D) This distance cannot be measured directly but can be inferred from the measurement of the diagonal conjugate, which can be done clinically. This is an estimated distance since the conjugate vera can seldom be reached, and the estimated distance varies depending on the examiner's experience and expertise.

756. (C) The classification of the female pelvis into gynecoid, android, platypelloid, or anthropoid is determined by the shape of the inlet. This upper limit begins at the terminal line demarcating the true pelvis.

757. (A) The diagonal conjugate can be measured clinically. It will normally be 1.5 to 2.0 cm longer than the true conjugate, which is from the top of the symphysis to the sacral promontory. The true conjugate is the actual room the fetus has in its passage.

758. (E) The pelvic outlet is bounded by the subpubic arch to the level of the ischial tuberosities (anterior triangle), while the posterior triangle is bounded by the tuberosities, lateral ligaments, and the sacrum posteriorly.

759. (E) The uterus often changes in its profile when the fetal head drops. In primigravidas, lightening usually occurs prior to the onset of labor, while in multigravidas it often occurs after the onset of labor. This engagement usually occurs after 37 weeks' gestation.

760. (A) This stage begins with the onset of true labor. Complete cervical dilation is one criterion that must be met for the application of forceps. No "pushing" should occur before full dilation.

761. (C) This stage ends with the delivery of the placenta. It includes placental separation and expulsion and should usually be accomplished within 20 minutes after the fetus is delivered. Otherwise, the cervix may partially close, entrapping the placenta.

762. (B) This stage covers that period of time during which the soft tissues of the perineum are distended by the fetus. It should not take longer than 2 hours or 20 normal uterine contractions, with good maternal voluntary effort. Prolongation is an indicator of fetal–pelvic disproportion.

763. (E) The four classic maneuvers give much information regarding the presentation of the fetus. One palpates successively the fundus, the small parts, the suprapubic area, and the area of the anterior inlet. Leopold's maneuvers should be performed from 36 weeks onward.

764. (C) External cephalic version is performed in an attempt to avoid vaginal breech delivery or cesarean section for malpresentation. It involves rotation of the fetus through the maternal abdomen. Reported success ranges from 60 to 75%.

765. **(A)** The McRoberts maneuver promotes delivery of the anterior shoulder. It involves hyperflexion of the maternal legs onto the maternal abdomen, which results in ventral rotation of her pelvis to maximize the size of the outlet.

766. **(B)** Some authorities recommend that a finger not be placed in the mouth at all because of the danger to the tongue and mandible. Two fingers can be placed on the malar eminences and some pressure exerted to maintain flexion of the head. This, along with gentle traction, should accomplish delivery.

767. **(D)** Control of the fetal head to prevent its rapid expulsion with concomitant perineal and dural tearing is important. Pushing is stopped and a gentle lift applied through the perineum to slowly deliver the head in a controlled fashion.

DIRECTIONS (Questions 768 through 799): Each of the numbered items or incomplete statements in this section is followed by answers or by completions of the statement. Select the ONE lettered answer or completion that is BEST in each case.

768. Maximum normal time for the second stage of labor in a primigravida, without anesthesia, is approximately

(A) 20 min
(B) 60 min
(C) 120 min
(D) 240 min
(E) there is no normal maximum

769. You are asked to consult on a 26-year-old woman (gravida 2, para 1) with a prior cesarean section for breech. She is at term. The nurse has plotted the labor curve (see Figure 11–1). The initial step in the evaluation and treatment of the most likely cause of this labor curve would be to

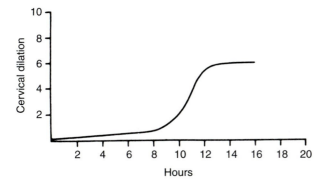

Figure 11–1.

(A) administer oxytocin
(B) assess pelvic adequacy
(C) give sympathetic block
(D) rupture membranes
(E) allow anesthesia to wear off

770. Of the following, the most common indication for primary cesarean section is

(A) dystocia
(B) prolapsed cord
(C) diabetes
(D) toxemia
(E) malpresentation

771. Preterm rupture of the membranes is most strictly defined as spontaneous rupture at any time prior to

(A) a stage of fetal viability
(B) the second stage of labor
(C) the 32nd week of gestation
(D) the onset of labor
(E) the 37th week of gestation

772. You are examining a term patient in the labor and delivery suite. Which of the following signs and symptoms is most likely to indicate ruptured membranes?

(A) vaginal pool pH of 6.5
(B) yellow-green color on nitrazine test
(C) ferning on a specimen from the vaginal pool
(D) superficial squamous cells in the vaginal pool
(E) copious leakage on pants or underwear

773. Which of the following factors tends to increase the average duration of labor?

    (A) increasing parity
    (B) increasing age of the mother
    (C) decreasing size of the baby
    (D) occiput posterior (OP) position of the baby
    (E) none of the above

774. An infant presents as a breech and is delivered without assistance as far as the umbilicus. The remainder of the body is manually assisted by the obstetrician. This is called

    (A) version and extraction
    (B) spontaneous breech delivery
    (C) partial breech extraction
    (D) total breech extraction
    (E) Pipers to the aftercoming head

775. At 39 weeks' gestation, a fetus was felt to be in breech presentation as judged by information gained through Leopold's maneuvers. The breech was well down in the pelvis, and the uterus was irritable. Pelvimetry was within normal limits and the estimated fetal weight was 7½ lb. Which of the following should be done?

    (A) cesarean section
    (B) external cephalic version
    (C) internal podalic version
    (D) oxytocin induction
    (E) expectant management

776. Transverse lie in a multipara at term in early labor is best treated by

    (A) external version
    (B) internal version and extraction
    (C) oxytocin induction
    (D) cesarean delivery
    (E) abdominal support to effect position change

777. Face presentations are common with

    (A) anencephaly
    (B) hydrocephaly

    (C) prematurity
    (D) placenta previa
    (E) oligohydramnios

778. You are checking a 34-year-old woman (gravida 3, para 2) at 38⅗ weeks' gestation. She is in early labor (1 cm). There is no fetal part in the pelvis. Ultrasound report notes a transverse lie with the fetal back toward the maternal legs. The procedure of choice is

    (A) expectant management anticipating spontaneous vaginal delivery
    (B) tocolysis
    (C) external version
    (D) cesarean delivery
    (E) expectant management expecting forceps rotation after complete dilation

779. A patient has entered spontaneous premature labor at 28 weeks' gestation. During the vertex delivery, one should

    (A) recommend epidural anesthesia to control delivery
    (B) perform an episiotomy
    (C) use prophylactic forceps
    (D) use vacuum extraction
    (E) allow spontaneous vaginal birth

780. The absolute diagnosis of amniotic fluid emboli is made by

    (A) chest pain
    (B) chest x-ray
    (C) amniotic debris in the pulmonary circulation
    (D) the presence of consumptive coagulopathy
    (E) electrocardiogram (ECG) changes

781. A contraindication to the use of oxytocin for stimulating labor is

    (A) fetal demise
    (B) hypertonic uterine dysfunction
    (C) hypotonic uterine dysfunction
    (D) twin gestation
    (E) estimated fetal weight less than 5 lb

782. In which of the following cases might internal podalic version be indicated?

(A) vertex delivery of the first twin and breech presentation of the second twin
(B) transverse lie with cervix completely dilated and membranes intact
(C) double footling breech
(D) impacted shoulder presentation
(E) compound presentation

783. You are delivering a 34-year-old woman (gravida 4, para 3) at 38½ weeks whose pregnancy is complicated by gestational diabetes. The head delivers, but the shoulders do not follow. An efficacious method of delivery for a shoulder dystocia includes McRoberts maneuver, which is

(A) fundal pressure
(B) extreme flexion of the maternal thighs
(C) rotation to an oblique position after delivery of posterior arm
(D) strong traction on the head
(E) rotation of the posterior shoulder to the anterior

784. A placenta accreta is most likely to cause bleeding

(A) during the first stage of labor
(B) prior to labor
(C) because of consumption coagulopathy
(D) after amniotic membrane rupture
(E) during attempts to remove it

785. The risk of serious infection transmitted by blood transfusion is greatest for

(A) hepatitis C
(B) Creutzfeldt–Jakob disease
(C) human immunodeficiency virus (HIV)
(D) syphilis
(E) hepatitis B

786. A fetomaternal transfusion of more than 30 mL has been found in what percentage of women at delivery?

(A) < 1%
(B) 5%

(C) 10%
(D) 15%
(E) 20%

787. If blood must be given without adequate crossmatching, the best type to use is

(A) AB Rh-positive
(B) AB Rh-negative
(C) O Rh-positive
(D) O Rh-negative
(E) A Rh-positive

788. Which of the following is associated with small infants?

(A) mothers with untreated gestational diabetes
(B) multiparity
(C) large parents
(D) maternal smoking
(E) postdate pregnancy

789. Rarely, a patient in labor engages the fetal head and effaces the cervix without dilation of the cervix. A dimple may be noted at the external os. Such a condition is called a

(A) uterine dystocia
(B) conglutinate cervix
(C) cervix condupulare
(D) sacculated uterus
(E) vasa previa

790. A 26-year-old woman is first seen at 28 weeks' gestation. Her history and physical are normal except for the presence of a 2-cm posterior cervical leiomyoma. The patient is relatively asymptomatic. Management should be

(A) myomectomy at 36 weeks
(B) myomectomy now with steroids and tocolysis
(C) progesterone therapy to decrease the myoma size
(D) elective cesarean delivery at term
(E) watchful waiting

791. Duhrssen's incisions are indicated

(A) in controlled situations after 36 weeks to initiate labor

(B) for placenta previa < 20 weeks

(C) after manual dilation of the cervix

(D) to hasten normal delivery in cases of fetal distress

(E) in extremely rare situations of a trapped fetal head

792. Which of the following locations is most likely to be the site of a vaginal laceration after an instrumented delivery?

(A) extending off the cervix

(B) anterior upper third under the pubic symphysis

(C) posterior upper third from an incompletely evacuated rectum

(D) lateral middle third over the ischial spines

(E) posterior middle third over the coccyx

793. A patient sustained a laceration of the perineum during delivery. It involved the muscles of the perineal body but not the anal sphincter. Such a laceration would be classified as

(A) first degree

(B) second degree

(C) third degree

(D) fourth degree

(E) fifth degree

794. Postpartum hemorrhage unresponsive to oxytocin and uterine massage is most likely due to

(A) laceration(s)

(B) placenta accreta

(C) retained placenta

(D) ruptured uterus

(E) coagulopathy

795. Couvelaire uterus is characterized by

(A) enlargement and invasion by placental tissue

(B) retroversion, retroflexion, and adherence to the cul-de-sac peritoneum

(C) a congenital anomalous development

(D) intramyometrial bleeding

(E) metabolic abnormalities

796. Which of the following situations has the greatest risk for the mother and infant?

(A) rupture of an intact uterus

(B) rupture of a previous uterine scar

(C) pathologic contraction ring

(D) dehiscence of a uterine scar

(E) cervical laceration

Questions 797 and 798

A 35-year-old woman (gravida 7, para 5, abortus 1) is in the active phase of labor with the vertex at −1 station. She complains of abdominal pain with the contractions. At the height of one contraction, the pain becomes very intense. Following this intense pain, uterine contractions cease. The maternal systolic BP drops 15 mm Hg.

797. You should

(A) immediately perform a pelvic examination

(B) place the patient on her side and reassure her

(C) manage expectantly

(D) begin oxytocin

(E) perform an ultrasound

798. On abdominal examination, you discover a firm mass in the pelvis. It does not feel like the presenting fetal part. The firm mass is most likely

(A) the placenta

(B) a uterine fibroid

(C) the contracted uterus

(D) the fetal head

(E) a pelvic kidney

799. A woman without prenatal care in labor at 38 weeks has a breech presentation. As the breech is expelled, a spina bifida is noted. The head does not deliver. With this history, the most likely possibility listed is

(A) hydrocephaly
(B) cephalopelvic disproportion (CPD)
(C) fetal goiter
(D) missed labor
(E) incompletely dilated cervix

DIRECTIONS (Questions 800 through 829): Each of the numbered items or incomplete statements in this section is followed by answers or by completions of the statement. Select the answers or completions that may apply.

800. In discussing reasons to use caudal anesthesia in your laboring patient, you mention which three of the following contraindications?

(A) pilonidal sinus
(B) thrombocytopenia
(C) maternal heart disease
(D) anticoagulant therapy
(E) premature labor

801. Which three of the following are recognized hazards of caudal anesthesia?

(A) maternal hypotension
(B) high spinal block
(C) fetal injection
(D) decrease in uterine contractions
(E) pudendal nerve palsy

802. A patient in labor with a systolic BP of 125 has just been given a saddle block. While lying on her back on the delivery table, the level of the block stabilized at T10, and labor showed decreased intensity of uterine contractions. However, her blood pressure dropped to 90 systolic. Which two of the following causes of these symptoms are most likely?

(A) high spinal block
(B) ruptured uterus
(C) cardiac failure
(D) acute vasodilation
(E) supine hypotensive syndrome

803. Maternal aspiration of gastric contents during labor may be caused by which of the following three conditions?

(A) gastric hypomotility
(B) pelvic pain
(C) pneumothorax
(D) anesthesia
(E) narcotics

804. Which three of the following are indications to anticipate doing a classic cesarean section rather than a traditional transverse lower uterine segment cesarean section?

(A) transverse lie at term
(B) vertical skin incision
(C) 24-week gestation with a breech presentation
(D) fundal myoma
(E) perimortem cesarean section

805. Which three of the following situations would be likely to have the complication of a contracted pelvis?

(A) floating head at term in early labor in a primigravida
(B) face presentation
(C) pendulous abdomen in a primigravida
(D) obese multigravida
(E) short maternal stature

806. The pathologic retraction ring of Bandl is associated with which two of the following?

(A) premature labor
(B) rupture of the uterine fundus
(C) obstructed labor
(D) precipitate labor

807. You are called to labor and delivery to consult on a 23-year-old primiparous patient. The labor curve at left has been plotted by the nurse. Which three of the following etiologies are likely?

    (A) cephalopelvic disproportion (CPD)
    (B) anesthesia
    (C) abnormal uterine contractions
    (D) prematurity
    (E) meconium

808. Which four of the following are factors predisposing to uterine atony?

    (A) deep anesthesia
    (B) high parity
    (C) prolonged labor
    (D) overdistended uterus
    (E) preterm fetus

809. The nurses in labor and delivery are discussing the labor curve shown in Figure 11–2. The mother, an 18-year-old gravida 1, para 1, delivered last night. The nurses ask you about possible causes. Which four of the following are possible causes?

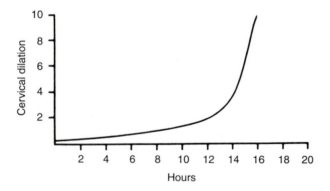

Figure 11–2.

    (A) early sedation
    (B) abnormal uterine contractions
    (C) cephalopelvic disproportion (CPD)
    (D) unripe cervix
    (E) anesthesia

810. Term labors lasting less than 3 hours are associated with which two conditions?

    (A) decreased fetal morbidity
    (B) increased maternal morbidity
    (C) increased fetal morbidity
    (D) primiparous labors
    (E) twins

811. You are delivering a 22-year-old woman's (gravida 2, para 0010) twin pregnancy at 38 weeks. The first baby is 6½ lb estimated fetal weight and vertex. The second is estimated at 6 lb and breech. In discussing complications of internal podalic version, you discuss which two of the following?

    (A) fecal contamination
    (B) rupture of the lower uterine segment
    (C) perineal tear
    (D) undiagnosed hydrocephaly
    (E) fetal trauma

812. Which two of the following define brow presentation?

    (A) is less common than face presentation
    (B) presents a small diameter of the head to the pelvic inlet
    (C) usually converts to a face or occiput
    (D) is recognized by vaginal palpation of the mouth
    (E) in a term infant usually results in vaginal delivery as a brow

813. The situations associated with premature labor include which four of the following?

    (A) bacterial vaginal infection
    (B) abruptio placentae
    (C) polyhydramnios
    (D) multiple pregnancy
    (E) anencephaly

814. Your patient has been in labor for over 12 hours and is febrile to 101.2°F. Pulse is 110 bpm. The fetal heart rate is 180 with good variability. The labor is progressing adequately. Appropriate steps may include which of the following?

(A) IV hydration

(B) antibiotics

(C) oxytocin

(D) fetal scalp sampling

(E) cesarean delivery

815. Abruptio placentae consists of which four of the following?

(A) occurs more frequently in hypertensive patients

(B) may lead to coagulopathy

(C) has a significant risk of recurrence in subsequent pregnancies

(D) reduces the effective nutrient exchange in the placenta

(E) presents as a consistent triad of uterine pain, bleeding, and abnormal fetal heart tones

816. A laboring patient receiving oxytocin for augmentation of labor suddenly clutches her chest in pain. Amniotic fluid embolus (AFE) is suspected. Signs and symptoms occurring with AFE include which three of the following?

(A) cyanosis

(B) pulmonary edema

(C) fever

(D) coagulopathy

(E) tumultuous labor and contractions

817. Treatment for AFE may include which three of the following?

(A) hysterectomy

(B) oxygen

(C) replacement of blood factors

(D) assisted ventilation

(E) corticosteroids

818. Conditions associated with a transverse lie of the fetus include which three of the following?

(A) placenta previa

(B) pelvic contraction

(C) placental abruption

(D) grand multiparity

(E) oligohydramnios

819. Which three of the following factors would predispose to a breech presentation?

(A) multiparity

(B) gestational diabetes

(C) uterine anomalies

(D) posterior implantation of the placenta

(E) fetal anomalies

820. Which three of the following may be associated with an increased incidence of abnormal fetal presentation?

(A) prematurity

(B) hypertensive disorders

(C) singleton infant

(D) soft tissue obstruction

(E) fetal malformation

821. You are checking a 22-year-old primigravida in active labor. Labor has lasted 14 hours. She is 8 cm dilated and at 0 station. As the fetal head has descended, the shape has changed. Which of the following may be causes?

(A) cephalohematoma

(B) molding

(C) subdural hematomas

(D) hydrocephalus

(E) caput succedaneum

822. Which four of the following factors increase the possibility of maternal aspiration of gastric contents during labor and delivery?

(A) high progesterone levels of pregnancy

(B) regional anesthesia causing sympathetic blockade

(C) increased gastric secretion

(D) IV analgesics

(E) pushing efforts in the second stage

823. Dystocia may be due to which three of the following?

- (A) maternal hypertensive disorders
- (B) ineffective uterine contractions
- (C) fetal abnormalities
- (D) abnormalities of the birth canal
- (E) electrolyte imbalance

824. Which three of the following are examples of soft tissue dystocia?

- (A) marked distention of the bladder
- (B) lower uterine segment myomas
- (C) bilateral pelvic kidneys
- (D) frozen hip joint secondary to motor vehicle accident
- (E) diagonal conjugate of 9 cm

825. Certain patients are more likely than others to have uterine atony and hemorrhage after delivery. Circumstances that allow one to anticipate increased bleeding postpartum are which two of the following?

- (A) prolonged labor
- (B) primigravidas
- (C) distended uterus
- (D) pudendal anesthesia for delivery
- (E) obesity

826. You have just delivered an 18-year-old woman (gravida 1, para 0). She is preeclamptic. Her uterus is soft with moderate bleeding. Examination reveals no laceration. You diagnose uterine atony. Of the following, which two options are the better choices?

- (A) 0.2 mg IM ergonovine (methergine)
- (B) 0.2 mg oral ergonovine
- (C) 10 units oral oxytocin
- (D) 250 μg prostaglandin F_2-alpha
- (E) 20 units oxytocin given IV

827. A 32-year-old woman (gravida 2, para 2) who has delivered by vaginal birth after cesarean (VBAC) is found bleeding heavily after delivery. At laparotomy you close the uterus easily, but a large, broad ligament hematoma and persistent bleeding are found. The site of the bleeding cannot be readily identified. Your best choices are which two of the following?

- (A) pack the uterus
- (B) take wide sutures in the broad ligament
- (C) ligate the external iliac artery
- (D) ligate the uterine artery
- (E) ligate the internal iliac artery

Questions 828 and 829

A 31-year-old healthy woman (gravida 3, para 2) is in normal labor at 40 weeks' gestation. Her first delivery was a low transverse cesarean for breech; the second was an uncomplicated VBAC. Her vital signs have been stable. Her epidural is functioning normally, and she is on her side. When the cervix was approximately 7 cm dilated and the fetus was at −1 station, she developed tachycardia to 120 and a drop in blood pressure from 115/60 to 70/30. She has become dizzy upon sitting up. Uterine contractions are continuing normally, and fetal heart tones (FHTs) are 130. No bleeding is evident.

828. The hematocrit is reported at 35%. Your differential diagnosis should include which three of the following?

- (A) vasa previa
- (B) pulmonary embolus
- (C) anesthetic complication
- (D) supine hypotensive syndrome
- (E) ruptured uterus

829. During an attempted VBAC, labor stops; the fetal parts are palpated abdominally on exam, and FHTs are heard at 80/min. You can feel fetal feet at −2 station. You should do which two of the following?

- (A) perform immediate laparotomy
- (B) give oxygen
- (C) given oxytocin to prevent maternal bleeding
- (D) perform breech extraction as soon as possible
- (E) give terbutaline to stop the contractions

DIRECTIONS (Questions 830 through 847): Each group of items in this section consists of lettered headings followed by a set of numbered words or phrases. For each numbered word or phrase, select the ONE lettered heading that is most closely associated with it. Each lettered heading may be selected once, more than once, or not at all.

Questions 830 and 831

    (A) prolonged latent phase
    (B) prolonged deceleration phase
    (C) prolonged active phase
    (D) arrest of labor
    (E) normal labor

830. Primiparous patient dilated 2 cm for 6 hours

831. Multiparous patient at 7 cm for 3 hours

Questions 832 through 834

    (A) occiput posterior
    (B) footling breech
    (C) mentum posterior
    (D) frank breech
    (E) mentum anterior

832. Has a high incidence of prolapsed cord

833. On pelvic examination, fetal bony prominences and a body orifice form a straight line; no extremities are palpated

834. Is undeliverable vaginally at term unless rotation occurs

Questions 835 through 839

    (A) breech
    (B) foot
    (C) face
    (D) anterior fontanel
    (E) compound

835. Bony prominences in line with an orifice.

836. Laterality can be determined by shaking hands.

837. Has both an anterior and posterior suture line.

838. Bony prominences and an orifice form a triangle.

839. Identified by a single bony prominence.

Questions 840 through 842

    (A) obliquely contracted pelvis
    (B) false promontory
    (C) chondroma
    (D) separation of the symphysis pubis
    (E) exostoses

840. Associated with lumbosacral kyphosis

841. Due to persistent unilateral leg deformity in early life

842. A nonbony lesion of the pelvis that may obstruct labor

Questions 843 through 847

Choose the most common listed cause of the problem in the cases presented.

    (A) rupture of a classic uterine scar
    (B) dehiscence of a uterine scar
    (C) spontaneous rupture of the intact uterus
    (D) cervical tear
    (E) traumatic rupture of the intact uterus

843. A patient develops severe hemorrhage during the third stage of an otherwise normal labor; the uterus is firmly contracted.

844. May be produced by injudicious use of Pitocin.

845. A prior, low transverse section scar is found to be paper thin and covered with only the peritoneum at the time of a repeat cesarean section.

846. Approximately one third occur prior to the onset of labor.

847. Tends to occur in the fundus during pregnancy and in the lower uterine segment during labor.

DIRECTIONS (Questions 848 through 851): Each group of items in this section consists of lettered headings followed by a set of numbered words or phrases. For each numbered word or phrase, select

    (A) if the item is associated with (A) only,

    (B) if the item is associated with (B) only,

    (C) if the item is associated with both (A) and (B),

    (D) if the item is associated with neither (A) nor (B).

Questions 848 through 851

    (A) hypotonic uterine dysfunction

    (B) hypertonic uterine dysfunction

    (C) both

    (D) neither

848. Has a synchronous pattern of myometrial activity.

849. Is aided by sedation.

850. Normally produces a rapid labor.

851. Oxytocin causes an increase in the dysfunction.

Answers and Explanations

768. (C) An exact time for optimum labor cannot be established, but prolonged labor leading to maternal exhaustion, often secondary to a disproportion can lead to increased fetal morbidity. The accepted time for the second stage is usually 2 hours. This makes observation of labor curves and fetal monitoring essential parts of the management.

769. (B) The pattern is one of secondary arrest of labor. Cephalopelvic disproportion (CPD) is the most likely cause. Therefore, the first step is the evaluation of the pelvis. Delivery through an inadequate pelvis is always contraindicated.

770. (A) The most common indications for primary cesarean section are CPD and uterine inertia, which are the reasons for dystocia. The most common reason for all cesarean sections is the history of a prior cesarean section.

771. (E) Preterm rupture of membranes refers to rupture before 37 weeks' gestation. Arguments exist as to the most appropriate therapy for preterm rupture of membranes. If it occurs early in gestation, one must balance the risk of infection against the risk of prematurity if labor is induced. The greatest risk is intrauterine or fetal infection. Premature rupture is prior to the onset of labor.

772. (C) The pH of amniotic fluid is alkaline, 7.0 to 7.5, and the nitrazine paper should turn blue or blue-green. However, blood will cause this reaction also. Superficial squamous cells are found in the normal vagina. Drainage on the patient's underwear could be vaginal secretion or urine.

773. (D) The length of labor generally lessens with increasing parity. The age of the mother alone does not affect labor. Smaller babies generally have a shorter second stage of labor. The occiput posterior position generally increases the total length of labor by 60 to 120 minutes.

774. (C) Partial breech extraction is a safe and effective means of delivering a breech. Piper forceps may also be applied to the aftercoming head for control. Spontaneous delivery is also possible.

775. (A) Current data suggest that a woman with breech presentation at term should be offered cesarean delivery. The Multisite Term Breech Delivery Study found higher morbidity to the fetus in this situation.

776. (D) Often, a classic or vertical uterine incision is the wisest choice, as extracting the infant through a low transverse incision may be extremely difficult. The purpose of abdominal delivery is to avoid fetal trauma. An inadequate uterine incision would defeat this intention.

777. (A) Anencephalics often have face presentation because of the lack of a cranium. Breeches are common with prematurity and hydrocephalus. Placenta previa does not allow a presenting part in the pelvis.

778. (D) Cesarean section is indicated for a transverse lie. The incision on the uterus will depend on assessment at surgery for ease of delivery.

779. (E) Vertex premature births may proceed spontaneously. In fact, use of a vacuum extraction may injure a premature infant presenting by vertex.

780. (C) Ready access to the pulmonary vessels is available while placing a Swan–Ganz catheter to monitor the patient. Another way of diagnosing amniotic fluid emboli is finding debris in blood from the right heart. However, presumptive diagnosis is made from suggestive signs and symptoms, and treatment is begun then.

781. (B) An absolute contraindication to the use of oxytocin is hypertonic uterine dysfunction. Oxytocin tends to increase hypertonic uterine dysfunction in the hypertonic uterus. Hypotonic uterine dysfunction is the principal indication for oxytocin. A dead fetus will obviously not be adversely affected. If the uterus can tolerate labor, oxytocin can be used judiciously with close monitoring in twin gestation.

782. (A) The only indication for internal podalic version that is at all likely to occur is the second twin. A transverse lie with a completely dilated cervix and intact membranes is extremely rare. A prolapsed cord with fully dilated cervix, unengaged vertex, and recently ruptured membranes is another possible indication, but this situation would be extremely rare also. Generally, cesarean section is a safer and more expeditious procedure.

783. (B) Shoulder dystocia creates an obstetric emergency. One must know what to do because no time will be available to read about it if it occurs. Many maneuvers have been described—all with fair success. You should know McRoberts maneuver, which is extreme flexion of the thighs. Others include suprapubic pressure and rotation of the posterior shoulders.

784. (E) A dictum in obstetrics is that a partially separated placenta bleeds. One that is not separated generally does not bleed. The bleeding occurs when attempts are made to deliver the placenta. Placenta accreta may require hysterectomy.

785. (A) Fortunately, the most feared infection (HIV) is the most rare, estimated at 1:300,000. Hepatitis is still the greatest risk for infection, although currently all blood for transfusion is checked for hepatitis B antigen.

786. (A) Since about 15% of white individuals in the United States are Rh-negative and as little as 0.1 mL of Rh-positive blood can sensitize an Rh-negative woman, it is amazing that less than 10% of all Rh-negative gravidas become sensitized to the Rh factor.

787. (D) O-negative blood should not have A or B antigens, nor should it sensitize or cause a reaction with the D antigen of the Rh system.

788. (D) Smoking tends to cause a decrease in fetal size. Although people with mild, uncontrolled diabetes have large children, severe diabetics tend to have "small-for-dates" infants. In multiparous patients, there is a tendency for subsequent children to be slightly larger. In postdate pregnancies, infants often continue to grow.

789. (B) One may start the cervical dilation by gently tearing the center of the cervix, after which dilation usually proceeds rapidly. This is a rare situation, and manual dilation is rarely indicated.

790. (E) In the absence of factors necessitating immediate action, the patient should be followed closely until the dangers of prematurity are past. Decision as to mode of delivery will depend on the position and size of the tumor. Myomectomy during pregnancy may precipitate labor and is almost always a contraindication. Myomas may also undergo red (hemorrhagic) infarction during pregnancy, causing pain and bleeding.

791. **(E)** Duhrssen's incisions are contraindicated in almost all cases. A trapped head of a small infant during breech delivery may be the only indication.

792. **(D)** Excluding perineal tears in the lower third, the most likely position for vaginal tears is over the ischial spines. This site should be specifically examined. Suburethral and high lateral fornix areas should also be routinely examined, as well as the cervix.

793. **(B)** The usual classifications do not include fifth-degree tears. Some use fourth degree as being through the rectal mucosa, while others use third degree with extension to the rectum to designate the most severe laceration. An anatomic repair in layers without devitalizing of tissue should ensure good healing.

794. **(A)** Massage and oxytocin is a good regimen for uterine atony, and may make even a ruptured uterus stop bleeding for a short time. After uterine atony, the next most common cause of bleeding postpartum is a laceration. Therefore, all postpartum bleeders should be reexamined to rule out such tears.

795. **(D)** The uterus can be enlarged due to extravasation of blood between the myometrial fibers. If severe, this bleeding may inhibit uterine contractions, though such severity is quite rare. If stable and not expanding, the intramyometrial hematoma is best left alone! Coagulopathy and lack of specific bleeding sites dictate conservative therapy.

796. **(A)** Maternal mortality from rupture of an intact uterus may be as much as 10%. The infant's prognosis is much worse. Obstruction or hyperstimulation is the most common etiology.

797. **(A)** This is a classic example of uterine rupture. If rupture has occurred, fetal mortality is very likely and one should anticipate the possibility of rapid onset of severe maternal shock. Delivery and mechanical methods will stop the bleeding. Massive vascular support is often necessary to save the mother's life.

798. **(C)** With the history of severe pain and cessation of contractions, the fetal head is probably no longer in the pelvis and the diagnosis of uterine rupture is more certain. Evaluation and treatment must be rapid.

799. **(A)** Spina bifida is noted in approximately one third of fetuses with hydrocephaly. Its presence in the situation described should immediately warn of the defect. This can become a very difficult problem if no further assessment of the degree of hydrocephalus has been made.

800. **(A, B, D)** Infections that are often found in pilonidal sinuses or deformities of the sacral area are contraindications to caudal anesthesia, as the infection may be spread or the spinal canal may be inaccessible. Thrombocytopenia and anticoagulant therapy are also contraindications. Caudal is a good choice in maternal heart disease and premature labor. It may also facilitate forceps delivery. Continuous administration avoids overdose and waning of the block.

801. **(A, B, D)** The pudendal nerve should not be damaged by caudal anesthesia, nor is the fetus affected. Maternal hypotension is the most significant common occurrence with caudal anesthesia. Hypotension can be avoided by fluid loading prior to anesthetic administration. Rarely, contractions may decrease.

802. **(D, E)** The supine hypotension can be relieved by putting the patient on her side or pushing the uterus off of the great vessels to allow adequate cardiac return and aortic flow. Increased fluid administration and medication can both be used to elevate blood pressure.

803. **(A, D, E)** Vomiting in labor is common, but aspiration is not—unless the patient is unconscious. Anesthesia ranks among the top four to six causes of maternal death. One of the mechanisms is by aspiration of vomitus with either food particle occlusion of the bronchioles or gastric acid burn of the alveoli

(Mendelson syndrome). The gastric hypo-motility leads to decreased gastric emptying. Maternal narcotics may lead to oversedation.

804. (A, C, E) The extraction of a fetus in a transverse lie through a low segment incision may be impossible without extending the incision. Anchor or T-shaped incisions do not heal well. Physical factors making lower segment dissection difficult or time consuming certainly favor vertical incisions. Time may also be important when forced to do a perimortem cesarean section. Premature breech fetuses may present with a poorly developed lower uterine segment.

805. (A, B, E) All the factors except obesity are danger signs warning the obstetrician to look for a small pelvis. Prior knowledge of borderline or absolute pelvic contraction can avert disaster. A good clue is an abnormal labor curve.

806. (B, C) If a prolonged obstructed labor is neglected, a thin and overdistended uterine segment may rupture. Cesarean section should be performed before a pathologic retraction ring has time to develop. In attended labor, Bandl's ring has become a rarity.

807. (A, B, C) Secondary arrest of labor of 2 hours' duration may be due to several factors, but meconium or prematurity should not affect the progress of dilation.

808. (A, B, C, D) All of the factors listed except the small fetus decrease the ability of the uterus to contract well and therefore add to the possibility of uterine bleeding. Poor contractions in the second stage often mean poor contractions postpartum. Anticipating atony can be helpful in having readily available appropriate medications, instruments, assistants, and blood.

809. (A, B, D, E) The curve has a prolonged latent phase that could be due to sedation, abnormal uterine contractions, an unripe cervix, or anesthesia given too early. CPD tends to

cause either a very slow increase or secondary arrest of cervical dilation. One would anticipate a normal delivery given this labor curve.

810. (B, C) Precipitate labors have an increased rate of fetal brain damage and hypoxia and an increased maternal morbidity.

811. (B, E) Fetal trauma can occur, but if the procedure is done only for indicated reasons, such as delivery of the second twin, it should not be a major factor. Rupture of the lower uterine segment is a potential danger, especially if the segment is thinned out.

812. (A, C) The brow presentation presents the largest diameter of the head to the pelvic inlet. Unless it converts spontaneously to a face or occiput in a term infant, the labor will usually be obstructed. Fortunately, brow is the least common type of presentation. It is recognized because one can feel the orbital ridges and eyes, but not the mouth or chin by vaginal examination.

813. (A, B, C, D) Anencephaly may result in post-term labor unless there is polyhydramnios due to inability of the fetus to swallow. The other situations often result in preterm labor. In more than half the cases, we cannot find an adequate explanation for the occurrence of premature labor. The treatment of preterm labor depends on the etiology and also is inadequate in many cases.

814. (A, B) Intervention with hydration and antibiotics may be indicated for infection. Cesarean delivery and oxytocin are not necessary if labor is progressing well.

815. (A, B, C, D) Obviously, less placental attachment provides less circulation and less nutrient exchange. Hypertension, coagulopathy, premature rupture of membranes, and multiparity are all associated with abruption, but the signs are quite variable. Uterine pain and abnormal fetal heart rate are common, but typically the bleeding is hidden.

816. **(A, B, D)** The sudden onset of dyspnea, cyanosis, and shock during labor should make one immediately consider amniotic fluid embolus, aspiration of gastric content, or heart failure. Immediate cardiorespiratory support should be given. The coagulopathy is almost pathognomonic for AFE.

817. **(B, C, D)** Hysterectomy is of no use and will only add operative insult. Immediate use of corticosteroids is also of minimal benefit. Positive end expiratory pressure–assisted respiration may be lifesaving in pulmonary edema from either cause, and replacement of blood products is usually indicated for the disseminated intravascular coagulopathy of AFE.

818. **(A, B, D)** If labor is in progress and the membranes are ruptured in the presence of a transverse lie, perinatal mortality is high, with complications of prolapsed cord and infection, as well as trauma. Immediate cesarean section is indicated. Placenta previa must always be considered as a possible complication even if one or more of the other etiologic factors are present. Pelvic contraction and grand multiparity are also associated with transverse lie.

819. **(A, C, E)** A posterior placental implantation does not predispose to breech presentation. Multiparity, low fluid volume, and uterine and fetal anomalies do.

820. **(A, D, E)** The normal single fetus provides the baseline for incidence of abnormal presentation. Other predisposing factors are lax uterine and abdominal muscles and uterine malformations. Any factor allowing increased or decreased fetal mobility can contribute to abnormal fetal position.

821. **(A, B, E)** Subdural hematomas, although they may occur, generally do not contribute to any marked change in shape. Cephalohematoma is a possibility, although it is unlikely to occur at this station. Molding and caput are normal changes in head shape to accommodate the birth canal and should not cause the head to change shape.

822. **(A, B, C, D)** Aspiration of gastric contents is most likely during inhalation anesthesia but can occur after any hypotensive episode. Vomiting is made more likely because of the relaxation of smooth muscle due to progesterone and the increased gastric secretion present during pregnancy. Increased intra-abdominal distention may also play a role. Intubation is protective, as is an empty stomach and preoperative administration of antacids. Pushing has no effect.

823. **(B, C, D)** One can think of dystocia as occurring because of some abnormality of the powers, the passenger, or the passage. Electrolyte imbalance and maternal hypertensive disease play no known direct role.

824. **(A, B, C)** The short diagonal conjugate is a bony pelvis problem. Hip joint trauma is also bony. The other soft tissue factors are all rare, but the obstetrician should be cognizant of their occurrence. Any entity that blocks the birth canal or could take up space in the pelvis is a possible cause. All need to be considered in dystocia.

825. **(A, C)** Other predictors of increased postpartum bleeding include past history of atony and high parity. Atony, injuries, and retained placental fragments are by far the most common. Obesity alone is not a significant cause.

826. **(D, E)** Ergot derivatives should not be given in patients with hypertension, and oxytocin is not effective orally, though it can be given by the buccal route.

827. **(D, E)** Packing is fruitless and wastes time since the broad ligament is bleeding. Deep sutures are apt to injure the ureter and not stop the bleeding. Both, therefore, are contraindicated. Often, ligation of the internal iliac artery on the affected side will decrease the blood flow. Occasionally, bilateral ligation is needed. Another choice, depending on conditions, is to ligate the uterine artery.

828. **(B, C, E)** Although it is unusual for labor to persist with a ruptured uterus, it must be included in the differential. Vasa previa would

cause immediate fetal distress. Pulmonary complication and anesthetic complication are also possibilities. Supine hypotension should not occur on her side.

829. **(A, B)** Obviously, some catastrophic event has occurred. Laparotomy is indicated. Oxygen should also be given.

830. **(A)** The latent phase is that initial time of labor during which effacement occurs but dilation is slow. Normal limits have been defined for its completion and therapies outlined for protraction disorders.

831. **(D)** In this case, cervical dilation was progressing normally when suddenly no further dilation occurred. If this happens in the active phase, it is called secondary arrest of labor. Assessment of fetal size, uterine contractility, and pelvic adequacy is indicated.

832. **(B)** The lack of a solid portion of fetal anatomy to occlude the pelvis allows the cord to prolapse.

833. **(D)** Because it is quite rare, a face presentation may be mistaken for a breech presentation. An important diagnostic differential between a face and a breech presentation is that the mouth and malar eminences form a triangle, while the ischial tuberosities and anus are in line.

834. **(C)** The head becomes wedged between the sacrum and symphysis and cannot extend without rotation. Small prematures may deliver from this position.

835. **(A)** The ischial tuberosities and the anus form a straight line across the breech. The face presents with the malar eminences and mouth in a triangular configuration.

836. **(E)** The hand will be identified as right or left if you grasp it as though shaking hands. The infant's right hand will fit with your right hand. This presentation does not preclude vaginal delivery.

837. **(D)** By sweeping the finger anterior to the anterior fontanel, another suture is palpated. Posterior to the posterior fontanel, one feels only the occipital bone. The Y shape of the posterior sutures meeting the sagittal sutures also aids in identification of position.

838. **(C)** A face presentation can be difficult to distinguish from a breech. Remember that the malar eminences and the mouth form a triangle, not a straight line.

839. **(B)** The heel allows one to distinguish the foot from the hand by palpation. The hand has no such bony protuberances. It also has an opposed thumb! Do not forget that a speculum can be used to visualize the presenting part. If doubt exists as to the fetal position, check it with ultrasound.

840. **(B)** This protuberance above the sacral curve may cause dystocia even if the diagonal conjugate is normal. The shortest anteroposterior (AP) diameter is one of most concern. This is referred to as the *pseudoconjugate*. Be aware that maternal skeletal malformations may cause change in size and shape of the pelvic birth canal.

841. **(A)** Weight is carried on the normal leg, and the pelvis becomes higher on the unaffected side with a compensatory scoliosis. Look for this deformity in patients with a long-standing limp.

842. **(C)** Other tumors of the pelvis are fibromas, osteomas, sarcomas, and carcinomas. Pelvic examination will discover their presence. Exostoses are bony outgrowths. Any space-occupying lesion can certainly prevent delivery.

843. **(D)** A deep cervical tear or vaginal laceration is the most likely cause of the bleeding in the situation described. Lower segment rupture can also cause bleeding during the third stage but is less common and tends to decrease if the uterus contracts firmly. Good visualization and assistance are often necessary to recognize and correct this problem.

844. **(E)** Poor use of oxytocin, fundal pressure, version and extraction, and forceps injury are other obstetric causes of traumatic uterine rupture. These should be used only when indicated and only when complications can be handled.

845. **(B)** Dehiscence is more common in low transverse than in classic scars. The fetal membranes remain intact and after labor can proceed normally if there is no obstruction. The risk of rupture is increased, however. Unless transvaginal examination is performed after normal delivery, these scar defects may never be found.

846. **(A)** In contrast, low segment scars seldom rupture until labor has occurred. The classic scar will usually hold up during normal labor, but the risk is still too high to leave it to chance.

847. **(C)** Spontaneous rupture is exceedingly rare in the absence of labor, but probably the greatest number of uterine ruptures presently fall into the spontaneous group. Predisposing factors include uterine overdistention and possible congenital defects.

848. **(A)** In essence, this type of contraction is weak but normal in its pattern of force application. Contractions often reach pressures above 15 mm Hg. The final assessment is effect on cervical dilation.

849. **(B)** Hypertonic contractions are often asynchronous and often painful but do not accomplish efficient cervical dilation. If sedation can break up this pattern, a normal progression may occur. Adequate hydration and positioning may also help.

850. **(D)** The hypotonic contractions are too weak and the hypertonic too inefficient to produce normal cervical dilation. Regular contractions of normal strength and frequency are best. Progression speed is often independent of strength, suggesting a cervical factor.

851. **(B)** Oxytocin simply causes an increase in the asynchronous, nonfundal-dominant contraction pattern. Clinically, if the contraction is painful with a hard uterus but the cervix is not put on stretch at the height of the contraction and no dilation is occurring, hypertonic dysfunction should be suspected. Oxytocin is contraindicated.

CHAPTER 12

Operative Obstetrics
Questions

DIRECTIONS (Questions 852 through 905): Each of the numbered items or incomplete statements in this section is followed by answers or by completions of the statement. Select the ONE lettered answer or completion that is BEST in each case.

852. A 23-year-old woman (gravida 1, para 0) comes to your office approximately 6 weeks' pregnant. A home pregnancy test was positive 1½ weeks ago. She has developed bleeding over the past 2 days. Which of the following is the most likely cause of the bleeding?

    (A) hydatidiform mole
    (B) abruptio placentae
    (C) ectopic pregnancy
    (D) abortion
    (E) uterine rupture

853. Hertig found that the average time for spontaneous expulsion of an abnormal fetus that aborted was about 10 to 11 weeks after the last menstrual period (LMP). If the embryo is present, it usually

    (A) is alive at the time of expulsion
    (B) died just prior to expulsion
    (C) had been dead for 1 to 2 days before expulsion
    (D) had been dead for 1 to 2 weeks before expulsion
    (E) had been dead for 5 to 6 weeks before expulsion

854. If a patient who has a threatened abortion does not abort, the risk of the fetus being abnormal is

    (A) the same as in patients without bleeding

    (B) slightly increased
    (C) moderately increased
    (D) markedly increased
    (E) 99 to 100%

855. Therapy for threatened abortion should include

    (A) progesterone IM
    (B) dilation and curettage (D&C)
    (C) prolonged bed rest
    (D) restricted activity
    (E) prostaglandin suppositories

856. You are in your office and a 19-year-old woman (gravida 1, para 0) with a positive pregnancy test 3 weeks ago at home has come in with complaints of mild cramping and light bleeding over the past 2 days. She does not believe that she has passed any tissue. During those 2 days, she has been at home on bed rest. Your first step is

    (A) thorough examination
    (B) D&C
    (C) give daily estrogen
    (D) give IM progesterone
    (E) advise continued bed rest

857. High doses of progesterone for threatened abortion may

    (A) save the fetus
    (B) keep the placenta alive
    (C) keep the corpus luteum functioning
    (D) cause habitual abortion
    (E) cause retention of a dead fetus

858. A major hazard of a fetal demise after 20 weeks is

(A) a positive human chorionic gonadotropin (hCG) titer

(B) systemic allergies

(C) bone marrow depression

(D) coagulopathy

(E) toxemia

859. Extrusion of an abortus from the fimbriated end of the tube is called

(A) spontaneous abortion

(B) delivery

(C) tubal abortion

(D) decidual cast

(E) Arias–Stella phenomenon

Questions 860 through 862

A 26-year-old woman whose last menstrual period (LMP) was 2½ months ago develops bleeding, uterine cramps, and passes tissue per vagina. Two hours later, she is still bleeding heavily.

860. The most likely diagnosis is

(A) twin pregnancy

(B) threatened abortion

(C) inevitable abortion

(D) premature labor

(E) incomplete abortion

861. Of the options listed, the bleeding is most likely due to

(A) retained products of conception

(B) ruptured uterus

(C) systemic coagulopathy

(D) vaginal lacerations

(E) bleeding hemorrhoids

862. The indicated procedure is

(A) hysterectomy

(B) vaginal packing

(C) compression of the hemorrhoids

(D) IV fibrinogen

(E) uterine curettage

Questions 863 through 865

A 24-year-old woman (gravida 2, para 0, abortus 1) is seen in the emergency department because of vaginal bleeding and abdominal cramps. Her LMP was 10 weeks ago. History is unrevealing except for an induced abortion 2 years ago without complications. She presently denies instrumentation for abortion. Physical examination reveals a BP of 110/70, pulse 120, and temperature 101.8°F. The abdomen is tender with slight rebound in the lower quadrants. The pelvic examination reveals blood in the vault and a foul-smelling discharge from the cervix, which is dilated to 2 cm. The uterus is 8- to 10-week size and tender, and no adnexal masses are palpated.

863. On the basis of the above information, the most likely diagnosis is

(A) choriocarcinoma

(B) hydatidiform mole

(C) pelvic inflammatory disease (PID)

(D) septic abortion

(E) twisted ovarian cyst

864. Ring forceps through the cervix removed necrotic-appearing tissue. Which of the following laboratory studies would you consider most important to obtain prior to instituting antibiotic therapy?

(A) white blood cell count (WBC) and hematocrit (Hct)

(B) type and Rh

(C) coagulation screen

(D) Gram stain and culture

(E) abdominal x-ray

865. Definitive initial therapy in this case is

(A) curettage after antibiotics

(B) hysterectomy

(C) bed rest and antibiotics

(D) hysterotomy

(E) outpatient antibiotics

866. Of the following women, which patient would be at greatest risk for ectopic pregnancy?

(A) a healthy woman on birth control pills

(B) a woman with past history of three incidents of PID

(C) a woman with history of endometriosis

(D) a healthy woman with irregular menses

(E) a woman with past history of several urinary tract infections (UTIs)

867. The most common implantation site for ectopic pregnancy is the

(A) external fallopian tube

(B) ovarian surface

(C) mesosalpinx

(D) ampulla of the fallopian tube

(E) interstitial portion of the fallopian tube

868. In a tubal ectopic pregnancy, the tube most commonly ruptures into the

(A) urachus

(B) bladder

(C) space of Retzius

(D) large bowel

(E) peritoneal cavity

869. The uterine cast sometimes shed when a patient has an ectopic pregnancy is made up of

(A) decidua capsularis

(B) decidua basalis

(C) decidua vera

(D) trophoblast

(E) blood

870. An interstitial ectopic pregnancy

(A) rarely exceeds 4 weeks' gestation

(B) is generally more dangerous than an ampullary ectopic pregnancy

(C) requires hysterectomy

(D) is quite common

(E) is extrauterine

871. Cervical pregnancy is rare and usually discovered before the fifth month of gestation because of bleeding. Of the following treatment options, the best therapy is

(A) immediate delivery per vagina

(B) transfuse as needed until viability of fetus is assured

(C) cesarean section

(D) chemotherapy with methotrexate

(E) estrogen injections and bed rest

872. The combination of an intrauterine and ectopic gestation (i.e., heterotopic pregnancy) is often considered, but the incidence in women who conceive spontaneously is about

(A) 1 in 1,000 births

(B) 1 in 7,000 births

(C) 1 in 15,000 births

(D) 1 in 30,000 births

(E) 1 in 60,000 births

873. You are called to the operating room. The general surgeons have operated on a woman to rule out appendicitis and they find signs of an abdominal pregnancy with an 18-week fetus and placenta attached to the omentum. The best course of action in this case is

(A) removal of both fetus and placenta

(B) laparoscopic ligation of umbilical cord

(C) removal of the fetus only

(D) closely follow until viability and then deliver by laparotomy

(E) IV methotrexate and removal of the fetus

874. Of the following, the BEST diagnostic sign indicating an abdominal pregnancy is

(A) positive pregnancy test

(B) ultrasound view not demonstrating uterine wall between fetus and bladder

(C) abnormal position of the fetus

(D) lateral x-rays showing fetal parts overlying the maternal spine

(E) uterine contractions with oxytocin administration

875. At laparotomy for a suspected ectopic pregnancy in a 24-year-old woman who wishes to bear children, you find a ruptured left tubal ectopic with about 400 mL of blood in the peritoneal cavity. The other tube appears normal, and the ovaries are uninvolved. The accepted treatment is

(A) bilateral salpingectomy
(B) left salpingectomy or salpingostomy
(C) bilateral salpingo-oophorectomy (BSO)
(D) hysterectomy and left salpingectomy
(E) right salpingectomy

876. The forceps designed for rotation of the fetal head in the midpelvis is the

(A) Barton
(B) Tucker–McLane
(C) Kielland
(D) Piper
(E) Simpson

877. Application of forceps is appropriate in which of the following situations?

(A) breech at +3 station, cervix completely dilated, membranes ruptured
(B) vertex at +1 station, cervix completely dilated, membranes intact
(C) mentum anterior, +3 station, cervix completely dilated, membranes ruptured
(D) transverse lie, +2 station, cervix completely dilated, membranes ruptured
(E) vertex at +2 station, cervix +8 cm dilated, membranes ruptured

878. Anticipating success, an operator has made a concerted attempt to deliver a patient using forceps. The attempt fails. The procedure is termed

(A) an incompelte delivery
(B) a trial of forceps
(C) malapplication of forceps
(D) failed forceps
(E) high forceps

879. You are delivering a woman (gravida 3, para 2) with two previous successful vaginal births. The woman has been in labor for 12 hours with a 10-hour first stage. The second stage of labor has lasted approximately 1 hour and 14 minutes. The baby is doing well without any evidence of distress. You feel that it is an appropriate size (approximately 8 lbs). The mother has had an epidural and is tired from pushing, and you decide to apply forceps. After pelvic examination, forceps are applied to the presenting part of a term pregnancy, but the lock does not properly articulate even with gentle maneuvering. You should

(A) rotate the forceps
(B) apply enough pressure to lock the forceps
(C) exert traction
(D) reapply the forceps

880. Relative contraindications to the use of vacuum extraction for delivery include

(A) nonvertex presentation
(B) fetal coagulopathies
(C) following fetal scalp sampling
(D) fetal prematurity
(E) all of the above

Questions 881 through 883

A 19-year-old primigravida at term has been in active labor for 4 hours. The membranes have just ruptured; the station is −3, fetal heart tones (FHTs) are 140 and regular, and the cervix is dilated 4 cm. Contractions are every 5 minutes and last approximately 40 seconds.

881. At this point, the BEST of the following plans of management is

(A) patient ambulation
(B) oxytocin augmentation
(C) cesarean section
(D) clinical pelvimetry and estimation of fetal size
(E) turn the patient on her side

882. The patient continues to have infrequent contractions. Your clinical pelvimetry is within normal limits. Estimated fetal size is 7½ lbs. Pelvic findings are unchanged. Of the following options, which is the BEST choice at this point?

    (A) determine the maternal hydration status
    (B) patient ambulation
    (C) oxytocin infusion
    (D) cesarean section
    (E) await vaginal delivery

883. Three hours later, the cervix is 5 cm dilated and the contraction pattern is irregular despite significant oxytocin infusion. The station is –2 and the head is molded. The FHTs are normal. Of the following, the BEST choice is

    (A) Duhrssen's incisions
    (B) forceps delivery
    (C) increased oxytocin
    (D) heavy sedation
    (E) cesarean section

884. A disadvantage of lower segment cesarean section over the classic incision is

    (A) ease of repair
    (B) decreased blood loss
    (C) lower probability of subsequent uterine rupture
    (D) decreased danger of bladder injury
    (E) ease of fetal delivery

885. Primary treatment of bleeding vulvar varices during pregnancy is

    (A) cautery
    (B) application of pressure
    (C) simple vulvectomy
    (D) sclerosing injection
    (E) nothing

886. Bleeding into the myometrium beneath the uterine serosa in severe cases of abruptio placentae is a cause of

    (A) uteroplacental apoplexy
    (B) uterine rupture
    (C) minimal effect on fetal heart rate
    (D) adnexal torsion

887. Vaginal examination is contraindicated in which of the following situations during pregnancy?

    (A) carcinoma of the cervix
    (B) gonorrhea
    (C) prolapsed cord
    (D) placenta previa
    (E) active labor

888. A 30-year-old woman (gravida 4, para 2, abortus 1) has been seen in the emergency department at 29 weeks' gestation because of the sudden onset of painless vaginal bleeding that soaked four perineal pads and has now ceased. The mother's vital signs and hematocrit are normal, and the FHTs are regular at 140 bpm. At this time, you should

    (A) perform a double setup examination
    (B) order an ultrasound examination
    (C) perform a cesarean section
    (D) send the patient home on bed rest

889. A 35-year-old married woman (gravida 4, para 3, abortus 0), who now is at approximately 36 weeks' gestation, developed copious, painless, vaginal bleeding 2 hours prior to admission. On examination, the uterus appeared soft and nontender. FHTs are 140 and regular, the vertex is floating, and there is no evident bleeding or signs of ruptured membranes. Maternal vital signs are stable. Of the following choices, the most likely diagnosis is

    (A) carcinoma of the cervix
    (B) placenta previa
    (C) abruptio placentae
    (D) vasa previa
    (E) hematuria

890. In the event of continued bleeding, requiring repeated transfusions, in a patient at 32 weeks' gestation with a possible posterior placenta previa on ultrasound, which of the following should be done next?

(A) vaginal packing

(B) oxytocin induction of labor

(C) rupture of membranes and application of Willett's forceps

(D) double setup examination

(E) expectant treatment until the fetus reaches 34 to 36 weeks' gestation

891. Which of the following patients would be most likely to have a placenta previa?

(A) 19-year-old gravida 1, para 0, vertex presentation

(B) 24-year-old gravida 2, para 1, breech presentation

(C) 34-year-old gravida 5, para 3, abortus 1, vertex presentation

(D) 36-year-old gravida 7, para 6, abortus 0, transverse lie

(E) 28-year-old gravida 3, para 1, abortus 1, breech presentation

892. Of the following options, the safest, most precise, and simplest method of placental localization is

(A) auscultation

(B) ultrasonography

(C) radioisotope study

(D) abnormal palpation

(E) soft tissue x-ray

893. Duhrssen's incisions classically are made at which of the following positions on the cervix?

(A) 8 o'clock

(B) 9 and 3 o'clock

(C) 10, 2, and 6 o'clock

(D) 12 and 6 o'clock

(E) anterior to the fetal chin and posterior to the occiput

894. A deep mediolateral episiotomy would be most likely to encounter the

(A) superficial transverse perineal muscle

(B) coccygeus muscle

(C) ischiorectal fossa

(D) crus of the clitoris

(E) anal sphincter

Questions 895 and 896

A walk-in patient has presented in labor with a double footling breech. As the buttocks are delivered, a meningomyelocele is seen. There is sudden arrest of progression, and the head cannot be delivered. Examination reveals a large mass above the pubis abdominally. Vaginal palpation confirms the impression of a grossly enlarged head.

895. The most probable diagnosis is

(A) anencephaly

(B) diabetic infant

(C) hydrocephaly

(D) huge goiter

(E) polycystic kidneys

896. Internal version and extraction at term is indicated in

(A) face presentation mentum posterior

(B) shoulder presentation in early labor

(C) persistent brow

(D) the second twin

(E) transverse lie

Questions 897 and 898

A pregnant patient at 37 weeks' gestation complains of nausea, anorexia, and upper midabdominal pain for 10 hours. Her physical examination is negative except for right upper quadrant tenderness. Her temperature is 102°F, pulse 90, BP 110/60, FHTs 140, Hct 38, and WBC 11,900. Urinalysis is negative for protein and red blood cells (RBCs) are present.

897. Of the following, the most likely diagnosis is

(A) appendicitis

(B) ureteral stone

(C) degeneration of a myoma

(D) eclampsia

(E) pyelonephritis

898. On further evaluation, probable appendicitis is diagnosed. The treatment is

(A) antibiotics and ice packs

(B) cesarean section at the time of appendectomy

(C) 24 to 48 hours of observation

(D) immediate laparotomy and appendectomy if appendicitis is found

899. A 25-year-old patient at 27 weeks' gestation has complained of nausea, dull right flank pain persistent for 2 days, and mild diarrhea. She presently complains of pain in the mid-right abdomen and flank. On examination, the pulse is 90, temperature is 100°F, and BP is 120/70. Her chest is clear, uterus is midway between the xiphoid and umbilicus and nontender, with FHTs at 140. Pelvic examination is within normal limits, as is the rest of the physical. Urinalysis reveals 50 to 100 white blood cells/high power field (HPF). HCT is 37, WBC is 11,800 with 70 P, 28 L, 2 M. On the basis of this information, which of the following is the BEST diagnosis?

(A) duodenal ulcer

(B) volvulus

(C) degenerating leiomyoma

(D) placental abruption

(E) pyelonephritis

900. A 36-year-old woman (gravida 5, para 3, abortus 1) is first seen for her present pregnancy at 21 weeks' gestation. History and examination are within normal limits. A routine Pap smear is taken, which returns as high-grade squamous intraepithelial lesion (SIL) (cervical intraepithelial neoplasia [CIN] III). You should

(A) repeat the Pap

(B) advise abortion with cone biopsy or hysterectomy in 4 to 6 weeks

(C) wait until after delivery and obtain another smear

(D) perform a cesarean hysterectomy with wide vaginal cuff

(E) perform colposcopy and biopsy

901. Colposcopically directed biopsies of the cervix show carcinoma in situ. The colposcopy was inadequate, and there was question of microinvasive cervical carcinoma. You should advise her to strongly consider

(A) expectant management until fetal viability

(B) a hysterectomy with a wide vaginal cuff now

(C) a cervical cone

(D) a radical hysterectomy at fetal viability

(E) being followed with Pap smears and colposcopy until after delivery at term

902. In a similar patient, a cone biopsy is performed. The cone specimen returns with the diagnosis of carcinoma in situ and free surgical margins. Your advice is to

(A) follow the patient to term

(B) perform a radical hysterectomy

(C) perform a cesarean hysterectomy with wide vaginal cuff

(D) give 6,000 rads whole-pelvic irradiation

(E) perform a cesarean section at term

903. A 32-year-old woman is seen at 12 weeks' gestation. History and physical are normal except for the presence of a 9- to 10-cm cystic adnexal mass. Of the following actions, your management should be

(A) immediate laparotomy and further indicated surgery

(B) follow the patient with repeat ultrasound

(C) immediate total abdominal hysterectomy (TAH) and BSO

(D) suppression of the cyst by estrogens

904. A pregnant patient is found by biopsy to have carcinoma of the breast. The most appropriate management is

(A) abortion and irradiation

(B) abortion and breast surgery

(C) abortion, surgery, and irradiation

(D) surgery on the breast node evaluation and irradiation following delivery

905. Treatment for severe abruptio placentae includes

(A) heparin

(B) blood replacement

(C) steroid therapy for pulmonary maturity

(D) monitoring of plasma fibrinogen and tocolysis

DIRECTIONS (Questions 906 through 912): Each of the numbered items or incomplete statements in this section is followed by answers or by completions of the statement. Select the answers or completions that may apply.

906. A 23-year-old sexually active woman is seen in the emergency department because of low abdominal pain of 6 hours' duration. She has used contraceptives intermittently. Her last vaginal bleeding was 2 weeks ago. It was scanty and prolonged, but came at the time of her expected menstrual period. She denies fever or prior similar pain and has no bowel or bladder symptoms. Pelvic examination revealed a tender uterus and adnexa (worse on the left) without masses. Hct is 39, WBC is 8,900, temperature is 98.4°F, BP is 120/80, pulse is 90, and urinalysis is within normal limits. Pregnancy test is positive. On the basis of this information, which three of the following might be likely diagnoses?

(A) twisted ovarian cyst

(B) ectopic pregnancy

(C) appendicitis

(D) incomplete abortion

(E) corpus luteum cyst

907. Which four of the following are good reasons for a cesarean section?

(A) prolapsed cord

(B) transverse lie at term

(C) placenta previa at term

(D) stabilized eclamptic at 38 weeks, after failed oxytocin induction

(E) dead hydrocephalic fetus

908. Which four of the following have been associated with placental abruption?

(A) postpartum hemorrhage

(B) consumptive coagulopathy

(C) fetal demise

(D) acute renal failure

(E) subsequent ectopic pregnancy

909. Which four of the following have been associated with abruptio placentae?

(A) concealed uterine bleeding

(B) toxemia of pregnancy

(C) consumptive coagulopathy

(D) multiparity

(E) erythroblastosis fetalis

910. During pregnancy, a medium-sized ovarian cyst may be subject to which three of the following?

(A) torsion

(B) necrosis

(C) infection

(D) rupture

(E) conversion from benign to malignant state

911. A 23-year-old woman (gravida 3, abortus 3) is in your office to discuss the possible causes of her miscarriage. Which three of the following options are significant possibilities?

(A) chromosomal abnormalities

(B) placental abnormalities

(C) high-level magnetic fields

(D) uterine abnormalities

(E) psychological stress

912. Match each labeled portion of the forceps in Figure 12–1 with its correct name.

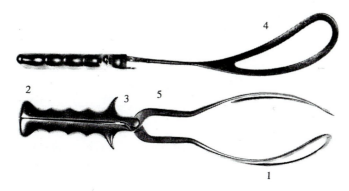

Figure 12–1.
(Reproduced, with permission, from Cunningham FG et al. *Williams Obstetrics*, 21st ed. New York: McGraw-Hill, 2001.)

(A) handle
(B) pelvic curves
(C) shank
(D) lock
(E) cephalic curve

DIRECTIONS (Questions 913 through 916): Each set of items in this section consists of lettered headings followed by several numbered words or phrases. For each numbered word or phrase, select the ONE lettered option that is most closely associated with it. Each lettered option may be selected once, more than once, or not at all.

Questions 913 through 916

Match the appropriate type of forceps or maneuver with the most appropriate descriptor.

(A) low forceps
(B) mid forceps
(C) high forceps
(D) outlet forceps

913. A patient is in labor and the cervix is completely dilated; the vertex is not molded and is occipito-anterior (OA) at a +2 station; forceps are applied.

914. The vertex is OA in the second stage of labor; the head is at a +4 station.

915. A patient is in the first stage of labor at a −1 station; fetal distress occurs and forceps are applied.

916. The head is on the perineum in a left occiput anterior (LOA) position; forceps are applied.

Answers and Explanations

852. (D) The bleeding from any of these options may be profuse or minimal. Abortion is the most common. Up to one third of all pregnancies are thought to end in early spontaneous abortion. Uterine rupture is very unlikely to cause bleeding in the first trimester.

853. (E) Often with abnormal gestations, there is no fetus at all (i.e., the "blighted ovum") and there is also a high incidence of hydropic degeneration of the placenta. If an embryo is present, it is usually a week smaller than the expected gestation, indicating embryonic death sometime earlier.

854. (B) There is a small but definite risk of fetal abnormality in any pregnancy. An early threatened abortion, as defined by bleeding only, does not appear to significantly increase the long-term risk of abnormality if an abortion does not occur. There is an increased risk of preterm delivery, low birth weight, and perinatal mortality. Bleeding after 16 weeks may be of greater significance.

855. (D) Reassurance and pelvic rest are the best modes of therapy. These modalities are not proven but are accepted care. Prolonged bed rest is not warranted. The patient should be followed to document continued uterine growth and viable products of conception. Ultrasound is of great help for this.

856. (A) If not examined before, a thorough pelvic examination to rule out bleeding, cervical polyps, cancer, varices, and so on should be performed. Life-threatening ectopic pregnancy needs to be excluded. The patient should have been seen when bleeding began. Any bleeding in pregnancy dictates prompt evaluation.

857. (E) Because pregnanediol drops when the fetoplacental unit dies, it was thought that progesterone was therapeutic. However, the true etiology was the death of the fetus. Giving more progesterone did not result in viability. It did inhibit myometrial activity, resulting in retained products of conception. If the fetus is alive, high doses of 19 norprogestins may be virilizing. Progestins are occasionally used to support a failing corpus luteum cyst.

858. (D) The ability of the blood to clot should be checked prior to performing a treatment for a fetal demise. Disseminated intravascular coagulopathy triggered by the release of tissue thromboplastins is usually a problem 3 to 4 weeks after fetal death.

859. (C) If the fetus and placenta are viable, the placenta may implant on some other peritoneal structure, and, rarely, an abdominal pregnancy may result. Many more ectopic gestations than realized may terminate as tubal abortions or simply be reabsorbed.

860. (E) An incomplete abortion is diagnosed if some, but not all, of the products of conception are passed. Often, bleeding can be severe. Evacuation should stop the bleeding and pain.

861. (A) A partially separated placenta will bleed profusely. If completely separated, the uterine contractions tend to occlude blood vessels and pass the tissue. Therapy is therefore directed at placental removal.

862. **(E)** The indicated therapy is to completely empty the uterus to allow the myometrium to contract. Vaginal packing will not often stop uterine bleeding, and hysterectomy would be used as a last resort. Suction is safer and more effective than sharp curettage.

863. **(D)** In the presence of missed menstrual periods; bleeding; cramping; enlarged, tender uterus; discharge; and fever, septic abortion is the first diagnostic possibility. Aggressive evacuation of the uterus and administration of intravenous antibiotics are indicated in this potentially life-threatening problem.

864. **(D)** Cultures should always be obtained prior to antibiotic therapy. Blood cultures from septic abortions often reveal anaerobes. The other tests should be ordered also, but their results will not be changed by antibiotics. Therapy, however, is begun on an empiric basis prior to the return of culture results.

865. **(A)** Early curettage after adequate antibiotics is the standard. Waiting for the patient to become afebrile to perform the curettage allows the infected material to remain in the uterus, and the patient may get worse instead of better. The infection must be evacuated promptly.

866. **(B)** Endosalpingitis, creating blind pockets in the tubal mucosa, is recognized as the leading predisposing factor for the development of ectopic pregnancies. Women on birth control pills or with irregular menses or endometriosis are not necessarily predisposed. The prompt and aggressive treatment of pelvic infection is designed to prevent tubal damage and maintain fertility.

867. **(D)** The ampulla is the most common site. Often, the ectopic embryo can be removed without removing the tube, but tubal function is occasionally compromised. After one ectopic pregnancy, the probability of having

another is about 10%. Future fertility also declines.

868. **(E)** Rupture into the peritoneal space may cause a hemoperitoneum. Less commonly, rupture into the broad ligament can also occur, resulting in a broad ligament hematoma without free blood in the peritoneal cavity. Tubal rupture generally will occur at about 8 to 10 weeks' gestation, producing rapidly progressive symptoms.

869. **(C)** Decidua capsularis and basalis come from above and below the developing chorionic sac. As the chorionic sac is in the tube, the only decidua available to slough is that found normally in the remainder of the endometrial cavity. Decidua vera is also called decidua parietalis. Passage of the uterine lining (cast) may be misinterpreted as passage of the products of conception.

870. **(B)** Interstitial pregnancies are rare—generally less than 2% of all ectopic pregnancies. However, because of their placement and large blood supply, they can grow quite a bit prior to rupture and then bleed massively. Because of the large uterine defect caused by rupture, hysterectomy may be (but is not always) necessary.

871. **(D)** The lower uterine segment and cervix do not constrict blood vessels well because they do not contract down, as does the fundus. Therefore, bleeding from the attempted surgical removal of a cervical gestation can be immense. Hysterectomy is a safe method of management but results in sterility. If the pregnancy is diagnosed early, other forms of management, including uterine artery embolization and chemotherapy, have been employed with success.

872. **(B)** The exact incidence is not as important as the recognition of its relative rarity, but it does occur and is becoming more common. With assisted reproductive technology, the incidence may be as high as 1%. Because of the rare occurrence, one is not likely to disrupt a normal gestation by doing a D&C in

the presence of an ectopic pregnancy. However, an intrauterine gestation may be mistaken for an ectopic pregnancy, in which case a D&C will cause an abortion. Ultrasound visualization of a fetal pole in the uterus with none in the adnexae is very good evidence against a heterotopic gestation.

873. **(C)** The maternal mortality from abdominal gestation is quite high. Usually, an abdominal fetus should be removed as soon as diagnosed. Removing the placenta adds to the risk of hemorrhage. Despite the complications, the placenta is best left in situ unless its entire blood supply can be visualized and occluded without harming the mother.

874. **(B)** Positive pregnancy tests and abnormal fetal positions are not specific. Uterine contractions should not be felt after oxytocin if the pregnancy is abdominal. X-rays may or may not help. One must be aware of oblique views, which may project the fetal skeleton over the maternal spine. Hysterograms may be definitive, but may be damaging if the fetus is in utero. Ultrasound is safer but subject to error also.

875. **(B)** Left salpingo-oophorectomy would also be acceptable, especially if the ovary is involved in the mass, or if there is a strong likelihood of compromising its blood supply by removing the tube and ectopic pregnancy. Every effort is now made to save the ovary and, many times, the tube. In many instances, the ectopic pregnancy can be "shelled out" and the tube repaired to preserve fertility.

876. **(C)** The Kielland forceps were specifically designed to rotate the fetal head. They have almost no pelvic curve and a sliding lock. Rotation of the fetal head should be done only by those with some experience and with absolute knowledge of the station and position of the fetal head and no evidence of cephalopelvic disproportion (CPD).

877. **(C)** For forceps to be applied, several criteria must be met, among them being that the head must be engaged (i.e., fetus must present by the vertex or by face with chin anterior; the cervix must be completely dilated and the membranes ruptured). Application of forceps in other situations is dangerous to both the mother and the fetus.

878. **(D)** Usually, such an event is traumatic for mother, child, and surgeon. A trial of forceps, which implies good application and moderate traction, is an acceptable procedure. If no progress is made, the trial is discontinued and a cesarean section performed. To persist with forceps constitutes poor judgment.

879. **(D)** If the forceps do not apply easily and lock securely without undue pressure, the probability exists that they are not properly applied. Position of the head should be rechecked and the forceps should be reapplied before any traction or maneuvers are attempted.

880. **(E)** The indications for vacuum extraction are the same as those for forceps delivery, namely (1) the head must be engaged; (2) it must be a vertex presentation; (3) the position of the fetal head must be precisely known; (4) the cervix must be completely dilated; (5) the membranes must be ruptured; and (6) there should be no CPD. Although forceps can be applied to a mentum anterior face presentation, the vacuum should not be used on the face for obvious reasons. If the fetus is very small, the vacuum does not fit well and there is increased risk of vascular rupture and bleeding, which is also a problem with fetal coagulopathies or after scalp sampling.

881. **(D)** With the head at a high station, one should be alert to the possibility of CPD and must also check for a prolapsed cord after membrane rupture. A primigravida in labor with an unengaged head is a high-risk patient. The pelvis should be evaluated. Clinical pelvimetry and evaluation of fetal size is indicated.

882. **(C)** Incoordinate uterine action may give rise to poor labor progression. Some authorities feel that oxytocin is contraindicated if the contractions do not have fundal dominance. Moving the patient about with a high head and ruptured membranes may lead to prolapse of the cord. Many, however, would attempt a trial of judicious oxytocin stimulation, especially as the contraction pattern is suboptimal.

883. **(E)** Forceps are contraindicated with an incompletely dilated cervix. Despite all efforts, the labor is not progressive. Abdominal delivery is indicated after these attempts have been made and progress is less than 1.2 cm/hr with no real descent.

884. **(E)** The first consideration should always be to achieve atraumatic delivery. Lower segment cesarean section is easier to repair, has less blood loss, and lower probability of subsequent uterine rupture than a classic incision. Adhesion formation after cesarean section is seldom a major problem.

885. **(B)** Pressure will not only relieve the symptoms of fullness and heaviness of vulvar varicosities but will also control their rare, spontaneous hemorrhage. A patient can be told over the telephone what to do to stop bleeding, but she should be examined to rule out other sources. Cautery is likely to cause more bleeding, as would vulvectomy. Sclerosing injections will not generally relieve acute bleeding.

886. **(A)** *Uteroplacental apoplexy* and *Couvelaire uterus* are terms used to describe the same process. The hematoma may spread via the broad ligament and tubes and, if extensive, may lead to decreased uterine muscle efficiency. The uterus may need to be removed. If hematomas are stable, they need not be evacuated. Such a degree of abruption would almost always result in fetal distress.

887. **(D)** No one believes how much a placenta previa can bleed until it happens. Ultrasound has helped immensely in the management of this difficult problem. Double setup examination may be used to diagnose the condition acutely in viable pregnancies. In other situations, such as premature pregnancies, ultrasound may allow time to temporize.

888. **(B)** Placenta previa must be ruled out, but this should not be done by pelvic examination at this time. If a previa is present, a pelvic exam may precipitate massive bleeding, making cesarean section mandatory. At 29 weeks' gestation, the fetus has a good chance of survival if further insults do not occur. The placenta should be localized by ultrasound and expectant treatment instituted if placenta previa is found and no further severe bleeding occurs. The limits of what constitutes acceptable blood loss are often hard to define and should be determined prospectively. Blood should be ordered and an IV started.

889. **(B)** The history is classic for placenta previa. An older, multiparous woman in late gestation with painless copious vaginal bleeding and a floating presenting part must be evaluated for placenta previa. Carcinoma of the cervix would be rare. Abruption often will have pain, and bleeding from vasa previa is statistically uncommon, especially with intact membranes.

890. **(D)** The continued severe bleeding contraindicates expectant therapy. A double setup examination allows you to make a definitive diagnosis of previa if this diagnosis could not be made by transvaginal ultrasound. If previa is present, one may proceed with a cesarean section. Vaginal packing is worthless and dangerous, and vaginal delivery should not be attempted until previa is ruled out.

891. **(D)** Both multiparity and increasing age tend to predispose to placenta previa, although age appears to be more important. Malpresentation, especially if no part of the fetus occupies the true pelvis, should also alert one to the possibility of previa. Ultrasound is the easiest way to make the diagnosis.

892. **(B)** Ultrasound has no radiation hazard, nor does it require intravascular injections. Ultrasound can also be used to determine fetal size and locate intraperitoneal masses. Most centers have ultrasound available in their labor and delivery areas.

893. **(C)** Classically, three incisions are made— one each at 2, 10, and 6 o'clock. These positions avoid the major blood supply and allow a vaginal repair. However, the use of Duhrssen's incisions should be extremely rare.

894. **(A)** A deep mediolateral episiotomy would be most likely to sever the superficial transverse perineal muscle. A deep midline episiotomy is likely to encounter the anal sphincter. Muscles transected should be repaired.

895. **(C)** The combination of breech presentation, meningomyelocele, and enlarged head make hydrocephaly the most likely diagnosis.

896. **(D)** Persistent face and brow, as well as transverse lie with shoulder presentations, can best be delivered by cesarean section. Internal version has few indications and is a difficult procedure, even for those with a great deal of experience.

897. **(A)** Eclampsia requires convulsions or coma, and even preeclampsia would most probably be ruled out by negative proteinuria and normal BP. The patient's fever points more to appendicitis. Increased WBC is not necessary to make the diagnosis. Pyelonephritis is possible but not as likely with no costo-vertebral angle (CVA) pain or pyuria. Pyelonephritis can cause gastrointestinal symptoms and is relatively common in pregnancy.

898. **(D)** The presence of pregnancy makes the diagnosis of appendicitis more difficult because many signs are changed. Pain, for example, may not be in the right lower quadrant. The treatment is immediate laparotomy and appendectomy.

899. **(E)** Early pyelonephritis can cause just such symptoms. There is no good evidence for abruptio placentae or degenerating myoma.

900. **(E)** Obtaining a histologic specimen is best done by colposcopically directed biopsy. Agreement exists as to the need for histologic examination in the immediate future. Directed biopsy is usually best when performed with colposcopic guidance. Small cervical biopsies pose no threat to the pregnancy.

901. **(C)** Invasion must be ruled out in any case with suspicion of microinvasion. Properly done, conization results in only a slightly higher incidence of abortion, but it does carry a moderate degree of risk. In experienced hands, colposcopically directed biopsies usually provide all the necessary information without the surgical and obstetrical risks of conization, but if there is question of microinvasion, a cone should be considered.

902. **(A)** If invasive disease is ruled out, vaginal delivery can be safely accomplished. Conization may predispose to cervical abnormalities of either premature dilation or lack of dilation, but such late complications are rare. Bleeding or premature labor may be a significant complication.

903. **(B)** There is a very slight risk that the cyst is a carcinoma or will obstruct labor. There is a greater risk that it will undergo torsion. Surgery early in pregnancy (first trimester) markedly increases the chance of abortion. If there is no immediate need to operate (i.e., the mass is unlikely to be cancer) the surgery may be done after 16 weeks. However, the mass may also be followed.

904. **(D)** Pregnancy does not seem to influence the long-term prognosis of breast carcinoma. Both surgery and radiation can be done prior to delivery, but radiation therapy is not recommended because of scatter, which may exceed the allowable fetal dose.

905. (B) Blood replacement should keep the patient out of shock and the urine output adequate. Delivery should occur within 6 hours, or sooner if the patient's condition is deteriorating. Coagulopathy is common, and replacement of blood products is often necessary. Fresh or freshly frozen serum contains coagulation factors. Cryoprecipitate is the major source of fibrinogen. Platelets may also be needed. Heparin is contraindicated, as is delay of delivery to give steroids.

906. (A, B, E) Although all the options are theoretic possibilities, ectopic pregnancy, if undiagnosed and untreated, poses the greatest immediate danger to life. If she is not bleeding now, incomplete abortion is incorrect. Appendicitis is unlikely given these signs and symptoms.

907. (A, B, C, D) All except option E are indications for a cesarean section. With a dead hydrocephalic fetus, transvaginal or transabdominal tapping of the fetal skull and withdrawal of the cerebrospinal fluid (CSF) will usually allow vaginal delivery. This should be done promptly if the hydrocephalic head is in the lower uterine segment because of increased risk of uterine rupture.

908. (A, B, C, D) Acute renal failure may occur with any prolonged and deep shock secondary to blood loss. Proteinuria may occur because of renal damage, and not only because of underlying toxemia. In any event, proteinuria at the time of vaginal bleeding and shock is a serious sign. Postpartum hemorrhage is rare, but the bleeding may not stop after the placenta is delivered if consumptive coagulopathy or severe Couvelaire uterus is present. Risk of subsequent ectopic pregnancy should not be affected.

909. (A, B, C, D) Hypertension and multiparity appear to have an etiologic relationship with abruptio placentae, and both concealed bleeding and coagulopathies may be a result of an abruption. Fetal vascular compromise may also be present. Monitoring of the fetus is essential to management. Usually, vaginal delivery is possible, but emergent cesarean section may be necessary if there is maternal or fetal compromise and vaginal delivery is not imminent. Erythroblastosis is not associated with placental abruption.

910. (A, B, D) Torsion is the most likely. Rupture and necrosis are possible. An ovarian cyst during pregnancy can have any of the complications found with ovarian cysts at any other time. Benign ovarian tumors are not known to convert to malignant ones. Fortunately, ovarian malignancy is extremely rare during pregnancy.

911. (A, B, D) Polyploidy and trisomies are often found in abortuses. Placental infarcts, maternal infections, and cervical incompetence can all result in abortion, but most frequently the cause is unknown. Stress and magnetic fields do not cause pregnancy loss.

912. (1-E, 2-A, 3-D, 4-B, 5-C) The handle of the forceps is obvious, and the lock holds the two branches together. The shank in the depicted Simpson's forceps is wide, and the blade has two curves. The cephalic curve fits around the fetal head; and the pelvic curve mimics the curve within the pelvic canal, which is transversed by the fetal head during delivery. When using the forceps, one must remember where the tips of the blades are in relation to the handle as firm rotation or lifting of the handles may cause a larger than anticipated movement of the tips of the blade, resulting in vaginal and perinatal lacerations.

913. (B) The biparietal diameter is through the inlet, but the presenting part is not at a +3 station. Mid forceps are not routinely used.

914. (A) This is a low forceps with the head at +4 station in an OA position. It requires no rotation.

915. **(C)** In this case, two cardinal rules have been violated. Cesarean section is much safer. Forceps should never be applied before the cervix is completely dilated and the head is engaged.

916. **(B)** The head is on the perineum (OA). It meets the criteria for outlet forceps.

CHAPTER 13

Puerperium
Questions

DIRECTIONS (Questions 917 through 956): Each of the numbered items or incomplete statements in this section is followed by answers or by completions of the statement. Select the ONE lettered answer or completion that is BEST in each case.

917. A previously energetic woman complains of crying, loss of appetite, difficulty in sleeping, and feeling of low self-worth, beginning approximately 3 days after a normal vaginal delivery. These feelings persisted for approximately 1 week and then progressively diminished. Her symptoms would be termed postpartum

    (A) manic depression
    (B) schizoid affective disorder
    (C) neurosis
    (D) psychosis
    (E) blues

918. A patient has just delivered her first child. She is anxious to breast-feed. As part of her postpartum discharge counseling, she should be told that few things interfere with lactation but she should avoid

    (A) high dose (≥ 50 µg estradiol) oral contraceptive pills
    (B) levonorgesterol implants
    (C) Depo-Provera
    (D) mini-pill
    (E) frequent suckling

919. At delivery, a perineal laceration tore through the skin of the fourchette, vaginal mucous membrane, and the fascia and perineal muscles of the perineal body but not the anal sphincter or mucosa. This should be recorded in the medical record as _____ laceration of the perineal body.

    (A) first-degree
    (B) second-degree
    (C) third-degree
    (D) fourth-degree
    (E) complete

920. A patient is being discharged from the hospital following an uncomplicated vaginal delivery. Discharge counseling and plans would include

    (A) no driving for 4 weeks
    (B) no coitus for 6 weeks
    (C) return to work only after 6 weeks of maternity leave
    (D) rubella immunization for nonimmune patients

Questions 921 through 923

A 24-year-old patient (gravida 2, para 2) has just delivered vaginally an infant weighing 4,300 g after a spontaneous uncomplicated labor. Her prior obstetric history was a low uterine segment transverse cesarean section for breech. She has had no problems during the pregnancy and labor. The placenta delivers spontaneously. There is immediate brisk vaginal bleeding of greater than 500 cc.

921. Although all of the following can be the cause for postpartum hemorrhage, which is the most frequent cause of immediate hemorrhage as seen in this patient?

(A) uterine atony

(B) vaginal and/or cervical lacerations

(C) uterine inversion

(D) coagulopathies

(E) uterine rupture

922. In this patient with a significant postpartum bleed, transfusions should be started

(A) after the loss of 750 cc of blood

(B) if the patient becomes hypotensive despite other volume expanders

(C) before using prostaglandin E_2 (PGE_2)-alpha

(D) before giving other volume expanders

(E) when packed cell volume (PCV) is < 30%

923. After a period of hypovolemic shock, the bleeding was controlled and the vascular volume replaced. Estimates of blood loss were over 2,000 cc. The patient apparently recovered well. However, she was unable to breast-feed and gradually noted breast atrophy and no resumption of menses. Later, she developed constipation, slurred speech, and moderate nonpitting edema. A likely diagnosis is

(A) acute tubular necrosis (ATN)

(B) amenorrhea–galactorrhea syndrome

(C) Sheehan syndrome

(D) Asherman syndrome

(E) Forbes–Albright syndrome

924. A patient calls your office complaining of continued heavy vaginal bleeding. She had an "uncomplicated" vaginal birth 2 weeks ago of her second child. The most likely diagnosis from the following differential is

(A) uterine atony

(B) uterine rupture

(C) retained placental fragments

(D) vaginal lacerations

(E) coagulopathies

925. The most efficacious treatment of persistent uterine hemorrhage in the second to fourth week of the puerperium, as described in Question 924, is

(A) high doses of estrogen

(B) uterine packing

(C) high doses of progesterone

(D) ergotrate

(E) dilation and curettage (D&C)

926. The postpartum nurse calls about a patient who had an uncomplicated vaginal delivery 12 hours ago. She is concerned about the patient who has the following findings. Which of them should be of most concern to you?

(A) proteinuria

(B) abdominal rigidity

(C) a pulse rate of 60

(D) leukocytosis of 16,000

(E) a single temperature of 100.4°F

927. A patient with a diagnosis of postpartum pelvic thrombophlebitis complains of chest pain and dyspnea. Which of the following tests will be most helpful to diagnose a pulmonary embolism?

(A) lung scan

(B) electrocardiogram (ECG)

(C) arterial blood gas

(D) auscultation of the chest

928. A patient develops a fever of 102°F, and a tender abdomen and uterus at 4 days postpartum. She also notices a dark brown urine, and when blood is drawn the serum is red. A flat plate x-ray of the abdomen shows air in the uterus. Gram-stain of uterine curettings reveals gram-positive plump rods. On the basis of this information, the most likely organism is

(A) gonococcus

(B) *Escherichia coli*

(C) *Bacteroides*

(D) *Enterococcus*

(E) *Clostridium perfringens*

Questions 929 through 932

An 18-year-old patient finally delivered a 4,000-g infant vaginally. Her prenatal course was complicated by anemia, poor weight gain, and maternal obesity. Her labor was protracted, including a 3-hour second stage, a mid-forceps delivery with a sulcus laceration, and a third-degree episiotomy.

929. Of the following, the greatest predisposing cause of puerperal infection in this patient is

    (A) tissue trauma
    (B) iron deficiency
    (C) coitus during late pregnancy
    (D) poor nutrition
    (E) maternal exhaustion

930. She develops a fever on the third day postpartum. What is the most likely etiology?

    (A) pneumonia
    (B) endometritis
    (C) mastitis
    (D) pyelonephritis
    (E) septic thrombophlebitis

931. If you were to culture this patient, you would likely find the most common bacteria isolated from cases of puerperal infection, which is

    (A) E. coli
    (B) anaerobic Streptococcus
    (C) anaerobic Staphylococcus
    (D) aerobic Streptococcus
    (E) Clostridium perfringens

932. If this infection spreads to include the areolar-supporting connective tissues of the uterus, it is called

    (A) thrombophlebitis
    (B) phlebothrombosis
    (C) peritonitis
    (D) pyemia
    (E) parametritis

933. Puerperal infection may be spread by several routes. The most common route that results in septic thrombophlebitis is

    (A) venous
    (B) lymphatic
    (C) arterial
    (D) direct extension
    (E) fomites

934. A patient develops severe parametritis secondary to vaginal and cervical lacerations during the delivery. The right broad ligament is severely involved and an abscess forms. Of the following choices, such an abscess is most likely to point

    (A) in the cul-de-sac
    (B) at the umbilicus
    (C) in the rectum
    (D) beneath the liver capsule
    (E) above the inguinal ligament

935. A patient who is 12 hours postpartum develops a temperature of 104°F, a tender uterus, and increased lochia without an odor. Your antibiotic choice needs to be sure to cover the most likely organism, which would be

    (A) E. coli
    (B) Bacteroides
    (C) beta-streptococcus
    (D) gonococcus
    (E) Staphylococcus

936. Bacteria can be cultured from most endometrial cavities 2 to 3 days postpartum in patients who are asymptomatic. The anaerobic organism most commonly found is

    (A) Peptococcus
    (B) Peptostreptococcus
    (C) Clostridium
    (D) E. coli
    (E) beta-streptococcus

937. During childbirth classes, a patient would be told which of the following regarding breast-feeding?

(A) Prolactin stimulates milk production and breast development.

(B) Mother's milk contains a large amount of iron.

(C) Most ingested drugs that are soluble in maternal blood do not cross into breast milk.

(D) The postpartum period of lactation is a time of above-normal fertility.

(E) Breast milk is a major source of immunoglobulin G (IgG).

938. A 16-year-old patient delivered a term infant yesterday. She does not want to breast-feed and asks for something to suppress lactation. The simplest and safest method of lactation suppression is

(A) bromocriptine

(B) breast binding, ice packs, and analgesics

(C) deladumone

(D) Depo-Provera

(E) oral contraceptive pills

939. A patient presents 1 week postpartum with complaints of her right breast being engorged, hot, red, and painful. She reports a fever of 101°F. If her breast were cultured, which of the following is the most likely organism to be found?

(A) anaerobic *Streptococcus*

(B) *E. coli*

(C) *Staphylococcus aureus*

(D) aerobic *Streptococcus*

(E) *Neisseria*

940. Given the diagnosis of a postpartum mastitis, you would initiate therapy. Of the following methods of management, the most controversial has been

(A) use of antibiotics

(B) identification of infectious organism

(C) drainage of abscesses

(D) discontinuance of nursing

941. A class C diabetic patient delivers at term. It is important to check her blood sugar levels immediately postpartum, since there may be a decrease in the insulin requirements of diabetic patients. This can be partly explained by

(A) increased food intake

(B) decreased activity

(C) decrease in plasma chorionic somatomammotropin

(D) decrease in plasma progesterone

(E) decrease in plasma estrogen

942. Immediately after the completion of a normal labor and delivery, the uterus should be

(A) firm and rounded

(B) at the level of the symphysis pubis

(C) immobile

(D) discoid

(E) boggy

943. Large blood vessels present in the uterus during pregnancy undergo changes postpartum. Which changes can be recognized years later?

(A) thrombosis

(B) slow reabsorption

(C) hyalinization

(D) necrosis

(E) fatty degeneration

944. A patient had a vaginal delivery of a 4,500-g infant after a prolonged second stage. She is now unable to void. Of the following, the most serious cause of inability to void in the immediate postpartum period is

(A) overdistention of the bladder

(B) edema

(C) hematoma

(D) anesthesia

(E) emotions

945. Average blood loss from vaginal delivery when carefully measured has been found to be

(A) < 100 mL
(B) approximately 250 mL
(C) approximately 600 mL
(D) approximately 750 mL
(E) approximately 1,000 mL

946. The decidual layer is divided into several parts, most of which are shed following pregnancy. The part that remains is the

(A) decidua capsularis
(B) decidua vera
(C) zona spongiosa
(D) zona basalis
(E) zona functionalis

947. The period of time from the end of delivery until the reproductive organs have returned to normal is called

(A) menopause
(B) puerperium
(C) perineum
(D) pachytene
(E) paravarium

948. Postpartum, the uterus involutes in 6 to 8 weeks. Its volume capacity goes from 5–10 L to 10–15 mL. Its weight decreases by how much?

(A) 100 g
(B) 500 g
(C) 900 g
(D) 1,300 g
(E) 1,700 g

949. Postpartum, the decidua becomes necrotic and is normally cast off within 5 to 6 days as

(A) decidual cast
(B) placental remnants
(C) lochia
(D) carunculae myrtiformes
(E) none of the above

Questions 950 and 951

A 20-year-old woman (gravida 1) has just delivered. After expression of the placenta, a red, raw surface is seen at the vaginal introitus. Simultaneously, the nurse states that the patient is pale and her BP is 70/40. External bleeding has been of normal amount.

950. Of the following, the most likely diagnosis would be

(A) ruptured uterus
(B) second twin
(C) ovarian cyst
(D) uterine inversion
(E) vaginal rupture

951. Treatment would consist of

(A) immediate hysterectomy
(B) delivery of the infant
(C) exploratory laparotomy
(D) immediate replacement of the fundus
(E) massive blood transfusion

Questions 952 through 954

A postpartum patient has been running a low-grade (100° to 101°F) fever of unknown origin. On her sixth postpartum day, she developed a tender area over the posterior right calf. The pain and fever increased, and tachycardia developed. Later, the leg became red and tender with edema, and groin pain became pronounced.

952. The most likely diagnosis is

(A) varicose veins
(B) pelvic cellulitis
(C) endometritis
(D) thrombophlebitis
(E) phlebothrombosis

953. This disease entity is most common in which of the following situations?

(A) nonpregnant middle-aged adult
(B) antepartum
(C) postpartum
(D) nonpregnant young adult
(E) intrapartum

954. Treatment of this disease would include

(A) heparin anticoagulation

(B) vigorous exercise

(C) tourniquets on the affected limb

(D) vitamin K

(E) incision of the affected vein

Questions 955 and 956

A 34-year-old patient developed an endometritis postpartum and was treated for 8 days in the hospital with bed rest, antibiotics, and fluids. She was improving when, on the eighth day, shortness of breath, anterior chest pain, and tachycardia occurred suddenly.

955. Of the following, the most likely diagnosis is

(A) myocardial infarction

(B) amniotic fluid emboli

(C) pelvic abscess

(D) Mendelson's syndrome

(E) pulmonary embolism

956. Chest film was negative. Ventilation–perfusion scan was intermediate, but spiral computed tomography (CT) scan was consistent with the diagnosis of pulmonary embolism. The most important therapy is

(A) vena cava ligation

(B) heparin

(C) hydrocortisone

(D) low-molecular-weight dextran

(E) warfarin

DIRECTIONS (Questions 957 through 959): Each of the numbered items or incomplete statements in this section is followed by answers or by completions of the statement. Select the answers or completions that may apply.

957. Immediate management of postpartum hemorrhage will involve many procedures almost simultaneously. Of the following interventions, which four are most likely to stop uterine bleeding in this setting?

(A) bimanual uterine compression

(B) oxytocin

(C) prostaglandin F$_2$ (PFG$_2$)-alpha

(D) packing the uterus

(E) ergotrate

958. A hospital is competing for an HMO contract. Part of the proposal is data on the puerperal infection rate. Which four of the following are included in the category of puerperal infection?

(A) endometritis

(B) pelvic thrombophlebitis

(C) parametritis

(D) pyelonephritis

(E) pelvic peritonitis

959. Subinvolution of the postpartum uterus may be due to which four of the following?

(A) retained secundae

(B) endometritis

(C) pelvic cellulitis

(D) myomas

(E) monilia

DIRECTIONS (Questions 960 and 961): Each group of items in this section consists of lettered headings followed by a set of numbered words or phrases. For each numbered word or phrase, select

(A) if the item is associated with (A) only,

(B) if the item is associated with (B) only,

(C) if the item is associated with both (A) and (B),

(D) if the item is associated with neither (A) nor (B).

Questions 960 and 961

(A) midline episiotomy

(B) mediolateral episiotomy

(C) both

(D) neither

960. Should be performed routinely

961. Little postpartum pain in most cases

Answers and Explanations

917. (E) Short-term feelings of depression, commonly called postpartum blues, occur in 85% of women for a short time in the immediate postpartum period. This is a mild disorder that is usually self-limited, but if it persists, it may represent postpartum depression. Medical intervention, including antidepressant therapy, is beneficial. If it is associated with severe symptoms of psychoses, suicidal thoughts, or delusions, consultation with a psychiatrist should be obtained immediately. In the situation of postpartum psychosis, both the woman and the infant are in danger of harm. If a woman has experienced postpartum depression or psychosis in a prior pregnancy or if she has depression or psychosis when not pregnant, she is at increased risk for a postpartum reoccurrence.

918. (A) Birth control pills containing high pharmacologic amounts of estrogens have been shown to decrease milk production, as has chronic smoking. Low doses of progestins alone do not appear to have this effect. Even higher doses of progestin as found in Depo-Provera given at 1 to 2 weeks postpartum do not seem to increase problems with breast-feeding. Estrogen is needed for milk production, but high levels are inhibiting. Suckling is a stimulus to milk production. However, the use of lower-dose combination oral contraceptive pills (≤ 30 μg estrogen) is an option once breast-feeding is well established.

919. (B) A second-degree tear does not involve the anal sphincter. Third-degree lacerations involve the anal sphincter, and fourth-degree lacerations include the sphincter and the rectal mucosa. Any laceration should be carefully repaired and examined after repair for the integrity of the anal sphincter and the rectal mucosa.

920. (D) The woman's comfort and desire should serve as the bases for resumption of coitus, although it is probably best to wait until the vaginal bleeding has stopped to decrease the risk of infection. After a vaginal delivery a patient should be able to resume normal activities within days. The recommendation for 4 to 6 weeks of maternity leave is more due to decreased energy levels and time to adjust to parenting role rather than true medical indications. Postpartum is an excellent time to immunize for rubella.

921. (A) Uterine atony accounts for by far the greater number of bleeding incidents. Potential trauma is obvious in the process of a delivery but usually does not cause this much bleeding. Also, in the case of lacerations, the bleeding is often evident prior to the delivery of the placenta. Coagulopathy is possible in cases of abruption or severe hypertension but typically does not cause immediate hemorrhage unless there are significant lacerations. Uterine rupture given this patient's history is a definite possibility but still is less common than atony. Uterine inversion is an uncommon event and is more likely to follow a delay in placenta separation with traction on the cord.

922. (B) A great danger exists in letting a patient become hypovolemic in the face of continued bleeding. Most deaths from maternal hemorrhage can be traced to inadequate blood replacement (too little, too late). Do not allow blood loss to get out of hand. By the same token, transfusion now involves many risks not previously present. It should be performed judiciously. Uterine massage and bimanual compression, ergotrate, dilute oxytocin IV, and PGF$_2$-alpha should all be tried for uterine atony. Surgical removal of placental fragments or repair of laceration should be done as needed.

923. **(C)** Anterior pituitary necrosis from postpartum hemorrhage results in loss of gonadotropins, thyroid-stimulating hormone (TSH), and adrenocorticotropic hormone (ACTH), generally in that order. Lack of breast milk is usually the first clue. Amenorrhea may be the second sign. Sheehan syndrome is a rare occurrence when good postpartum management prevents or adequately treats blood loss. ATN would have presented early postpartum with extremely dilute urine and evidence of hypovolemia. Asherman syndrome is the scarring of the endometrial cavity after a D&C, especially in the situation of a postpartum hemorrhage. The symptoms are confined to postpartum amenorrhea with or without cramping, depending on whether it is only an outlet obstruction. Forbes–Albright syndrome (amenorrhea–galactorrhea syndrome) is usually associated with a pituitary tumor and not with pregnancy. Galactorrhea is also associated with this syndrome.

924. **(C)** Early bleeding is most often due to atony or lacerations. Late continued profuse bleeding, even several weeks following delivery, may be due to retained placenta. Other causes may be subinvolution of the uterus, infection, and/or choriocarcinoma.

925. **(E)** Retained placenta and subinvolution of the placental sites are common causes of late puerperal bleeding. Ergotrate causes cramping, but does not often resolve the problem. Severe hemorrhage can occur during a D&C and should be anticipated in high-parity women possibly because the placenta is implanted lower in the uterus with each subse-

quent pregnancy. The possibility of removing all of the endometrium and creating Asherman syndrome must be kept in mind, especially if there is an infection. Placental polyps and gestational trophoblastic disease are rare causes that should be remembered.

926. **(B)** A leukocytosis of up to 25,000 may occur immediately postpartum with no other signs of infection. A low pulse rate is normally seen, and proteinuria can be expected, especially following a difficult labor. Abdominal rigidity is not normal during the puerperium.

927. **(A)** Of the tests listed, ventilation–perfusion lung scan is the best. Pulmonary emboli usually cause decreased PO_2 and may cause cardiac right-axis shift, pulmonary avascular areas, and pleural effusion. Blood gases and auscultation are not very specific or sensitive for PE. Pulmonary angiography, which will usually reveal filling defects from embolic phenomena, is more specific but is costly and takes longer. Spiral CT is rapidly becoming the diagnostic test of choice since it is accurate, low risk for the patient, and relatively quick to obtain. Anticoagulation is the mainstay of therapy. About one half of the pulmonary emboli during pregnancy originate in the pelvic veins.

928. **(E)** *Clostridium perfringens* is a club-shaped, gram-positive rod that produces a potent lecithinase toxin causing intravascular hemolysis. Other enzymes cause hydrolysis of glycogen, releasing hydrogen and causing gas gangrene. *Bacteroides* and *Clostridium* are both anaerobes, and only *Clostridium* and *Enterococcus* are gram-positive.

929. **(A)** Devitalized tissue forms an excellent culture medium for bacteria, especially anaerobic forms. Meticulous surgical technique will help to decrease the incidence of infection, as will careful selection of surgical materials.

930. **(B)** One must look at the wound if a fever arises following surgery. After a delivery, the wound or raw surface always includes the uterus, and infection there must be actively ruled out. Mastitis may occur but is usually later. Urinary tract infection (UTI) is another very likely source of the fever. Finally, any vaginal laceration must be evaluated for infection.

931. **(B)** *Peptostreptococcus* is the organism most commonly found. Anaerobic organisms are difficult to culture, and special media and techniques should be employed if valid information is to be obtained.

932. **(E)** Parametritis, or pelvic cellulitis, may be secondary to genital tract lacerations, thrombophlebitis, or direct invasion by pathogenic bacteria. It is treated in a similar fashion to nonpuerperal pelvic infection.

933. **(A)** Thrombophlebitis is associated with about 40% of fatal cases of puerperal sepsis. Fomites are objects not in themselves infected, but they can carry an infecting organism from one place to another. Direct extension is always a possibility but not the most likely one.

934. **(E)** Fortunately, this is a rare occurrence in modern obstetrics. Following tissue planes such an abscess can easily point just above Poupart's ligament. It can be drained by incision, which is usually the most important step in abscess treatment.

935. **(C)** Although puerperal infectious morbidity definition states to "ignore" the first 24 hours, high temperatures such as 104°F must be addressed. This may be associated with a very aggressive infectious source. The lack of foul odor would imply aerobic bacteria. Coverage for group A and group B streptococcus is critical. Also, pediatrics should be notified of this development since it may alter their management of the newborn.

936. **(B)** Most endometrial bacteria appear to be contaminants rather than causing a clinical infection, as patients tend to remain asymptomatic and have a normal postpartum course. However, if a fever occurs, the most likely cause is metritis. Anaerobic bacteria re-

quire meticulous culture technique be recovered. *E. coli* and streptococci are facultative bacteria.

937. **(A)** Prolactin stimulates milk production. Breast milk is very low in iron, and supplementation is needed for breast-fed babies. Anemia can also be present in babies fed only cow's milk. Although the time of lactation is one of subnormal fertility, breast-feeding cannot be claimed as a highly effective method of birth control. Most drugs will enter breast milk; therefore, one must consider this when counseling and prescribing for breast-feeding mothers. IgA is the primary antibody contained in breast milk and appears to prevent many gastrointestinal infectious complications for newborns.

938. **(B)** Multiple hormonal interventions have been tried. These predispose to thromboembolic phenomena and have a significant occurrence of rebound engorgement as the hormonal influence decreases. Bromocriptine, via a decrease in prolactin levels, was tried, but there was an association with hypertension, stroke, and seizure with its use. The safest treatment is a binder of the breast, ice packs, and analgesics for the first week postpartum.

939. **(C)** *Staphylococcus aureus* is the most common etiologic agent in postpartum mastitis. Mastitis is rare in the non-nursing mother. It is usually transmitted by the nursing infant who is already colonized.

940. **(D)** Treatment of mastitis includes antibiotics, continuance of nursing, and drainage of any abscess. Argument exists as to the method of skin incision for drainage of breast abscesses. Circumareolar skin incisions following Langer's skin lines are advocated by some for cosmetic reasons. A deep abscess can be opened radially after the skin incision is made. Identification of possible nosocomial infection is important since infants may be colonized by nursery staff in the hospital who are carriers of resistant strains of *Staphylococcus* and other organisms. Fewer authorities now recommend the discontinuance of nursing, although the need to empty the breast is still emphasized.

941. **(C)** Both human chorionic somatomammotropin (hCS), often called placental lactogen, and pituitary somatomammotropin levels are low immediately postpartum. As they have marked anti-insulin effects, the rapid loss may account for part of the decrease in the insulin requirement often seen in postpartum diabetic patients. Also, placental insulinase is no longer present. One should be careful not to give too large an insulin dose, which might precipitate insulin shock in the postpartum patient.

942. **(A)** The uterus may be discoid prior to the separation of the placenta, but after the third stage of labor, it should be rounded and firm at the level of the umbilicus. A soft or boggy uterus usually signifies lack of tonus and the diagnosis of atony.

943. **(C)** Thrombosis occurs in the placental site, and hyalinization that slowly resorbs occurs elsewhere. The reabsorption is so slow that one can identify a parous uterus years later by finding such hyaline remains.

944. **(C)** Trauma causing hematoma large enough to cause inability to void is potentially a serious complication postpartum. A pelvic examination should be done whenever there is urinary retention postpartum. Delivery usually causes some trauma to the base of the bladder and trigone, and edema and ecchymosis are common. Anesthesia and/or overdistention may result in poor bladder function for varying periods of time, but all of these will usually resolve with a short time of catheterization. Prolonged bladder distention can cause pain, detrussor injury, and uterine atony with delayed hemorrhage.

945. **(C)** Estimates of blood loss are often 250 mL. However, measurements have shown that a blood loss of 500 to 600 mL is quite common. This amount will not result in a hematocrit drop in most women. This is because the ex-

panded blood volume during pregnancy is like having two autologous units for transfusion. Immediate postpartum hemodynamic changes provide rapid compensation.

946. **(D)** The zona basalis remains to give rise to new endometrium. Some of the basal endometrium is located between myometrial fibers and will usually remain, even after a D&C. This layer rapidly regenerates. If it is removed in a vigorous D&C, one will have Asherman syndrome.

947. **(B)** Usually, the period of involution is complete by 6 weeks, but there is nothing magic about that duration. The healing of the placental site takes the longest time. Some physical changes are not readily reversible.

948. **(C)** The normal uterus postpartum weighs about 1,000 g (2 lb) and drops to 60 g (2 oz) at 8 weeks.

949. **(C)** Lochia is the discharge from a postpartum uterus. Its character normally changes from red and heavy to white and light over 2 to 3 weeks.

950. **(D)** Uterine inversion is a rare occurrence, and shock is often out of proportion to blood loss. Immediate recognition is important in the treatment.

951. **(D)** Immediate replacement is the quickest and most effective therapy. If recognized early before administering postpartum oxytocin or contraction of the lower uterine segment, replacement is easy. If it is allowed to persist, surgical repair may be required. Bleeding and hypotension out of proportion to blood loss are the greatest dangers. If there is a delay in replacement, aggressive volume expansion is necessary.

952. **(D)** Thrombophlebitis usually occurs 5 to 10 days postpartum with fairly rapid onset of fever, chills, and severe pain in the affected extremity. It can also occur in pelvic veins without the obvious external swelling and pain. The diagnosis of a pelvic clot can be

very difficult and sometimes is made only after a trial of anticoagulants.

953. **(C)** Most cases occur postpartum and are associated with either trauma or infection, though thrombophlebitis can arise spontaneously. Stasis, endothelial damage, and a hypercoagulation state (pregnancy) are all risk factors. The greatest risk factor is hereditary thrombophilia.

954. **(A)** Heat, bed rest, elevation, and heparin anticoagulation are basic to the treatment of this disease.

955. **(E)** Chest pain, tachycardia, and dyspnea of sudden onset 7 to 10 days postpartum must be regarded as resulting from a pulmonary embolus until proven otherwise. Immediate tests to confirm the diagnosis should be done.

956. **(B)** Heparin is anti-inflammatory, anticoagulant, and lipid clearing. It will prevent progression of thrombus formation and further emboli in the majority of cases.

957. **(A, B, C, E)** Uterine packing has little place in modern obstetrics as a first-line treatment for early postpartum hemorrhage. It causes uterine distention when the desired effect is contraction of the muscle fibers to occlude bleeding vessels. The other methods are quite effective. Bimanual compression is always available until other modalities can be employed. Packing may be appropriate for delayed postpartum hemorrhage from the placenta site around 1 to 4 weeks postpartum.

958. **(A, B, C, E)** Pyelonephritis is not included in puerperal infection statistics. Blood cultures are often positive in pylonephritis, as well as in pelvic thrombophlebitis and peritonitis, and the differential diagnosis may be difficult. Broad-spectrum antibiotics are the most common and effective therapy.

959. **(A, B, C, D)** The usual symptoms of subinvolution include prolonged lochial discharge or frank bleeding, as well as a uterus larger than expected for the time postpartum. Subinvolution allows venous channels that usually regress to remain open. Another rare entity that should be kept in mind that produces the same symptoms is choriocarcinoma. Monilia does not cause subinvolution.

960. **(D)** Episiotomy should not be done routinely but reserved for appropriate situations, such as unusual presentations or significant dystocias. The major reason advocated for performing an episiotomy is to prevent tears and give more space for delivery. However, this approach is under challenge. Most individuals are advocating allowing the tears to occur since they are less likely to extend to damage the rectum or perirectal tissues with the result of incontinence.

961. **(A)** Healing with a midline episiotomy is usually better, and dyspareunia is unusual. The anatomic result is usually better also. Some clinicians prefer mediolateral episiotomy in high-risk situations, such as forceps delivery, because of lower likelihood of rectal tears.

CHAPTER 14

Newborn Assessment and Care
Questions

DIRECTIONS (Questions 962 through 1006): Each of the numbered items or incomplete statements in this section is followed by answers or by completions of the statement. Select the ONE lettered answer or completion that is BEST in each case.

962. An infant is born with a vigorous cry, a heart rate of 105, movement of all four extremities, grimacing, and with bluish hands and feet. The Apgar score is

(A) 10
(B) 9
(C) 8
(D) 7
(E) 6

963. The normal infant after delivery will have a normal adult pH in about

(A) 5 minutes
(B) 1 hour
(C) 12 hours
(D) 3 days
(E) 1 month

964. Newborns who are immediately exposed to room temperature are at risk for the development of

(A) metabolic acidosis
(B) metabolic alkalosis
(C) respiratory acidosis
(D) respiratory alkalosis
(E) pneumonia

965. The most common cause of failure to establish effective respiratory effort in the newborn is

(A) fetal acidosis
(B) fetal immaturity
(C) upper airway obstruction
(D) congenital laryngeal stenosis
(E) infection

966. For statistical purposes, a premature birth has been defined as a fetus born

(A) before 37 weeks of gestation
(B) before 25 weeks of gestation
(C) prior to the viability
(D) weighing < 1,000 g
(E) weighing > 1,000 g but < 2,500 g

967. A patient presents in labor claiming to be at 43 weeks of gestation. Which of the following neonatal findings would support the diagnosis of a postmature infant?

(A) anemia
(B) increased subcutaneous fat
(C) long fingernails
(D) vernix
(E) fusion of the fetal eyelids

968. Which of the following newborns would be classified as high risk?

(A) 3,500 g, 39 weeks' gestation, Apgar 8/9
(B) 2,650 g, 41 weeks' gestation, Apgar 7/8
(C) 3,800 g, 41 weeks' gestation, Apgar 7/8
(D) 3,100 g, 38 weeks' gestation, Apgar 7/9
(E) 2,650 g, 38 weeks' gestation, Apgar 7/8

969. You have just delivered a term infant who is the product of a normal pregnancy. The umbilical cord has yet to be cut. The baby has not yet cried. The most appropriate next step is

(A) to place the baby on the maternal abdomen
(B) to vigorously slap the baby to stimulate respiration
(C) deep bulb suctioning of the posterior oropharynx
(D) to maintain the baby in a head down position while you cut the umbilical cord
(E) to begin gentle mask ventilation with oxygen

970. Mild degrees of hyperbilirubinemia in the newborn should be treated by

(A) exchange transfusion
(B) exposing the infant to light
(C) O-negative packed red blood cells (RBCs) given as an exchange transfusion
(D) spinal tap
(E) soy-based formula feeding

971. On the fifth day of life, the weight of a normal infant would be expected to have

(A) increased 6 to 8 oz
(B) increased 2 oz
(C) remained the same
(D) decreased 2 oz
(E) decreased 6 to 7 oz

972. The umbilical cord stump of a newborn most frequently sloughs off about the

(A) second day after delivery
(B) fifth day after delivery
(C) 10th day after delivery
(D) 15th day after delivery
(E) 21st day after delivery

973. A term infant is delivered as a double-footling breech. It is noted to have an Apgar of 3 at 1 minute and later to be irritable and restless. The infant's muscles are rigid, and the anterior fontanel bulges. The infant develops progressive bradycardia. The most likely diagnosis is

(A) brain stem injury
(B) infection
(C) congenital abnormality
(D) neonatal sepsis
(E) intracranial hemorrhage

974. The most likely finding in a neonate with asphyxia is

(A) alkalemia
(B) hypoxia
(C) hypocapnia
(D) tachycardia
(E) increased anal sphincter tone

975. After a difficult delivery due to a shoulder dystocia, a newborn is found to have paralysis of one arm with the forearm extended and rotated inward next to the trunk. This is most likely due to

(A) damage to the C8–T1 nerve roots
(B) neonatal asphyxia
(C) damage to the brachial plexus
(D) fracture of the clavicle
(E) comminuted fracture of the humerus

976. Traumatic brain hemorrhage is most commonly associated with

(A) vacuum extraction at the pelvic outlet
(B) outlet forceps
(C) mid-forceps deliveries
(D) neonatal coagulopathy
(E) spontaneous vertex deliveries

977. A large swelling in one of the sternomastoid muscles is noted in a newborn 2 days after delivery. This most likely represents a

(A) lipoma
(B) hematoma
(C) thymoma
(D) cystic hygroma
(E) neonatal lymphoma

978. Within a short time after delivery, the baby does not breathe spontaneously. The heart rate is 80 to 90. There is some movement and questionable irritability. The most appropriate next step is to

(A) dry and warm the newborn
(B) slap the baby's back gently at first, then vigorously if necessary
(C) ventilate the infant by mask
(D) do external cardiac massage
(E) administer intravenous bicarbonate ($NaHCO_3$) via umbilical vein

979. An infant has an Apgar score of 0 at 1 minute despite clearing the airway and gentle stimulation. The next best step is to

(A) immediately intubate
(B) dry and warm the baby
(C) administer intracardiac epinephrine
(D) administer a narcotic antagonist
(E) initiate electrical cardioversion

980. When faced with the delivery of a premature newborn, the normal resuscitation should be altered to routinely include

(A) assisted ventilation
(B) minimal handling
(C) systemic antibiotic prophylaxis
(D) nikethamide
(E) intravenous bicarbonate ($NaHCO_3$)

981. Apnea in the newborn most often results from

(A) maternal infection
(B) epidural anesthesia
(C) central nervous system (CNS) depression
(D) maternal hyperventilation
(E) naloxone administration

982. The tidal volume of the normal newborn is about

(A) 5 mL
(B) 20 mL
(C) 50 mL

(D) 70 mL
(E) 150 mL

983. A baby is delivered with an Apgar score of 2 at 5 minutes. Oxygen should be administered by mask at a pressure of

(A) 0 to 5 cm of water
(B) 10 to 20 cm of water
(C) 20 to 35 cm of water
(D) 40 to 80 cm of water
(E) 80 to 100 cm of water

984. If utilized during infant resuscitation, the amount of $NaHCO_3$ given (per infant body weight) should be approximately

(A) 1 mEq/kg
(B) 3 mEq/kg
(C) 7 mEq/kg
(D) 10 mEq/kg
(E) 20 mEq/kg

985. The most common factor associated with neonatal death is

(A) birth injury
(B) prematurity
(C) congenital malformations
(D) metabolic diseases
(E) intrauterine growth restriction

986. A premature newborn exhibits rapid grunting respiration, chest retraction, and a diffuse infiltrate in the lung fields demonstrated on chest x-ray. The most likely diagnosis is

(A) pneumococcal pneumonia
(B) neonatal sepsis
(C) respiratory distress syndrome (RDS)
(D) congestive heart failure (CHF)
(E) hypoglycemia

987. The remnant of fetal circulation that normally remains patent during adult life is the

(A) ductus arteriosus
(B) umbilical arteries
(C) ductus venosus
(D) hepatic portal vein
(E) umbilical vein

988. After a normal labor and delivery of monozygotic twins at 35 weeks of gestation, one is found to be polycythemic, and the other small and markedly anemic. The most likely etiology of this phenomenon is

(A) acute fetal bleeding
(B) fetal cardiac failure
(C) poor maternal iron intake
(D) placental anastomosis
(E) Rh incompatibility

989. Approximately 2 days after delivery, an apparently healthy newborn male infant develops an intracranial hemorrhage. Vital signs are normal. His hematocrit and white blood count (WBC) are normal, but platelets are slightly decreased. The bleeding time is normal for age, but the prothrombin time is greatly prolonged. Blood type is A, Rh-negative. The most likely diagnosis is

(A) unrecognized birth trauma
(B) sepsis
(C) erythroblastosis fetalis
(D) hemophilia
(E) hemorrhagic disease of the newborn

990. Vitamin K administered to the newborn is given to prevent

(A) erythroblastosis fetalis
(B) hemophilia
(C) hemorrhagic disease of the newborn
(D) idiopathic thrombocytopenia

991. A premature newborn is found to have abdominal distention, ileus, and bloody stools. An abdominal x-ray shows excessive gas in the bowel and free air under the diaphragm. The most likely diagnosis is

(A) appendicitis
(B) toxic megacolon
(C) peptic ulcer disease
(D) necrotizing enterocolitis
(E) diabetic enteropathy

992. A male infant is delivered with very little amniotic fluid. He is noted to have low-set ears, contractures of the extremities, and prominent epicanthal folds. He does not void and dies during the first day of life. The most likely diagnosis is

(A) glycogen storage disease
(B) renal agenesis
(C) talipes equinovarus
(D) iniencephalus
(E) trisomy 18

993. Fetal anencephaly is commonly associated with

(A) pituitary hyperplasia
(B) oligohydramnios
(C) bradycardia
(D) adrenal hypertrophy
(E) post-term labor

994. The most common manifestation of fetal anoxic brain injury is

(A) choroid plexus hemorrhage
(B) rupture of the cerebral vein at the junction of the falx and tentorium
(C) mental retardation
(D) cerebral palsy

995. Neurologic abnormalities are found in greatest proportion in infants with

(A) high Apgars and normal birth weight
(B) low Apgars and normal birth weight
(C) low Apgars and low birth weight
(D) high Apgars and high birth weight
(E) low Apgars and high birth weight

996. It is estimated currently that intrapartum events account for what proportion of individuals with cerebral palsy (CP)?

(A) essentially 0%
(B) < 10%
(C) 20 to 40%
(D) 60 to 70%
(E) nearly 100%

997. An infant was born 10 hours previously to a mother whose membranes ruptured 27 hours prior to delivery. The mother was febrile in labor. The infant develops respiratory distress, apnea, and an unstable blood pressure. The most likely explanation of this infant's symptoms is

(A) group A streptococcus

(B) group B streptococcus

(C) listeriosis

(D) herpetic encephalopathy

(E) infant rubella

998. The most common sequela of a fetal toxoplasmosis infection is

(A) phocomelia

(B) anencephaly

(C) mental retardation

(D) ambiguous genitalia

(E) respiratory distress in the first 24 hours of life

999. A general figure for the incidence of significant fetal malformations (birth defects) is

(A) < 1%

(B) 3 to 5%

(C) 10 to 15%

(D) 25 to 30%

(E) > 40%

1000. Phocomelia is

(A) an error in color vision

(B) supernumerary digits

(C) defects in the long bones

(D) a two-vessel umbilical cord

(E) an inborn error of metabolism

1001. A child is born with genital ambiguity. The genital folds (scrotum and labia minora) are adherent in the midline, and there is severe hypospadias. The parents ask you about the gender of their child. Your best response, based on the information given above, is that

(A) the child has female pseudohermaphrodism and should be raised as female

(B) the diagnosis is most likely testicular feminization and the child should be raised as a male

(C) this is called an incomplete scrotal raphe and the child should be raised as a male

(D) it is likely the child has vaginal atresia, but should be raised as a female

(E) while the sex of rearing will most likely be female, assignment must await further investigation

1002. Alcohol abuse during pregnancy is associated with

(A) fetal hypospadias

(B) postmaturity

(C) midfacial hypoplasia

(D) macrosomia

(E) congenital cataracts

1003. The perinatal death rate is defined as

(A) deaths in utero of fetuses weighing 500 g or more per 1,000 population

(B) the sum of the fetal death rate and neonatal death rate per 1,000 live births

(C) infant deaths (under 1 year of age) per 1,000 live births

(D) deaths in utero of fetuses weighing 1,000 g or more per 1,000 births

(E) fetal and neonatal deaths occurring after 36 weeks' gestation and until 3 months of life, expressed per 1,000 population

1004. The most common cause of neonatal mortality is

(A) diabetes

(B) hypoxia

(C) erythroblastosis

(D) birth trauma

(E) premature placental separation

1005. A patient delivers shortly after arriving in the labor and delivery suite. Fetal prematurity would be suggested by finding

- (A) labia majora that are in contact with one another
- (B) one or both testes in the scrotum
- (C) fingernails that extend to or beyond the fingertips
- (D) breast tissue palpable
- (E) lanugo hair

1006. The most common cause of a "large-for-dates" (LGA) infant is

- (A) maternal diabetes
- (B) congenital abnormalities
- (C) in utero infections
- (D) erroneous last menstrual period (LMP)
- (E) maternal hypertension

DIRECTIONS (Questions 1007 through 1013): Each set of items in this section consists of lettered headings followed by several numbered words or phrases. For each numbered word or phrase, select the ONE lettered option that is most closely associated with it. Each lettered option may be selected once, more than once, or not at all.

Questions 1007 through 1009

Match the appropriate Apgar score to the description of the infant.

- (A) 0
- (B) 2
- (C) 5
- (D) 9
- (E) unable to give a score with this information

1007. Alert infant with good tone and color

1008. Pale infant with poor cry, flexed extremities, irregular respiration, and heart rate of 90

1009. Pink body, blue fingers, vigorous cry and active motion, good respiration, and heart rate of 120

Questions 1010 through 1013

Match the appropriate syndrome with the corresponding physical finding in the newborn.

- (A) Turner syndrome
- (B) Down syndrome
- (C) cri du chat syndrome
- (D) Klinefelter syndrome
- (E) trisomy 13

1010. Simian line or crease

1011. Lymphedema of hands and feet

1012. Microcephaly, catlike cry, micrognathism, low birth weight

1013. Genital atrophy may be present, but is generally not noticeable until after puberty

Answers and Explanations

962. (B) The Apgar scoring system, described by pediatrician Virginia Apgar in 1952, is a technique to assess the well-being of a newborn. An Apgar score is awarded to the infant at 1 and 5 minutes of life. In some cases, the Apgar score may be assessed again at 10 minutes of life or beyond. The infant gets a score of 0, 1, or 2 points in each of five categories: heart rate, respiratory effort, reflex irritability, muscle tone, and color. An Apgar score of 3 or less at 5 minutes in infants with a complicated birth is associated with an increased risk of cerebral palsy (goes from 0.3 to 1%). The change from 1 to 5 minutes is a good indicator of the successful neonatal resuscitation. See Table 14–1.

TABLE 14–1. Apgar Scoring

Signs	0	1	2
		Points Scored	
Heartbeats per minute	Absent	Slow (< 100)	Over 100
Respiratory effort	Absent	Slow, irregular	Good, crying
Muscle tone	Limp	Some flexion of extremities	Active motion
Reflex irritability	No response	Grimace	Cry or cough
Color	Blue or pale	Body pink, extremities blue	Completely pink

963. (B) All infants have a low pH at birth. If the infant is depressed or asphyxiated, it takes much longer to develop a normal pH. Changes in fetal circulation demonstrate the greatest effect in raising pH.

964. (A) The normal infant who is cool will resist metabolic acidosis and maintain pH by compensatory respiratory alkalosis. If the infant is in trouble from asphyxia, it may be unable to compensate, and the acidosis is accentuated. Ventilation will usually restore normal function. A common error in the resuscitation of infants is to do the resuscitation on a cold table rather than in an infant warmer.

965. (C) In the majority of infants, respiratory effort will be initiated between 30 and 60 seconds after birth. Fetal acidosis, drugs given to the mother, upper airway obstruction, a premature infant, pneumothorax, congenital anomalies, infection, and trauma can all be severe enough to inhibit an infant's respiratory effort. The cause must be sought and corrected. Most often, the cause is upper airway obstruction by fluids and mucus, which may be easily cleared by bulb suction.

966. (A) Prematurity has been defined for statistical purposes. There is no marked change in survival at 37 weeks or 2,500 g, and some infants who are mature but undergrown may be much more mature in terms of survival. There is no good single definition, and the recent obstetric terminology refers only to preterm infants as born before the 37th week of gestation.

967. (C) Other identifying features are decreased subcutaneous fat, wrinkled skin, decreased vernix, polycythemia, dehydration, and meconium staining. Such infants are classically described as having the features of "a little old man." If good nutrition is maintained throughout pregnancy, an infant of a long gestation can be macrosomic. Fusion of the eyelids is characteristic of a very immature fetus (26 to 27 weeks of gestation).

968. **(B)** This infant is undergrown or small for dates. He has grown too slowly in utero and may have been nutritionally compromised for some time. Postmaturity and growth retardation are risks often found together, often with poor infant outcomes.

969. **(D)** The normal newborn should breathe spontaneously and not have acid–base problems. The baby should be maintained in a head-down position to allow amniotic fluid and mucus to drain while the umbilical cord is cut. Slapping is unnecessary and dangerous and any attempt at full resuscitation (such as bag and mask ventilation) will be impractical until the baby can be moved to a warmed bed. Placing the infant on the maternal abdomen provides bonding and warmth, but this should be delayed until it is certain that the baby has established spontaneous respiration and is stable.

970. **(B)** As bilirubin pigment appears to break down in ultraviolet light, such treatment may keep the bilirubin from reaching a dangerous level that could necessitate an exchange transfusion. Putting the bassinet in daylight is treatment enough for some; others will need a special treatment system exposing them to higher levels of ultraviolet light.

971. **(D)** The normal newborn will lose 6 to 7 oz of his birth weight after delivery and gain it back by 10 days postpartum. He should then continue to gain weight rapidly. Feeding generally does not go well at first, accounting for the weight loss.

972. **(C)** Mothers often ask how long the umbilical stump will remain and what to do to care for it. Leaving it open and washing the area with soap and water seems to be adequate care. The umbilical stump should be cultured in cases of neonatal sepsis.

973. **(E)** The breech delivery, bulging fontanel, and progressive worsening of the condition all point to CNS bleeding. A subdural hematoma should be treated by immediate aspiration. The breech places the newborn at greater risk for head entrapment and resultant trauma. Also, it has been noted that infants that are breech at term have a higher risk of congenital anomalies.

974. **(B)** Asphyxia is a condition in which the arterial blood is hypoxic, acidotic, and hypercapnic. The heart rate is decreased and the anal sphincter may relax, causing loss of meconium. It is often associated with cooling of the infant, narcosis, brain hemorrhage, or metabolic acidosis.

975. **(C)** In the newborn, both Erb's and Klumpke's paralysis usually result from trauma to the brachial plexus during a difficult delivery. The brachial plexus is made of C5,6,7,8, and T1,2. Klumpke's paralysis affects only the hand and involves C7,8 and T1. Ptosis and miosis can also occur if sympathetic fibers of these nerves are involved in the injury. The injury most often occurs when pressure on the fetal head and neck (and therefore the brachial plexus) is too great. Lateral pressure on the head during vertex delivery (especially with shoulder dystocia) or hyperextension of the arms over the head during breech birth may cause this injury. This is also called Duchenne's paralysis.

976. **(C)** By eliminating the major causes of trauma, the incidence of brain damage at the time of delivery can be markedly reduced. The object of delivery is to do what is safest for mother and child. Mid-forceps delivery, especially when associated with an arrest disorder in labor, is associated with an increased incidence of intracranial hemorrhage.

977. **(B)** The injury is rare and results in bleeding from the muscle bed secondary to excessive traction, usually from breech delivery. There are generally no adverse long-term effects, and this will resolve.

978. (C) This is a moderately to severely depressed infant (estimated Apgar score 2 to 4). Respiration must be established. Gentle or rough handling is unlikely to help. If the baby is hypoxic, respiration by assisted ventilation is the key to helping the neonate. Establishing effective ventilation will speed the heart, and acidosis will correct with ventilation.

979. (A) Ventilation, base replacement, and cardiac massage must all be done simultaneously in the depressed, apneic infant with a very slow or absent heartbeat. If no blood circulates, neither oxygen nor base will get to the peripheral cells, where metabolism occurs. Anything short of successful ventilation and circulation will result in a severely damaged or dead baby.

980. (B) Minimal handling, a warm environment, and supplemental oxygen are indicated for any premature newborn, with more vigorous resuscitation and treatment utilized only as indicated by the fetal condition. Drugs to stimulate respiration have not proven to be effective and may be dangerous.

981. (C) Drugs, fetal immaturity, fetal trauma, fetal anomalies, fetal infection, and fetal hypoxia are the major causes of newborn apnea. Most of these result in depression of the fetal CNS. Naloxone, stimulation, and assisted ventilation are all used to overcome apnea.

982. (B) The tidal volume is that amount of air that is moved with each breath. This amount must be sufficient to clear the dead space of the upper respiratory tract and ventilate the periphery of the lung. Therefore, moving less than 20 mL of air back and forth during ventilation may not provide adequate air exchange in a newborn.

983. (C) If the pressure at which oxygen is given is too low, the lung will not expand, and if it is too high, the danger of ruptured alveoli and pneumothorax exists. Special masks and bags should be available for infants.

984. (A) The $NaHCO_3$ can be given in a 7.5% solution slowly through the umbilical vein. Be sure there is an adequate (> 80) heart rate so that the solution is properly distributed. Liver damage can occur if the $NaHCO_3$ remains in the liver parenchyma because of poor circulation.

985. (B) Prematurity from whatever etiology is the most common factor associated with neonatal death. Respiratory difficulty is often the major problem with these infants. However, many organs can fail in these small infants. While intrauterine growth restriction is often associated with premature delivery or pregnancies with poor outcomes, growth restriction by itself does not appear to be an independent factor in neonatal death. The second most common cause of neonatal death is congenital malformations.

986. (C) RDS is most common in premature infants and is due to a decreased amount of phospholipid surfactants in the alveoli. It is treated with assisted ventilation. Artificial surfactant is now available for use.

987. (D) The portal vein persists into adult life. If the ductus arteriosus persists, severe circulatory compromise occurs. Surgery is often necessary to close this defect.

988. (D) One twin can get a progressively larger amount of blood than the other because of placenta anastomoses. This is called twin–twin transfusion and classically results in one small, anemic twin and one large, plethoric twin who is subject to CHF. Acute fetal bleeding could cause anemia but should not result in significant size discrepancy. Poor maternal iron stores or an Rh incompatibility would affect both infants.

989. (E) The time to onset of the bleeding associated with a normal bleeding time and with a prolonged prothrombin time points to hemorrhagic disease of the newborn. The infant has hypoprothrombinemia as a result of low placental transport of vitamin K. Infants of mothers with epilepsy are at an increased risk for this disease. Infants of those mothers should be given supplemental vitamin K at birth. Routine administration of vitamin K is recommended for all neonates. Vitamin K in small doses given to the mother in labor or the infant at the time of delivery is prophylactic for hemorrhagic disease of the newborn. One milligram of vitamin K given to the infant is also used in therapy of hemolytic disease of the newborn.

990. **(C)** Vitamin K is routinely given to newborns to prevent hemolytic disease of the newborn.

991. **(D)** Necrotizing enterocolitis is a disease seen in both low-birth-weight and premature infants. The cause is unknown, but it is thought that the cause is related to immaturity of the gastrointestinal system rather than ischemia, as previously thought. It can be prevented by administration of immunoglobulin. In mild forms, the disease can be treated by dietary restriction; in severe forms, the bowel may need to be resected.

992. **(B)** Defects in the urinary system are associated with defects in the genital tract, low-set ears, and other anomalies. Low-set ears and cardiac defects are also seen in trisomy 18. Ultrasound studies performed during pregnancy will reveal oligohydramnios.

993. **(E)** In fetuses with anencephaly, the pituitary is either absent or markedly hypoplastic. Whether the lack of adrenocorticotropic hormone (ACTH) causes the associated adrenal atrophy is disputed. Lack of an intact CNS delays the onset of labor. There is no effect on fetal heart rate. Face presentations are common with anencephaly; because of the lack of a cranium, the head will not stay flexed. Fetal CNS malformations tend to occur with pregnancies in very young or very old mothers. Diabetics also are at increased risk, unless the hydramnios caused by the fetal inability to swallow prompts labor earlier.

994. **(A)** Ventricular hemorrhages from the choroid plexus are the result of hypoxia. Rupture of the great cerebral vein at the junction of the

falx and tentorium is more likely to occur from mechanical trauma and to result in subdural hematomas and/or dural tears. Studies suggest that the majority of cases of cerebral palsy occur before birth or are acquired after birth as a result of factors such as sepsis or fever. Cerebral palsy due to birth anoxia is much less common than choroid plexus hemorrhage.

995. **(C)** This concept is both important and logical. The premature or undergrown infant who is depressed at birth has a higher incidence of neurologic abnormalities than term normal-weight, high-Apgar infants. In some cases, both the newborn's low birth weight and poor Apgar scores are the result of an underlying process that results in neurologic abnormalities as well. That is, the low Apgar and birth weight are the result, not the cause, of the infant's developmental problems. Long-term follow-up is needed.

996. **(C)** Myers demonstrated that prolonged partial asphyxia in monkeys is more likely to result in CP than is acute hypoxia. This situation may occur at times other than labor, although labor may be a cause. Neurologic damage can occur as the result of many factors other than hypoxia. Currently, this is a subject of great controversy and ongoing study.

997. **(B)** Mothers are often asymptomatic carriers (urine, rectum, or vagina) of group B beta-hemolytic streptococci. Half of newborns are colonized at the time of delivery. Early overwhelming sepsis occurs in about 1 in every 100 of the infants of colonized mothers. This is the reason why authorities recommend antibiotic prophylaxis in culture-positive or high-risk mothers during labor. Listeriosis and *Salmonella* can cause infant sepsis but are very rare. Rubella is not associated with sepsis at birth but of serious indolent infectious sequelae both before and after birth.

998. **(C)** Cerebral calcification, chorioretinitis, and head size abnormalities are also found in infants following a toxoplasmosis infection.

Fortunately, not all infants of infected mothers are affected. Some also show only mild effects.

999. (B) About 3 to 5% have clinically significant malformations, and about 1% die. Congenital malformations account for a significant proportion of perinatal deaths.

1000. (C) The defects in the extremities may be of varying severity. Most of the infants are of normal intelligence and survive. Thalidomide made the public aware of this drug-induced anomaly. It is the most potent human teratogen known.

1001. (E) Sex assignment can be very difficult in the case of the infant with ambiguous genitalia. Generally, three categories of children fit this problem: female pseudohermaphrodites, male pseudohermaphrodites, and those with genetic or metabolic gonadal abnormalities. When the abnormality is severe, the female sex is usually assigned because the female pseudohermaphrodite can often have normal fertility and sexual function; the male pseudohermaphrodites in most cases can have neither. While there is great pressure to assign a gender in the delivery room, further investigation of the genital structures present, as well as the infant's chromosomal makeup, must be established before the optimal sex of rearing is assigned.

1002. (C) When one drug is abused, it is likely two or more are used. In illicit drug users, the incidence of polydrug abuse has been estimated as up to 75% of all users. From the aspect of neonatal malformation, alcohol abuse is most commonly associated with midfacial hypoplasia and behavioral/social problems. It has also been associated with brain, spine, and cardiac defects. Prematurity and growth restriction are also common. Congenital cataracts are more typical of infants exposed to viral infections early in gestation.

1003. (B) Perinatal deaths refer to both fetal and neonatal deaths, and the rate is calculated per 1,000 live births. It has been often proposed as an indirect measure of the quality of perinatal care.

1004. (B) Prematurity, with its attendant greater risk of pulmonary malfunction, malpresentation, and birth injury, greatly increases the risk of death from hypoxia. Very immature infants can be impossible to ventilate because of poor lung compliance.

1005. (E) Preterm infants have lanugo hair, rudimentary nails, no palpable breast tissue, gaping labia, and undescended testes. Dubowitz's scale utilizing these and other characteristics is accurate to about ±2 weeks.

1006. (A) Large for dates implies that the infant who has been in utero for whatever length of time has grown more than normally during that period. Diabetes in the mother will result in episodes of excessive increased glucose available for fetal growth, but the mother does not have much, if any, small vessel disease that may adversely affect placental transport and fetal growth. Thus, the overall effect is likely an LGA infant. Congenital anomalies, intrauterine infection, and maternal hypertension will cause small-for-dates (SGA) infants.

1007. (E) Inadequate data is given to derive an Apgar score. Heart rate, respiratory effort, muscle tone, reflex irritability, and color must be described. Each area must be scored.

1008. (C) This infant is in a high-risk category and needs close attention and respiratory assistance. The Apgar score could be as low as 3, suggesting severe CNS depression.

1009. (D) Given the high hematocrit of most newborns, it is very difficult for them to saturate it all with oxygen to make their fingers pink. There is no prognostic difference between an Apgar of 9 and an Apgar of 10.

1010. (B) Trisomy 21 is more common with older mothers. The children also have hypotonia, epicanthal folds, Brushfield spots, a furrowed tongue, and a distal axial triradius. The retardation may be mild to severe.

1011. (A) This finding is recognizable at birth and should be evaluated carefully. Though not commonly known, Turner syndrome involves in utero blocked lymphatics. It is this blockage that results in the webbed neck.

1012. (C) A deletion of the short arm of chromosome 5, cri du chat, is characterized by all of the signs mentioned, along with hypertelorism with epicanthus and abnormal dermatoglyphics. The phrase itself means "cry of the cat."

1013. (D) Klinefelter syndrome is an XXY male, characterized therefore by the presence of a Y chromosome and chromatin positivity. Many times, this syndrome has been described as a phenotypic male, often overweight and with testicular atrophy. Testicular atrophy is present in some cases but is not the general case, nor is the often ascribed gynecomastia. The syndrome occurs in about 2 to 3:1,000 live male births.

Infertility
Questions

1014. What percentage of reproductive-age couples are unable to conceive after 1 year of coitus without contraception?

(A) 1 to 2%

(B) 15%

(C) 30%

(D) 50%

(E) 75%

1015. A 31-year-old infertility patient with regular ovulatory menstrual cycles has begun therapy with clomiphene citrate. Before she starts therapy, what information should you provide her regarding the medication?

(A) Typically, the timing of ovulation is increased by a week.

(B) Approximately 40% of patients will respond to clomiphene citrate with increased endometrial thickness.

(C) The risk of multiple gestation is 25%.

(D) Clomiphene citrate improves the fecundity rate principally through its effect on the endometrial lining.

(E) Risk and side effects of clomiphene citrate include nausea, hot flushes, weight gain, and mood swings.

1016. Which of the following statements regarding basal body temperatures is TRUE?

(A) An oral temperature is taken prior to bedtime.

(B) A rise of 0.2°F between 2 consecutive days reflects ovulation.

(C) A biphasic temperature shift reflects estrogen action on the hypothalamus.

(D) Absence of a biphasic temperature shift suggests pregnancy.

(E) none of the above

1017. Which of the following is the BEST method to time intercourse for procreative means?

(A) thermogenic shift in basal body temperature

(B) urinary luteinizing hormone (LH) kit testing

(C) serum progesterone level

(D) profuse, thin, acellular cervical mucus

(E) mittelschmerz

1018. In a young, obese, chronically anovulatory woman with an elevated LH:FSH (follicle-stimulating hormone) ratio and polycystic-appearing ovaries, which of the following is the preferred initial method of ovulation induction?

(A) metformin

(B) human menopausal gonadotropins (hMGs)

(C) pulsatile gonadotropin-releasing hormone (GnRH)

(D) clomiphene citrate

(E) bromocriptine mesylate

1019. The initial treatment of choice in a patient with hypogonadotropic hypogonadism when ovulation is desired is

(A) low-dose estrogen therapy

(B) human menopausal gonadotropin (hMG) therapy

(C) bromocriptine mesylate

(D) cyclic progesterone

(E) clomiphene citrate

1020. A woman who suffers from anterior pituitary failure (Sheehan syndrome) can be induced to ovulate using which of the following hormonal therapies?

(A) low-dose estrogen therapy

(B) hMG injections

(C) pulsatile GnRH

(D) clomiphene citrate

(E) bromocriptine mesylate

1021. Which of the following statements BEST describes estrogen action on cervical mucus?

(A) It decreases the water content of cervical mucus.

(B) It decreases the palm-leaf crystallization pattern of mucus upon drying (ferning).

(C) It decreases formation of glycoprotein channels favoring sperm penetration.

(D) It increases cervical mucus stretchability (spinnbarkeit).

(E) It increases the amount of potassium chloride in the cervical mucus.

1022. Which of the following statements regarding the postcoital test (PCT) is TRUE?

(A) It predicts whether pregnancy can occur.

(B) It is performed 1 to 2 days after ovulation.

(C) It correlates the number of sperm in the cervical mucus with the pregnancy rate.

(D) It examines the ability of sperm to reach and survive in the mucus.

(E) It is performed within 1 hour of coitus.

1023. A 31-year-old patient is preparing to start in vitro fertilization (IVF) because of obstructed fallopian tubes. On hysterosalpingogram (HSG), it is noted that she has large dilated hydrosalpinges present bilaterally. What should be the next step?

(A) The patient should begin her IVF treatment cycle.

(B) The patient should repeat the HSG to confirm the result.

(C) The patient should not be offered the opportunity to have IVF.

(D) The patient should be recommended bilateral tubal ligation prior to starting IVF.

(E) The patient should be counseled to have her hydrosalpinges drained via transvaginal aspiration.

1024. An infertile patient with regular menses has a biphasic basal body temperature. The temperature rise during the luteal phase is 9 days in length (normal luteal phase, 10 to 14 days' duration). Which of the following tests should be performed to further evaluate the shortened luteal phase?

(A) serum LH

(B) diagnostic laparoscopy

(C) serum estradiol

(D) serum FSH

(E) serum prolactin

1025. Besides infertility, the most common symptom of a luteal-phase defect is

(A) vaginal dryness

(B) spontaneous miscarriage

(C) tubal occlusion

(D) breast tenderness

(E) ovarian enlargement

1026. Which of the following may be implied by an HSG but commonly represents a problem with the procedure technique?

(A) unicornuate uterus

(B) distal tubal obstruction

(C) proximal tubal obstruction

(D) hydrosalpinx

(E) intrauterine synechiae

1027. A 31-year-old infertile woman requests surgical tuboplasty for correction of tubal occlusion. You advise her that the pregnancy rate after surgical tuboplasty depends on the location of the fallopian tube occlusion. Three areas of tubal occlusion correctable by surgical tuboplasty, in decreasing prognosis for pregnancy, are

(A) isthmic–cornual (endometriosis), isthmic–isthmic (sterilization), infundibular (salpingitis)

(B) isthmic–isthmic (sterilization), isthmic–cornual (endometriosis), infundibular (salpingitis)

(C) infundibular (salpingitis), isthmic–cornual (endometriosis), isthmic–isthmic (sterilization)

(D) isthmic–isthmic (sterilization), infundibular (salpingitis), isthmic–cornual (endometriosis)

(E) isthmic–cornual (endometriosis), infundibular (salpingitis), isthmic–isthmic (sterilization)

1028. A 33-year-old Scottish woman complains of pelvic pain and amenorrhea associated with low-grade fever and weight loss. Physical examination demonstrates a tender pelvic mass. Surgical findings include dense pelvic adhesions, segmental dilatation of the fallopian tubes, and everted fimbria. Microscopic examination of the right fallopian tube shows proliferation of tubal folds with giant cells within the tube. These findings should lead to the diagnosis of

(A) endometriosis

(B) adenocarcinoma

(C) tuberculosis

(D) gonorrheal salpingitis

(E) salpingitis isthmica nodosa

1029. Which of the following cell types undergoes the first meiotic division to form haploid cells?

(A) spermatogonia

(B) primary spermatocyte

(C) secondary spermatocyte

(D) spermatid

(E) spermatozoa

1030. A 27-year-old azoospermic male undergoes a testicular biopsy revealing normal seminiferous tubules. He has been diagnosed with hypogonadotropic hypogonadism and receives FSH and human chorionic gonadotropin (hCG) injections. What is the minimal time required before repeating the semen analysis for spermatogenesis response?

(A) 15 days

(B) 30 days

(C) 60 days

(D) 90 days

(E) 120 days

1031. Sperm capacitation refers to a process by which spermatozoa become capable of

(A) stimulating meiosis of the ovum

(B) dispersing the zona radiata

(C) penetrating the cervical mucus

(D) producing acrosomal enzymes

(E) fertilizing the ovum

1032. Which of the following statements BEST decribes regulation of testicular function?

(A) LH stimulates inhibin production by the Leydig cells.

(B) LH stimulates androgen-binding protein by Sertoli cells.

(C) FSH stimulates spermatogenesis by the seminiferous tubules.

(D) FSH stimulates testosterone synthesis by Leydig cells.

(E) LH stimulates spermatogenesis by the seminiferous tubules.

1033. Which of the following tests should be considered primarily in infertile males with previous vasectomy reversal?

(A) Sims–Huhner test

(B) hamster egg sperm penetration assay

(C) sperm antibody testing

(D) semen analysis

(E) split ejaculate analysis

1034. Which of the following semen parameters requires more sophisticated testing than semen analysis?

    (A) sperm motility

    (B) sperm concentration

    (C) sperm morphology

    (D) sperm penetration

    (E) seminal fluid viscosity

1035. A couple with male infertility characterized by a semen analysis with a sperm count of 14 million/mL, 25% motility, and 23% normal forms presents to your clinic. The husband's physical examination and hormone studies are normal. The appropriate initial therapy is

    (A) clomiphene citrate

    (B) varicocelectomy

    (C) in vitro fertilization (IVF)

    (D) intrauterine insemination with washed husband's sperm

    (E) insemination with donor sperm

1036. A 32-year-old male with oligospermia (low sperm count) has a history of fever accompanying painful swelling of the parotid gland and right testicle during high school. The most likely etiology of this condition is

    (A) cytomegalovirus

    (B) herpes simplex

    (C) varicella-zoster

    (D) mumps

    (E) influenza

1037. A 43-year-old woman and her husband report to you a history of pelvic adhesions and bilateral distal occlusion of both fallopian tubes with large hydrosalpinges. Both ovaries are buried in thick vascular adhesions. Adoption is not a consideration for the couple. What is the appropriate recommended therapy for this couple?

    (A) gamete intrafallopian transfer (GIFT)

    (B) IVF using her own eggs

    (C) lysis of adhesions and surgical mobilization of the ovaries

    (D) ovulation induction using gonadotropins with intrauterine inseminations

    (E) IVF using donor eggs

1038. Which of the following causes for infertility may be treatable by assisted reproductive technology?

    (A) fallopian tube obstruction

    (B) low sperm count

    (C) cervical mucus abnormalities

    (D) unexplained infertility

    (E) all of the above

1039. Which of the following studies would be more appropriate for a 36-year-old woman who is G0P0 with 2 years of infertility, than for one who is G3P0030?

    (A) hysterosalpingogram

    (B) endometrial biopsy

    (C) karyotype with banding

    (D) lupus anticoagulant assay

    (E) diagnostic laparoscopy

1040. The risk of first-trimester spontaneous abortion after three successive abortions is about

    (A) 0 to 5%

    (B) 10 to 20%

    (C) 30 to 50%

    (D) 55 to 70%

    (E) 75 to 90%

1041. Which of the following statements regarding the incompetent cervix is TRUE?

    (A) It is associated with first-trimester spontaneous abortions.

    (B) It is easily diagnosed by precise measurement of cervical resistance to dilatation.

    (C) It is characterized by painless dilatation of the cervix after the first trimester of pregnancy.

    (D) It is inherited as an autosomal recessive disease.

    (E) It is primarily treated by medical therapy.

DIRECTIONS (Questions 1042 through 1051): Each of the numbered items or incomplete statements in this section is followed by answers or by completions of the statement. Select the answers or completions that may apply.

1042. Which four of the factors listed below contribute to the increased number of infertility evaluations in the United States?

(A) a rise in pelvic inflammatory disease (PID) in women aged 20 to 24 years

(B) an increased incidence of male factor infertility

(C) the greater number of people born during 1946–1964 who are now infertile

(D) the delay in childbirth to ages at which women are less likely to conceive

(E) a greater public awareness of modern infertility therapies

1043. Which four of the following statements regarding the function of cervical mucus are true?

(A) It provides a barrier to vaginal microorganisms.

(B) It provides an acid environment for prevention of uterine infection.

(C) It provides a conducive environment for spermatozoa survival.

(D) It provides glucose as energy substrate for spermatozoa.

(E) It provides an environment for spermatozoa capacitation.

1044. Which two patient situations are suggested by a profuse, thin, acellular cervical mucus with a high degree of stretchability and a palm-leaf crystallization pattern upon drying?

(A) late follicular phase of the menstrual cycle

(B) anovulatory

(C) on birth control pills

(D) postmenopausal

1045. In completing the infertility workup in a 36-year-old patient with secondary infertility of 2 years' duration, you perform an HSG that demonstrates a uterine filling defect consistent with intrauterine synechiae. You elect to perform an operative hysteroscopic resection of these synechiae using nonelectrolyte distention media. Which four of the following statements are true?

(A) Nonelectrolyte solutions do not conduct electrical current and can be used safely with electrosurgery during hysteroscopy.

(B) Intravenous absorption of nonelectrolyte solutions can result in fluid overload.

(C) Intrauterine synechiae typically appear after operative trauma to the uterine cavity or infection.

(D) Hysteroscopic resection of intrauterine synechiae can result in restoration of normal menstruation in the majority of patients.

(E) Term pregnancies after hysteroscopic resection of intrauterine synechiae are rare.

1046. Infertility from endometriosis may be due to which four of the following abnormalities?

(A) pelvic adhesions

(B) altered fallopian tube motility

(C) sperm phagocytosis by peritoneal macrophages

(D) defective embryo implantation

(E) pituitary failure

1047. Which four of the following are causes of abnormal spermatogenesis?

(A) cold environment

(B) cryptorchidism

(C) genetic abnormalities

(D) varicocele

(E) marijuana

1048. Which four of the following environmental factors adversely affect spermatogenesis?

(A) swimming

(B) prolonged sitting

(C) febrile illness

(D) use of jockey shorts

(E) hot bath

1049. Which four of the following statements regarding a testicular varicocele are true?

(A) It is an abnormal dilation of the pampiniform plexus within the spermatic cord.

(B) It results from defective valves within the internal spermatic vein.

(C) It causes abnormal spermatogenesis by raising intratesticular temperature.

(D) It occurs in 10 to 15% of the general population.

(E) It occurs more frequently on the right side.

1050. Which four of the following immunologic factors are associated with recurrent abortion?

(A) lupus anticoagulant

(B) anticardiolipin antibody

(C) antinuclear antibodies

(D) antiovarian antibodies

(E) human lymphocyte antigen (HLA) compatibility

1051. What test(s) is/are most predictive of diminished ovarian reserve as a result of age-related changes?

(A) serum early follicular phase FSH and estradiol levels

(B) serum early follicular phase FSH and LH levels

(C) serum progesterone during the late luteal phase

(D) serum inhibin B levels during the late luteal phase

(E) none of the above

DIRECTIONS (Questions 1052 through 1060): Each set of items in this section consists of lettered headings followed by several numbered words or phrases. For each numbered word or phrase, select the ONE lettered option that is most closely associated with it. Each lettered option may be selected once, more than once, or not at all.

Questions 1052 through 1055

(A) clomiphene citrate

(B) bromocriptine mesylate

(C) hMGs

(D) GnRH

(E) dexamethasone

(F) GnRH analog

(G) none of the above

1052. Lysergic acid derivative

1053. Antiestrogen

1054. Urinary metabolites of postmenopausal women

1055. Ovulatory agent for hypergonadotropic hypogonadism

Questions 1056 through 1060

(A) colposcopy

(B) laparoscopy

(C) hysteroscopy

(D) HSG

(E) ultrasound

(F) more than one of the above

1056. A procedure that asesses both uterine cavity and tubal lumen

1057. A procedure that visualizes pelvic endometriosis

1058. A procedure that visualizes the uterine cavity

1059. A procedure that assesses tubal patency

1060. A procedure that detects ovum release from the follicle

Answers and Explanations

1014. (B) About 15% of reproductive-age couples are unable to conceive after 1 year of coitus without contraception. Eighty percent of couples achieve conception within 1 year, with 25% conceiving during the first month of unprotected coitus.

1015. (E) The risks and side effects of clomiphene citrate include nausea, hot flushes, weight gain, and emotional lability. These side effects occur with relative frequency in 10 to 25% of patients. The risk of multiple gestation with clomiphene citrate is 7%. Clomiphene citrate acts on the hypothalamus as an antiestrogen to blunt the negative feedback of estrogen. It may also have negative effects on endometrial proliferation, thus causing a decrease in endometrial thickness. Typically, ovulation takes place at the expected time for an ovulatory woman.

1016. (E) Basal body temperatures (BBTs) rely on the presence of circulating progesterone to identify ovulation. The oral temperature is taken upon awakening and a rise of 0.4° to 0.6°F between 2 consecutive days reflects the thermogenic action of progesterone on the hypothalamus. High circulating progesterone levels during pregnancy cause a persistent elevation in temperature after the biphasic temperature shift (see Figure 15–1).

1017. (B) When used by a motivated individual, the urinary LH surge predicts ovulation within 24 hours in 87% of menstrual cycles. BBTs and endometrial decidualization rely on progesterone action to retrospectively identify ovulation. Profuse, thin, acellular cervical mucus results from high circulating estrogen levels unopposed by progesterone. It cannot distinguish between the presence of a dominant follicle or chronic anovulation. Mittelschmerz, the transient abdominal pain accompanying bleeding from the ovulatory follicle, does not occur in all women.

1018. (A) Metformin is rapidly gaining acceptance as the initial method of spontaneous ovulation induction. It is an insulin-sensitizing agent that induces spontaneous ovulatory cycles in ~33% of women with insulin-resistant polycystic ovary syndrome (PCOS). Intramuscular administration of hMGs and intravenous pulsatile GnRH therapy is expensive and inconvenient. They are not the drugs of choice in a woman with an intact pituitary and functioning ovaries. Under these conditions, clomiphene citrate is easy to use and comparatively inexpensive, but has an increased risk of multiple pregnancy.

1019. (B) Absence of ovarian function due to hypothalamic dysfunction is characterized by low-normal circulating gonadotropin levels and is referred to as hypogonadotropic hypogonadism. Anovulation accompanying hypogonadotropic hypogonadism is associated with low circulating estrogen levels and is therefore unresponsive to clomiphene citrate. Ovulation can be established with pulsatile GnRH therapy or hMG administration.

1020. (B) Sheehan syndrome is a condition in which the cells of the anterior pituitary responsible for FSH and LH production are no longer viable. Thus, the remnant pituitary

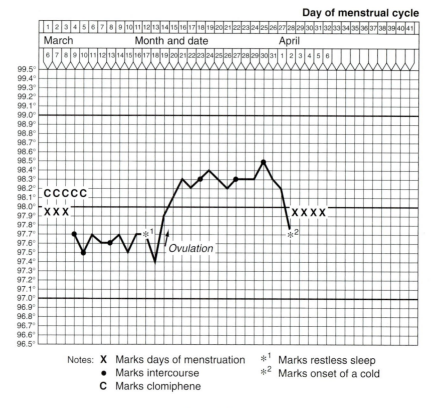

Figure 15–1.

will be unresponsive to increases in endogenous (clomiphene citrate) or exogenous (pulsatile) GnRH. These women undergo successful ovulation with daily injections of hMG (a combination of 75 IU FSH and 75 IU LH) for an average length of time of 10 to 12 days, which directly stimulates folliculogenesis to create mature follicles and oocytes.

1021. **(D)** Cervical mucus consists of multiple cross-linked glycoproteins. Although amounts vary with the menstrual cycle, 90% of cervical mucus consists of water and sodium chloride (NaCl). In the early follicular phase, a scant amount of cervical mucus is present. During the late follicular phase, a rise in circulating estrogen levels alters vascular epithelial permeability and increases the water content of cervical secretions. The mucus becomes profuse, thin, acellular, and clear, resulting in a high degree of stretchability (8 to 10 cm), referred to as spinnbarkeit, when pulled from the cervix, or stretched between a slide and a cover slip. The NaCl content of

the mucus allows it to form a palm-leaf crystallization pattern upon drying, a phenomenon referred to as *ferning*. These properties of estrogen-stimulated mucus promote formation of glycoprotein channels favoring sperm penetration.

1022. **(D)** The PCT, or Simms–Huhner test, examines sperm survival in cervical mucus and determines whether sperm are migrating into the female reproductive system. It does not predict whether pregnancy can occur. The test is performed after 2 days of sexual abstinence and 1 to 2 days before ovulation, when estrogen-stimulated cervical mucus is abundant. BBTs or the midcycle LH surge may be used to determine the timing of the PCT. Mucus is withdrawn from the endocervical canal within 8 hours of coitus and examined. The presence of any forwardly motile sperm in alkaline mucus suggests adequate coital technique and a normal cervical mucus–sperm interaction.

1023. (D) The bulk of the evidence in the current literature suggests that the presence of large hydrosalpinges decreased the pregnancy success rate of IVF by ~50%. Thus, it is now standard practice to recommend bilateral tubal ligation prior to initiating IVF to increase the couple's chances of success. Aspirating the hydrosalpinges will simply result in refilling of the fallopian tubes with fluid.

1024. (E) Luteal phase deficiency should be considered in women with a shortened luteal phase as detected by a rise in BBT of less than 11 days' duration. Hyperprolactinemia is often associated with luteal-phase deficiency and is treatable with bromocriptine.

1025. (B) Besides its effect on fertility, luteal-phase deficiency is associated with an increased incidence of recurrent first-trimester abortion.

1026. (C) Hysterosalpingography entails injection of radiopaque dye through the uterus with fluoroscopic visualization of the uterine cavity and tubal lumen. The resulting HSG is useful in detecting uterine anomalies and fallopian tube occlusion in women with histories of repetitive spontaneous abortion and infertility. Proximal occlusion of the tube may frequently occur during an HSG due to intermittent tubal spasm. While the presence of hydrosalpinx, distal tubal occlusion, uterine synechiae, and müllerian anomalies can be confirmed by HSG, one must be careful not to overinterpret an HSG with unilateral or bilateral proximal tubal obstruction. When proximal tubal obstruction is found, one should either repeat the HSG or perform a diagnostic laparoscopy with chromotubation.

1027. (B) About 60 to 80% of women achieve pregnancy after reversal of sterilization due to isthmic–isthmic obstruction. For isthmic–cornual occlusion due to disease such as endometriosis, proximal tubal reanastomosis is associated with a 40 to 50% pregnancy rate. (Isthmic–cornual occlusion due to inspissated cellular debris may be correctable by retrograde tubal cannulation.) Correction of fimbrial occlusion (neosalpingostomy) due to

salpingitis has only a 10 to 20% pregnancy rate.

1028. (C) *Mycobacterium tuberculosis* is prevalent in several parts of the world, including the southeastern United States, Asia, Mexico, and Scotland. Pelvic tuberculosis usually represents a secondary invasion, occurring by lymphohematogenous spread from a primary lung infection. Pelvic tuberculosis occurs in about 5% of patients with pulmonary disease. The tube may be studded with miliary implants, which should not be mistaken for Walthard rests or metastatic cancer. Distinguishing features of this disease are extremely dense pelvic adhesions, segmental dilatation of the fallopian tubes, and everted fimbria, giving the tube the appearance of a "tobacco pouch." Peritoneal disease may cause ascites, while endometrial involvement may lead to amenorrhea.

1029. (B) Spermatogonia divide by mitosis to form primary spermatocytes. The primary spermatocyte undergoes the first meiotic division, producing two secondary spermatocytes, each of which contains 23 double-stranded chromosomes. Each secondary spermatocyte completes the second meiotic division, yielding two spermatids, each of which contains 23 single-stranded chromosomes. Therefore, every primary spermatocyte gives rise to four spermatids (two with 22 + 1 X chromosomes and two with 22 + 1 Y chromosomes) that develop into mature spermatozoa.

1030. (D) Spermatogenesis occurs over 72 days. Therefore, the earliest time period that sperm can be detected is 90 days but frequently requires longer observation periods.

1031. (E) Within the female reproductive tract, spermatozoa undergo capacitation, a process by which spermatozoa become capable of fertilizing an ovum. Capacitation is normally inhibited by substances within the seminal plasma and is induced in vitro by separating spermatozoa from seminal plasma. Capacitation is associated with the removal of glycoproteins from the plasma membrane overlying the acrosomal region of the spermatozoa. Acrosomal enzymes released locally and/or bound to the remaining inner acrosomal membrane play a crucial role in sperm penetration of the ovum.

1032. **(C)** FSH, in conjunction with testosterone, stimulates spermatogenesis by the seminiferous tubules. FSH also stimulates Sertoli cells to synthesize androgen-binding protein (which maintains high gonadal testosterone levels) and inhibin. The primary effect of LH is to stimulate testosterone synthesis by Leydig cells.

1033. **(D)** The most important part of the male infertility evaluation is a semen analysis. A semen specimen is obtained by masturbation after 3 to 7 days of abstinence, or through intercourse using nonspermicidal silicon condoms. The sample must be kept warm and received by the laboratory within 1 hour. Occasionally, it is important to examine subtle aspects of sperm function by other methods. The sperm penetration assay evaluates the ability of human sperm to penetrate golden hamster eggs prepared to accept foreign sperm. A split ejaculate may be useful for some types of inseminations and collects the semen in two portions: the first portion containing the sperm-rich fraction and prostatic fluid, and the second portion containing seminal vesicle fluid with less sperm numbers. Detection of antibodies directed against sperm is helpful for rare cases of immunologic infertility. The sperm penetration assay of cervical mucus in vitro was developed to study sperm–mucus interactions but is rarely performed today.

1034. **(D)** Normal values for semen analysis are: volume, 2 to 6 mL; liquefaction (conversion of semen from a gelatinous to a liquid form), within 1 hour; pH, 7 to 8; count, 20 million/mL or more; motility, 50% or more; morphology, 60% or more. Sperm density less than 20 million spermatozoa per milliliter is associated with a five- to tenfold increased risk of infertility but also occurs in some fertile men. To assess the sperm's ability to pen-

etrate the ovum requires a hamster egg sperm penetration assay.

1035. **(D)** Appropriate initial therapy is intrauterine inseminations with husband's sperm. With mild to moderate male factor infertility, the success of inseminations is lower (5–15% per cycle). However, this method should be attempted before proceeding to donor sperm or IVF. If the couple requires IVF to successfully conceive, then the recommended procedure for IVF is intracytoplasmic sperm injection (ICSI). This is a procedure that involves the injection of single sperm into an oocyte to achieve fertilization. Varicocelectomy is helpful only after documentation of a varicocele.

1036. **(D)** The RNA virus, paramyxovirus, is responsible for mumps. It causes parotid gland inflammation, which is occasionally accompanied by pancreatitis, orchitis, and encephalitis. Mumps orchitis can produce abnormalities in sperm quality and quantity, particularly if it occurs postpuberty.

1037. **(E)** Maternal aging and decreased ovarian reserve at age 43 precludes the use of GIFT or IVF as a reasonable therapeutic approach for this couple. Ovulation induction is not indicated due to the presence of severe tubal factor with bilateral hydrosalpinges. There is no need for lysis of adhesions due to the poor prognosis with this couple using the patient's own tubes and ovaries. Donor egg IVF would offer a 1 in 2 chance for pregnancy success in this couple.

1038. **(E)** Assisted reproductive technology is used for many causes for infertility when lesser therapies are unsuccessful or associated with a poor prognosis.

1039. **(E)** Diagnostic laparoscopy is not indicated in patients with recurrent abortion but would be appropriate after a negative infertility workup. Immunologic testing with anticardiolipin antibodies, lupus anticoagulant assay, and antiphospholipid antibodies should be performed. A hysterosalpingogram may reveal an intracavitary lesion as a cause of recurrent pregnancy loss as well as tubal occlusion. Luteal phase deficiency can be detected with endometrial biopsy performed later in the luteal phase. Finally, karyotype analysis may reveal balanced translocations in either parent that would increase the risk of genetically imbalanced offspring.

1040. (C) The risk of first-trimester spontaneous abortion after three successive abortions is about 32% (30 to 55%). Inaccurate theoretical calculations performed over 50 years ago stated that a woman with a history of three successive abortions had a 73 to 84% chance of aborting a subsequent pregnancy. The use of these inaccurate, pessimistic projections led to several empirical therapies for the treatment of recurrent abortion.

1041. (C) The term incompetent cervix refers to the painless dilatation of the cervix during the second trimester or early third trimester of pregnancy. Prolapse of fetal membranes through the cervix is usually followed by expulsion of a living fetus that is too immature to survive. A careful history to determine whether these events occurred previously is required since precise methods to diagnose an incompetent cervix do not exist. The most common cause of incompetent cervix is trauma (e.g., dilatation and curettage, conization, cervical amputation), although exposure to stilbestrol in utero has also been associated with this disorder. An incompetent cervix is usually treated by surgical cerclage (e.g., McDonald, Shirodkar), a procedure designed to restore the competency of the cervix.

1042. (A, C, D, E) Although the proportion of infertile couples has not changed significantly over the past 20 years, several factors contribute to the rising number of infertility investigations in the United States. The threefold increase from 1965 to 1982 in the percentage of infertile women aged 20 to 24 years probably reflects the rise in PID in this age group. The greater number of people born during the baby boom (1946–1964) who are now infertile also increases infertility investigation. In addition, many women have delayed childbirth to ages at which they are less likely to conceive. Many couples have greater knowledge of modern therapies for infertility and financial resources for health care at a time when the supply of infants for adoption is limited.

1043. (A, C, D, E) The cervix consists of an endocervical canal, which is bounded caudally by the ectocervix. Mucus secreted by the endocervical epithelium prevents ascent of vaginal microorganisms while providing a conducive environment for spermatozoa survival. In the early follicular phase, a scant amount of cervical mucus containing leukocytes acts as a barrier to sperm and bacteria. Midcycle cervical mucus offers an alkaline environment (pH 8.5) for spermatozoa protection from vaginal acidity (pH 3 to 5), and provides energy substances to spermatozoa. Although some reach the tubal ampulla within 5 to 10 minutes after coitus, most spermatozoa remain within the cervical mucus and undergo capacitation, a process by which they attain the ability to fertilize ova. They continuously ascend the female reproductive tract over the next 48 hours or longer.

1044. (A, B) Profuse, thin, acellular cervical mucus reflects high circulating estrogen levels unopposed by progesterone. In ovulatory women, this cervical mucus pattern can be used to detect the presence of a developing ovarian follicle. If the patient is postmenopausal, there is no estrogen. If she is pregnant or on birth control pills, there is a high level of progesterone, which prevents this type of mucus.

1045. (A, B, C, D) Hysteroscopic resection of intrauterine synechiae, which occur after uterine trauma or infection is currently considered the standard of therapy for Asherman's syndrome. In these patients, normal menstruation can be restored and pregnancy can occur. Since 0.2% glycine and hyskon are commonly used as distention media in hysteroscopic procedures that require nonconducting media, intravenous absorption can induce fluid overload.

1046. (A, B, C, D) One third of women with endometriosis experience infertility. Conversely, up to 60% of women undergoing laparoscopy for infertility have this disease. Severe endometriosis causes pelvic adhesions leading to damage of pelvic viscera. Lesser amounts of endometriosis may also diminish the probability of conception. A reduction in pregnancy rate has been shown in women with mild endometriosis undergoing donor insemination. Since many of these women have anatomically normal pelvic viscera, subfertility under these conditions may reflect altered tubal motility due to prostaglandin release by endometriosis, phagocytosis of sperm by activated peritoneal macrophages, or defective embryo implantation resulting from immunologic phenomena. Endometriosis should not affect hypothalamic or pituitary function.

1047. (B, C, D, E) Male infertility may be due to: (1) defective spermatogenesis, (2) genital duct obstruction, (3) retrograde ejaculation (ejaculation into the urinary bladder), or (4) antibody formation against sperm. Abnormal spermatogenesis accompanies:

- Endocrine diseases (hypothalamic/pituitary failure, hypothyroidism, hyperprolactinemia)
- Cryptorchidism (undescended testes)
- Genetic abnormalities (Klinefelter syndrome [47,XXY])
- Infections (mumps orchitis, prostatitis)
- Surgery and/or trauma to the genitals or spermatic cord (inguinal canal)
- Drugs (excessive use of alcohol, tobacco, marijuana)
- Environmental toxins (lead, radiation, chemotherapy)
- Increased intratesticular temperature (cold environment does not cause defects)

1048. (B, C, D, E) Several environmental factors, including occupations with prolonged sitting (truck drivers), febrile illness, use of jockey shorts, and hot baths or saunas may adversely affect spermatogenesis by increasing intratesticular temperature. Attempts to reduce scrotal temperature (e.g., use of boxer shorts) is commonly advised as part of the treatment of male infertility. Swimming should not harm spermatogenesis.

1049. (A, B, C, D) The testes are located outside the abdomen because the optimal temperature for spermatozoa production is 1°F less than body temperature. An elevation in intratesticular temperature can adversely affect sperm function. Forty percent of infertile men have a varicocele, defined as dilation of the pampiniform plexus above the testis. It is caused by defective valves within the internal spermatic vein and usually occurs on the left side because of the direct insertion of the spermatic vein into the renal vein. Retrograde blood flow increases scrotal temperature and disturbs spermatogenesis. A varicocele also occurs in approximately 10 to 15% of the general population.

1050. (A, B, C, E) Recurrent abortion has been associated with abnormal maternal immune responses directed against maternal (autoimmunity) or fetal (alloimmunity) tissues. Abnormalities of autoimmunity include lupus anticoagulant (antibodies directed against thromboplastin), anticardiolipin antibody, and antinuclear antibodies. The lupus anticoagulant is associated with placental thrombosis, leading to recurrent abortion, fetal growth retardation, and fetal death. In addition, pregnancy maintenance may require immunologic recognition of the fetus by the mother, causing antibody–antigen complex formation (blocking factors) that prevents maternal rejection of the fetus. Sharing of human lymphocyte antigens between husband and wife may accompany an alloimmune etiology of recurrent abortion.

1051. (A) The most predictive test of diminishing ovarian reserve in a woman are the early follicular phase FSH and estradiol levels. Serum LH is not helpful. There is no evidence that luteal progesterone is predictive of ovarian reserve. Serum inhibin B levels have been implicated but remain less predictive than FSH and estradiol.

1052. (B) Bromocriptine, a lysergic acid derivative, acts as a dopamine agonist, to inhibit prolactin release. In most women with elevated serum prolactin levels and amenorrhea–galactorrhea, bromocriptine restores normal menstruation within 6 weeks and causes cessation of galactorrhea by 13 weeks. Bromocriptine therapy also may diminish the size and symptoms of prolactin-secreting pituitary adenomas. Approximately 5% of patients terminate bromocriptine therapy due to nausea, headache, and faintness. These side effects may be minimized by taking the medication with food and by gradually increasing the bromocriptine dose to the appropriate level for the patient.

1053. (A) Clomiphene citrate is an oral antiestrogen that binds to estrogen receptors in the reproductive tract and hypothalamus. By inhibiting estrogen-negative feedback on FSH, clomiphene induces an elevation in circulating FSH levels, which stimulates folliculogenesis. Clomiphene therapy may be combined with midcycle hCG administration and luteal-phase progesterone supplementation. Its use may cause a reduction in cervical mucus and an abnormal endometrial biopsy due to antiestrogenic actions on the cervix and endometrium. The multiple birth rate associated with clomiphene therapy is about 5%, and most of these pregnancies are twin gestations.

1054. (C) Human menopausal gonadotropins are derived from the urine of postmenopausal women. Commercially available ampules contain about equal amounts of LH and FSH. Intramuscular administration of hMGs is expensive and associated with a multiple birth rate of about 10%. Purified FSH, separated from urinary LH by immunochromatography, has become available.

1055. (G) Primary ovarian failure characterized by elevated serum gonadotropin levels and low serum estradiol levels is referred to as hypergonadotropic hypogonadism. This condition usually is unresponsive to any ovulatory agent.

1056. (D) Hysterosalpingography detects intrauterine pathology and confirms tubal patency by spill of dye from the tube into the peritoneal cavity. Radiopaque dye is used for the HSG and may be either oil or water soluble. Oil-soluble media produce a sharp image and transiently increase fertility in some women, perhaps by decreasing local macrophage activation or enhancing tubal ciliary action. Their use may be associated with granuloma formation and a 1% rise of pulmonary embolism that is usually asymptomatic. Water-soluble media are used when there is a history suggestive of tubal disease. Hysterosalpingography is performed shortly after menstruation to avoid radiation exposure to an early pregnancy. It should be postponed in women with suspected pelvic infection due to a 1 to 3% risk of exacerbating the disease.

1057. (B) Laparoscopy refers to the endoscopic visualization of the pelvic viscera. It can directly visualize pelvic disease and assess tubal patency by confirming spill of methylene blue dye from the tubal fimbria after its intrauterine injection (chromotubation). Laparoscopy identifies unsuspected pathology such as pelvic endometriosis in up to 50% of asymptomatic women with no other cause for infertility.

1058. (C) The uterine cavity can be assessed directly by hysteroscopy. Surgical instruments may be used during hysteroscopy to treat abnormalities of the uterine cavity.

1059. (F) Both hysterosalpingography and laparoscopy are capable of assessing tubal patency.

1060. (E) Ultrasound can detect ovum release from the follicle. Unfortunately, no procedure currently exists to detect ovum transfer into the fallopian tube.

CHAPTER 16

Clinical Endocrinology
Questions

DIRECTIONS (Question 1061 through 1085): Each of the numbered items or incomplete statements in this section is followed by answers or by completions of the statement. Select the ONE lettered answer or completion that is BEST in each case.

1061. A 21-year-old diabetic athletic woman on a low-dose oral contraceptive comes to your clinic with irregular menses and galactorrhea. On examination, galactorrhea is confirmed, with fat globules seen microscopically. She currently takes metoclopramide (Reglan) for delayed gastric emptying. A random serum prolactin level is 65 ng/mL. Which of the following is most likely responsible for her hyperprolactinemia?

(A) metoclopramide
(B) pregnancy
(C) oral contraceptive
(D) pituitary adenoma
(E) exercise

1062. Which of the following hormones decreases after the first trimester of pregnancy?

(A) progesterone
(B) prolactin
(C) human chorionic gonadotropin (hCG)
(D) human placental lactogen (hPL)
(E) estriol

1063. A 25-year-old woman who underwent menarche at 11 years of age presents with a history of irregular menstrual cylces over the last 12 months, increased weight gain, and bilateral pelvic pain. Transvaginal ultrasound shows large cystic adnexa, with cysts measuring 7 to 9 cm in size. A urine pregnancy test is negative. Her thyroid stimulating hormone (TSH) level is 17 mIU/mL and prolactin level is 10 ng/mL. What is the treatment of choice for this patient to regain normal menstrual cycles?

(A) monophasic birth control pills
(B) triphasic birth control pills
(C) levothyroxine treatment
(D) bromocriptine treatment
(E) none of the above

1064. A 22-year-old woman with amenorrhea of 6 weeks' duration undergoes surgery for acute appendicitis. At the time of surgery, a 3-cm semisolid left ovarian cyst is discovered. It is vascular and appears to contain a blood-filled central cavity. A serum pregnancy test is positive. Which of the following procedures should be done?

(A) ovarian cystectomy
(B) ovarian wedge resection
(C) oophorectomy
(D) salpingo-oophorectomy
(E) none of the above

1065. A 25-year-old woman suffers a severe intrapartum hemorrhage. Which of the following symptoms is evidence of pituitary infarction?

(A) infrequent urination
(B) diarrhea
(C) easy bruisability
(D) lactation failure
(E) perspiration

1066. A 16-year-old girl has not experienced menarche. Examination shows absence of breast development and small but otherwise normal female pelvic organs. Which of the following diagnostic tests is most useful in determining the etiology of the amenorrhea?

(A) serum follicle-stimulating hormone (FSH)
(B) serum estradiol
(C) serum testosterone
(D) magnetic resonance imaging (MRI) of the head
(E) ovarian biopsy

1067. An 18-year-old patient has not experienced menarche. Examination shows normal breast development and absence of a uterus. Which of the following diagnostic tests is most useful in determining the etiology of the amenorrhea?

(A) serum FSH
(B) serum estradiol
(C) serum testosterone
(D) MRI of the head
(E) ovarian biopsy

1068. Congenital androgen insensitivity syndrome (testicular feminization) is secondary to defective androgen

(A) synthesis
(B) metabolism
(C) receptor action
(D) excretion
(E) aromatization

1069. An adult genetic male with 17-alpha-hydroxylase deficiency would have which of the following findings?

(A) no breast development, uterus present, hypertension
(B) no breast development, uterus present, hypotension
(C) breast development, uterus absent, hypotension

(D) no breast development, uterus absent, hypertension
(E) breast development, uterus present, hypertension

1070. A 28-year-old patient complains of amenorrhea after dilation and curettage (D&C) for postpartum bleeding. The most likely diagnosis is

(A) gonadal dysgenesis
(B) Sheehan syndrome
(C) Kallmann syndrome
(D) Mayer–Rokitansky–Küster–Hauser syndrome
(E) Asherman's syndrome

1071. A 25-year-old woman experiences galactorrhea and amenorrhea of 8 weeks' duration with irregular spotting. Which of the following serum assays should initially be performed?

(A) hCG
(B) progesterone
(C) prolactin
(D) FSH
(E) luteinizing hormone (LH)

1072. Anovulatory bleeding (dysfunctional uterine bleeding) is usually associated with

(A) bloating
(B) mood changes
(C) breast tenderness
(D) unpredictable vaginal bleeding
(E) uterine cramping

1073. Anovulatory bleeding (dysfunctional uterine bleeding) is

(A) common in prepubertal girls
(B) common in the early teens
(C) usually suggestive of a steroid-producing ovarian tumor

(D) uncommon during the perimenopausal years

(E) dependent on the presence of progesterone

1074. A 14-year-old girl complains of irregular vaginal bleeding. Her general examination and pelvic organs are normal. The most likely cause of anovulatory bleeding (dysfunctional uterine bleeding) in this patient is

(A) hypothyroidism

(B) pituitary adenoma

(C) polycystic ovary syndrome (PCOS)

(D) congenital adrenal hyperplasia

(E) none of the above

1075. A 15-year-old girl is seen in the emergency department. She has a sudden onset of heavy vaginal bleeding. She has noted irregular, painless vaginal bleeding of 6 months' duration. Her past medical history is unremarkable, and she is not sexually active. Her local physician has previously determined that serum prolactin and thyroid-stimulating hormone (TSH) levels are normal. Physical and pelvic examinations are normal, but blood is coming through the cervical os. A serum pregnancy test is negative, and hematocrit is 37% (normal, 35 to 45%). The BEST course of immediate action is

(A) observation

(B) estrogen therapy

(C) clomiphene citrate therapy

(D) D&C

(E) hysterectomy

1076. An 18-year-old woman comes to your clinic with irregular cycles since menarche and mild hirsutism. She is not interested in pregnancy or contraception. Her serum TSH, prolactin, and hehydroepiandrosterone sulfate (DHEAS) levels are normal, with a slightly elevated serum testosterone level of 80 ng/dL. Which of the following is the most appropriate next step for this patient?

(A) oral contraceptive treatment

(B) endometrial biopsy

(C) gonadotropin-releasing hormone (GnRH) stimulation test

(D) clomiphene citrate

(E) bromocriptine

1077. A 25-year-old healthy woman complains of breast tenderness and amenorrhea of 6 weeks' duration. She uses condoms for birth control and does not take any medication. Examination demonstrates a whitish breast discharge with milk-containing fat droplets on microscopic examination. A pregnancy test is negative, and a serum TSH level is normal. A serum prolactin is 80 ng/mL (normal, < 20 ng/mL). The next action would be to obtain radiologic assessment of the

(A) kidneys

(B) lumbar spine

(C) sella turcica

(D) chest

(E) none of the above

1078. The growth of coarse hair in androgen-dependent body regions is referred to as

(A) masculinization

(B) defeminization

(C) virilization

(D) hirsutism

(E) androgenization

1079. Congenital adrenal hyperplasia (CAH) is BEST treated with

(A) cyclic progesterone

(B) cyclic estrogen

(C) daily glucocorticoids

(D) daily GnRH analogue

(E) daily oral contraceptives

1080. A 23-year-old woman with irregular menses complains of facial hair increasing in amount over several years. She is sexually active but does not wish to conceive. Examination demonstrates hirsutism, obesity, and hyperpigmentation of the neck and axillae. The ovaries are bilaterally enlarged and cystic. A serum testosterone value is 1.2 ng/mL (normal, < 0.8 ng/mL). Serum levels of DHEAS, 17-hydroxyprogesterone (17-OHP), and prolactin are normal. The BEST single therapeutic agent for this patient is

(A) oral contraceptives (OCs)
(B) glucocorticoids
(C) clomiphene citrate
(D) antiandrogens
(E) GnRH analogue

1081. A 4-year-old girl is brought in by her mother for evaluation of clitoral enlargement. She is tall for her age, with no breast or axillary hair development. There is slight pubic hair growth on examination and an enlarged clitoris with a single perineal opening. Karyotype is 46,XX. The 17-OHP level is 108 ng/mL. What is the most likely diagnosis?

(A) testicular insensitivity syndrome
(B) PCOS
(C) CAH with 21-hydroxylase deficiency
(D) none of the above

1082. Female pseudohermaphroditism refers to individuals who have

(A) ovaries, an XX karyotype, and varying degrees of masculinization
(B) testes, an XY karyotype, and varying degrees of masculinization failure
(C) ovaries, an XY karyotype, and varying degrees of masculinization failure
(D) testes, an XX karyotype, and severe masculinization
(E) both ovarian and testicular tissue

1083. An infant with ambiguous genitalia is found to have testes and an XY karyotype. Seminal vesicles, ejaculatory ducts, epididymis, and vas deferens (wolffian duct derivatives) are

present. There is no uterus, fallopian tubes, or upper vagina. The ratio of circulating testosterone to dihydrotestosterone (DHT) is elevated compared to normal male infants. The most likely diagnosis is

(A) 20,22 desmolase deficiency
(B) 21-hydroxylase deficiency
(C) testicular feminization
(D) 5-alpha-reductase deficiency
(E) embryonic testicular regression

1084. Prolactin-secreting pituitary adenomas (prolactinomas) usually

(A) diminish in size during pregnancy
(B) increase in size over time
(C) are symptomatic during lactation
(D) impinge on the olfactory nerve
(E) respond to medical therapy

1085. A 17-year-old boy presents for delayed sexual development. He is 6'5" tall with a weight of 152 lbs. There is a reduced amount of pubic hair with a small phallus and small testicles. Endocrine testing reveals increased FSH and LH levels and a low testosterone level. What is the most likely diagnosis?

(A) Kallmann syndrome
(B) Klinefelter syndrome
(C) Savage syndrome
(D) Beckwith–Wiedemann syndrome
(E) Turner syndrome

DIRECTIONS (Questions 1086 through 1098): Each of the numbered items or incomplete statements in this section is followed by answers or by completions of the statement. Select the answers or completions that may apply.

1086. Which three of the following are true statements regarding thyroid function during pregnancy?

(A) Maternal thyroxine-binding globulin (TBG) levels rise.
(B) Maternal total thyroxine (T_4) and total triiodothyronine (T_3) levels rise.

(C) The secretion of fetal thyroid hormone begins in midgestation.

(D) Propylthiouracil and methimazole do not cross the placenta.

(E) Maternal antithyroid antibodies do not cross the placenta.

1087. Which four of the following effects is attributed to hCG?

(A) maintenance of corpus luteum during early pregnancy

(B) regulation of fetal adrenal androgen production

(C) regulation of fetal testicular androgen production

(D) stimulation of thyroid activity

(E) inhibition of peripheral glucose uptake

1088. Which four of the following substances are placental protein hormones?

(A) dopamine

(B) inhibin

(C) GnRH

(D) human chorionic thyrotropin (hCT)

(E) thyroid-releasing hormone (TRH)

1089. Which three of the following statements are TRUE about pregnancy?

(A) Luteectomy after 7 weeks of gestation can interfere with gestation.

(B) Luteectomy before 42 days results in a decrease in levels of serum progesterone and estradiol, followed by spontaneous miscarriage.

(C) The elevation of basal body temperature (BBT) during pregnancy is thought to be mediated by progesterone via interleukins.

(D) Decidua is the endometrium of pregnancy.

(E) A combination of hCG, alpha-fetoprotein, and progesterone levels can be used to detect fetal Down syndrome with high sensitivity and specificity.

1090. Which four of the following conditions are associated with low circulating maternal estriol (E_3) levels?

(A) corticosteroid therapy

(B) anencephaly

(C) placental sulfatase deficiency

(D) antibiotic therapy

(E) maternal renal disease

1091. Which three of the following statements are TRUE about estrogen production during pregnancy?

(A) The key step in estriol synthesis is 16-alpha-hydroxylation of fetal DHEAS.

(B) The ovary is capable of producing estriol via conversion of 16-alpha-hydroxy-DHEAS.

(C) Fetal DHEAS is converted by placental sulfatase to DHEA.

(D) Estrogen is necessary for the maintenance of pregnancy.

(E) Serum estriol may reflect the well-being of the fetus.

1092. Which four of the following statements regarding lactation are TRUE?

(A) Estrogen stimulates mammary ductal proliferation.

(B) Progesterone stimulates mammary alveolar development.

(C) High circulating sex steroid levels during pregnancy inhibit lactation.

(D) The gestational mammary gland produces a transudate containing casein and alpha-lactalbumin.

(E) The postpartum decline in circulating sex steroid levels initiates lactation.

1093. Amenorrhea, estrogen deficiency, and elevated circulating gonadotropin levels are noted in a normal-appearing 27-year-old woman. Which four of the following conditions are associated with these findings?

(A) X chromosome abnormalities

(B) polyglandular autoimmune syndrome

(C) Kallmann syndrome

(D) alkylating antineoplastic drugs

(E) pelvic irradiation

1094. A 33-year-old woman who underwent normal puberty describes an 18-month history of secondary amenorrhea and hot flashes. A pregnancy test was negative. A progesterone withdrawal challenge test revealed no bleeding. Her FSH was 94 mIU/mL, and her LH level was 68 mIU/mL. She desires to be pregnant with her current partner. Which two of the following are considered appropriate steps in the management of this individual?

(A) karyotype

(B) assessment of thyroid, adrenal, and ovarian antibodies

(C) clomiphene citrate therapy

(D) gonadotropin stimulation therapy

(E) estrogen replacement therapy

1095. Management of anovulatory bleeding (dysfunctional uterine bleeding) depends on which four of the following conditions?

(A) age of the patient

(B) desire for fertility

(C) size of the cervical os

(D) amount of bleeding

(E) cause of bleeding

1096. Treatment of hyperprolactinemia results in which four of the following?

(A) elimination of galactorrhea

(B) prevention of acne

(C) establishment of normal estrogen production

(D) treatment of prolactin-secreting pituitary adenomas

(E) induction of ovulation

1097. Hirsutism is associated with which four of the following conditions?

(A) PCOS

(B) CAH

(C) Cushing syndrome

(D) increased androgen utilization by skin

(E) hyperprolactinemia

1098. Which four of the following statements regarding PCOS are true?

(A) Elevated androgen production decreases sex hormone–binding globulin (SHBG) synthesis.

(B) Elevated androgen production increases peripheral aromatization.

(C) Acyclic estrogen production increases LH secretion.

(D) Acyclic estrogen production decreases bone mineralization.

(E) Acyclic estrogen production increases endometrial proliferation.

DIRECTIONS (Questions 1099 through 1110): Each set of items in this section consists of a list of lettered headings followed by several numbered words or phrases. For each numbered word or phrase, select the ONE lettered option that is most closely associated with it. Each lettered option may be selected once, more than once, or not at all.

Questions 1099 through 1102

(A) estrone

(B) estradiol

(C) estriol

(D) androstenedione

(E) testosterone

(F) DHEAS

(G) aldosterone

(H) cortisol

(I) thyroxine

(J) parathyroid hormone (PTH)

(K) insulin

1099. Principal androgen used for placental estrogen synthesis

1100. Principal estrogen produced during pregnancy

1101. Principal hormone produced by the maternal zona gomerulosa

1102. Principal hormone responsible for 1,25-dihydroxy vitamin D_3 synthesis

Questions 1103 through 1105

    (A) spontaneous menses

    (B) menses only after progesterone administration

    (C) menses only after estrogen administration

    (D) menses after sequential estrogen/progesterone administration

    (E) none of the above

1103. Destruction of endometrium

1104. Hypothalamic failure

1105. Ovarian failure

Questions 1106 through 1110

    (A) 20,22-desmolase deficiency

    (B) 3-beta-hydroxysteroid dehydrogenase (3-n HSD) deficiency

    (C) 21-hydroxylase deficiency

    (D) 11-beta-hydroxylase deficiency

    (E) Cushing syndrome

    (F) adrenal tumor

    (G) PCOS

    (H) arrhenoblastoma

    (I) theca-lutein cysts

1106. Hirsutism, ovarian androgen excess, elevated serum luteinizing hormone levels

1107. Hirsutism, adrenal androgen excess, elevated 17-OHP

1108. Hirsutism, hypertension, diabetes mellitus

1109. Hirsutism, multiple gestation

1110. Virilization, serum testosterone level 2.8 ng/mL (normal, < 0.8 ng/mL)

Answers and Explanations

1061. (A) Pregnancy increases prolactin levels; however, this patient is unlikely to be pregnant because she was taking the oral contraceptive. The oral contraceptive rarely increases prolactin to such high levels. Metoclopramide is a potent dopamine antagonist that can act on the lactotroph to ramp up secretion of prolactin. A prolactin-producing pituitary adenoma is unlikely since most tumors present with serum prolactin levels greater than 100 ng/mL.

1062. (C) Maternal serum levels of progesterone rise to term to peak at 190 ng/mL. Maternal prolactin levels continue a steady increase throughout pregnancy to a third-trimester peak level of 200 ng/mL. Maternal hPL levels also increase during the entirety of the pregnancy. However, hCG peaks at 10 weeks and decreases to a lower plateau through the second and third trimesters. Estriol, estradiol, and estrone all increase steadily during pregnancy.

1063. (C) Ovarian cysts and irregular menstrual cycles can both arise from compensated hypothyroidism, which is revealed by this patient's elevated TSH level. Levothyroxine is the treatment of choice. Monophasic or triphasic birth control pills would only mask the underlying problem despite the fact that regular withdrawal bleeding can be achieved. This patient has a normal serum prolactin level, and thus bromocriptine is not indicated.

1064. (E) Blood often accumulates within a vascularized corpus luteum. A corpus luteum cyst may develop as the blood reabsorbs, causing a physiologic ovarian enlargement. Since progesterone production by the corpus luteum maintains pregnancy until the seventh gestational week, removal of the corpus luteum (luteectomy) before this time will terminate pregnancy. There is a transitional period between the seventh and tenth gestational weeks when the corpus luteum and placenta contribute to circulating progesterone levels. After the tenth week, the placenta is the major source of progesterone.

1065. (D) Pituitary infarction (Sheehan syndrome) due to severe intrapartum hemorrhage is associated with low serum prolactin levels and postpartum lactation failure.

1066. (A) Primary amenorrhea is defined as absence of menarche by age 16 years with appearance of secondary sex characteristics, or by age 14 years without appearance of secondary sex characteristics. A practical approach used by some investigators assigns patients with normal female external genitalia and primary amenorrhea into one of four groups based on physical examination. A series of diagnostic steps unique to each category determines the etiology of amenorrhea. The four groups of patients with primary amenorrhea are: (1) no breast development and uterus present; (2) breast development and uterus absent; (3) no breast development and uterus absent; and, (4) breast development and uterus present. In the evaluation of a patient from group 1 (as described in this problem), a serum FSH level can distinguish between absence of gonadal function (elevated FSH) or diminished pulsatile GnRH release (suppressed FSH). Further investigation is similar to that of delayed puberty. All individuals with secondary amenorrhea are included in group four.

1067. (C) This patient belongs in group two (breast development and uterus absent) from answer 1066. The two disorders in this group are (1) abnormal müllerian duct development in females, and (2) defective androgen action in males. These disorders are distinguished by measuring serum testosterone levels, which are in the female range in women with abnormal müllerian duct development. Mayer–Rokitansky–Küster–Hauser syndrome is a disorder of müllerian duct development in which the uterus and vagina are congenitally absent. Ovarian function is preserved, and ovulation occurs during the reproductive years. In contrast, circulating testosterone levels are in the male range in men with defective androgen action. These individuals commonly have congenital androgen insensitivity syndrome (testicular feminization) due to defective androgen action and should have a karyotype performed to confirm genetic sex.

1068. (C) Congenital androgen insensitivity syndrome (testicular feminization) occurs in men and is due to defective androgen receptor action. It is an X-linked recessive disorder of androgen receptor function and is characterized by lack of masculinization. Androgen insensitivity of target tissues causes failure of male sexual differentiation (female-appearing external genitalia), absence of wolffian duct development, and lack of pubertal hair growth in the axillary and pubic regions. During puberty, testicular androgen production is normal and provides androgenic precursors for peripheral aromatization to estrogen. Consequently, abundant breast tissue develops at puberty due to estrogen production uninhibited by androgen action. However, müllerian duct regression in response to testicular müllerian inhibitory factor (MIF) causes the vagina to end as a blind pouch, resulting in primary amenorrhea. The testes are located in the pelvis or within an inguinal hernia and contain immature seminiferous tubules. Gonadectomy is performed to avoid the risk of malignant gonadal degeneration but is delayed until after puberty in order to allow hormone-dependent pubertal changes. These individuals have a female gender identity and should receive postoperative estrogen replacement therapy.

1069. (D) Genetic males (46,XY) with enzymatic defects in the early pathways of steroidogenesis (20,22 desmolase 17-alpha-hydroxylase, 17,20 desmolase) are extremely rare (group 3 from answer 1066). Absence of sex steroid production accounts for elevated gonadotropins, low circulating testosterone levels, and lack of breast development. Müllerian duct regression due to testicular MIF causes absence of uterine development. Neonates with these disorders often die from cortisol deficiency. Adults with 17-alpha-hydroxylase deficiency have hypertension and hypokalemic alkalosis and should undergo gonadectomy to prevent the risk of developing a malignant gonadal tumor.

1070. (E) Asherman syndrome refers to the presence of intrauterine scarring (synechiae). The most common cause of this disorder is uterine curettage for postpartum hemorrhage or abortion. It may also accompany myomectomy, metroplasty, cesarean section, uterine infection due to intrauterine device use, tuberculosis, and schistosomiasis. Intrauterine synechiae are diagnosed either by injecting radiographic dye into the uterus under fluoroscopic view (hysterosalpingography) or by directly visualizing the uterine cavity (hysteroscopy). The latter technique also may be used therapeutically to lyse adhesions. About 70% of patients treated for Asherman syndrome have a subsequent successful pregnancy. Many experience difficulties with placental–uterine separation after birth, leading to an increased risk of postpartum hemorrhage.

1071. (A) The first diagnostic step in a reproductive-aged woman with amenorrhea is to exclude pregnancy with a serum hCG determination. After excluding pregnancy, serum prolactin and TSH levels should also be measured because abnormalities of prolactin secretion and thyroid function disrupt ovulation. Hyperprolactinemia occurs in about 20% of amenorrheic individuals without galactorrhea and should be evaluated further if present.

1072. (D) Ovulatory menstrual cycles occur at monthly intervals of 21 to 45 days and result in blood loss of 30 to 40 mL per menses over 3 to 7 days (approximately 10 to 15 soaked tampons or pads per cycle). Premenstrual symptomatology refers to the breast tenderness, mood change, bloating, and uterine cramping (primary dysmenorrhea) that commonly accompanies ovulatory menstruation. These symptoms are collectively known as molimina and reflect progesterone action on target tissues. Severe premenstrual symptomatology resulting from cyclical ovarian activity is referred to as premenstrual syndrome (PMS). Without progesterone production by the corpus luteum, anovulatory cycles usually lack moliminal symptoms and occur at irregular intervals.

1073. (B) Anovulatory bleeding is common during the early teens and the perimenopausal years. Absence of progesterone production at these times causes menstrual irregularity. Steroid-producing ovarian tumors are rare but can disrupt ovulation, causing anovulatory bleeding.

1074. (E) In the absence of androgen and prolactin excess, most anovulatory women with normal circulating gonadotropin levels have hypothalamic dysfunction. This condition may be due to suppression of hypothalamic GnRH release. The resulting decline in circulating estradiol (E_2) levels is insufficient to induce the ovulatory LH surge but is able to stimulate endometrial proliferation. Hypothalamic dysfunction may be idiopathic in origin or induced by medication (narcotics), ethanol, stress, and weight loss.

1075. (B) For severe dysfunctional uterine bleeding (DUB), estrogen therapy inhibits endometrial desquamation and provides prompt but transient relief. Conjugated estrogens may be administered orally (2.5 to 3.75 mg daily) or intravenously (25 mg at 4-hour intervals), depending on the amount of bleeding. Bleeding should be controlled within 24 hours of estrogen therapy. Addition of a progestin after bleeding has ceased allows for withdrawal menstruation when the patient is hemodynamically stable. Administration of estrogen-dominant oral contraceptives (containing 50 mg ethinyl estradiol) three times daily for 7 days also controls heavy DUB when gaining cycle control is not urgent. Failure of hormonal management to control DUB requires D&C. Hysterectomy is indicated for patients found to have endometrial carcinoma and also may be necessary for individuals no longer desiring fertility.

1076. (A) This patient most likely suffers from PCOS and does not desire to conceive at this time. Thus, clomiphene citrate is not indicated as an ovulation-inducing agent. Since her prolactin level is normal, bromocriptine treatment is not appropriate. An endometrial biopsy might be indicated if she were older or obese with a long period of exposure to unopposed estrogen. A GnRH stimulation test is reserved primarily for patients with hypothalamic disorders. The oral contraceptive is the appropriate therapy for her to reduce androgen levels, provide contraception, and control irregular bleeding.

1077. (C) All women with galactorrhea and amenorrhea should be questioned regarding the use of birth control and lactotropic medication. Reproductive-aged women should be considered pregnant until proven otherwise, by measuring urinary or serum hCG. In the absence of pregnancy, evaluation of galactorrhea also includes determination of serum prolactin, TSH, and thyroid function studies. A serum creatinine with blood urea nitrogen (BUN) and chest radiogram also may be indicated if renal or pulmonary disease is suspected. The presence of hyperprolactinemia requires radiologic assessment of the hypothalamus and pituitary.

1078. (D) Hirsutism is defined as growth of coarse hair in androgen-dependent body regions, such as the sideburn area, chin, upper lip, periareolar area, chest, lower abdominal midline, and thighs. It should be distinguished from masculinization, which refers to development of male secondary sex characteristics (e.g., temporal balding, deepening of the voice, masculinization of body habitus, and clitoromegaly). Defeminization is the loss of female secondary sex characteristics (e.g., decreased breast size). Virilization refers to the combination of defeminization and masculinization. These definitions describe disorders of androgen excess. Since the ovary and adrenal are the major sources of circulating androgens in women, the diagnostic approach to hirsutism and virilization includes investigation of these organs for benign and malignant diseases.

1079. (C) Women with CAH should receive glucocorticoids to replace cortisol deficiency. Exogenous glucocorticoids restore negative feedback on adrenocorticotropic hormone (ACTH) and decrease circulating androgen levels. Judicious surveillance is required when prescribing glucocorticoids since their excessive use is associated with bone demineralization, adrenal atrophy, fluid retention, and mood changes.

1080. (A) The presence of ovarian hyperandrogenism (HA), insulin resistance (IR), and hyperpigmentation of the neck, axillae, and skin folds (acanthosis nigricans [AR]) constitutes the HAIR-AN syndrome, a variant of PCOS. Normal values of serum DHEAS and 17-hydroxy-progesterone exclude a primary adrenal disorder (CAH) or a neoplastic process. The treatment of hirsutism under these conditions depends on the desires of the patient. Women with PCOS-induced hirsutism who do not wish to conceive should receive OCs to suppress gonadotropin secretion and ovarian androgen production. The estrogen component of the oral contraceptive also stimulates hepatic SHBG synthesis. As SHBG-bound testosterone (T) levels increase, the amount of biologically active T in the circulation decreases. The progestin component

of the OC opposes estrogen-induced endometrial stimulation. GnRH analogues also have been used for treatment of PCOS-related hirsutism, but the risk of bone demineralization and the complaints of menopausal side effects (e.g., hot flashes and vaginal dryness) limit the usefulness of this therapy unless it is combined with exogenous hormones. Antiandrogens block T action by competing with T for its skin receptors but may also inhibit steroidogenic enzymes, causing menstrual irregularity. Antiandrogens are contraindicated during pregnancy because they may enter the fetal circulation and antagonize T action during sexual differentiation. For these reasons, antiandrogens are usually combined with OCs for treatment of hirsutism. Anovulatory women with PCOS who wish to conceive should receive ovulation-inducing agents (e.g., clomiphene citrate). Estrogen increases bone formation.

1081. (C) Congenital adrenal hyperplasia accounts for the majority of cases of congenital sexual ambiguity with enlarged clitorides. These patients have normal 46,XX karyotypes and elevated adrenal androgens, which are responsible for the external genitalia changes.

1082. (A) True hermaphroditism occurs when ovarian and testicular tissue coexist in the same individual. Pseudohermaphroditism is defined as variance between the gonadal and genital sex of an individual. The term male or female denotes the corresponding gonadal, and therefore genetic, sex. Male pseudohermaphroditism refers to an individual who has testes, an XY karyotype, and varying degrees of masculinization failure. Female pseudohermaphroditism refers to an individual who has ovaries, an XX karyotype, and varying degrees of masculinization.

1083. (D) Male pseudohermaphrodites generally produce müllerian inhibitory factor and therefore have no uterus, fallopian tubes, or upper vagina. Inadequate androgen stimulation in males reflects either deficient androgen formation or defective androgen action. The former condition accompanies inheritable enzyme deficiencies in testosterone synthesis. Defective androgen action is caused by either androgen receptor abnormalities or failure of DHT formation in androgen-dependent target tissues. Androgen receptor defects may be total or partial, causing complete absence of testosterone (T) action (testicular feminization) or ambiguous genitalia. Deficiency of 5-alpha-reductase causes failure of T conversion to DHT. Under this condition, structures derived from the urogenital sinus and external genital anlagen are partially masculinized, while those derived from wolffian ducts are male in character. Ambiguous genitalia occasionally results from embryonic testicular regression at a time in which müllerian duct regression has occurred but masculinization is in progress. The elevated serum T/DHT ratio (combined with the presence of wolffian duct derivatives) supports the diagnosis of 5-alpha-reductase deficiency in this infant.

1084. **(E)** Most prolactin-secreting pituitary adenomas (prolactinomas) grow slowly, if at all, and may undergo infarction with resorption. Pituitary adenomas may grow during pregnancy. Fewer than 2% of prolactinomas smaller than 1 cm in diameter (microadenomas) and less than 15% of prolactinomas larger than 1 cm in size (macroadenomas) cause symptoms suggestive of growth during pregnancy. Upward expansion of some adenomas into the optic nerve can be associated with headache and visual field defects (bitemporal hemianopsia). Breast-feeding does not adversely affect the natural course of the adenoma. Malignant degeneration of pituitary adenomas is rare. Although medical therapy does not eliminate the tumor, the use of bromocriptine (a dopamine agonist) decreases tumor size and circulating prolactin levels.

1085. **(B)** A karyotype should be ordered and most likely will reveal 47,XXY, or Klinefelter syndrome. The phenotype is classic with assicated degrees of gynecomastia and azoospermia. They are tall due to the lack of estrogen exposure, leading to appropriate closure of epiphyseal plates. They require testosterone replacement due to the lack of endogenous androgen production from the testicles.

1086. **(A, B, C)** Both maternal TBG and total T_4 and T_3 levels rise during pregnancy. The rise in TBG is due to estrogen-induced hepatic glycosylation of TBG with N-acetylgalactosamine, which prolongs the metabolic clearance rate of TBG. There is a concomitant rise in total T_4 and T_3 levels but not free T_4 and T_3 levels. The secretion of thyroid hormone in the fetus begins at 18 to 20 weeks' gestation. Maternal antithyroid antibodies and propylthiouracil and methimazole all cross the placenta to affect fetal thyroid function.

1087. **(A, B, C, D)** The function of circulating hCG is to maintain corpus luteum function until the placenta synthesizes progesterone, to stimulate androgen production by the fetal adrenal and testes, and to inhibit local lymphocyte function, preventing pregnancy rejection by the mother. hCG also stimulates thyroid activity by competing with TSH for thyroid receptors. The thyrotropic activity of hCG is approximately 1/4,000th that of TSH, and may contribute to thyroid hyperactivity in patients with high circulating hCG values (e.g., trophoblastic disease and multiple gestation). Human chorionic somatomammotropin (hCS) inhibits peripheral uptake of glucose and amino acids.

1088. **(B, C, D, E)** Each placental protein hormone has a hypothalamic or pituitary analogue of similar biological action. The cytotrophoblast and syncytiotrophoblast probably act together as a miniature hypothalamus and pituitary to produce peptide hormones that regulate placental function. This concept of endogenous placental regulation is referred to as placental autoregulation. Placental protein hormones include TRH, hCT, corticotropin-releasing factor (CRF), human chorionic corticotropin (hCC), GnRH, and inhibin. Dopamine is an aminergic neurotransmitter.

1089. **(B, C, D)** Luteectomy (removal of the corpus luteum of pregnancy) before 42 days will result in spontaneous miscarriage with a dra-

CHAPTER 17

Contraception
Questions

DIRECTIONS (Questions 1111 through 1137): Each of the numbered items or incomplete statements in this section is followed by answers or by completions of the statement. Select the ONE lettered answer or completion that is BEST in each case.

1111. The most direct public health or socioeconomic effect of contraceptive use is

(A) improved socioeconomic status

(B) stabilized world population growth

(C) reduced maternal morbidity

(D) diminished incidence of fetal abnormalities

(E) decreased prevalence of sexually transmitted diseases (STDs)

1112. Which contraceptive method has the lowest pregnancy rate in 100 women using the method for 1 year (100 woman-years of use)?

(A) intrauterine device (IUD)

(B) long-acting progestins (Depo-Provera, Norplant)

(C) diaphragm

(D) oral contraceptives (OCs)

(E) spermicidal cream

1113. A 23-year-old woman and her husband use natural family planning as their contraceptive method. Her menstrual cycle length is variable, ranging from 26 to 32 days. She does not measure her basal body temperature (BBT). The time of her maximum fertility, with the first day of menses defined as day 1, would be between cycle days

(A) 1 and 14

(B) 6 and 14

(C) 6 and 21

(D) 14 and 21

(E) 14 and 28

1114. A couple is using "natural family planning" for contraception. Figure 17–1 shows the basal temperature graph made by the couple the previous month. Which letter most closely identifies when ovulation may occur?

(A) point A

(B) point B

(C) point C

(D) point D

(E) point E

1115. Spermicides destroy spermatozoa primarily by

(A) activating acrosomal enzymes

(B) disrupting cell membranes

(C) inhibiting glucose transport

(D) altering vaginal enzymes

(E) increasing vaginal pH

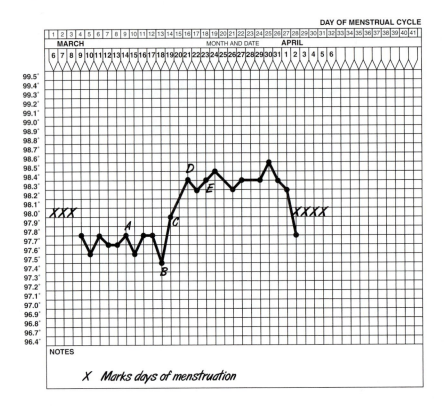

Figure 17–1.

1116. A 19-year-old woman and her boyfriend wish to use condoms as a barrier contraceptive method. This couple should be advised that male condoms should be used

   (A) when the possibility of an STD is suspected
   (B) for every act of coitus
   (C) when a female condom is not available
   (D) without spermicidal creams, which may weaken the condom
   (E) in conjunction with the female condom

1117. An 18-year-old woman complains that a condom broke during sexual intercourse. Coitus occurred 1 day ago when she was at midcycle. She does not wish to be pregnant and will terminate the pregnancy if menses does not occur. You advise her that

   (A) unprotected midcycle coitus has a 5% risk of pregnancy
   (B) little can be done, since sperm have already entered the cervical mucus

   (C) postcoital douching is effective in preventing pregnancy
   (D) postcoital brief course of oral contraception is usually effective in preventing pregnancy
   (E) postcoital contraception is usually ineffective when given more than 24 hours after coitus

1118. A 42-year-old patient (G3P3003) requests a diaphragm for contraception. When fitting the contraceptive diaphragm, it should sit comfortably between the

   (A) anterior and posterior vaginal fornices
   (B) anterior vaginal fornix and posterior urethrovesical angle
   (C) pubic symphysis and anterior vaginal fornix
   (D) pubic symphysis and posterior vaginal fornix
   (E) pubic symphysis and posterior urethrovesical angle

1119. IUDs are associated with an increase in

(A) salpingitis in the first few weeks of use
(B) salpingitis in long-term users
(C) the number of ectopic pregnancies
(D) dysmenorrhea in multiparous patients
(E) the rate of pelvic inflammatory disease (PID)

1120. A 23-year-old patient is considering contraceptive methods but is devoutly religious and will not accept a method that may "cause an abortion." The primary mechanism by which IUDs prevent pregnancy is

(A) creating chronic endometritis
(B) preventing fertilization
(C) inhibiting ovulation
(D) altering tubal motility
(E) destroying sperm

1121. A 35-year-old woman wearing an IUD complains of amenorrhea of 5 weeks' duration. A serum pregnancy test is positive. Because of the presence of the IUD, this patient is at significantly increased likelihood of

(A) ectopic pregnancy
(B) fetal malformations
(C) spontaneous abortion
(D) septic abortion
(E) placental abruption

1122. The primary mechanism by which OCs prevent pregnancy is by

(A) inhibiting serum follicle-stimulating hormone (FSH) levels
(B) inhibiting serum luteinizing hormone (LH) levels
(C) inducing endometrial atrophy
(D) inducing lymphocytic endometritis
(E) increasing cervical mucus viscosity

1123. Reducing the estrogen content of OCs results in an increase in the rate of

(A) pregnancy
(B) breakthrough bleeding
(C) thromboembolic complications
(D) insulin resistance
(E) premenstrual symptoms

1124. A 37-year-old obese woman wishes to use OCs for birth control. Her past medical history is unremarkable. She smokes one pack of cigarettes daily. Her blood pressure is 140/90. Physical and pelvic examinations are normal. Total serum cholesterol is 275 mg/dL (normal, < 200 mg/dL). You advise her that combined OCs are primarily contraindicated because of her

(A) age
(B) cholesterol
(C) hypertension
(D) smoking

1125. The use of OCs may increase the risk of which of the following conditions?

(A) fibrocystic breast disease
(B) hepatic adenoma
(C) salpingitis
(D) ovarian cancer
(E) endometrial cancer

1126. An 18-year-old woman requests OCs for birth control. She is healthy but occasionally experiences severe migraine headaches. Her menses occur at monthly intervals. A grandmother has recently been treated for breast cancer. Her brother has juvenile-onset diabetes mellitus. Her physical and pelvic examinations are normal. A serum total cholesterol level is 195 mg/dL (normal, < 200 mg/dL). You advise her that OC use will increase her risk of

(A) breast cancer
(B) migraine headache
(C) diabetes mellitus
(D) fetal malformations
(E) "post-pill" amenorrhea

1127. A 36-year-old obese woman comes to your clinic for an annual examination. She has no complaints and is sexually active with multiple partners. She uses OCs for birth control. There is a strong family history of heart disease. Based on risk factors present in this patient, which of the following is indicated?

(A) prophylactic antibiotic treatment for possible infection by *Chlamydia trachomatis*
(B) fasting serum cholesterol
(C) 3-hour glucose tolerance test
(D) electrocardiogram (ECG)
(E) screening colposcopy

1128. Compared to users of combination OCs, users of progestin-only OCs are less likely to experience

(A) intrauterine pregnancy
(B) irregular vaginal bleeding
(C) gonadotropin suppression
(D) ectopic pregnancies
(E) mood swings

1129. A 36-year-old multiparous woman and her husband request information regarding permanent sterilization. You advise them that when compared to female sterilization, vasectomy

(A) has a lower failure rate
(B) requires a longer stay in the hospital
(C) is effective immediately
(D) carries a higher mortality rate
(E) is less reversible than tubal ligation

1130. Which of the following surgical approaches for a sterilization procedure is associated with the highest failure rate?

(A) postpartum mini-laparotomy
(B) interval mini-laparotomy
(C) laparoscopy
(D) hysteroscopy
(E) vaginal colpotomy

1131. A 35-year-old man requests a vasectomy. He has been married for 10 years and has three children. You advise him that vasectomy may

(A) increase his risk for developing testicular cancer
(B) decrease his risk for developing prostatic cancer
(C) increase his risk for developing cardiovascular disease
(D) decrease his circulating testosterone levels
(E) decrease his fertility even after vasectomy reversal

1132. The number of pregnancies worldwide that are terminated electively by abortion is

(A) 1 of every 4
(B) 1 of every 8
(C) 1 of every 16
(D) 1 of every 32
(E) 1 of every 64

1133. The risk of maternal death from legal first-trimester abortion is

(A) greater than that of second-trimester terminations
(B) greater than that from birth at some maternal ages
(C) increased with maternal age
(D) lowest when termination is performed during the first 8 weeks of gestation

1134. The administration of RU 486 results in

(A) abortion when given in early pregnancy
(B) delayed menses when given during the midluteal phase
(C) menses when given during the follicular phase
(D) resistance to prostaglandin inhibitors
(E) induction of progesterone receptors in the endometrium

1135. A 28-year-old woman is seen for her first obstetrical visit. Her last menstrual period (LMP) was 8 weeks ago. Her history is significant for infertility due to chronic salpingitis and she required in vitro fertilization (IVF) with multiple embryo transfer. A serum pregnancy test is positive. A transabdominal ultrasound shows an enlarged uterus containing five viable fetuses. You advise her that the optimal outcome can be achieved only with

(A) close supervision

(B) embryo reduction

(C) intramuscular prostaglandin

(D) progestin therapy

(E) termination of the pregnancy

1136. A 33-year-old woman cannot feel the string of her IUD. Her LMP was 1 week ago. A serum pregnancy test is negative. The BEST immediate action is to

(A) obtain an abdominal radiogram

(B) probe the cervical canal gently to pull down the string

(C) obtain a pelvic ultrasound

(D) perform a hysterosalpingogram

(E) insert another IUD to replace the lost one

1137. A 32-year-old woman has an intrauterine fetal demise at 25 weeks' gestation. The highest rate of complications is associated with second-trimester pregnancy termination using

(A) intravenous oxytocin

(B) intravenous prostaglandin

(C) intravaginal prostaglandin

(D) intramuscular prostaglandin

(E) dilation and evacuation (D&E)

DIRECTIONS (Questions 1138 through 1149): Each set of items in this section consists of a list of lettered headings followed by several numbered words or phrases. For each numbered word or phrase, select the ONE lettered option that is most closely associated with it. Each lettered option may be selected once, more than once, or not at all.

Questions 1138 through 1145

Match the following contraceptive methods with the most likely associated condition.

(A) OCs

(B) progestin-only pill (the mini-pill)

(C) male condoms

(D) cervical cap

(E) IUD

(F) coitus interruptus

(G) female condom

(H) long-acting progestin (Depo-Provera, Norplant)

(I) female sterilization

(J) male sterilization

1138. Toxic shock syndrome

1139. Cholelithiasis

1140. *Actinomyces israelii*

1141. Highest risk of contraceptive failure

1142. Lowest risk of contraceptive failure

1143. Dysmenorrhea

1144. Reliability must be tested prior to use

1145. Highest protection from STDs

Questions 1146 through 1149

For each patient, select the contraceptive method that would be relatively or absolutely contraindicated.

(A) OCs

(B) progestin-only pill (the mini-pill)

(C) levonorgestrel implant

(D) condoms

(E) diaphragm

(F) IUD

1146. A 17-year-old woman with a history of ectopic pregnancy

1147. A 25-year-old woman who is nursing

1148. A 38-year-old woman who smokes more than 20 cigarettes daily

1149. A 37-year-old woman with a large cystocele

Answers and Explanations

1111. (C) Family planning refers to the use of contraceptive methods to defer or prevent reproduction. The goals of family planning include: fertility regulation; reduction in maternal, infant, and childhood morbidity and mortality; decrease in the prevalence of STDs; and stabilization of population growth. Growth of the world population from less than 300 million people at the beginning of the Christian era to nearly 10 billion people today emphasizes the importance of contraception as a worldwide issue. The availability of effective contraception does not directly translate to a stabilization of world populations because of sporadic use and imperfect accessibility. Contraception will have no direct effect on socioeconomic status, though allowing pregnancies to be planned and wanted increases the chance that the birth of an infant will not exceed the family's ability to care for the child. Three to 5% of all infants have a birth defect, most of which are multifactorial in origin. The incidence of fetal abnormalities is not affected by the contraceptive method. The availability of reliable contraception may increase the number of sexual partners, thereby potentially increasing the prevalence of STDs.

1112. (B) Method effectiveness refers to the pregnancy rate of 100 women using a particular contraceptive method correctly for 1 year (100 woman-years of use). Use effectiveness reflects failure due to patient misuse of the contraceptive method and is less than method effectiveness (Table 17–1). The lowest rate of pregnancy is accomplished by the long-acting progestin-based methods such as

Depo-Provera and Norplant. These methods actually have failure rates that are comparable to, or lower than, those achieved by sterilization procedures. The copper-containing IUD, however, is very close and over a 5-year period probably has a better effectiveness rate due to the low patient compliance needs.

Table 17–1. Contraceptive Failure Rate per 100 Women Using the Method for 1 Year (100 Woman-Years of Use)

Type of Birth Control	Method Effectiveness	Use Effectiveness
Oral contraceptives	0.1	2.5
Intrauterine device	1.5	4.0
Condoms	3.0	10.0
Diaphragm	3.0	18.0
Spermicidal cream	10.0	20.0
Rhythm	10.0	24.0

From Speroff, Glass, and Kase, 1994, with permission.

1113. (C) Natural family planning (the rhythm method) involves abstinence during the periovulatory period. The 1% of women using this birth control method must be able to identify lower abdominal discomfort from the dominant follicle (mittelschmerz); thin, clear, sticky characteristics of estrogenized cervical mucus; and/or the progesterone-induced biphasic shift in BBTs (sympto-thermal method). The average method and use effectiveness of natural family planning is low. In women with variable cycle lengths (e.g., 26 to 32 days), the time of maximal fertility can be calculated, assuming that (1) ovulation occurs 14 ± 2 days before menses, (2) spermatozoa survive in the cervical mucus approximately 2 to 4 days, and (3) the ovulated ovum survives for 1 day. The earliest ovulatory time is the shortest cycle length (26) minus earliest ovulatory day (14 + 2) minus survival time for sperm (2 to 4 days); or 26 − 16 − 4 = 6. The latest time of fertility is the longest cycle length (32) minus latest ovulation (14 − 2) plus survival of the ovum (+1); or 32 − 12 + 1 = 21.

1114. (C) The slight dip in the BBT is correlated ±1 day with the LH surge. Since the LH surge precedes ovulation by 1 day, point C is probably the better estimate of the day of ovulation. The rise in temperature after ovulation (due to the production of progesterone by the corpus luteum) is an even more reliable indicator of ovulation. The rising temperatures on days C and D, and the maintained elevated temperature by day E, would support the estimate of ovulation on day C.

1115. (B) Spermicides are surfactant agents that immobilize and destroy sperm by disrupting cell membranes. Nonoxynol-9 and octoxynol-9 are two spermicidal agents that are available in suppositories, creams, foams, and gels. They are placed high in the vagina shortly before coitus (within 20 minutes) and are commonly used in conjunction with barrier methods.

1116. (B) Barrier methods (e.g., male and female condoms, cervical caps, vaginal diaphragms, and vaginal sponges) inhibit sperm entry into the uterus. The use of these methods is safe and does not need a prescription but has to be timed with sexual activity. Latex male condoms are placed over the erect penis prior to coitus and are commonly coated on the inner and outer surfaces with a spermicidal cream, though additional spermicide may also be used. Male condoms may be purchased lubricated or nonlubricated. The ability of male condoms to protect against STDs has increased condom use in men from 9% in the early 1980s to 16% of contraceptive users in 1991. While no barrier method provides protection from all STDs, the partial protection afforded by these methods means that any sexually active couple who are not known to be disease free and mutually monogamous should use condoms for their disease protection alone. Although the incidence of male condom breakage is 1 to 2% or less, inconsistent condom use by men is probably a major reason for the difference between optimal and actual effectiveness. Spermicidal creams placed within the vagina or male condom provide greater contraceptive effectiveness in the event the condom breaks during intercourse. Men may notice a reduction in sensation with the male condom, and both sexes may experience allergic reactions to the latex or spermicide. A polyurethane female condom, approved by the FDA in 1992, is designed as a vaginal pouch with an internal diaphragm-like ring to facilitate placement (Figure 17–2). It has a 0.6% breakage

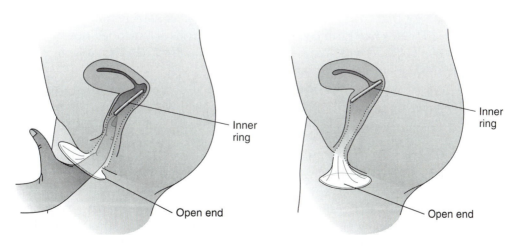

Figure 17–2.

rate and is impermeable to human immuno-deficiency virus (HIV), cytomegalovirus, and hepatitis B virus.

1117. **(D)** Unprotected, midcycle coitus has a 15 to 30% risk of pregnancy. Postcoital contraception may be used after any unprotected coitus. Several emergency contraceptive products are available and offer comparable efficacy. When these are not available, two oral contraceptive pills, containing 50 mg ethinyl estradiol and 50 mg norgestrel, are given within 3 days (72 hours) of coitus and repeated in 12 hours. The apparent effectiveness of the treatment is ≥ 95%.

1118. **(D)** The diaphragm is a latex cup that is stretched across a flat or arching spring. It is available in various sizes and is fitted by a health care provider to cover the cervix. Prior to coitus, a spermicidal agent is placed into the diaphragm, which is then inserted behind the pubic symphysis to fit into the posterior vaginal fornix. The diaphragm is left in place for 6 to 8 hours after ejaculation. Additional spermicide may be inserted vaginally without removing the diaphragm if coitus occurs again within this time. Diaphragm use has been associated with cystitis, vaginal lesions (posing a threat of toxic shock syndrome), and vaginal colonization with *Staphylococcus aureus*, particularly if the diaphragm is left in place for lengthy intervals. It should not be used in women with sensitivity to latex or spermicide, and may fit improperly in individuals with significant pelvic relaxation.

1119. **(B)** The IUD is a highly effective birth control method consisting of a plastic device that is inserted into the uterus. The device may contain a progestin, be wrapped with copper, or simply be plastic. It is identified by a string passing through the cervical os. The IUD failure rate is only slightly higher than that of OCs (see Table 17–1 on page 280). Unfortunately, medical litigation has forced the removal of most IUDs from the U.S. market, except for a progesterone-containing IUD (Progestasert), a copper-containing IUD (ParaGard), and a recently approved levonorgestrel-releasing in-trauterine system (Mirena). The progesterone-containing IUDs require periodic replacement (because the progesterone is completely absorbed in 14 months to 5 years) but are associated with less menstrual blood loss. Copper enhances the contraceptive effectiveness in inert devices, and copper-containing IUDs may be used continuously for up to 10 years. The IUD does not protect against pelvic infection or STDs, but it does not appear to directly increase the rate either; this is a function of patterns of sexual behavior. The risk of salpingitis in IUD wearers is greatest within the first weeks after insertion and in individuals with histories of recent insertion, previous STD, or multiple sexual partners. Pelvic infection may involve only one adnexa, a finding perhaps unique to the IUD. While the likelihood of having an ectopic pregnancy is greater in IUD users if a pregnancy occurs, the rate of pregnancy overall is reduced, leading to an overall decrease in the number of ectopic pregnancies. Dysmenorrhea and intermenstrual bleeding are more common in nulliparous IUD wearers.

1120. **(B)** Recent evidence suggests that the primary mechanism by which the IUD prevents pregnancy is by altering the sperm's ability to fertilize the ovum. It is true that the IUD creates a chronic endometritis that could interfere with embryo implantation. The progesterone-releasing IUD also exerts additional contraceptive effects by altering tubal motility, inducing endometrial atrophy, and altering cervical mucus. The copper-releasing IUD is detrimental to sperm capacitation and survival but does not destroy sperm per se. The IUD does not interfere with ovulation.

1121. **(C)** Pregnancy must be considered in any IUD user with amenorrhea. The IUD is more effective in preventing an intrauterine pregnancy compared to an extrauterine pregnancy. Therefore, IUD users who become pregnant have a fivefold increase (1 in 20 to 50 pregnancies) in the risk of having an ectopic pregnancy compared to normal women. While this is a significant increase in rate, the greatest probability is that the pregnancy is intrauterine. The IUD should be removed, if possible, as soon as the patient is found to be pregnant. Pregnant IUD users have a 25% chance of spontaneous abortion if the IUD is removed. However, failure to remove the IUD during pregnancy increases the risk of spontaneous abortion to 50% and also increases the chance of septic abortion and premature birth. IUD users who are pregnant are not at risk for fetal malformations but must consider pregnancy termination in the event of uterine infection. Patients desiring pregnancy termination can have the IUD removed at the time of the procedure. If the IUD remains in place and the pregnancy continues, there is no change in the risk of placental abruption.

1122. **(A)** OCs inhibit ovulation through gonadotropin suppression. While both FSH and LH are suppressed, the suppression of FSH results in the lack of induction of any primordial follicles. As a result, no follicles develop and ovulation does not take place. OCs also induce endometrial atrophy and alter cervical mucus viscosity, making it less penetrable by sperm. These additional mechanisms serve to bolster the efficacy of these medications but are not their primary mechanism of action.

1123. **(C)** In the United States, OCs (birth control pills) are the most common form of temporary contraception. They are used by 20 to 30% of sexually active women. Ethinyl estradiol (EE_2) is the most commonly used estrogen in oral contraceptives. (Mestranol is an alternative contraceptive estrogen, which requires hepatic conversion to EE_2.) Progestins, derived from 19-carbon androgens (19-nortestosterone derivatives), are also present in OCs. Recognition that hormonal side effects are dose dependent led to development of "low-dose pills" containing 20 to 35 mg (rather than 50 mg) EE_2 and lower amounts and new forms of progestins. Newer multiphasic pills deliver a low estrogen dose and varying progestin amounts over two (biphasic) and three (triphasic) portions of the cycle. Thromboembolic diseases (e.g., venous throm-

bosis and pulmonary embolism) are related to the dose-dependent effect of estrogen on blood clotting. Estrogen increases blood coagulation factors and decreases circulating levels of antithrombin III. The use of "low-dose pills" has decreased the relative risk of thromboembolic disease from 3–11 (70 per 100,000 users) to 2.8 (3 per 100,000 users) times the nonuser rate so that death from OC use is less than that from pregnancy (25 per 100,000 users). The increased risk of these conditions disappears after OCs are discontinued. Carbohydrate metabolism is affected mainly by the progestin component of the pill, which promotes insulin resistance by decreasing insulin receptor number. This is unchanged by reducing the level of estrogen. Low-dose and multiphasic pills have minimal effects on carbohydrate metabolism. The estrogen does help control the amount of breakthrough bleeding (BTB) so formulations with lower estrogen may have more BTB, but the incidence is very low. Any preparation seems to decrease premenstrual complaints. The contraceptive effectiveness of multiphasic and low-dose OCs is similar to that of 50-mg EE_2 pills and is used initially whenever possible.

1124. **(D)** The risk of myocardial infarction in users of OCs occurs primarily in smokers and in women with other risk factors for coronary heart disease, including hypertension, hypercholesterolemia, obesity, diabetes, and age beyond 35 years. Low-dose and multiphasic preparations have little effect on circulating lipid levels and carbohydrate metabolism. Hypertension occurs in less than 5% of current OC users and is mediated by increased circulating angiotensinogen levels. Smoking, which has no positive effects, potentiates all these complications. Thus, using a non–estrogen-containing hormonal preparation and encouraging smoking cessation is best. While this patient is at increased risk of cardiovascular disease due to a number of factors, a low-dose OC may still be considered if no other method is an option because the risk of these agents is still significantly less than that associated with pregnancy. Other, alternate methods of contraception still should be strongly encouraged as well.

1125. (B) OCs regulate menses in anovulatory women, decrease dysmenorrhea, improve hirsutism from polycystic ovarian disease, and reduce menstrual bleeding and iron-deficiency anemia. Oral contraceptives also reduce the risk of benign breast lesions (e.g., fibroadenomas and fibrocystic changes), benign and malignant ovarian tumors, endometrial carcinoma, and pelvic inflammatory disease. OCs increase the risk of hepatic adenoma. Estimated annual risk is 3 to 4/100,000 women. These benign tumors can rupture, causing severe intraperitoneal hemorrhage, and may regress when the OCs are stopped.

1126. (B) OCs may increase the frequency and intensity of migraine headaches, though this does not always occur. Because migraine symptoms may mimic those of stroke, many physicians consider the history of migraine headaches as a relative contraindication to OC use. After discontinuation of OCs, ovulation is usually reestablished within 2 to 3 months. The incidence of amenorrhea for up to 1 year after OC use (mistakenly called "post-pill" amenorrhea) is about 0.8%. It usually occurs in women with a history of anovulation. There is no conclusive evidence that OCs significantly increase the risk of breast cancer, even in women with benign breast disease or a family history of breast cancer. OCs reduce the incidence of benign breast disease. OC use during early unrecognized pregnancy does not appear to adversely affect the fetus. Although impaired glucose metabolism may occur (see question 1123), OC users with a family history for diabetes mellitus do not alter their risk of developing the disease. Low-dose OCs contain insufficient amounts of progestin to adversely affect circulating lipoprotein levels.

1127. (B) Young healthy women using OCs are seen annually for exclusion of problems by history, blood pressure measurement, and physical examination. A serum cholesterol and 2-hour postprandial blood glucose should be considered in high-risk individuals (e.g., age beyond 35 years, diabetes mellitus, previous gestational diabetes mellitus, obesity, xanthomatosis, strong family history of heart disease, or hyperlipidemia). This patient is at risk for cardiovascular disease by virtue of her age and weight, warranting a screening cholesterol measurement. Without other indications of risk for diabetes, a 3-hour glucose tolerance test is probably not indicated. In the absence of symptoms, an ECG is unlikely to show any abnormality. With a history of multiple sexual partners, a Papanicolaou smear should be performed to rule out cervical pathology and appropriate cervical cultures and serum tests for STDs should be carried out. Prophylactic or therapeutic antibiotic administrations should be reserved for known exposure or infections confirmed by laboratory testing.

1128. (C) Progestin therapy may be used for contraception by women who are nursing or unable to take estrogen (e.g., older women who smoke or who have other risk factors). The progestin-only pill (the mini-pill) contains either norethindrone (0.35 mg) or norgestrel (0.075 mg). Gonadotropin suppression is not as complete as that associated with OCs and use effectiveness is 2 to 3 pregnancies per 100 woman-years. Ectopic pregnancy is not prevented as effectively as intrauterine pregnancy. Its use is associated with irregular vaginal bleeding, mood change, headache, amenorrhea, and weight gain. Other progestin-only contraception methods include intramuscular medroxyprogesterone acetate, subcutaneous levonorgestrel implants, and progestin-containing vaginal rings.

1129. (A) Surgical sterilization (permanent contraception) is the most frequently used contraceptive method in the United States. One third of couples practicing birth control use some type of sterilization procedure. Twice as many females as males undergo surgical sterilization, and the mortality rate from female sterilization is about 3 deaths per 100,000 procedures. Female sterilization has a failure rate of less than 1% and may be performed immediately postpartum (postpartum tubal ligation), or at a time other than after childbirth (interval procedure). The failure rate of tubal occlusion performed puerperally is slightly higher than that of interval procedures. About 1% of women who undergo tubal ligation request reversal. Successful reversal of tubal ligation is possible if tubal damage is minimal and normal fimbria are present. The ability to reverse either male or female sterilization procedures is poor, and all patients should be counseled that the procedure is considered to be permanent. Male sterilization (vasectomy) is a simple procedure in which a segment of vas deferens is ligated and excised through a scrotal incision. The procedure has a failure rate of less than 1%. Since sperm may be stored in the reproductive tract beyond the ligated vas deferens, sterility is not immediate. Semen analysis must be monitored for several months after vasectomy to confirm the absence of sperm in the ejaculate. Because of this, a failure of the vasectomy can be detected before a pregnancy occurs.

1130. **(D)** Postpartum tubal ligation is performed within 24 hours of vaginal delivery and utilizes a 2- to 3-cm incision (mini-laparotomy)

under the umbilicus to visualize the fallopian tubes. A knuckle of tube usually is created by ligating the middle portion of the tube, which is then excised (Pomeroy technique, Figure 17–3). Tubal ligation may be performed by mini-laparotomy or laparoscopy. Although the Pomeroy technique is the most common interval procedure used during mini-laparotomy, other techniques include:

- Irving technique: A 1- to 2-cm segment of tube is removed and each end is ligated. The proximal portion of the tube is buried underneath the uterine peritoneum.
- Kroener fimbriectomy: The fimbriated portion of the tube is removed.
- Parkland technique: The tube is ligated in two places approximately 2 cm apart, and the segment between the ligatures is excised.
- Uchida technique: A 1- to 2-cm segment of tube is removed and the proximal portion of the tube is buried between the leaves of the broad ligament.

Laparoscopic tubal ligation is performed through 1-cm subumbilical and 0.5-cm suprapubic incisions and is less painful than mini-laparotomy. Electrocoagulation (fulguration) or mechanical methods are used to occlude

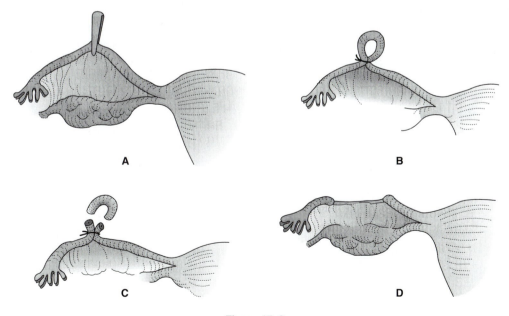

A

B

C

D

Figure 17–3.

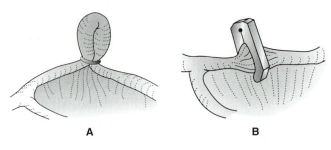

Figure 17–4.

the tube at the junction of the isthmus and ampulla (Figure 17–4). Both techniques have comparable failure rates. Mechanical occlusive devices damage a smaller tubal area compared to electrocoagulation, but are slightly more painful because of tubal ischemia within the occlusive device. Although rare, mortality from laparoscopic sterilization is generally due to general anesthesia complications occurring in obese women. Vaginal colpotomy (incision through the posterior fornix into the pouch of Douglas) with partial salpingectomy is an effective method of female sterilization but is associated with a 10% incidence of infection at the incision site unless prophylactic antibiotics are used at the time of surgery. Hysteroscopic tubal occlusion with electrocautery or silicon plugs has a significant failure rate and for that reason is still considered experimental by most physicians.

1131. (E) Apart from local complications of the procedure (hematoma formation, skin infection), vasectomy may be associated with a local inflammatory response to sperm leakage (sperm granuloma). It does not alter the risk of developing testicular cancer, prostatic cancer, or cardiovascular disease. Circulating hormone levels are unaffected by the procedure. Although 75 to 90% patency rates have been reported after vasectomy reversal (microsurgical vasovasostomy), pregnancy rates are only 33 to 70%. This discrepancy between patency and pregnancy rates reflects alterations in sperm quality influenced by duration of vas deferens occlusion and development of sperm autoantibodies.

1132. (A) Approximately 1 of every 4 pregnancies in the world is terminated electively by abortion, making this technique one of the most common methods of fertility control.

1133. (D) The risk of death from legal abortion is lowest when it is performed within the first 8 weeks of gestation (Table 17–2). First-trimester legal abortions are consistently safer for women of all ages than if they gave birth. Although the maternal morality rate from birth increases with age, the risk of death from first-trimester legal abortion is not age-related.

Table 17–2. Maternal Mortality per 100,000 Women Annually in Developed Countries

Type of Birth Control	Maternal Age (Years)					
	15–19	20–24	25–29	30–34	35–39	40–44
None (birth-related)	5.6	6.1	7.4	13.9	20.8	22.6
First-trimester legal abortion	1.2	1.6	1.8	1.7	1.9	1.2

Adapted from Tietze C. Induced abortion: 1977 supplement (Table 11). *Rep Popul Fam Plann* 14(2nd ed. Suppl): 16 Dec 1977.

1134. (A) RU 486 is a 19-norsteroid derivative that acts as an antiprogesterone by binding strongly to progesterone receptors. The major target tissue of RU 486 is the endometrium. RU 486 induces menses within 3 days when given during the midluteal phase. It does not induce menses without luteal-phase levels of progesterone (e.g., follicular phase). It induces abortion (abortifacient) with an 85% success rate when given before 6 weeks' gestation. The addition of prostaglandins to RU 486 therapy increases the abortion rate to over 95%. Although side effects of RU 486 include nausea, vomiting, and gastrointestinal cramping, the major risk accompanying therapy is severe hemorrhage resulting from partial expulsion of products of conception.

1135. (B) The incidence of multifetal pregnancies has risen dramatically with increased use of agents for ovulation induction and transfer of multiple embryos during IVF. Generally, the number of fetuses is inversely related to pregnancy duration and birth weight. This patient has a grand multifetal pregnancy, defined as four or more embryos. She has a significant risk of developing pregnancy complications (including preterm delivery and pregnancy-induced hypertension) leading to low-birth-weight infants and high perinatal mortality. Although this case presents several ethical dilemmas, the patient should be offered selective termination, a technique in which the number of fetuses is reduced. It is commonly performed by ultrasound-directed transcervical injection of potassium chloride into the fetal thoracic cavity.

1136. (B) The IUD string may retract into the cervical canal so that it is not palpable. It may also become displaced because of pregnancy, uterine malposition, expulsion, and perforation. The latter complication accompanies about 1 in 1,000 IUD insertions and occurs more frequently with insertions performed postpartum when uterine involution is incomplete. The IUD string can often be found by gently probing the cervical canal. If cervical probing is unsuccessful, further studies, including colposcopy with an endocervical speculum, pelvic ultrasound, abdominal radiography, or hysteroscopy may be necessary (generally in that order).

1137. (E) Second-trimester pregnancy termination may be accomplished by either surgical evacuation of the uterus or induction of labor. D&E is a surgical procedure in which the cervix is dilated and the intrauterine contents are removed with a forceps and blunt curet. Unlike the evacuation of the uterus employed with early (first-trimester) terminations, evacuating the contents of a pregnancy at 25 weeks is associated with a much increased risk of perforation, sepsis, and retained products (incomplete removal). Labor may be induced by parenteral, vaginal, or intra-amniotic administration of prostaglandins. Intravenous oxytocin administration is less effective in inducing labor, although it is frequently used in conjunction with prostaglandin therapy.

1138. (D) The cervical cap is a small diaphragm that is held in place over the cervix by suction. Its prolonged use of 1 to 2 days' duration can cause cervical erosions, which may predispose to toxic shock syndrome. Rare cases of toxic shock syndrome have been reported with the use of the vaginal diaphragm as well.

1139. (A) OCs increase the risk of cholelithiasis in susceptible women. Estrogen induces alteration of bile composition. Some studies suggest that the increase in cholelithiasis is actually an acceleration in detection in the first few years of use and that long-term risk is not increased.

1140. (E) *Actinomyces israelii* is an anaerobic, gram-positive bacterium that occasionally causes pelvic inflammatory disease. Prolonged IUD use has been associated with an increased risk of cervical *Actinomyces,* as identified by Papanicolaou smear. Cervical *Actinomyces* usually persists until the IUD is removed. Although most individuals with cervical *Actinomyces* are asymptomatic, a Pap smear positive for *Actinomyces* in an asymptomatic woman may be managed by IUD removal or by treating with antibiotics and then repeating the Pap smear. Penicillin therapy may be necessary for those individuals with persistently positive smears or clinical evidence of salpingitis despite IUD removal.

1141. (F) Coitus interruptus is an unreliable contraceptive method in which the penis is withdrawn from the vagina before ejaculation.

1142. (H) Long-acting progesterone-based contraception is associated with failure rates that rival or are less than sterilization if used correctly. The copper-containing IUD is close behind, with use effectiveness rates that can equal or surpass sterilization over a 5- to 10-year period.

1143. (E) About 15% of women discontinue IUD use during the first year because of dysmenorrhea and abnormal menstrual bleeding.

1144. (J) The efficacy of male sterilization must be confirmed by semen analysis before a couple may use it for reliable contraception. Even though the vas deferens may have been blocked by the surgical procedure, sperm that are stored in the upper portions of the genital tract must be either flushed out by ejaculations or reach their life span before contraceptive efficacy will be achieved.

1145. (G) Both the male and female condom provide some degree of protection from STDs. Neither is perfect, and neither can absolve risky behavior. Because of the larger surface area covered by the female condom (including portions of the vulva), it should provide slightly greater protection, though studies to confirm this are lacking.

1146. (F) The IUD is best suited for older, parous women who wish to use a temporary method of contraception; do not have a history of salpingitis; have a stable, monogamous relationship; and have a normally shaped uterus. IUD use should be discouraged in nulli- parous individuals or women with a history of ectopic pregnancy or a medical condition (e.g., corticosteroid therapy or valvular heart disease) that increases the incidence of infection.

1147. (A) The use of oral contraceptives in a nursing woman may diminish milk production. Progestin-only pills, barrier methods, chemical contraceptives, and IUD use have no effect on nursing.

1148. (A) OCs are relatively contraindicated in smokers (more than 15 cigarettes daily) over the age of 35 years. Other contraindications to OC use are confirmed or suspected pregnancy, thromboembolic disease, impaired liver function, known or suspected pelvic and/or estrogen-dependent malignancy, undiagnosed vaginal bleeding, known or suspected pelvic infection, and congenital hyperlipidemia.

1149. (E) A diaphragm may not fit properly in women with significant pelvic relaxation.

CHAPTER 18

Gynecology: Common Lesions of the Vulva, Vagina, Cervix, and Uterus; Gynecologic Pain Syndromes; Imaging in Obstetrics and Gynecology
Questions

DIRECTIONS (Questions 1150 through 1186): Each of the numbered items or incomplete statements in this section is followed by answers or by completions of the statement. Select the ONE lettered answer or completion that is BEST in each case.

1150. A 63-year-old patient is seen for routine examination. An excoriated 2-cm lesion is found on her left labium majus, which, she states, has been present for at least 3 months. The next best step is to

   (A) prescribe hydrocortisone cream
   (B) schedule colposcopy
   (C) perform excisional biopsy
   (D) prescribe Burow's solution soaks
   (E) paint the area with toluidine blue stain

1151. The most common skin disease or condition to affect the vulva is

   (A) lichen planus
   (B) psoriasis
   (C) seborrheic dermatitis
   (D) contact dermatitis
   (E) hidradenitis suppurativa

1152. An 18-year-old woman consults you for a painful swelling of her left labium that has progressively worsened over the past 3 days. She has been treating the discomfort with over-the-counter analgesics and warm sitz baths. On examination, a 6-cm swollen, red, tender, tense cystic mass is present in the base of the left labium majus. The most appropriate next step in the care of this patient is

   (A) excision of the mass
   (B) dry heat
   (C) oral antibiotics
   (D) intramuscular or intravenous antibiotics
   (E) incision and drainage of the mass

1153. Which of the following is most likely to cause vulvar pruritus?

   (A) vaginal trichomaniasis
   (B) leukemia
   (C) personal hygiene products
   (D) secondary syphilis
   (E) hidradenitis suppurativa

1154. A 79-year-old woman presents to your office with a 1-cm fleshy outgrowth from her urethra. It has a slightly infected appearance and bleeds on contact. You perform a biopsy, and the report states "transitional and stratified squamous epithelium with underlying loose connective tissue." The most likely diagnosis is

(A) urethral leiomyoma

(B) hidradenitis suppurativa

(C) senile urethritis

(D) urethral caruncle

(E) urethral carcinoma

1155. A patient consults you with complaints of recurrent, painful, draining vulvar lesions. Examination shows multiple abscesses and deep scars in the labia. A foul-smelling discharge from the lesions is noted. During the review of systems, the patient reports the occasional appearance of similar lesions in the axilla. The most likely diagnosis is

(A) herpetic vulvitis

(B) hidradenitis suppurativa

(C) lymphogranuloma venereum

(D) granuloma inguinale

(E) secondary syphilis

1156. A 20-year-old patient complains of painful vulvar ulcers present for 72 hours. Examination reveals three tender, punched-out lesions with a yellow exudate but no induration. The most likely diagnosis is

(A) chancroid

(B) granuloma inguinale

(C) herpes

(D) lymphogranuloma venereum

(E) syphilis

1157. Large cysts lined with cuboidal, nonciliated epithelium, most commonly found on the lateral vaginal wall, are most likely to be

(A) paramesonephric duct remnants

(B) mesonephric duct remnants

(C) epidermoid inclusion cysts

(D) endometrial implants

(E) adenomatous hyperplasia

1158. The most common cause of vaginal adenosis is

(A) in utero exposure to thalidomide

(B) in utero exposure to diethylstilbestrol (DES)

(C) in utero exposure to progesterone

(D) chronic tampon use

(E) elevated hormone levels during late pregnancy

1159. A 17-year-old girl is seen at a local clinic desiring contraception because she thinks she will soon become sexually active. During her examination, an ulcerative lesion is seen in the vaginal fornix. It has a rolled, irregular edge with a reddish-appearing granular base. The lesion is mildly tender to palpation. This lesion is most likely

(A) vaginal intraepithelial neoplasia

(B) vulvar carcinoma

(C) syphilis

(D) an ulcer caused by the use of tampons

(E) genital herpes

1160. The most common vaginal complaint or problem seen in practice is

(A) vaginal intraepithelial neoplasia

(B) herpes infection

(C) human papillomavirus (HPV)

(D) vaginitis

(E) traumatic vulvitis

1161. The most common benign neoplasm of the cervix and endocervix is a

(A) polyp

(B) leiomyoma

(C) nabothian cyst

(D) endometriosis

(E) Gartner's duct cyst

1162. The most likely complication of cervical stenosis is

(A) pyometra

(B) adenomyosis

(C) primary dysmenorrhea

(D) cervical polyps

(E) uterus didelphys

1163. The most likely cause of abnormal genital bleeding in a 13-year-old girl is

(A) uterine cancer

(B) ectopic pregnancy

(C) anovulation

(D) systemic bleeding diatheses

(E) threatened abortion

1164. The most likely cause of abnormal genital bleeding in a 22-year-old woman is

(A) uterine cancer

(B) ectopic pregnancy

(C) anovulation

(D) systemic bleeding diatheses

(E) threatened abortion

1165. A 15-year-old patient has had menstrual bleeding every 2 to 4 weeks since menarche 1 year ago. The bleeding can be both heavy and light. It sometimes lasts as long as 2 weeks. The best next step in the management of her problem is to

(A) obtain a pregnancy test

(B) perform an endometrial biopsy

(C) obtain pelvic ultrasonography

(D) initiate oral contraceptives (OCs)

(E) initiate cyclic progestin therapy

1166. A 47-year-old woman complains of postcoital bleeding, nearly as heavy as menses. The most likely origin of her bleeding would be cervical

(A) polyps

(B) ectropion

(C) carcinoma

(D) nabothian cysts

(E) infection

1167. An obese 63-year-old woman presents with a 3-month history of continuous scanty vaginal bleeding. She denies use of hormone replacement therapy. Adequate history and physical examination in the office reveals no other ab-

normalities. A Pap smear is negative. The next most appropriate step in her management is to

(A) begin estrogen replacement therapy

(B) sample the endometrium

(C) perform colposcopic evaluation of the cervix

(D) obtain random biopsies of the cervix

(E) obtain serum follicle-stimulating hormone (FSH), luteinizing hormone (LH), estradiol, and prolactin levels

1168. A patient being treated for prothrombin deficiency develops abnormal uterine bleeding. An anatomic lesion has been ruled out. Further management to control the bleeding should begin with

(A) gonadotropin-releasing hormone (GnRH) antagonists

(B) medroxyprogesterone acetate

(C) conjugated equine estrogens

(D) OCs

(E) transdermal estradiol

1169. A patient complains of heavy but regular menstrual periods. An anatomic cause of the magnitude of her flow has been ruled out. Which of the following has been shown to be most effective in reducing her menstrual flow?

(A) tanexamic acid

(B) formal dilation and curettage

(C) depo-medroxyprogesterone acetate

(D) misoprostol

(E) ergonovine maleate

1170. An endometrial sampling is likely to be reported as showing endometrial hyperplasia in a patient who is

(A) obese

(B) postmenopausal

(C) using cyclic combination OCs

(D) using depo-medroxyprogesterone acetate

(E) using an intrauterine device (IUD)

1171. Primary dysmenorrhea is caused by

  (A) uterine hypercontractility
  (B) uterine ischemia
  (C) high levels of estrogen
  (D) coitus during menses
  (E) ovulation

1172. Of the following, the best therapy for secondary dysmenorrhea thought to be due to adenomyosis is

  (A) cervical dilation
  (B) cylic OCs
  (C) analgesics
  (D) hysterectomy
  (E) testosterone injections

1173. A 35-year-old accountant complains of episodic bloating, breast tenderness, dyspareunia, irritability, and depression, which leave her with "only 1 good week a month." She is currently using condoms and foam for birth control because she "felt terrible" on OCs.

Pelvic examination is normal. Your best diagnostic course is to

  (A) begin a prospective diary of symptoms for the next 2 months
  (B) obtain a serum progesterone level during the last half of her menstrual cycle
  (C) obtain a serum estrogen level during the first half of her menstrual cycle
  (D) perform an transvaginal ultrasound examination of the posterior cul-de-sac
  (E) begin basal body temperature (BBT) recording

1174. Which of the following symptom patterns suggest true premenstrual syndrome (PMS) (see Figure 18–1)?

  (A) graph A
  (B) graph B
  (C) graph C
  (D) graph D
  (E) graph E

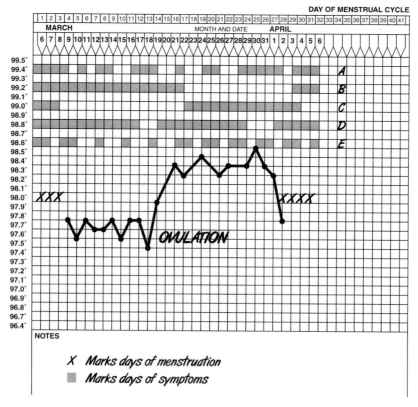

Figure 18–1.

1175. A 33-year-old patient has been diagnosed as having adenomyosis. Which of the following is most consistent with this diagnosis?

(A) dyspareunia
(B) mood swings
(C) painful defecation
(D) dysmenorrhea
(E) infertility

1176. The diagnosis of endometriosis is confirmed histologically by identifying extragenital implants containing

(A) endometrial glands and stroma
(B) hypertrophic smooth muscle
(C) hemorrhage and iron pigment deposits
(D) fibrosis
(E) stromal decidualization

1177. Adenomyosis may be associated with which of the following clinical or histologic changes?

(A) stromal hypertrophy
(B) an irregular uterus
(C) atrophy of the overlying endometrium
(D) deformation of the basal endometrium into folds that dip into the myometrium
(E) myometrial hypertrophy

1178. The most common indication for treatment of uterine leiomyomata in a 42-year-old woman is

(A) interference with reproductive function
(B) rapid enlargement
(C) pain
(D) excessive uterine bleeding
(E) impingement on another organ

1179. A 45-year-old patient with uterine leiomyomata found on pelvic examination complains of excessive uterine bleeding. The next step in the management of this patient should be

(A) myomectomy
(B) hysterectomy
(C) ultrasonography
(D) endometrial biopsy
(E) hysterosalpingography

1180. A 26-year-old patient is found to have an 8-week-size, irregular uterus. She does not complain of pain or excessive menstrual bleeding. Her Pap smear is normal. The best next step in the management of this patient is

(A) continued observation
(B) endometrial biopsy
(C) cervical conization
(D) hysterectomy
(E) pelvic ultrasonography

1181. A 23-year-old woman complains of heavy, painful menstrual periods every 2 weeks. On further questioning, you find that every other bleed is actually very brief, consisting of only 2 days of spotting. At these times, the pain is also only an occasional twinge. During the heavy bleeding, the pain is crampy, nearly constant, located centrally in the pelvis, and lasts 3 days. A BBT curve is biphasic, compatible with normal ovulatory cycles 28 days in length. Her physical examination is normal. In addition to dysmenorrhea, the most likely diagnosis would be

(A) anovulatory bleeding
(B) progressive endometriosis
(C) chronic constipation
(D) mittelschmerz
(E) Halban's disease

Questions 1182 and 1183

A 25-year-old patient with her last menstrual period (LMP) 3 weeks ago is being followed for a 5 × 4 × 4-cm right ovarian cystic mass. She comes to the emergency department complaining of sudden right-sided low abdominal pain and nausea that has been constant for 2 hours. She had intermittent spasms of pain for a week preceding this episode (when you first felt the cyst). All these pain episodes resolved within minutes. The patient denies fever or recent coitus (none in 6 months). Examination demonstrates a 10 × 8 × 6-cm right pelvic mass that is very tender. White blood cell count (WBC) is 12,500/mL and temperature is 100.2°F. She has had no prior surgery.

1182. Of the following options, the most likely diagnosis is

  (A) appendiceal abscess
  (B) torsion of an ovarian cyst
  (C) diverticulitis
  (D) ectopic pregnancy
  (E) pelvic inflammatory disease (PID)

1183. The patient undergoes diagnostic laparoscopy, and a black mass is seen replacing the entire right ovary. The most appropriate management of this patient is

  (A) removal of the ovary
  (B) antibiotic therapy
  (C) *Clostridium* antitoxin
  (D) reverse torsion and oophoropexy
  (E) anticoagulation

1184. Computed tomography (CT) scans currently can detect pelvic masses larger than (lowest limit of reliable identification)

  (A) 0.02 mm
  (B) 0.5 mm
  (C) 5 mm
  (D) 2 cm
  (E) 5 cm

1185. A 36-year-old virgin with a low-grade fever complains of pelvic and flank pain. No irregular bleeding has occurred. Her past history is unremarkable with the exception of mi-

graine headaches that are well controlled by medication. Pelvic examination demonstrates slight induration posteriorly but is otherwise normal. The Pap smear is normal. Intravenous pyelogram (IVP) shows "medial displacement of the ureters with moderate bilateral obstruction." The most likely diagnosis is

  (A) stage II cervical cancer
  (B) PID
  (C) idiopathic retroperitoneal fibrosis
  (D) uterine fibroids
  (E) endometriosis

1186. The most effective treatment of vulvar pruritus associated with atrophic vulvitis is

  (A) antihistamines
  (B) hydrocortisone
  (C) alcohol injections
  (D) tranquilizers
  (E) topical estrogen therapy

DIRECTIONS (Questions 1187 through 1206): Each set of items in this section consists of a list of lettered headings followed by several numbered words or phrases. For each numbered word or phrase, select the ONE lettered option that is most closely associated with it. Each lettered option may be selected once, more than once, or not at all.

Questions 1187 through 1189

Match the clinical menopausal problem with the most appropriate medication.

  (A) orally administered DES 0.2 to 2 mg/day for the first 25 days of each month
  (B) vaginal estrogen cream daily
  (C) orally administered progesterone 5 to 10 mg daily for 10 days
  (D) testosterone tablets 10 mg/day
  (E) estrogen 20 mg administered intravenously

1187. Anovulatory dysfunctional bleeding

1188. Senile vaginitis

1189. Postmenopausal vasomotor symptoms

Questions 1190 through 1194

Match the appropriate signs or symptoms with the most appropriate diagnosis.

    (A) ectopic pregnancy

    (B) PID

    (C) endometriosis

    (D) appendicitis

    (E) urinary tract infection (UTI)

    (F) ruptured corpus luteum cyst of the ovary

1190. Amenorrhea for 8 weeks, 1 week of unilateral adnexal pain, acute abdomen on examination, rapidly falling hematocrit, positive pregnancy test

1191. Bilaterally equal adnexal pain, cervical motion tenderness, direct abdominal tenderness, temperature 101.3°F, WBC 12,000/mL

1192. Flank pain, temperature 100.9°F, WBC 14,000/mL

1193. Increasingly severe dysmenorrhea

1194. Delayed onset of menses, sudden onset of severe pain, syncope, negative pregnancy test

Questions 1195 through 1206

Match the disease, diagnosis, or test with the most likely finding.

    (A) teeth in a pelvic cyst

    (B) paralytic ileus and edema of the bowel

    (C) extrinsic pressure defect of the bowel with intact mucosa

    (D) gas in the uterine soft tissues

    (E) stippled calcifications in the area of the ovaries

    (F) ring of echoes around the fetal head on ultrasonography

    (G) double bubble on ultrasonography

    (H) enlarged iliac lymph nodes on magnetic resonance imaging (MRI)

    (I) CT demonstrating sellar enlargement

    (J) unicornuate uterus

    (K) lack of filling on hysterosalpingography

    (L) echogenic ring 9.6 cm in diameter seen on ultrasonography

    (M) acetowhite changes

    (N) echogenic mass with "shadowing" behind

1195. Acute PID

1196. Ovarian carcinoma

1197. *Clostridium* endometritis

1198. Endometriosis

1199. Teratoma

1200. Term pregnancy

1201. Duodenal atresia

1202. Cervical carcinoma

1203. Prolactinoma

1204. Asherman syndrome

1205. Abnormal Pap smear

1206. Increased incidence of renal anomalies

Answers and Explanations

1150. (C) Any vulvar ulcer in a woman of this age should be biopsied and, if benign, evaluated at regular intervals for change. If invasive carcinoma is found, radical vulvectomy and inguinal lymphadenectomy are generally the treatment of choice.

1151. (D) The most common dermatologic condition found to affect the skin of the vulva is contact dermatitis. The vulva is subjected to a wide variety of irritants, many of which can induce contact dermatitis. The vulva is subject to virtually any of the diseases of skin elsewhere on the body. Biopsy is necessary in most cases to confirm the diagnosis, primarily because of the possible appearance of vulvar cancer.

1152. (E) The patient described presents a typical history of a Bartholin's gland abscess. In the acute phase, incision and drainage via some form of catheter or by marsupialization is most appropriate. Since the duct of the Bartholin's gland has become obstructed, allowing the formation of an abscess, a neocystostomy must be created. This may be done by placing a short catheter with an inflatable bulb (Word catheter) into the abscess and leaving it there for 10 to 14 days, or constructing a new duct by marsupialization of the abscess wall. Simple incision and drainage is ineffective in creating a long-term cure and allows for reformation of the abscess. The etiology of a Bartholin duct abscess is unknown. Rest, hot soaks to the area, analgesics, and antibiotics for associated infection may all help speed healing. Cystectomy (or excision of the gland) is used to treat only re-

calcitrant cases or cases suspected of malignancy.

1153. (C) An accurate and careful history may yield information that will solve the problem of vulvar pruritus. Obviously, vaginitis, diabetes, and uncleanliness may be contributing factors. A wet prep from the vagina will yield the etiology in many cases. The most common vaginitis to cause vulvar pruritus is *Monilia* infection. Bacterial vaginosis may cause itching, as may trichomoniasis, but itching is not their major symptom. Systemic diseases, including leukemia, may cause vulvar symptoms, but these are rare. Hidradenitis suppurativa causes vulvar pain and suppurative lesions, but generally not itching. The most likely source of pruritus of those listed are feminine hygiene products. These agents very commonly cause a contact dermatitis that can result in skin changes and itching.

1154. (D) Small, fleshy, polypoid growths from the urethra are most likely urethral caruncles. They are most common in postmenopausal women but also occur in children. Topical estrogen cream will usually allay any symptoms. In postmenopausal women, a biopsy must be done prior to treatment in order to rule out the main differential diagnosis, urethral carcinoma. When these caruncles are found in children, prompt recognition will prevent these lesions from being misinterpreted as evidence of sexual abuse.

1155. (B) Hidradenitis suppurativa is a refractory infection of the apocrine sweat glands, usually caused by staphylococci or streptococci. Treatment early in the disease consists of drainage and antibiotic therapy. Severe chronic infections may not respond to medical therapy and require extensive surgery. Multiple, recurrent, infected-appearing ulcers occurring bilaterally on the labia should suggest hidradenitis suppurativa. Herpetic vulvitis presents as a maculopapular rash with vesical formation. Lymphogranuloma venereum and granuloma inguinale are both uncommon sexually transmitted diseases (STDs) and present with limited but characteristic ulcers (Table 18–1). Secondary syphilis generally does not present with vulvar symptoms, but rather with a "money spot" rash over the torso, palms, and soles of the feet.

1156. (A) Very painful punched-out lesions with a yellow exudate but no induration surrounded by an erythematous halo should suggest chancroid. Each of the other conditions listed present with significantly different symptoms and findings (see Table 18–1).

1157. (B) Such cysts, though rare, can cause technical difficulties during examination, during intercourse, or during tampon insertion. The cysts are invariably benign and need to be re-

moved only when they cause problems for the patient.

1158. (B) The first 8 weeks of gestation is the period of organogenesis. The use of estrogen supplementation (specifically DES) during the first few weeks of pregnancy may induce vaginal adenosis and morphologic changes in the cervix. Many feel that beyond the first 42 days after conception, there is little risk of teratogenesis. The use of DES during the first trimester was common in the 1950s and 1960s when a woman was threatening to miscarry. In utero exposure is rare for women born after 1965.

1159. (D) Tampon ulcers may cause vaginal discharge or spotting but may also be asymptomatic. When seen on examination, they have the characteristic appearance described in the question; rolled-edge ulcers with a granular base. They are found in the vaginal fornices and go away after the discontinuation of tampon use. A herpetic lesion does not have this appearance. A syphilitic lesion is also unlikely if the woman has not been sexually active, but it would be wise to screen with a rapid plasma reagin (RPR) or Venereal Disease Research Laboratory (VDRL). The other diseases mentioned are less likely because

Table 18–1. Minor Sexually Transmitted Diseases

Disease	Causative Agent	Main Symptom	Diagnosis	Treatment
Chancroid	*Hemophilus ducreyi*	Painful "soft chancres," adenopathy	Clinical smears, culture	Erythromycin 500 mg q.i.d. for 10 days
Granuloma inguinale	*Calymmatobacterium granulomatis*	Raised, red lesions	Clinical smears	Tetracyclin 500 mg q6h for 3 weeks
Lymphogranuloma venereum (LGV)	*Chlamydia trachomatis*	Vesicle, progressing to bubo	Clinical complement fixation test	Tetracycline 500 mg q6h for 3 weeks
Molluscum contagiosum	*Molluscum contagiosum* (DNA virus)	Raised papule with waxy core	Clinical inclusion bodies	Desiccation, cryotherapy, curettage
Parasites	*Pediculosis pubis,* scabies	Itching	Inspection	Lindane 1%
Enteric infections	*Neisseria gonorrhoeae, Chlamydia trachomatis, Shigella* sp., *Salmonella,* protozoa	Diarrhea	Culture	Based on agent
Vaginitis (sexually transmitted)*	*Trichomonas*	Odor, irritation	Microscopic examination of secretions	Metronidazole 500 mg b.i.d. for 7 days

* Debate persists about the sexual transmission of bacterial vaginosis.

From: Sexually Transmitted Disease, in Beckman CRB, Ling FW, Barzansky BM, et al., eds. *Obstetrics and Gynecology*, 2nd ed. Baltimore: Williams & Wilkins, 1995;309.

they are sexually transmitted or are extremely unlikely in a woman this age.

1160. **(D)** By far the most common vaginal disease is vaginitis, with the most common causes being bacterial vaginosis (*Gardnerella* vaginitis), candidiasis, and trichomoniasis. Herpes and HPV may cause a discharge and viral vaginitis, but they are much less common than the other forms of vaginal infection. Trauma to the vulva may occur during sexual intercourse or through daily activities or tight clothing. These are uncommon and the diagnosis is generally self-evident.

1161. **(A)** Benign endocervical or cervical polyps have been reported in up to 4% of patients in some series. They are most common in multiparous women in the 40- to 50-year-old age group. The main clinical symptom is intermenstrual bleeding. Though uncertain, their etiology is thought to be some type of inflammation. Nabothian cysts arise at areas of active metaplasia of the cervix, resulting in a squamous cell covering of a mucus-secreting gland. This causes a mucus-filled cyst on the cervix but they do not involve the endocervical canal. Gartner's duct cysts are lateral on the vaginal wall and represent remnants of the wolffian duct.

1162. **(A)** Blood, pus, or a sterile, clear fluid may accumulate within the uterus in response to narrowing of the cervix or upper vagina. Cervical stenosis in elderly women should always prompt the consideration of malignancy. It is also a relatively common complication after radiotherapy to the lower genital tract. The backup of blood or secretions can cause massive enlargement of the vagina and uterus. Primary dysmenorrhea is menstrual pain that is not associated with a clinically apparent cause and is based on increased prostaglandin (F2$_a$) production by the endometrium.

1163. **(C)** The first consideration in the evaluation of abnormal bleeding is the age of the patient: prereproductive, reproductive, and postreproductive. Prereproductive-age bleeding

may signal precocious puberty or neoplasia, though both are rare. Do not forget the rare, but serious, systemic coagulopathies that may present at menarche. In a 13-year-old patient, anovulation is common and can often present in the form of irregular vaginal bleeding. Though less likely, pregnancy can occur, especially if she has been having regular menses. A urine pregnancy test is always indicated any time pregnancy is a possibility.

1164. **(E)** Reproductive-age bleeding is most likely to be pregnancy-related. Contraceptive-induced bleeding (breakthrough, IUD, etc.) is also a common etiology in the reproductive-age woman. Perimenopausal women are most likely to suffer from benign neoplasia in the form of polyps or leiomyomata. Postmenopausal women are at the greatest risk for cancer, especially endometrial cancer—the most common gynecologic malignancy.

1165. **(A)** In nearly every patient, abnormal uterine bleeding is either from an organic lesion or a hormonal imbalance. In a patient of this age, diagnostic and therapeutic alternatives may be altered by her level of maturity and social situation, but the most common causes for her abnormal bleeding will be anovulation followed by pregnancy. A pregnancy test is always the first step in the evaluation and management of abnormal bleeding for reproductive-age patients. While it is probable that this patient has anovulatory or oligo-ovulatory bleeding that could be treated with cyclic progestin therapy, no therapy should be instituted until pregnancy has been ruled out. Organic lesions need to be ruled out by pelvic examination, but neoplasia is so unlikely that only under unusual circumstances would a biopsy of any kind be indicated. Ultrasonography is indicated only if the pelvic examination is inadequate or to further evaluate adnexal abnormalities. Every patient, regardless of age, should receive an explanation of the problem and a discussion of therapeutic alternatives.

1166. **(C)** Organic lesions, such as endocervical polyp, cervical ectropion, and infection, may all be the origin of bleeding in a woman of this age. Of these, the most significant bleeding is generally found with cervical lesions associated with carcinoma. Bleeding from cervical polyps may be heavy, but when sufficient to cause heavy postcoital bleeding, they will generally cause bleeding at other times as well. In contrast, cervical carcinoma may present with heavy postcoital bleeding alone in the early stages of its growth. Therefore, malignancy must always be ruled out. Nabothian cysts of the cervix are not associated with abnormal bleeding.

1167. **(B)** Amenorrhea for at least 6 months establishes the diagnosis of menopause. Uterine bleeding thereafter must be aggressively investigated to rule out neoplasia. Assessment of the endometrium can be accomplished by means of endometrial sampling, for which disposable plastic cannulas are available. Ultrasound evaluation of the endometrial stripe is another method of determining the risk of neoplasia. A stripe of less than 5 mm is very infrequently associated with neoplasia and, with other clinical findings, may be a useful adjunct to patient management. The larger the thickness of the endometrial stripe, the more likely it is that an endometrial neoplasm is present. Given this patient's history, endometrial sampling is indicated no matter what thickness of endometrium might be found.

1168. **(D)** Initially, medical management should be attempted with surgery as a last resort. At times, severe bleeding can be controlled with either OC or cyclic/continuous progestational agents. OC agents offer convenience and a high degree of efficacy in these patients, making them a good first choice unless contraindications to their use exist. They also offer a good method of birth control. In cases in which the endometrium has been denuded, the patient may initially require estrogen to stop her bleeding.

1169. **(A)** Epsilon-aminocaproic acid (EACA), tanexamic acid (AMCA), and para-aminomethylbenzoic acid (PAMBA) are po-

tent inhibitors of fibrinolysis. They have been shown to decrease menstrual blood loss by 50% or more in cases of severe menstrual bleeding. Nonsteroidal anti-inflammatory drugs (NSAIDs) such as mefenamic acid (Ponstel) have been shown to provide significant reductions in menstrual blood loss. The reduction caused by these agents is proportional to the severity of the menorrhagia: The heavier the flow, the greater the reduction. Use of ergot alkaloids to control uterine bleeding is clinically ineffective. Although misoprostol, a prostaglandin E analogue used to prevent gastric ulcers in patients taking NSAIDs, has uterotonic effects, it is not recommended for the treatment of menorrhagia. Long-acting progestins should eliminate rather than decrease menstrual blood loss because their inhibitory effect is at the pituitary level. Unopposed estrogen is the cause of much profuse irregular bleeding and seldom offers a cure unless the bleeding is from atrophy, which is unlikely in an ovulatory woman. Progesterone tends to decrease flow in anovulatory patients, if taken cyclically, but evidence is lacking for its effect in the ovulatory patient.

1170. **(A)** The obese, diabetic, hypertensive, anovulatory, nulliparous woman is at risk for both endometrial hyperplasia and adenocarcinoma. Progesterone decreases the incidence of, and in some cases can reverse the changes of, endometrial hyperplasia. IUDs are associated with varying degrees of chronic endometritis.

1171. **(A)** Prostaglandins (PGs) released at the time of menstruation cause increased myometrial contractions, which are painful. They are known to be direct causes of end-organ pain in other pain syndromes. This is likely also to be true in dysmenorrhea. Studies indicate that pressure inside the uterus during a dysmenorrheic cramp may exceed 400 mm Hg.

1172. **(B)** In primary dysmenorrhea, there is no apparent lesion associated with the pain. In secondary dysmenorrhea, there is, and it might include processes within the uterus, within the uterine wall, or external to the uterus (Table 18–2). The best therapy for secondary dysmenorrhea is always directed toward the underlying cause. In this case, the most appropriate alternative of those given would be OC therapy based on the ability of these agents to produce a thin, atrophic endometrium, even in ectopic endometrial implants. Testosterone in high enough dosage will stop ovulation but causes hirsutism and acne, and its use is generally avoided. Many patients will be helped by one of many prostaglandin inhibitors during episodes of dysmenorrhea, but again, OCs are more effective by preventing the cause of the pain.

1173. (A) The patient's symptoms point to PMS as the most likely diagnosis. Because the diagnosis of PMS is based solely on the timing of symptoms, the only way to establish the diagnosis for this, or any other, patient is to begin a prospective symptom diary. Studies have shown that retrospective assessments of symptom timing and severity are consistently inaccurate, making a prospective diary the only reliable method available. No consistent hormonal alterations have been demonstrated to be associated with PMS.

1174. (C) To establish the existence of a true PMS, the patient must experience distressing symptoms during the luteal phase of the cy-

cle and an absence of symptoms during the follicular phase of the menstrual cycle (Table 18–3). Some patients may experience a worsening of ongoing, cycle-independent symptoms referred to as premenstrual magnification (PMM). Patients with PMM experience variable symptoms that persist throughout the cycle, but undergo significant worsening just prior to menses. PMS and PMM are part of a continuum of menstrually related symptoms (Figure 18–2).

1175. (D) While anyone can have mood swings concurrent with other problems, psychological symptoms are not a characteristic of adenomyosis. Pain and heavy menses are the most common complaints. The pain is typically limited to menses, unlike endometriosis, which begins with menses and often ex-

Table 18–2. Possible Causes of Secondary Dysmenorrhea

Uterine Causes	Extrauterine Causes
Adenomyosis	Endometriosis
Cervical stenosis and cervical lesions	Inflammation and scarring (adhesions)
Congenital abnormalities (outflow obstructions, uterine anomalies)	Nongynecologic causes: Musculoskeletal, gastrointestinal, urinary
Infection (chronic endometritis)	"Pelvic congestive syndrome" (debated)
Intrauterine contraceptive devices (IUDs)	Psychogenic (rare)
Myomas (generally intracavitary or intramural)	Tumors: Myomas, benign or malignant tumors of ovary, bowel, or bladder
Polyps	

Reproduced, with permission, from Smith RP. *Gynecology in Primary Care*. Baltimore: Williams & Wilkins, 1996;390.

Table 18–3. Diagnostic Criteria for Premenstrual Dysphoric Disorder

All of the following:
  Symptoms NOT an exacerbation of another underlying psychiatric disorder
  Symptoms clustered in luteal phase; absent within first few days of the follicular phase
  Symptoms cause significant disability
Plus, five or more of the following:
  At least one:
    Marked affective lability
    Marked anxiety, tension, feelings of being "keyed up" or "on edge"
    Markedly depressed mood, feelings of hopelessness, or self-deprecating thoughts
    Persistent and marked anger or irritability
  One or more of the following:
    Avoidance of social activities
    Decreased interest in usual activities
    Decreased productivity and efficiency
    Increased sensitivity to rejection
    Interpersonal conflicts
    Lethargy, easy fatigability, lack of energy
    Marked change in appetite, cravings
    Physical symptoms (reproducible pattern of complaints)
    Sleep symptoms (hypersomnia, insomnia)
    Subjective sense of being "out of control"
    Subjective sense of being overwhelmed
    Subjective sense of difficulty in concentration

Modified from Reid RL, Yen SSC. Premenstrual syndrome. *Am J Obstet Gynecol* 1981;139:85.

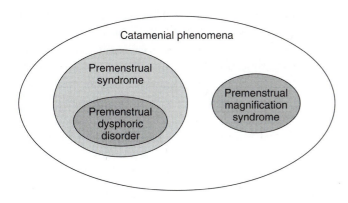

Figure 18–2. Summary of menstrually related diagnoses. All menstrually related diagnoses fall into the broad classification of "catamenial" phenomena. Within this grouping are the premenstrual syndromes (PMS and premenstrual dysphoric disorder) and premenstrual magnification syndrome. (Areas shown do not reflect the relative frequency of occurrence.)

(Reproduced, with permission, from Smith RP. *Gynecology in Primary Care.* Baltimore: Williams & Wilkins, 1996;428.)

tends to include most or all of the menstrual cycle. Since the definition of adenomyosis is endometrial glandular tissue within the myometrium, there is no pelvic involvement. Pelvic involvement with endometriosis, especially in the posterior cul-de-sac and uterosacral ligaments, may cause pain with intercourse, defecation, and/or pain on examination. Getting rid of or suppressing the endometrial implants is the only way to get rid of the pain in either adenomyosis (endometriosis interna) or endometriosis. With adenomyosis, since it typically occurs in women who have had children, the simplest therapy is after a hysterectomy.

1176. (A) Glands and stroma are all that are necessary for the diagnosis, but the other choices are commonly associated findings, though nondiagnostic. Visualization of the lesions alone without biopsy is often an unreliable means to make a diagnosis.

1177. (E) Muscle hypertrophy may or may not occur in adenomyosis and is not a criterion for diagnosis, though it is often present. Adenomyosis presents on examination as an enlarged, boggy, but symmetrical uterus associated with menorrhagia and severe dysmenorrhea. It has no effect on the overlying

endometrium. Care must be taken when making the microscopic diagnosis of adenomyosis that natural folds of the endometrium that may be cut tangentially are not confused with the free-lying islands of glands and stroma within the myometrium necessary to establish the diagnosis.

1178. (D) Uterine leiomyomata are the most common pelvic tumors and are generally asymptomatic. While the other options offered may be indications for treatment, they are less common. At one time removal of any uterus greater than 12 weeks' size was recommended, but the ability to evaluate the uterus and adnexa with ultrasonography has mitigated against this practice.

1179. (D) Endometrial biopsy is needed to rule out other etiologies for bleeding. All bleeding from a myomatous uterus is not due to the myomas. Laparoscopy or hysteroscopy allows for better external and internal uterine examination to rule out other causes of bleeding, but is not indicated for initial evaluations.

1180. (A) In the absence of symptoms, the patient should be told of the findings and periodic examinations done to detect any change in uterine size or symptomatology. Therapeutic interventions or further evaluations are not appropriate.

1181. (D) Bleeding and pain at midcycle occurs regularly in some women and is associated with ovulation. The bleeding may be due to decreased estrogen with endometrial sloughing and/or the rupture of the corpus luteum. The pain associated with ovulation itself is called mittelschmerz (from the German for "middle pain"). The pain at the time of menstrual bleeding is consistent with dysmenorrhea. The patient actually has these problems in combination (which is not unusual). Prostaglandin inhibitors or OCs are likely to help.

1182. (B) The history of a known cyst and the sudden onset should make one think of torsion of an ovarian cyst (there is no verb "torsed").

The enlargement of the cyst occurs when the venous blood outflow is stopped by the torsion, but the degree of torsion is insufficient to stop the arterial blood inflow. (Remember that masses that increase quickly in size suggest internal hemorrhage of some type.) The intermittent nature of this pain prior to the terminal episode also is characteristic of adnexal torsion. Certainly, there is a surgical indication for laparoscopy or exploratory laparotomy for treatment as well as diagnosis.

1183. **(A)** The severity of symptoms and the black adnexal mass (an infarcted ovary) indicate that excision is imperative. If the ovarian pedicle is twisted tightly so as to completely infarct the ovary, it should be resected without untwisting it to avoid emboli and thromboplastin release with the possibility of resultant disseminated intravascular coagulation (DIC). If the ovary looked viable (not black), it could be untwisted and the cyst removed. This, however, relies solely on the judgment of the surgeon.

1184. **(D)** Both ultrasound and CT scans will miss lesions of the pelvis that can be detected by clinical pelvic examination. However, they will occasionally find lesions that are otherwise unsuspected due to both their great resolution and their ability to examine patients you cannot (secondary to obesity, pain, guarding, lack of cooperation). They must be used as tools in combination with physical examination and clinical judgment. It must also be remembered that very few gynecologic lesions of significance will be less than 4 cm in diameter. Not everything the radiologist finds is pathologic.

1185. **(C)** Posterior pelvic induration and obstructed, medially deviated ureters are highly suggestive of retroperitoneal fibrosis. Most diseases move the ureters laterally. Methysergide (a drug used to prevent migraine headaches) causes this condition.

1186. **(E)** As with most things in medicine, the most effective therapy for any complaint will be tailored to the underlying cause present.

Alcohol injections are used only when all else fails, since its use risks the sloughing of vulvar skin. Local testosterone can be very helpful when thinning of the vulvar skin is present, such as in lichen sclerosis. Antihistamines, steroids, and tranquilizers may help decrease symptoms. These approaches are symptomatic only. The most appropriate treatment is estrogen replacement therapy. This can take the form of systemic therapy or local therapy in the form of creams or medicated rings. Systemic therapy offers additional benefits of cardioprotection, reduced osteoporosis, improved sleep, reduced skin wrinkling, improved libido, and other changes. For these reasons, many experts recommend systemic treatment over topical therapy alone.

1187. **(C)** As the patient usually has adequate estrogen, the use of progesterone alone administered in monthly cycles will often stop the bleeding. Ten-day courses have been shown to be the minimum effective dosage required to prevent or reverse hyperplasia.

1188. **(B)** A local symptom can often be well-treated with the local administration of medication. Often, associated urinary symptoms will decrease as well. Systemic estrogen can also be used to relieve these symptoms and provide additional benefits. Since long-term therapy is required, IV therapy is clearly inappropriate.

1189. **(A)** You must provide a dosage of estrogen high enough to stop symptoms but low enough to keep the patient from bleeding. Often, conjugated estrogens are better tolerated than DES (less nausea). Progesterone should be given for 10 to 14 days each month if the patient still has her uterus. Though conjugated estrogens are more commonly used, DES is still an excellent choice for therapy.

1190. **(A)** Intraperitoneal bleeding may be of a sudden or insidious nature. If pelvic pain exists concomitantly with a falling hematocrit, ectopic pregnancy must be ruled out. Very sensitive, rapid, and specific urine pregnancy tests have now been developed to assist in this diagnostic problem. Still, amenorrhea, pain, bleeding, and an adnexal mass is an ectopic pregnancy until proven otherwise.

1191. **(B)** Although pelvic pain will be present in all the diagnoses listed, PID is most likely to produce symmetric, bilateral adnexal pain, abdominal pain, and cervical motion tenderness, along with an elevated temperature and WBC. The others tend to produce pain that is more severe on the affected side.

1192. **(E)** Costovertebral angle pain may be present with pyelonephritis or more simply, if the kidney is infected, it should hurt over the kidney. With lower urinary tract disease, the symptoms of dysuria and frequency may predominate. Pregnancy predisposes to pyelonephritis.

1193. **(C)** Endometriosis is also associated with sterility, severe dysmenorrhea, chronic abdominal–pelvic pain, and dyspareunia. In some cases, pain, leukocytosis, and masses may closely mimic PID. The diagnosis can be confirmed only by direct observation.

1194. **(F)** The sudden, severe pain is often associated with the rupture of a corpus luteum cyst. It may be accompanied by intra-abdominal hemorrhage. Syncope is not uncommon. Observation is generally all that is necessary for the patient.

1195. **(B)** A diagnosis of small bowel obstruction may be erroneously made from a flat plate radiogram of the abdomen during an episode of acute PID. PID may also cause paralytic ileus. Laparoscopy may be needed to make the correct diagnosis.

1196. **(E)** Stippled calcifications can occur in leiomyomata, as well as in ovarian serous cystadenocarcinoma (psammoma bodies). Ultrasound can aid in differentiating these entities.

1197. **(D)** In overwhelming *Clostridium* infections, gas can sometimes be found in the soft tissues. Other signs of severe infection are invariably present by this time. The treatment includes rapid hysterectomy to remove the infected site. Surgery to debride the infected tissue is followed by broad-spectrum antibiotics.

1198. **(C)** Any space-occupying lesion extrinsic to the bowel may produce an indentation without involvement of the bowel mucosa. This may easily be mistaken for an intrinsic bowel lesion. Endometriosis must be considered in such cases if the patient is of menstrual age.

1199. **(A)** Occasionally, fat layers can be seen within the cyst as well as teeth (actually appropriately sized, irregular deposits of calcium). One must rule out the possibility of swallowed teeth, but these are usually passed quickly and are not associated with a pelvic mass. Only a small proportion of dermoid cysts have well-formed teeth, but most have calcium.

1200. **(L)** Ultrasound is the most widely used technique to determine fetal gestation age. The biparietal diameter is the most widely used ultrasonic measurement for "dating." The most accurate single measurements of the biparietal diameter occur from 20 to 24 weeks' gestation. A biparietal diameter of 9.5 is typical of a term fetus.

1201. **(G)** Duodenal atresia is an anomaly seen more frequently in male fetuses. It is seen as a "double bubble" on ultrasound. In the newborn, it often presents with projectile vomiting. It can be surgically corrected.

1202. **(H)** Cervical cancer begins as a central cervical lesion and spreads to the lymph nodes of the parametria and pelvic sidewalls. CT is probably the best nonsurgical method for the evaluation of the lymph nodes on the pelvic sidewall and along the aorta. It can isolate nodes as small as 1.5 to 2 cm. It is poor at locating enlarged nodes in the parametrial tissue.

1203. (I) The most common tumor of the pituitary is the prolactin-secreting adenoma. A tumor as small as 2 mm in the pituitary (not in the pelvis) can be detected using these specialized techniques (CT). Although MRI can image the pituitary even better, there is rarely need for the accuracy provided given the much higher cost for MRI than for CT.

1204. (K) Asherman syndrome is amenorrhea resulting from intrauterine adhesions formed after the trauma of uterine curettage associated with pregnancy. The injection of dye into the uterus fails to show filling. Office hysteroscopy is also diagnostic.

1205. (M) A cervigram is a method of taking pictures of the cervix that are eventually sent to experts for evaluation. Some studies have shown it to be equally effective as colposcopy in some settings. Others have found it generally to produce too many false-positive results.

1206. (J) Renal anomalies are many times found when there is a müllerian anomaly, especially if there is the lack of müllerian development on one side resulting in a uterus formed from a single müllerian duct.

CHAPTER 19

Pelvic Floor Dysfunction: Genital Prolapse and Urogynecology
Questions

DIRECTIONS (Questions 1207 through 1233): Each of the numbered items or incomplete statements in this section is followed by answers or by completions of the statement. Select the ONE lettered answer or completion that is BEST in each case.

1207. A 44-year-old woman (gravida 5, para 5) comes in complaining that she has noticed a bulge protruding out her vagina. Her other medical problems include hypertension treated with medication, diabetes mellitus, and alcoholism. She stands at work as a grocery clerk. She has a family history of genital prolapse. On examination, you notice a uterine prolapse, cystocele, and rectocele. Her major risk factor for her pelvic support disorder is

(A) childbirth
(B) hypertension
(C) diabetes mellitus
(D) positive family history
(E) environmental factors—job

1208. A 49-year-old parous woman comes in complaining that over the last several years it feels as though "her organs are progressively falling out her vagina." Along with this, she complains of losing urine with coughing, occasional urgency, and sometimes a feeling of incomplete emptying of her bladder with voiding. On further examination, you will most likely find a(n)

(A) cystocele
(B) rectocele
(C) enterocele

(D) complete uterine prolapse
(E) urinary tract infection (UTI)

1209. A 56-year-old woman complains that she is "sitting on a ball." She says constipation is a significant problem for her and that sometimes she needs to push stool out of her rectum by inserting a finger in the vagina and pressing on a bulge. On further examination, you will most likely find a(n)

(A) cystocele
(B) rectocele
(C) enterocele
(D) complete uterine prolapse
(E) hemorrhoid

1210. A 68-year-old woman complains of something falling out of her vagina, and she thinks it causes a constant backache. The backache is least symptomatic when she gets up in the morning and worsens as the day goes on. She says she cannot understand why she has this, because 4 years ago she had an abdominal hysterectomy and urethral suspension (Burch procedure) to correct the "falling out" and some problem with urine loss. Her ability to hold her urine is excellent since the first surgery. Given her history, on examination you expect to find a(n)

(A) cystocele
(B) rectocele
(C) enterocele
(D) complete uterine prolapse
(E) hemorrhoid

1211. A 90-year-old woman comes to your office complaining that she feels as though she is "sitting on a ball." On examination, you find that the vagina is essentially turned inside out, and the entire uterus lies outside the vaginal introitus. This condition is known as

(A) first-degree prolapse

(B) second-degree prolapse

(C) third-degree prolapse

(D) fourth-degree prolapse or procidentia

(E) vaginal evisceration

1212. Study Figure 19–1. The letter A represents

(A) rectocele

(B) uterine prolapse

(C) cystocele

(D) sigmoidocele

(E) enterocele

1213. An 18-year-old nulliparous woman comes into your office complaining of a 24-hour history of urinary frequency, urgency, and suprapubic pain. She had intercourse for the first time earlier this week. She is using a diaphragm for birth control. Which of the following statements is true?

(A) Cystitis occurs two times more commonly in men than in women.

(B) In a freshly voided, clean-catch urine specimen, the finding of bacteria and 6 to 20 white blood cells (WBCs)/hpf is strongly indicative of an infection.

(C) Use of a diaphragm helps prevent the development of UTIs.

(D) A teenager is more likely to have asymptomatic bacteriuria than is a postmenopausal woman.

(E) In women who have frequent urinary tract infections related to coitus, infection can be prevented by voiding immediately before coitus.

1214. A woman complains of postvoid dribbling of urine when she stands, painful intercourse, and dysuria. She has no other symptoms. She is most likely to have

(A) a urinary fistula

(B) detrusor instability

(C) female prostatism

(D) genuine urinary stress incontinence

(E) a urethral diverticulum

1215. A 38-year-old multigravid woman complains of the painless loss of urine, beginning immediately with coughing, laughing, lifting, or straining. Immediate cessation of the activity stops the urine loss after only a few drops. This history is most suggestive of

(A) fistula

(B) stress incontinence

(C) urge incontinence

(D) urethral diverticulum

(E) UTI

1216. Kegel exercises were designed to

(A) strengthen the abdominal muscles after childbirth

(B) increase the blood flow to the perineum to speed the healing of an episiotomy

(C) improve the tone of the muscles surrounding the bladder base and proximal bladder neck

(D) prevent denervation of pelvic muscles after childbirth

(E) decrease the muscle atrophy associated with aging

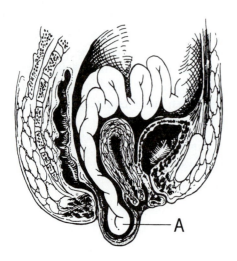

Figure 19–1.

1217. An 88-year-old woman who lives in a nursing home and is in poor general health complains of difficulty initiating urination and with defecation. On examination, she has fourth-degree uterovaginal prolapse. What is your recommendation?

(A) transabdominal uterine suspension operation

(B) transvaginal uterine suspension operation

(C) trial of a pessary

(D) the use of diapers and tight-fitting underclothing for support

(E) surgical closure of the vaginal introitus

1218. A 10-year-old patient's mother gives a history of the child constantly wetting herself, requiring the continuous use of diapers since birth. The child is otherwise very healthy and happy and does well in school. Which of the following diagnoses would most closely fit this clinical history?

(A) maternal anxiety

(B) ectopic ureter

(C) stress incontinence

(D) urethral diverticula

(E) vesicovaginal fistula

1219. A 52-year-old postmenopausal woman complains of urinary frequency, urgency, and urge incontinence. She is otherwise healthy. You recommend behavioral treatment that includes

(A) relaxation techniques

(B) anticholinergic medication

(C) voiding every hour during the daytime

(D) bladder retraining

(E) incontinence pad testing

1220. A 35-year-old woman (gravida 4, para 4) complains that she loses urine intermittently and without warning. At other times, she cannot get to the bathroom in time when she first feels the urge to void and also loses urine. She denies dysuria or loss of urine with exercise. Pelvic examination is normal, except for a first-degree cystocele. Postvoid residual is 150 mL. Of the following options, the BEST plan would be to

(A) instruct in Kegel exercises

(B) teach clean intermittent self-catheterization

(C) do an intravenous pyelogram (IVP) looking for a urinary fistula

(D) perform urodynamic testing looking for a neurogenic bladder

(E) give her a trial of anticholinergic medication

1221. Ten days after an abdominal hysterectomy for abnormal bleeding, a woman begins to have continuous drainage of urine from the vagina. She wants this condition repaired as soon as possible. You advise her that the best time for repair is

(A) immediately

(B) within 2 weeks

(C) not before 1 to 3 months

(D) not before 6 to 8 months

(E) not before 12 months

1222. The most common cause of rectovaginal fistula is

(A) obstetrical delivery

(B) irradiation to the pelvis

(C) carcinoma

(D) hemorrhoidectomy

(E) Crohn's disease

1223. If a rectovaginal fistula is identified, initial treatment should include

(A) diverting colostomy

(B) bowel resection

(C) rectal pull-through operation

(D) vaginal repair of the fistula

(E) systemic steroids and antibiotics

1224. Fecal incontinence may be related to

(A) interplay between the pubococcygeus muscle and rectum

(B) innervation of the pelvic floor and the anal sphincters

(C) normal colonic transit time

(D) nulliparity

(E) urinary retention

1225. When performing retropubic urethropexy (like the Burch or Marshall–Marchetti–Krantz [MMK] procedure) for stress urinary incontinence in a woman with moderate cystocele, the goal of the procedure is to

(A) strengthen the levator ani muscles

(B) correct the posterior urethrovesicle angle

(C) lengthen the urethra

(D) place the urethra in a high retropubic position

(E) plicate the endopelvic fascia under the bladder neck

1226. When performing a vaginal hysterectomy for any indication, prevention of future enterocele or vaginal vault prolapse is aided by

(A) reattachment of the round ligaments to the vaginal cuff

(B) closing the vaginal mucosa

(C) reattachment of the cardinal and uterosacral ligaments to the vaginal cuff

(D) complete a purse string suture closure of the cul-de-sac peritoneum

(E) placing a vaginal pack for 24 hours postoperatively

1227. A 35-year-old woman (gravida 3, para 3) returns for her 6 weeks' postpartum visit. She had an uncomplicated spontaneous vaginal delivery with no lacerations. She had mild stress incontinence symptoms during her pregnancy, but they are much worse now. You instruct her in starting a Kegel exercise program

(A) whenever she voids

(B) while waiting at stoplights

(C) 20 minutes three times per day

(D) 10 times twice a day

(E) 10 times four times a day

Questions 1228 through 1230

A 30-year-old woman complains of 36 hours of urinary frequency, dysuria, and pelvic pain. She has never had a UTI and has no medical problems.

1228. The most likely pathogen is

(A) *Escherichia coli*

(B) *Staphylococcus saprophyticus*

(C) *Klebsiella pneumonia*

(D) *Proteus mirabilis*

(E) enterococci

1229. The recommended treatment regimen is a

(A) 7-day course of tetracycline

(B) 3-day course of trimethoprim–sulfamethoxazole

(C) 7-day course of ciprofloxacin

(D) 3-day course of amoxicillin

(E) 7-day course of erythromycin

1230. If the patient is diabetic or pregnant, the appropriate therapy is a

(A) 3-day course of ciprofloxacin

(B) 3-day course of trimethoprim–sulfamethoxazole

(C) 7-day course of ciprofloxacin

(D) 3-day course of nitrofurantoin

(E) 7-day course of trimethoprim–sulfamethoxazole

Questions 1231 through 1233

A 49-year-old woman had a radical hysterectomy and lymph node sampling for stage 1B squamous cell cancer of the cervix. A suprapubic catheter was placed at the time of surgery. She is now 8 weeks postoperative and has not been able to void. She is also leaking urine with activity, coughing, and sneezing.

1231. What is the most likely reason for voiding difficulty?

(A) spasm of the pelvic floor muscles

(B) outflow obstruction

(C) postoperative swelling around the bladder

(D) innervation to the lower urinary tract was transected

(E) overdistention of the bladder

1232. The most likely etiology of her incontinence is

(A) urge incontinence

(B) stress incontinence

(C) overflow incontinence

(D) ureterovaginal fistula

(E) urethral diverticulum

1233. Which of the following is a normal urologic consequence of aging?

(A) incontinence

(B) elevated postvoid residual to 50 to 100 mL

(C) increased daytime diuresis

(D) increased bladder capacity

(E) delayed sensation of first desire to void

DIRECTIONS (Questions 1234 through 1279): Each set of items in this section consists of a list of lettered headings followed by several numbered words or phrases. For each numbered word or phrase, select the ONE lettered option that is most closely associated with it. Each lettered option may be selected once, more than once, or not at all.

Questions 1234 through 1245

Abnormalities of pelvic support are often associated with other types of support disorders, including hernias.

(A) cystocele

(B) direct inguinal hernia

(C) enterocele

(D) femoral hernia

(E) incarcerated hernia

(F) incisional hernia

(G) indirect inguinal hernia

(H) rectocele

(I) Rokitansky's hernia

(J) sliding hernia

(K) Spigelian hernia

(L) strangulated hernia

(M) umbilical hernia

(N) urethrocele

1234. Results from injury to the pubourethral ligaments.

1235. A true hernia into the potential space of the vagina.

1236. The organ protruding makes up a portion of the wall of the hernia sac.

1237. Herniation where the vertical linea semilunaris joins the lateral border of the rectus muscle.

1238. Results from a defect in the posterior levator ani musculofascial attachments.

1239. The contents of the hernia sac cannot be easily reduced.

1240. Comes through Hesselbach's triangle.

1241. Closes during the first 3 years of life in many people.

1242. Much more common hernia in the female than the male.

1243. Associated with absorbable suture material.

1244. Can be closed more tightly in the female than the male.

1245. Acute pain, possible surgical emergency.

Questions 1246 through 1253

Using the following items, match the type of incontinence with the most appropriate description of incontinence.

(A) detrusor instability (or overactivity)

(B) genuine stress incontinence (or urodynamic stress incontinence)

(C) incontinence

(D) overflow incontinence

(E) urethral syndrome

(F) urinary urge incontinence

(G) enuresis

(H) sudden onset urinary incontinence, frequency, and urgency

1246. Loss of urine secondary to involuntary bladder detrusor contractions

1247. An inflammatory condition with negative bacterial cultures, sometimes associated with positive chlamydial cultures

1248. Involuntary urine loss accompanied by or immediately preceded by a strong desire to void

1249. Involuntary loss of urine when intravesical pressure exceeds intraurethral pressure in the absence of a detrusor contraction

1250. Incontinence that occurs during sleep

1251. Urine loss in association with bladder distention in the absence of bladder contractions

1252. All involuntary urine loss

1253. Cystitis

Questions 1254 through 1259

Match the name of the stress incontinence operation with the most appropriate description.

(A) Kelly plication

(B) MMK procedure

(C) Burch procedure

(D) Pereyra procedure

(E) TVT (tension-free vaginal tape) sling

(F) pubovaginal sling procedure

1254. Attaches the paraurethral tissue on each side to the back of the pubic symphysis.

1255. Permanent suture is used to grasp the pubourethral ligaments, and the suture is fixed to the anterior abdominal wall using a special needle.

1256. Synthetic material or fascia encircles the urethra while held in place by sutures to the anterior abdominal wall.

1257. Metal needles attached to a prolene tape sling are passed from the vagina to the abdomen and a "U"-shaped sling loops around the midurethra.

1258. Lateral edges of the vagina are sutured to Cooper's ligaments.

1259. The pubocervical fascia is reinforced beneath the bladder base and bladder neck.

Questions 1260 through 1268

Match the following urodynamic and urologic tests with their intended purpose.

(A) Bonney or Marshall test

(B) cystometrogram

(C) endoscopy

(D) IVP

(E) measurement of residual urine

(F) pad test

(G) positive pressure urethrography

(H) Q-tip test

(I) urethral pressure profile study

(J) urinalysis and/or urine culture

(K) standing cough stress test

1260. A simple test of urethral hypermobility.

1261. An indirect test of the neurologic function of the bladder.

1262. Screens for infection.

1263. Evaluation of cystocele and overflow incontinence.

1264. Identifies and quantifies incontinence outside the office setting.

1265. Identifies noninfectious inflammation, malignancy, and abnormal anatomy.

1266. A low pressure predicts failure of standard incontinence procedures.

1267. A means of predicting the likelihood of surgical success in patients with stress incontinence.

1268. A means of noninvasively confirming the clinical diagnosis of stress incontinence in the office.

Questions 1269 through 1275

Select the most likely diagnosis for each patient with a bladder disorder.

   (A) acute cystitis
   (B) acute urethritis (often due to *Chlamydia*)
   (C) interstitial cystitis
   (D) painful bladder syndrome of unknown etiology
   (E) postural diuresis
   (F) sensory urgency
   (G) urethral diverticulum
   (H) urethral syndrome
   (I) vaginitis

1269. An 18-year-old female with acute onset frequency, dysuria, suprapubic pain, and a new sexual partner. Office leukocyte esterase dipstick is positive.

1270. An 18-year-old female with frequency, urgency, and suprapubic pain. The pain increases with bladder filling and is temporar-

ily relieved with voiding. Multiple urine cultures over 6 months have been negative and antibiotics have not improved her symptoms. Cystoscopy under anesthesia is negative.

1271. An 80-year-old female with nocturia three to five times a night that disrupts her sleep. She voids every 2 to 3 hours during the daytime. Her medical history is complicated by mild congestive heart failure and hypertension.

1272. An 18-year-old female with frequency, urgency, nocturia, and suprapubic pain. She voids every 30 minutes because it temporarily reduces her symptoms. Urine cultures have been negative. Cystoscopy under anesthesia reveals petechial hemorrhages after bladder distention.

1273. An 80-year-old female with frequency, urgency, and nocturia. Urine culture is negative and postvoid residual is 30 mL. Office cystometrics shows no uninhibited detrusor contractions.

1274. An 18-year-old female with acute onset frequency, urgency, dysuria, vaginal discharge, and a new sexual partner. Microscopic urine evaluation shows pyuria. Urine culture is negative.

1275. An 18-year-old female with acute onset of vaginal discharge, external dysuria, and a new sexual partner. No pyuria is seen on microscopic urine evaluation.

Questions 1276 through 1279

Match the part of the nervous system with the function.

(A) adrenergic receptors

(B) cerebral cortex

(C) muscarinic receptors

(D) parasympathetic nervous system

(E) pontine micturition center

(F) sacral spinal cord

(G) somatic nervous system

(H) sympathetic nervous system

1276. Contains the detrusor motor neurons

1277. Regulates the storage phase of micturition cycle

1278. Stimulation causes relaxation of the detrusor muscle

1279. Controls the voiding phase of the micturition cycle

Answers and Explanations

1207. (A) Risk factors for pelvic support disorders are increasing parity, increases in intra-abdominal pressure (chronic coughing or straining at stool and possibly obesity), pelvic trauma from radical surgery or pelvic fractures, aging, estrogen deprivation, heredity, or connective tissue disorders.

1208. (A) The sensation of pressure, fullness, or falling out is probably the most common symptom of anterior vaginal prolapse or cystocele formation. Mild urine loss with coughing, sneezing, straining (urinary stress incontinence), some urinary urgency, and incomplete emptying are also common complaints.

1209. (B) The sensation of pressure, fullness, or falling out is probably the most common symptom of any uterovaginal prolapse. The rectal symptoms that she has with defecation, however, are pathognomonic for a rectocele. When symptoms are this severe, the treatment of choice is surgical repair.

1210. (C) The sensation of pressure, fullness, or falling out is probably the most common symptom of any uterovaginal prolapse, as we have seen in the preceding examples. The point to be made here is that this patient has supposedly had a repair of her prolapse and incontinence. Two things contribute to the development of an enterocele: (1) She has had a prior hysterectomy; and (2) she has had a transabdominal urethral suspension, which contributes to enterocele formation in about 1 in 6 to 7 patients. The history of symptoms worsening throughout the day and getting better with rest is characteristic for genital prolapse and especially so for any enterocele. The most common treatment for enterocele is surgical repair. Pessaries or exercises are of little value with severe prolapse. The pessary is unlikely to be retained in the vagina.

1211. (D) Uterovaginal prolapse describes the position of the cystocele, rectocele, enterocele, or uterus. It is usually described as a "degree" of prolapse. First-degree prolapse is when the leading edge of the prolapsed organ (cervix or vagina) extends below the ischial spines (or into the distal one third of the vagina); second-degree prolapse is just to the vaginal introitus; third-degree prolapse is when the organ readily passes through the introitus; and fourth-degree (or total procidentia) is when the entire body of the prolapsing organ (uterus or vagina) lies outside the vaginal introitus. The more advanced the prolapse, the more difficult is the therapeutic task of restoring comfort and/or function. At patient age 90, it can be a tremendously difficult task for the clinician.

1212. (E) The marked prolapse in Figure 19–1 shows an enterocele protruding posterior to the uterus. The figure also shows a uterine prolapse. A sigmoidocele is not seen as no sigmoid colon is depicted in the picture; instead, small bowel is depicted.

1213. (B) Urinary tract infections are rare in men less than 50 years of age. In contrast, 40 to 50% of women will have a UTI in their lifetime. The use of diaphragms and spermicides has been associated with recurrence of UTIs, probably because the vaginal flora is altered by the spermicide. Voiding immediately after coitus is thought to provide some protection from coitus-related infections. The bacteria are washed from the urethra by the passage of urine. Voiding prior to coitus would not do this.

1214. (E) A small outpouching of the urethra can contain enough urine to dribble after voiding. Such a diverticulum may be very difficult to demonstrate. A specialized urethrogram, urethroscopy, MRI, or examination by a very experienced examiner may allow diagnosis to be made. If suspicion is strong enough, surgical exploration is indicated. The classic history is dribbling, dysuria, and dyspareunia. A urinary fistula usually leads to continuous incontinence. Detrusor instability is a urodynamic diagnosis with incontinence symptoms associated with a strong urge to void.

1215. (B) Stress incontinence is precipitated by anything that increases intra-abdominal pressure. The patient is able to suppress this loss after a few drops in most cases. Patients with mild stress incontinence lose only a small spurt of urine that stops when not straining.

1216. (C) Kegel first described these isometric exercises to improve the strength of the levator ani and pubococcygeus muscles after childbirth. These exercises can improve the condition in many women with mild stress incontinence. The exercises may work better to prevent stress incontinence, if done regularly and properly, than to cure it. The addition of pelvic floor physical therapy with biofeedback can help women strengthen these muscles, particularly in women who have trouble contracting these muscles.

1217. (C) This woman has symptoms and findings completely consistent with obstruction of her urethra and rectum secondary to uterovaginal prolapse. She is a poor candidate for surgery of any kind. There are mechanical devices called pessaries that can be fitted to hold the prolapsed organs within the vagina.

A trial of pessary support preceding surgery to treat uterine malposition or stress incontinence may be a good predictor of the success of the contemplated procedure (mimics surgical results). In this patient, it may relieve her symptoms. The pessary may be a good alternative to improve continence or correct prolapse in patients who for medical reasons are poor surgical risks.

1218. (B) With any congenital incontinence, anatomic defects must be considered. If the child is neurologically normal, an ectopic ureter (one that opens into the vagina) is the most likely cause. A congenital vesicovaginal fistula is unlikely. A test that would help delineate the etiolgy of this problem would be an intravenous dye (indigo carmine or methylene blue) study with follow-up examination to see where the dye is extruded. An IVP might also be helpful.

1219. (D) Behavioral therapy benefits many patients and encompasses bladder retraining, pelvic muscle rehabilitation, and timed/prompted voiding. Bladder retraining involves increasing the time between voiding episodes gradually, so that the patient relearns to suppress the micturition reflex. Eventually, this leads to a larger functional bladder capacity and fewer incontinence episodes. Medications could be helpful for this patient, but that is not a behavioral treatment. Timed voiding is a behavioral treatment, but it is generally used for neurologically impaired patients and voiding every hour would not be appropriate for treating this patient.

1220. (D) The urgency and unheralded loss of urine are classic symptoms of a neurologically abnormal bladder. The different types of incontinence that could cause this problem must be distinguished from one another, as the treatments are different. Standard urodynamic testing should be performed.

1221. (C) Ideally, the injury is noted at the time of the surgery and repaired while still in the operating room. If the injury is not noted at the time of the surgery or arises subsequent to an operative procedure, time should be given for the edema and induration to resolve. Many small fistulae will close spontaneously if drainage is provided and infection is avoided. There have been several reports supporting closure immediately after the patient presents with fair results.

1222. **(A)** Symptoms include passing flatus per vagina with or without fecal passage. Air can enter the vagina under other circumstances and be passed later, such as when a patient gets up from a knee–chest position. Spontaneous fistulization has not been reported. The most common cause of rectovaginal fistula is obstetrical delivery.

1223. **(D)** Fistula repair should be postponed until all inflammatory reaction around the fistula has resolved (8 to 12 weeks in most cases). The initial repair should be definitive; feeble attempts at repair, because the hole is small, are apt to result in a larger defect. A complete bowel preparation before surgery is mandatory.

1224. **(B)** Fecal continence requires normal stool consistency and volume, intact innervation of the pelvic floor and anal sphincters, and coordination of the puborectalis muscle, rectum, and anal sphincters. Increased colonic transit time can lead to fecal incontinence. Over 30% of women reporting urinary incontinence also report fecal incontinence. Vaginal delivery is the most common cause of fecal incontinence.

1225. **(D)** The goal of retropubic urethropexy is to restore the hypermobile bladder neck to a location behind the pubic symphysis in order to improve the pressure transmission to the bladder neck during stress (like coughing or Valsalva's maneuver). The urethrovesicle angle may be altered with surgery and the urethra may lengthen slightly, but neither is thought to be the important factor in treating incontinence. Plicating the endopelvic fascia under the bladder and bladder neck are anterior colporrhaphy techniques for cystocele re-

pair and not recommended for correction of stress urinary incontinence.

1226. **(C)** Isolating the uterosacral and cardinal ligaments during the hysterectomy is important so they can be used in the support of the vaginal vault. Many people suture the uterosacral ligaments together to decrease the opening in the pouch of Douglas. The vaginal mucosa has no inherent strength, but it is important to close the pubocervical and rectovaginal fascia underlying the vaginal mucosa. The round ligaments are not considered a major support structure to the vaginal vault. While the peritoneum is often closed and is described in enterocele repairs, it is not the best procedure for reducing later prolapse.

1227. **(C)** Patients are often told to do Kegels, but with few other instructions. Arnold Kegel reported outstanding success rates (84%), but these women were doing exercises for 20 minutes three times a day. Exercises are not effective if done infrequently or for short time periods (probably 4 to 6 weeks is necessary for a response). Furthermore, if women are given verbal instructions only, up to a third will do the exercises incorrectly. It is simple to check technique during a pelvic examination.

1228. **(A)** In acute uncomplicated cystitis, *E. coli* is seen 80% of the time, *S. saprophyticus* 5 to 15% of the time, and occasionally *Klebsiella* or *Proteus* species are seen. This is a predictable and narrow group of pathogens.

1229. **(B)** Because the pathogens and antimicrobial susceptibilities are so predictable in acute uncomplicated cystitis, therapy has been evaluated extensively. About a third of strains are resistant to amoxicillin and sulfonamides. Resistance to trimethoprim–sulfamethoxazole is 5 to 15% and may be rising. Three-day regimens are optimal. Single-dose therapy can be used, although lower cure rates are seen. A three-day course of a fluoroquinolone would also be acceptable, and resistance is closer to 5%. Tetracycline and erythromycin are not appropriate regimens.

1230. (E) Three-day courses of antibiotics are not adequate in pregnancy, diabetes, age over 65, or if symptoms have been present more than a week. Fluoroquinolones should not be used in pregnancy. Trimethoprim–sulfamethoxazole, although not approved in pregnancy, has been widely used.

1231. (D) Transaction of the nerves supplying the lower urinary tract can result in a denervated, atonic bladder. Some women can learn to void by Valsalva or pelvic floor muscle relaxation, while others will require clean, intermittent self-catheterization. Spasm of the pelvic floor muscles can cause voiding difficulty after pelvic operations or even pelvic infections, but would not usually persist for 8 weeks. Outflow obstruction is usually seen after anti-incontinence procedures. Overdistention would cause voiding difficulty, but she has had a catheter in place.

1232. (B) If she has denervation injury to her bladder, she most likely would not have urge incontinence. She may have denervation to the urethra and reduced urethral pressure, leading to stress incontinence. Overflow would be unlikely while catheterized. A ureterovaginal fistula is a well-documented risk in radical pelvic surgery, but she would usually have continuous leakage.

1233. (B) There are many normal changes in the lower urinary tract with aging—increased nocturnal diuresis, nocturia 1 to 2 times per night, urogenital atrophy, increased postvoid residual, decreased capacity, earlier first desire to void, and decreased urine flow rates. However, incontinence is not a normal part of aging!

1234. (N) A urethrocele probably never exists without some component of cystocele. It results from detachment, attenuation, or atrophy of the pubocervical fascia known as the pubourethral ligaments. The primary symptom involved is urinary incontinence in the presence of increased intra-abdominal pressure (urinary stress incontinence).

1235. (C) An enterocele is a true hernia into the potential space of the vagina with bowel pushing peritoneum between the uterosacral ligaments and down the plane dividing the rectovaginal septum. It is most common after hysterectomy. Its main symptom is an uncomfortable, pressure-like sensation. The associated "bulge" emanates from the vaginal apex.

1236. (J) In a sliding hernia, the organ protruding makes up a portion of the wall of the hernia sac.

1237. (K) In this rare type of hernia (Spigelian), the herniation occurs where the vertical linea semilunaris joins the lateral border of the rectus muscle. This is also called a lateral ventral hernia.

1238. (H) A rectocele is not a true hernia but rather results from a defect in the posterior levator ani musculofascial attachments or covering of the rectum. It allows the rectum to bulge into and sometimes out of the vagina. It is associated with the symptoms of a falling-out feeling, retention of stool in the rectal reservoir, and sometimes pushing stool out the rectum by applying posterior, transvaginal pressure with the finger (splinting).

1239. (E) In an incarcerated hernia, the contents of the hernia sac cannot be easily reduced but are not strangulated. This condition can be acute or chronic, asymptomatic, or very painful.

1240. (B) In a direct inguinal hernia, the hernia sac comes through the area known as Hesselbach's triangle (with borders formed by the lateral margin of the rectus muscle, the inguinal ligament, and the lateral epigastric artery).

1241. (M) A large percentage of infants are born with umbilical hernias (more African-American than Caucasian infants). Most infants will have a spontaneous resolution of small umbilical hernias. Pregnancy also predisposes to the formation of umbilical hernia.

1242. (D) Femoral hernias occur more frequently in women. They often pass beneath the inguinal ligament and require division of this ligament, with later repair of the ligament in order to mobilize structures sufficiently to correct the hernia.

1243. (F) Incisional hernias are those that occur after surgery. While the patient may have inherently weak fascia, many experts feel that the use of absorbable suture of low tensile strength and short half-life may predispose to incisional hernia formation. Several operations through the same wound, as well as diabetes, steroid use, and malignancy all contribute to the formation of incisional hernias.

1244. (G) An indirect hernia passes through the inguinal ring. In the male, the inguinal ring is the passage for the spermatic cord. If repaired too tightly, damage to the spermatic cord and pain will result. This hernia can be repaired more tightly in women because only the round ligament passes through the canal, and it is not easily damaged.

1245. (L) A strangulated hernia is generally a surgical emergency. The blood supply becomes compromised by the neck of the hernia sac, and without relief the involved organ may undergo necrosis.

1246. (A) Involuntary bladder contractions with or without incontinence is called detrusor instability. The bladder with involuntary contractions is neurologically impaired, but the etiology of the impairment is seldom known. It is the second most common cause of incontinence in women. Involuntary contractions are also a common cause of urgency without incontinence.

1247. (E) Urethral syndrome, an inflammatory condition with negative bacterial cultures, most often has no known etiology but sometimes is associated with positive chlamydial cultures. The urethra has a reddened, inflamed appearance on cystoscopy.

1248. (F) Involuntary urine loss associated with a strong desire to void is a symptom called urinary urge incontinence. The diagnosis of detrusor instability or detrusor overactivity requires urodynamic testing to show involuntary detrusor contractions.

1249. (B) Involuntary loss of urine when intravesical pressure exceeds intraurethral pressure in the absence of a detrusor contraction is called genuine stress incontinence. This is a physical problem in which the proximal urethra and bladder base are not adequately supported anatomically. To treat it, intraurethral pressure must be increased, usually by performing Kegel exercises or by stabilizing the urethra surgically.

1250. (G) Incontinence during sleep is enuresis. The proper term is *nocturnal enuresis*. This may be a form of bladder instability. Adults with this problem often report a history of childhood bedwetting.

1251. (D) Urine loss in association with bladder distention in the absence of bladder contractions is called overflow incontinence. The underlying problem is urinary retention. It can have neurologic causes, such as diabetes or lower motor neuron disease; pharmacologic causes, such as anticholinergic or antipsychotic drugs; obstructive causes, such as massive prolapse; or may even be psychogenic.

1252. (C) All involuntary urine loss is referred to as incontinence. Incontinence, however, is the symptom, not the disease; an underlying cause must be sought.

1253. (H) Cystitis or lower urinary tract infection is a common problem. It may result in incontinence until it is either treated or spontaneously resolves.

1254. (B) The MMK procedure is a retropubic urethrovesical suspension operation for urinary stress incontinence. It attaches the paraurethral tissue on each side to the back of the pubic symphysis.

1255. (D) The Pereyra procedure was the first operation to use a special needle to enable the blind placement of a suture from the abdomen out into the vagina. The procedure has since been modified, now using an endoscope to check for proper suture placement. Transvaginal dissection is carried into the space of Retzius on each side of the urethra and bladder base, then permanent suture is used to grasp the pubourethral ligaments, and suture is fixed to the anterior abdominal wall. The long-term success rate of the needle suspension procedures (like the Stamey or Pereyra) have been poorer than the MMK, Burch, or sling procedures and have largely been abandoned for stress incontinence surgery.

1256. (F) A sling operation is usually used for recurrent incontinence after a prior surgical repair when the urethral support is still good but the urethral function is poor. Synthetic material or fascia is used to fashion a strap that encircles the urethra, while being held in place by sutures to the anterior abdominal wall. A sling may be used as the primary surgical procedure for a type of stress incontinence called intrinsic sphincter deficiency.

1257. (E) The TVT sling is a new technique for treating female stress incontinence that can be performed under local anesthesia as an outpatient procedure. It differs from the traditional pubovaginal sling as it is placed around the midurethra. An 84% 2-year cure rate is reported.

1258. (C) The Burch procedure is a modification of the MMK procedure that suspends the urethra and bladder base by suspending the lateral vagina by suturing it to Cooper's ligaments in the space of Retzius. It can be performed laparoscopically.

1259. (A) The Kelly plication should no longer be used for the treatment of stress incontinence. Though modified considerably from Kelly's initial description, it is basically a transvaginal operation in which the pubocervical fascia is reinforced beneath the bladder base and

the bladder neck. It is associated with a higher failure rate in most series than retropubic suspensions and slings for incontinence. It is an effective surgical procedure for cystocele defects without incontinence (with an anterior colporrhaphy).

1260. (H) The Q-tip test is abnormal in the great majority of patients with urinary stress incontinence. It demonstrates urethral hypermobility. Without urethral hypermobility, stress incontinence should be suspected as a diagnosis. Simply, a sterile cotton-tipped applicator lubricated with anesthetic jelly is placed into the urethra to the level of the vesical junction. When the patient strains, if the wooden tail portends an arc of more than 30 degrees when measured from the horizontal, hypermobility is present.

1261. (B) A cystometrogram is an indirect test of the neurologic function of the bladder. It evaluates bladder sensation, identifies any evidence of detrusor instability (involuntary contraction), and measures capacity.

1262. (J) Urinalysis and urine culture are both tests for infection. When infection of the bladder is present, function can be greatly altered. Testing or instrumenting the infected bladder is inaccurate and may be harmful to the patient.

1263. (E) Measurement of residual urine helps in the evaluation of cystocele and overflow incontinence. The patient voids, and then a catheter is inserted in the bladder to see if urine remains. Under normal circumstances, at least 150 mL should be voided and less than 50 mL remain. Ultrasound scanning is now readily available and can be used as a noninvasive means to determine residual urine volume.

1264. (F) Some women lose urine quite readily in their normal settings, but in clinical settings they may lose none. The pad test is performed to identify incontinence outside the office setting, or it may be used to objectify amounts of urine loss. Simply, the patient puts on a menstrual napkin that has been weighed. After normal activity the napkin is removed and may be checked to make sure urine is present and weighed to determine the amount of urine loss. This test may also be combined with administration of a urinary dye to check for small amounts of loss.

1265. **(C)** Endoscopy of the urethra and bladder identifies noninfectious inflammation, malignancy, and abnormal anatomy. It also allows the examiner to observe anatomic changes with strain, cough, Valsalva, and so on.

1266. **(I)** Urethral pressure profile testing is used to measure pressures within the urethra and may demonstrate a low pressure in the condition of intrinsic urethral sphincter deficiency. A low-pressure urethra, in the opinion of many authorities, predicts failure when standard incontinence procedures are performed. Many feel a suburethral sling is the only correct choice of operation for these patients.

1267. **(A)** The Bonney or Marshall test was designed to predict the likelihood of surgical success in patients with stress incontinence. When the patient with a full bladder strains, the patient with stress incontinence should spurt urine. The bladder neck is then gently elevated and the patient asked to cough again. If no urine is lost, many examiners feel this is a good sign that reparative surgery will be successful. Many authorities question the value of this test because overelevation of the bladder neck can cause obstruction, and give falsely reasurring results.

1268. **(K)** The standing cough stress test is a simple, inexpensive way to confirm stress incontinence. The patient is asked to come to clinic with a full bladder. She stands with legs apart and is asked to cough. An immediate loss of urine confirms stress incontinence. Delayed leakage might signify cough-induced detrusor instability.

1269. **(A)** Leukocyte esterase dipstick rapidly identifies pyuria and has a sensitivity of 75 to 96%. Women with acute, uncomplicated cys-

titis symptoms can be safely treated based on detection of pyuria on leukocyte esterase dipstick or on microscopy.

1270. **(D)** This patient has an unexplained painful bladder syndrome. Her symptoms are distinguished from sensory urgency due to the pain component. Treatment might include bladder training, fluid management, avoidance of dietary irritants, or medications.

1271. **(E)** A normal consequence of aging is increased nighttime diuresis. Additive to her problem may be dependent fluid excretion at night when supine because of her congestive heart failure. Treatment might include altering her fluid consumption time to avoid drinking fluids in the evening, avoiding diuretic use at bedtime, or trying medications like desmopressin or anticholinergics.

1272. **(C)** The symptoms mentioned for interstitial cystitis are often severe and the pain may be varied in location. Complete remissions are rare and the symptoms may be quite disabling. The etiology is not known and the diagnosis is generally by history and at cystoscopy with distention. The classic findings are Hunner's ulcers, fissures and linear scars, small bladder capacity, and glomerulations (petechial hemorrhages).

1273. **(F)** Sensory urgency is defined as a strong desire to void in the absence of a detrusor contraction. In an elderly woman, especially if a smoker, bladder cancer must be ruled out with urine cytology and cystoscopy. If the workup is negative, treatment with bladder retraining, fluid management, and avoidance of dietary irritants can be useful.

1274. **(B)** Differentiating infectious causes of acute dysuria in women is best done by evaluating for pyuria and hematuria, performing a wet mount and obtaining urine culture if needed and STD cultures when appropriate. Acute urethritis with chlamydia, gonorrhea, or herpes usually causes pyuria, rarely hematuria and negative urine culture. Cervicitis or herpetic lesions may be seen.

1275. **(I)** Vaginitis symptoms may include external dysuria and discomfort, but rarely frequency or urgency. Vaginal wet mount preparation often is most helpful in making the diagnosis in the absence of pyuria and hematuria. STD cultures should be obtained as well.

1276. **(E)** The pontine micturition center is thought to be the origin of the neurons that are excitatory to sacral parasympathetic neurons to produce bladder contraction.

1277. **(H)** The sympathetic nervous system acts to prevent micturition by inhibiting detrusor activity.

1278. **(A)** Adrenergic receptors are separated into alpha receptors and beta receptors. Alpha receptors are primarily found in the urethra and bladder neck and cause smooth muscle contraction. Beta receptors are found in the bladder muscle and when stimulated lead to smooth muscle relaxation.

1279. **(D)** Parasympathetic cholinergic receptors are numerous in the bladder and when stimulated lead to bladder contraction. This is almost exclusively muscarinic receptors. Anticholinergic medications are the primary drugs for treating detrusor overactivity.

CHAPTER 20

The Pelvic Mass
Questions

DIRECTIONS (Questions 1280 through 1299): Each of the numbered items or incomplete statements in this section is followed by answers or by completions of the statement. Select the ONE lettered answer or completion that is BEST in each case.

1280. Examination of an asymptomatic 2-day-old infant girl shows a distended abdomen. The urinary bladder and rectal ampulla are empty. A solitary unilocular cyst is visualized with ultrasonography. The best next step in the management of this patient is

   (A) observation
   (B) intravenous pyelogram (IVP)
   (C) cystoscopy
   (D) barium enema
   (E) exploratory surgery

1281. You are called to the operating room to evaluate a pelvic mass in an infant girl. Laparoscopy shows a 3-cm cystic mass in the broad ligament between the fallopian tube and ovarian hilum. The best next step is

   (A) observation
   (B) cyst aspiration
   (C) cystectomy
   (D) adnexectomy
   (E) laparotomy

1282. Childhood neoplastic ovarian masses most commonly originate from

   (A) gonadal epithelium
   (B) gonadal stroma
   (C) germ cells
   (D) sex cords
   (E) metastatic disease

1283. A 6-year-old girl has a history of 2 weeks of abdominal pain. She is significantly taller than her peers. Physical examination shows early breast development and abdominal distention. Blood is present at the introitus, and pelvic examination is attempted but cannot be accomplished. Serum gonadotropin levels are in the prepubertal range and do not change after gonadotropin-releasing hormone (GnRH) administration. Abdominal sonography shows a 6-cm solid right adnexal mass. The most likely diagnosis is a(n)

   (A) epoöphoron
   (B) granulosa cell tumor
   (C) corpus luteum cyst
   (D) endometrioma
   (E) fibroma

1284. A colleague asks you to evaluate a 5-year-old Caucasian girl with sexual precocity. Areas of mucocutaneous pigmentation are present. Rectal examination demonstrates a 4-cm pelvic mass. Prepubertal levels of serum gonadotropins do not change after GnRH administration. In addition to the findings noted above, the patient is most likely to have

   (A) dextrocardia
   (B) renal agenesis
   (C) gastrointestinal polyps
   (D) skeletal anomalies
   (E) müllerian anomalies

1285. An 8-year-old girl has acute right lower abdominal pain. The pain began last night in the periumbilical area and shifted this morning to the right lower abdomen. She noted a loss of appetite over the past day and has vomited three times since yesterday. She has not had a bowel movement today. Vital signs are: blood pressure, 120/60; pulse, 90 bpm; and temperature, 101.8°F. Abdominal examination demonstrates tenderness halfway between the umbilicus and the right anterior superior iliac spine. Bowel sounds are absent. Rectal examination shows a fluctuant, fixed, ill-defined right pelvic mass. A hematocrit is 34% (normal, 35 to 45%); white blood count, 23,000/mL (normal, 3 to 10,000/mL). Stool guaiac is negative for occult blood. Abdominal radiogram shows a calcified fecalith in the right lower quadrant. The most likely diagnosis is

(A) regional enteritis
(B) ulcerative colitis
(C) Meckel's diverticulum
(D) appendicitis
(E) ovarian torsion

1286. The most common pelvic mass associated with amenorrhea in a reproductive-age woman is a

(A) follicular cyst
(B) corpus luteum cyst
(C) benign cystic teratoma
(D) leiomyoma
(E) pregnancy

1287. A 14-year-old girl has had progressively increasing cyclic left pelvic pain since menarche. She is not sexually active. Menses occur at monthly intervals. Pelvic examination demonstrates a uterus deviated to the right. An elongated left adnexal structure is palpable above a left-sided vaginal mass. You should suspect the presence of

(A) an ovarian cyst
(B) a uterine anomaly
(C) cervical stenosis

(D) vaginal adenosis
(E) a pelvic kidney

1288. A 23-year-old woman desiring conception has amenorrhea of 5 weeks' duration. She noticed an elevation in her basal body temperatures (BBTs) since unprotected coitus 3 weeks ago. Her vital signs are: blood pressure, 120/80 mm Hg; pulse, 80 bpm; and temperature, 98.6°F. Physical examination is normal with the exception of the pelvic examination, which demonstrates a tender 3-cm right adnexal mass. A hematocrit is 38% (normal, 35 to 45%). A serum pregnancy test is negative. The best next step is

(A) observation
(B) estrogen therapy
(C) progesterone therapy
(D) RU 486 therapy
(E) laparoscopy

1289. You are asked to evaluate a 28-year-old unconscious woman involved in a motor vehicle accident. An abdominal radiogram shows two teeth in the right pelvis. Pelvic examination demonstrates a 7-cm semisolid mass in the right adnexa. The most likely diagnosis is

(A) severe head and facial trauma
(B) fetal demise
(C) fetus papyraceus
(D) calcified leiomyoma
(E) mature teratoma

1290. A 39-year-old woman with acute right lower abdominal pain is seen in the emergency department. She is nauseated and has vomited four times today. She is monogamous and uses a diaphragm for contraception. Vital signs are: blood pressure, 90/40 mm Hg; pulse, 110 bpm; and temperature, 102.4°F. Physical examination demonstrates a rigid abdomen with rebound tenderness. Pelvic examination shows a fluctuant 3-cm right adnexal mass. A hematocrit is 35% (normal, 35 to 45%); white blood count, 28,000/mL (normal 3 to 10,000/mL). At laparotomy, you find a pelvic abscess and a ruptured fingerlike pouch arising 40 cm proximal to the ileocecal junction. The most likely diagnosis is

(A) regional enteritis
(B) diverticulitis
(C) Meckel's diverticulum
(D) chronic appendicitis
(E) Walthard rest

1291. You are asked to see a 34-year-old woman with intermittent abdominal pain and bloody diarrhea. She has experienced similar symptoms previously but has always recovered. She is married and uses a diaphragm for contraception. Vital signs are: blood pressure, 130/80 mm Hg; pulse, 90 bpm; and temperature, 101.0°F. A localized area of tenderness is present in the right lower abdominal quadrant. Pelvic examination shows a fluctuant 4-cm right adnexal mass. A hematocrit is 35% (normal, 35 to 45%); white blood count, 27,000/mL (normal, 3 to 10,000/mL). Stool testing shows blood intermixed with white blood cells (WBCs). Gastrointestinal studies show mucosal changes and narrowing of the terminal ileum. The best next step is

(A) corticosteroid therapy
(B) estrogen therapy
(C) appendectomy
(D) colectomy
(E) salpingo-oophorectomy

1292. A 23-year-old woman has left lower abdominal pain of 1 week's duration. Her last menstrual period (LMP) was 8 weeks ago. Vital signs are: blood pressure, 130/72 mm Hg; pulse, 76 bpm; and temperature 98.6°F. Abdominal examination is unremarkable. Pelvic examination demonstrates an enlarged uterus and a tender 4.5-cm left adnexal mass. A serum human chorionic gonadotropin (hCG) level is 3,500 mIU/mL. Transvaginal sonography shows a single viable intrauterine pregnancy and a left echogenic adnexal mass. The cyst most likely represents a

(A) heterotopic ectopic pregnancy
(B) follicular cyst
(C) hemorrhagic corpus luteum

(D) cystic teratoma
(E) leiomyoma

1293. A 21-year-old woman has amenorrhea, transient late-cycle spotting, and pelvic pain. Her vital signs are: blood pressure, 100/50 mm Hg; pulse, 110 bpm; and temperature 98.6°F. Abdominal examination shows left lower quadrant tenderness with rebound. Pelvic examination demonstrates a painful 4-cm left adnexal mass. A serum pregnancy test is positive. A hematocrit is 22% (normal, 35 to 45%). The best next step is

(A) observation
(B) estrogen therapy
(C) progesterone therapy
(D) methotrexate therapy
(E) surgery

1294. A 38-year-old healthy woman comes for prenatal care. Her past medical history is unremarkable. General physical and pelvic examinations before conception were normal. She undergoes chorionic villus sampling, which shows a 46,XX karyotype. She has noticed progressive hirsutism during pregnancy. She eventually delivers an infant with ambiguous genitalia. A maternal pelvic examination in the delivery room confirms a 6-cm left adnexal mass. The most likely diagnosis is a

(A) luteoma
(B) theca lutein cyst
(C) persistent corpus luteum
(D) luteinized unruptured follicle
(E) luteinized endometrioma

1295. A large cystic ovarian tumor is detected during routine prenatal examination. The most common complication of such a tumor during the first trimester of pregnancy is

(A) torsion
(B) rupture
(C) intracystic hemorrhage
(D) solid degeneration
(E) luteinization

1296. The most common pelvic mass in a post-menopausal woman is a(n)

(A) follicular cyst

(B) corpus luteum cyst

(C) germ cell tumor

(D) leiomyoma

(E) endometrioma

1297. Most neoplastic ovarian masses in post-menopausal women originate from

(A) ovarian epithelium

(B) ovarian stroma

(C) ovarian germ cells

(D) ovarian sex cords

(E) metastatic disease

1298. Signet ring cells are characteristic findings in which tumor of the ovary?

(A) Brenner tumor

(B) Krukenberg's tumor

(C) dermoid cyst

(D) endometrioid carcinoma

(E) dysgerminoma

1299. A 1-year-old girl has an abdominal mass. Rectal examination demonstrates a mass extending into the right pelvis. The cervix is not palpable. Abdominal sonography shows that the uterus and vagina are absent. Both ovaries appear normal. The origin of the mass is most likely

(A) gastrointestinal

(B) renal

(C) musculoskeletal

(D) hepatic

(E) pancreatic

DIRECTIONS (Questions 1300 through 1316): Each set of items in this section consists of a list of lettered headings followed by several numbered words or phrases. For each numbered word or phrase, select the ONE lettered option that is most closely associated with it. Each lettered heading may be selected once, more than once, or not at all.

Questions 1300 through 1304

(A) diverticulitis

(B) phlegmon

(C) pyosalpinx

(D) hydrosalpinx

(E) endometritis

(F) chronic salpingitis

(G) appendicitis

(H) follicular cyst

(I) corpus luteum cyst

(J) endometrioma

(K) benign cystic teratoma

(L) ovarian malignancy

(M) endometrioid tumor

(N) adnexal torsion

(O) endometrial carcinoma

(P) endosalpingiosis

(Q) leiomyoma

1300. A 23-year-old woman with right-sided lower abdominal pain and chills is seen in the emergency department. The pain began 3 days ago and is associated with a vaginal discharge. Her last menstrual period was 5 days ago. She uses an intrauterine device for contraception and had coitus 1 week ago with her new boyfriend. There is no history of nausea, vomiting, or diarrhea. Her vital signs are: blood pressure, 120/80 mm Hg; pulse, 100 bpm; and temperature, 101.4°F. Abdominal examination shows bilateral lower quadrant guarding with rebound tenderness on the right side. Pelvic examination shows pus at the cervical os and a tender 6-cm right adnexal mass. Laboratory data are: hematocrit, 38% (normal, 35 to 45%); white blood count, 25,000/mL (normal, 3 to 10,000/mL); and serum pregnancy test, negative. Transvaginal sonography shows a 6-cm complex right adnexal mass. The uterus and left adnexa are normal.

1301. A 35-year-old woman complains of constant, deep, pelvic pain. It worsens during menstruation, sexual intercourse, and bowel movements. Her LMP was 1 week ago. Vital signs are: blood pressure, 110/70 mm Hg; pulse, 80 bpm; and temperature, 98.6°F. Abdominal examination elicits bilateral lower quadrant tenderness without rebound. Pelvic examination demonstrates a tender 6-cm left adnexal mass and fixation of the uterus and uterosacral ligaments. Laboratory data are: hematocrit, 40% (normal, 35 to 45%); white blood count, 7,000/mL (normal, 3 to 10,000/mL); and serum pregnancy test, negative. Transvaginal sonography shows a 6-cm echogenic left adnexal mass. The uterus and right adnexa are normal.

1302. A 25-year-old woman has had intense right lower abdominal pain and nausea since jogging yesterday afternoon. Intermittent episodes of similar pain have occurred over the past several days. She has vomited twice today, but her bowel movements are normal. Her vital signs are: blood pressure, 108/60; pulse, 90 bpm; and temperature, 100.4°F. Abdominal examination shows right lower quadrant tenderness. Pelvic examination demonstrates a tender 5-cm right adnexal mass anterior to the uterus. The uterus and left adnexa are normal. Laboratory data are: hematocrit, 39% (normal, 35 to 45%); white blood count, 11,000/mL (normal, 3 to 10,000/mL); and serum pregnancy test, negative.

1303. A 35-year-old woman is seen for annual examination. Her LMP was 1 week ago. Menses occur at 30-day intervals but are heavier than they were 5 years ago. She has experienced three spontaneous abortions over the past 5 years. Abdominal examination is normal. Pelvic examination demonstrates an enlarged, firm, irregular uterus and a 4-cm left adnexal mass fixed to the uterus. A complete blood count (CBC) is normal, and a serum pregnancy test is negative. Transvaginal sonography shows a solid left adnexal mass.

1304. A 4-cm right rudimentary uterus is present in a 16-year-old girl with a left unicornuate uterus. The right uterus does not communicate with the adjacent left uterine cavity. She has symptoms of cyclic ovarian function (e.g., breast tenderness, bloating, mood changes) and experiences severe abdominal cramping at the time of menses. Pelvic examination shows a single cervix and an 8-cm right adnexal mass. There is fixation of the uterus and uterosacral ligaments. A CBC is normal, and a serum pregnancy test is negative. Transvaginal sonography shows a right uterine cavity and an echogenic right adnexal mass.

Questions 1305 through 1311

(A) distended bladder
(B) follicular cyst
(C) corpus luteum cyst
(D) ectopic pregnancy
(E) theca lutein cysts
(F) luteoma
(G) multiple subcapsular follicles
(H) endometrioma
(I) Gartner's duct cyst
(J) rudimentary uterine horn
(K) ovarian fibroma

1305. A 7-year-old child with sexual precocity, cystic bone lesions, and café au lait spots

1306. A 23-year-old obese woman with hirsutism and anovulation

1307. A 28-year-old woman with a twin gestation and bilateral adnexal masses

1308. An 18-year-old woman with a left unicornuate uterus and a right solid adnexal mass

1309. A 1-day-old female neonate with an anterior abdominal mass after breech delivery

1310. A 45-year-old woman with an adnexal mass, ascites, and pleural effusions

1311. A 22-year-old woman with anovulation and a 4-cm unilocular ovarian cyst

Questions 1312 through 1314

    (A) fallopian tube carcinoma

    (B) ovarian carcinoma

    (C) uterine leiomyoma

    (D) uterine sarcoma

    (E) endometrial carcinoma

    (F) cervical carcinoma

    (G) breast carcinoma

    (H) gastric carcinoma

    (I) colorectal carcinoma

    (J) lymphoma

    (K) fibroma

1312. A 58-year-old postmenopausal woman has pelvic pain of 3 months' duration. She has recently noticed irregular vaginal bleeding, urinary frequency, and rectal pressure. Last year a physician remarked that her uterus was 12 gestational weeks in size. Physical and pelvic examination shows a firm, irregular, midline abdominal mass approximately 20 gestational weeks in size. Stool guaiac is negative for occult blood. An endometrial biopsy demonstrates atrophic endometrium.

1313. A 63-year-old woman has bloating associated with tightening of her clothing around her abdomen. She recently has developed dyspepsia and has lost 15 pounds unintentionally. She is short of breath. Pulmonary auscultation shows loss of breath sound. Abdominal percussion causes a wavelike movement of fluid around a central tympanitic area. Pelvic examination demonstrates a fixed, irregular nodular adnexal mass with cul-de-sac nodularity. A chest radiogram shows bilateral pleural effusions.

1314. A 51-year-old woman is hospitalized for treatment of right pyelonephritis. An IVP shows right-sided hydronephrosis and a dilated ureter. Physical examination is unre-markable. During pelvic examination, you observe a malodorous vaginal discharge. A firm, irregular right adnexal mass extends to the pelvic side wall. The patient experiences vaginal bleeding after examination.

Questions 1315 and 1316

    (A) regional enteritis

    (B) ulcerative colitis

    (C) Meckel's diverticulum

    (D) appendicitis

    (E) diverticulitis

    (F) colorectal carcinoma

    (G) endometrial carcinoma

    (H) ovarian carcinoma

1315. A 75-year-old woman has long-standing, self-limited episodes of left lower abdominal pain. An episode of pain occurred yesterday and has progressed to severe left lower abdominal pain. She vomited once this morning. Vital signs are: blood pressure, 150/90 mm Hg; pulse, 90 bpm; and temperature, 102.4°F. Abdominal examination demonstrates guarding over the left lower quadrant. There is no rebound tenderness. Pelvic examination shows a fluctuant, fixed, ill-defined left adnexal mass. A hematocrit is 38% (normal, 35 to 45%), and white blood count, 15,000/mL (normal 3 to 10,000/mL). Stool guaiac is positive for occult blood.

1316. A 69-year-old woman noticed a reduction in the size of her stool over 6 months. Abdominal examination elicits left-sided abdominal tenderness. Pelvic examination shows a hard, tubular mass with a transverse orientation behind the left adnexa. The patient is afebrile, and her vital signs are normal. A CBC is unremarkable. Stool guaiac is positive for occult blood.

Answers and Explanations

1280. (A) Age is one of the best predictors of the etiology of an adnexal mass. During infancy the most common adnexal mass is an ovarian cyst. It arises in response to a transient elevation in circulating gonadotropins after birth. Unilocular ovarian cysts usually regress as serum gonadotropin levels decline.

1281. (B) Mesonephric (wolffian) duct remnants may persist after fetal life as cystic structures adjacent to the fallopian tube, uterus, or cervix. Parovarian cysts develop from the cranial portion of the mesonephric duct and are found in the broad ligament between the fallopian tube and ovarian hilum (Figure 20–1). Gartner's duct cysts develop from the caudal portion of the mesonephric duct and are located lateral to the uterus or vagina. While these cysts are benign and could be merely followed, in the situation given with the patient already in the midst of an operation, most would aspirate and decompress the cyst.

1282. (C) Most childhood pelvic masses in females are either neoplastic or endocrinologic in origin. Two to five percent of malignant pediatric tumors involve the female reproductive organs, most commonly the ovary. Childhood neoplastic ovarian masses originate from the germ cell component in about 80% of cases.

1283. (B) Abdominal distention with signs of pseudosexual precocity is suggestive of an endocrinologically active tumor. Estrogen-producing ovarian neoplasms are most commonly granulosa cell tumors. These low-grade malignant tumors are usually solid and unilateral. They are capable of recurring 15 to 20 years after initial diagnosis and apparently successful treatment.

1284. (C) Peutz–Jeghers syndrome is characterized by the presence of an estrogen-secreting ovarian tumor (causing pseudoprecocious puberty), gastrointestinal polyposis, and mucocutaneous pigmentation. The ovarian tumor is composed of sex cord and stromal elements, which are arranged in annular tubules. Granulosa–theca cell tumors are also associated with this syndrome.

1285. (D) Appendicitis occurs in 10% of the general population, most commonly during

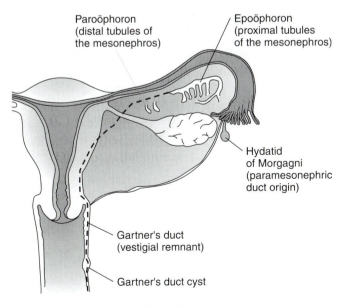

Paroöphoron (distal tubules of the mesonephros)

Epoöphoron (proximal tubules of the mesonephros)

Hydatid of Morgagni (paramesonephric duct origin)

Gartner's duct (vestigial remnant)

Gartner's duct cyst

Figure 20–1.

childhood. Nausea, vomiting, and loss of appetite occur early in the disease process. The abdominal pain often begins in the periumbilical area and shifts to the right lower abdomen, halfway between the umbilicus and the right anterior superior iliac spine (McBurney's point). Several intestinal disorders, including periappendiceal abscess, regional enteritis, colitis, and diverticulitis, may produce a local inflammatory mass (phlegmon) that is palpable on pelvic examination. Torsion of an ovarian mass causes acute pain but is not associated with a fever or the laboratory findings present in this case.

1286. (E) In reproductive-age women, pregnancy is the most common cause of a pelvic mass associated with amenorrhea. Any reproductive-age woman who experiences amenorrhea must be considered pregnant until proven otherwise.

1287. (B) Defective müllerian duct fusion causes varying degrees of uterine duplication. Fusion failure involving the entire müllerian duct results in a double uterus and cervix (uterine didelphys), occasionally accompanied by a longitudinal septum of the upper vagina (double vagina). If one of the reproductive tracts does not communicate with the outside (obstructive anomaly), menstrual blood accumulates in the portion of the tract preceding the obstruction (e.g., vagina and uterus), causing abdominal pain and a pelvic mass. Surgery is required to drain blood from the obstruction site. Endometriosis secondary to retrograde seeding from these obstructed structures is common. Uterus didelphys, with one of two vaginas ending in a blind pouch, is associated with renal agenesis on the side of the pouch.

1288. (A) A corpus luteum cyst may occur as a result of hemorrhage or cyst formation. Delayed involution of the corpus luteum cyst (Halban's syndrome) causes prolonged progesterone secretion, leading to persistently elevated BBTs, amenorrhea, and pelvic pain. Luteolysis is eventually accompanied by the onset of spontaneous menses. Symptoms of Halban's syndrome are similar to those of ectopic pregnancy but are distinguished from the latter by a negative serum pregnancy test.

1289. (E) The mature teratoma, or dermoid cyst, is the most common germ-cell tumor. It is composed of the three germ-cell layers: ectoderm, mesoderm, and endoderm. It commonly occurs in young women and has a bilaterality rate of 15 to 25%. Ectodermal derivatives (e.g., hair, skin elements) predominate, causing accumulation of a greasy, sebaceous fluid within the cyst. Bone fragments, teeth, and gastrointestinal mucosa are often present and located adjacent to projections within the cyst cavity, referred to as Rokitansky's protuberances. These protuberances are the sites from which 1 to 3% of benign cystic teratomas undergo malignant transformation in postmenopausal women, most commonly a squamous carcinoma.

1290. (C) During human development, the midgut communicates with the yolk sac via the yolk stalk or vitelline duct. The intra-abdominal portion of the yolk stalk connecting the umbilicus to the intestine usually atrophies but may persist as a Meckel's diverticulum in 2 to 4% of persons, more commonly in males. It appears as a 3- to 6-cm-long fingerlike pouch arising 40 to 50 cm from the ileocecal junction. It may be attached to the umbilicus by a fibrous cord or fistula. Twenty percent of Meckel's diverticula contain secretory gastric mucosa that may ulcerate, leading to intra-abdominal bleeding. Meckel's diverticulum also may cause symptoms mimicking appendicitis and intestinal obstruction (due to intussusception or volvulus of the diverticulum).

1291. (A) Inflammatory bowel disease commonly occurs during reproductive life and includes ulcerative colitis and regional enteritis (Crohn's disease). The former refers to inflammation confined to the colon, while the latter is characterized by multiple sites of small bowel or colonic inflammation. The symptoms of regional enteritis mimic those of appendicitis but often can be distinguished from the latter by the presence of bloody diarrhea, blood and white blood cells in stool specimens, and bowel mucosal changes on gastrointestinal studies. Acute inflammatory bowel disease generally responds to corticosteroid therapy and is associated wth poor healing and fistula formation after surgery.

1292. (C) A hemorrhagic corpus luteum may accompany an intrauterine pregnancy. It may cause pelvic pain indistinguishable from that of an ectopic pregnancy. The corpus luteum cyst generally persists for the first 8 to 12 gestational weeks and then regresses spontaneously as progesterone production is shifted to the placenta. A heterotopic ectopic pregnancy refers to the coexistence of an ectopic pregnancy and an intrauterine pregnancy. Heterotopic ectopic pregnancies occur in about 1 in 7,000 pregnancies and increase in frequency to 1 in 900 pregnancies after ovulation induction therapies.

1293. (E) This woman has a ruptured ectopic pregnancy. The intra-abdominal bleeding is potentially life threatening and requires immediate surgery.

1294. (A) A luteoma results from extensive luteinization of ovarian thecal cells during normal pregnancy. The benign tumor is solid, occurs bilaterally in 45% of cases, and produces significant amounts of androgens. It is associated with a 25% risk of maternal virilization with concurrent, female, fetal masculinization in many of the newborns. Luteomas regress spontaneously after delivery.

1295. (A) Most ovarian tumors detected during pregnancy are cystic. The most common complication of ovarian tumors during pregnancy is adnexal torsion during the first trimester. Cystic ovarian tumors may rupture, causing intra-abdominal hemorrhage and extrusion of cyst contents into the peritoneal cavity. A large tumor also may obstruct labor, leading to uterine rupture if labor is prolonged.

1296. (D) Uterine leiomyomas are the most common pelvic masses in postmenopausal women. Most authors report a prevalence of up to 45 percent for postmenopausal women. Uterine leiomyomata are also the most common indication for major surgery in women.

1297. (A) Ovarian tumors derived from capsular epithelium are the most common neoplastic ovarian tumors in reproductive- and postreproductive-age women.

1298. (B) Signet ring cells are characteristic findings in Krukenberg's tumors. These tumors arise in the gastrointestinal tract (most often the stomach) and spread to the ovary. It is characterized by areas of mucoid degeneration and the presence of signet ring cells.

1299. (B) Forty percent of abdominal masses in children under the age of 2 years are renal in origin. An ectopic pelvic kidney occurs in up to 15% of girls without a uterus or vagina. The pelvic kidney may be palpable abdominally or rectally.

1300. (C) In reproductive-age women, infections of the adnexa may result from sexually transmitted diseases and may be more common when associated with intrauterine device (IUD) use. The patient commonly gives a history of recent sexual activity, multiple sexual partners, or a new sexual partner. She usually experiences fever, chills, low bilateral abdominal pain, and vaginal discharge. During acute salpingitis, the tube becomes distended with purulent material, causing a tender tubal abscess (pyosalpinx). As chronic salpingitis develops, peritubal adhesions obstruct the fimbriated ends of the fallopian tubes, leading to hydrosalpinges and infertility. In contrast to most cases, pelvic infection associated with IUD use may involve only one adnexa.

1301. (J) Endometriosis should be suspected when pelvic examination in a reproductive-age woman shows tenderness, an ovarian mass, or fixation of the uterus with nodularity of the uterosacral ligaments. An ovarian collection of endometriosis large enough to form a tumor is called an endometrioma. Endometriomas contain hemorrhagic debris, which give them an echogenic appearance by ultrasound. They are often called "chocolate cysts" because their contents have a chocolate-like appearance.

1302. (N) Adnexal torsion results from twisting of the fallopian tube and ovary around their long axes. Torsion commonly occurs in reproductive-age women and often is precipitated by abrupt pelvic movement. The right adnexa has a greater tendency to twist than the left adnexa (perhaps because the sigmoid colon fills the left pelvis). The most frequent findings of torsion are lower abdominal pain and a tender adnexal mass located anterior to the uterus. Two thirds of patients with adnexal torsion have nausea, vomiting, and episodes of previous intermittent abdominal pain (presumably due to incomplete torsion). Conditions associated with an increased risk of adnexal torsion are pregnancy and ovarian tumors, particularly benign cystic teratomas. During early torsion, venous and lymphatic obstruction causes ovarian cyanosis and edema. The adnexa can be untwisted, and the ovarian tumor can be removed if necessary. Prolonged adnexal torsion interrupts the arterial blood supply to the ovary, causing necrosis, low-grade fever, and temperature elevation. Salpingo-oophorectomy removes necrotic tissue and avoids the risks of infection, intra-abdominal hemorrhage, and embolization of necrotic tissue into the circulation.

1303. (Q) Uterine leiomyomas, also called "fibroids" and myomas, are benign smooth muscle tumors (Figure 20–2). They are the most common solid pelvic tumor, occurring in at least 20% of all women by age 40 years, 50% of black women, and 25% of Caucasian women. Myomas are round, firm, myometrial tumors and may extend from the uterine wall into the broad ligament (intraligamentous leiomyoma), giving the impression of an adnexal mass. Although most women with uterine leiomyomas are asymptomatic, some

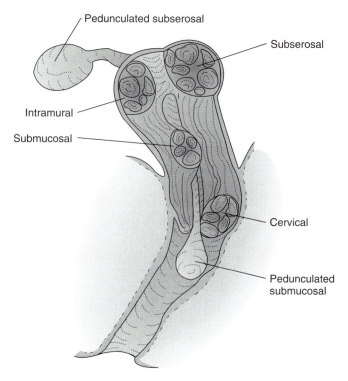

Figure 20–2.

women experience abnormal vaginal bleeding (metrorrhagia and/or menorrhagia). Distortion of the uterine cavity may interfere with embryo implantation, leading to spontaneous abortion. Leiomyomata may undergo degeneration, infarction, or infection, causing abdominal pain. Rarely sarcomatous changes within the leiomyomata cause rapid enlargement of the uterus.

1304. (J) Endometriosis occurs commonly in reproductive-age women with obstructive uterine anomalies. The retrograde menstruation theory described by J. A. Sampson probably explains the most common cause of endometriosis. This theory postulates that viable epithelial and stromal cells of the endometrium regurgitate through the fallopian tubes during menstruation and implant on the peritoneal surface. This hypothesis is supported by the following observations:

- Hemorrhagic fluid containing endometrium is recoverable from the abdomen of most menstruating women.

- Viable endometrium obtained from menses is transplantable to in vivo abdominal wall fascia and in vitro tissue culture.
- The location of peritoneal endometriosis follows the principle of retrograde menstruation. Disease occurs in gravity-dependent areas of the pelvis and adjacent to the tubal ostia. The ovary is the most common site of endometriosis (55% of affected women), followed in descending order by the posterior broad ligament (35%), the anterior or posterior pouch of Douglas (each 34%), and the uterosacral ligaments (28%).

1305. **(B)** The McCune–Albright syndrome is a rare disease in which pseudosexual precocity results from an estrogen-secreting ovarian follicular cyst. Multiple cystic bone lesions (polyostotic fibrous dysplasia), and café au lait spots are also present in these children.

1306. **(G)** Polycystic ovary syndrome (PCOS) is characterized by bilateral ovarian enlargement associated with hirsutism, anovulation, and obesity. Ovaries are two to five times normal size and have a smooth, thickened capsule covering numerous subcapsular follicles (2 to 7 mm in diameter) arrested in the mid-antral stage of development.

1307. **(E)** Theca lutein cysts occur in response to high circulating hCG levels (e.g., gestational trophoblastic disease, multifetal pregnancy) and ovulation-inducing medication. Bilateral, smooth, thin-walled, cysts contain clear, straw-colored fluid and are surrounded by extensively luteinized stroma. The cysts generally disappear after termination of pregnancy or discontinuation of medication.

1308. **(J)** Absence of an entire müllerian duct results in a hemiuterus (unicornuate uterus). If the cephalic (proximal) portion of the defective müllerian duct is present, a rudimentary uterus (rudimentary uterine horn) often lies adjacent to the unicornuate uterus. If a rudimentary horn containing endometrium does not communicate with the adjacent uterine cavity (obstructive anomaly), hematometra develops during menarche, causing a painful adnexal mass.

1309. **(A)** Voiding usually occurs shortly after birth but may be delayed until the second day of life. A female infant delivered in a breech presentation may develop swelling of periurethral soft tissues. Inability to void causes bladder distention that is alleviated by catheterization.

1310. **(K)** Fibromas are benign ovarian tumors derived from stromal mesenchyme. They are solid, irregular, and mobile (ranging in size from small to several thousand grams). Fibromas contain spindle cells that form collagen but do not produce hormones. Meigs' syndrome refers to the findings of ascites and pleural effusions in combination with an ovarian fibroma. Peritoneal fluid accumulates intra-abdominally and traverses diaphragmatic lymphatics into the pleural cavities.

1311. **(B)** Some anovulatory women develop ovarian follicular cysts lined by granulosa cells. Most of the cysts are unilocular (less than 4 cm in diameter), contain clear fluid, and spontaneously regress in 2 to 3 weeks.

1312. **(D)** Leiomyomas enlarging after menopause are suspicious for malignancy, most commonly sarcoma. Leiomyosarcomas consist of malignant mesenchymal (sarcomatous) tissue originating from stromal components of the uterus (e.g., endometrial stroma, myometrium, or connective tissue). The risk of a uterine leiomyoma transforming to a malignant leiomyosarcoma is 0.1 to 0.5%. Less than 10% of leiomyosarcomas originate in a leiomyoma. Most women with a leiomyosarcoma experience symptoms of short-term duration. Symptoms commonly include abdominal bloating. Pressure on adjacent organs may cause urinary symptoms (e.g., urinary frequency, retention, and incontinence), backache (due to ureteral obstruction with hydronephrosis), and rectal pressure (e.g., constipation and/or tenesmus).

1313. **(B)** Most women with ovarian carcinoma have a palpable abdominal or pelvic mass. Twenty to thirty percent of these individuals have clinically detectable malignant ascites, defined as accumulation of serous fluid–containing cancerous cells within the abdominal cavity. Abdominal percussion of ascites causes a wavelike movement of fluid around a central tympanitic area of bowel. Malignant pleural effusions may be detected as a loss of breath sounds by pulmonary auscultation. The pelvic examination remains the cornerstone for detection of ovarian neoplasia, and the presence of a fixed, irregular nodular adnexal mass with cul-de-sac nodularity or a palpable postmenopausal ovary should be considered an ovarian carcinoma until proven otherwise.

1314. **(F)** The most common symptoms of cervical cancer are abnormal vaginal bleeding and vaginal discharge. The cervix is friable and may bleed with examination. The discharge may be serous, mucoid, or purulent. The tumor usually spreads by direct extension through the parametrium. About 30 to 50% of women with advanced disease suffer ureteral obstruction, with death occurring by uremia.

1315. **(E)** Colonic diverticula, formed by herniation of bowel mucosa through weaknesses in the colonic muscularis, occur in up to one third of postmenopausal women. Disruption of the mucosa may lead to episode bleeding and local infection (diverticulitis), causing self-limited left lower abdominal pain. The pain usually subsides as the mucosa heals. Severe diverticulitis causes intense left lower abdominal pain, fever, and leukocytosis. The local inflammatory process may produce a palpable adnexal phlegmon.

1316. **(F)** In the United States, colorectal cancer is the second most common malignancy in women of all ages. Colorectal carcinoma should be suspected when a hard, tubular, pelvic mass with a transverse orientation is palpable in an elderly patient or in any individual with a family history of colorectal cancer or polyposis.

CHAPTER 21

Gynecologic Oncology: Premalignant and Malignant Diseases of the Lower Genital Tract—Vulva, Vagina, and Cervix
Questions

DIRECTIONS (Questions 1317 through 1365): Each of the numbered items or incomplete statements in this section is followed by answers or by completions of the statement. Select the ONE lettered answer or completion that is BEST in each case.

1317. The etiologic agent (or immediate precursor lesion) for vulvar cancer is

   (A) squamous cell hyperplasia
   (B) atrophic dystrophy
   (C) chronic granulomatous diseases
   (D) chronic irritation
   (E) unknown

1318. Vulvar intraepithelial neoplasia (VIN) has also been called

   (A) carcinoma in situ
   (B) erythroplasia of Queyrat
   (C) Bowen's disease
   (D) Paget's disease
   (E) all of the above

1319. A 56-year-old woman has a biopsy-proven VIN III. She undergoes a wide excision and returns three months later with vulvar pruritis. You advise her that

   (A) steroid cream on the vulva will reduce the itching
   (B) she may need a repeat biopsy
   (C) there is no chance of cancer
   (D) there is no chance of recurrence
   (E) if there is a recurrence, it will regress spontaneously

1320. Paget's disease is associated with

   (A) epidermoid immaturity
   (B) a high incidence of other primary carcinomas
   (C) sharply demarcated borders
   (D) brown melanin pigment
   (E) unifocal spread

1321. Which of the following types of vulvar cancer occurs most commonly?

   (A) Paget's
   (B) epidermoid
   (C) melanoma
   (D) adenocarcinoma
   (E) basal cell

1322. A 48-year-old woman has a large verrucous lesion of her vulva. Such a lesion is most likely

(A) clear cell carcinoma
(B) condyloma acuminata
(C) adenocarcinoma
(D) hidradenoma
(E) urethral caruncles

1323. The most common symptom of vulvar carcinoma in elderly women is

(A) abnormal bleeding
(B) a foul smell
(C) pruritus
(D) vulvar atrophy
(E) painful intercourse

1324. A blue swelling on the vulva is most likely to be

(A) a melanoma
(B) a varicosity
(C) endometriosis
(D) a cyst of the canal of Nuck
(E) a hemangioma

1325. A vulvar carcinoma with tumor-positive unilateral nodes and no distant spread would be which FIGO (International Federation of Gynecology and Obstetrics) stage?

(A) I
(B) II
(C) III
(D) IV
(E) cannot be staged without further information

1326. A 58-year-old woman has a 2-cm vulvar ulcer. A biopsy shows invasive squamous cell carcinoma. The preferred treatment would be

(A) Burow's soaks
(B) 5-fluorouracil (5-FU) cream
(C) radiotherapy

(D) hemivulvectomy and regional lymphadenectomy
(E) radical hysterectomy and node dissection

1327. If the lymph nodes in the preceding case are negative, the 5-year survival should be about

(A) 12%
(B) 25%
(C) 52%
(D) 78%
(E) > 90%

1328. The most common complication of radical vulvectomy is

(A) debilitating edema of the lower extremities
(B) pulmonary embolism
(C) necrotizing fasciitis
(D) breakdown of the surgical wound
(E) urinary and rectal incontinence

1329. A 72-year-old woman has had a radical vulvectomy for stage II squamous cell vulvar cancer. She wants to know the most likely site of recurrence if the tumor comes back. You can correctly tell her

(A) at the site of tumor resection
(B) in the bladder or rectum
(C) in the scalene lymph nodes
(D) the chest
(E) the upper leg

1330. Which of the following tumors of the vulva has the best prognosis?

(A) stage I verrucous carcinoma
(B) melanoma
(C) stage I squamous cell cancer of vulva
(D) basal cell carcinoma
(E) rhabdomyosarcoma

1331. The most common method of diagnosing carcinoma of the vagina is

(A) bleeding from the tumor bed
(B) pain with intercourse

(C) Papanicolaou smear screening

(D) incidental discovery on bimanual examination of the pelvis

(E) colposcopic prophylaxis in high-risk patients

1332. Which of the following would be classified as vaginal carcinoma?

(A) a large tumor involving the lateral edge of the cervix and the upper two thirds of the vagina

(B) a tumor extending from the right labium minus into the vagina all the way to the right vaginal fornix

(C) an isolated vaginal nodule of adenocarcinoma in a patient with previously diagnosed endometrial carcinoma

(D) all of the above

(E) none of the above

1333. The offspring of women who were exposed to diethylstilbestrol (DES) during gestation have an increased risk of

(A) vaginal agenesis

(B) adenocarcinoma of the endometrium

(C) clear cell carcinoma of the vagina

(D) squamous carcinoma of the vagina

(E) more than one of the above

1334. Which of the following malignancies tends to metastasize to the vagina most frequently?

(A) ovarian

(B) endometrial

(C) bowel

(D) bladder

(E) melanomas

1335. A malignant tumor of the vagina of young children that appears clinically as a mass of grape-like edematous polyps is

(A) emphysematous vaginitis

(B) squamous cell carcinoma

(C) sarcoma botryoides

(D) adenocarcinoma

(E) choriocarcinoma

1336. A 72-year-old woman has carcinoma of the vagina that has reached the lateral pelvic wall. The stage is

(A) 0

(B) I

(C) II

(D) III

(E) IV

1337. The most likely histology of vaginal carcinoma in this woman is

(A) melanoma

(B) verrucous

(C) clear cell

(D) adenocarcinoma

(E) squamous cell

1338. A 72-year-old woman with vaginal cancer is found on physical examination to have tumor extending from the lateral vaginal wall to the pelvic side wall. The BEST treatment for her would be

(A) total vaginectomy

(B) upper vaginectomy

(C) chemotherapy

(D) radiation therapy

(E) exenteration

1339. A frail 82-year-old woman has stage III vaginal squamous cell cancer. The best initial treatment would be

(A) radical hysterectomy, partial vaginectomy, and lymphadenectomy

(B) chemotherapy

(C) external radiation with additional implants

(D) radial vaginectomy and radiation therapy

(E) simple vaginectomy, radiation, and chemotherapy

1340. The most common method used to diagnose cervical intraepithelial neoplasia (CIN) is

(A) complaints of abnormal discharge

(B) postcoital bleeding

(C) chronic pelvic pain

(D) vaginal wet preparation

(E) abnormal Pap smears

1341. Which of the following is most TRUE concerning the etiology of cervical dysplasia and cervical cancer?

(A) They are both directly caused by human papillomavirus (HPV).

(B) Both are associated with venereal diseases.

(C) They are associated with obesity and nulliparity.

(D) There is a strong genetic component to the development of cervical cancer.

(E) The most strongly associated risk factor is cigarette smoking.

1342. A 40-year-old woman is seen for a routine examination. Her menses have been regular, and she has no complaints. Findings, including those on pelvic examination, are normal. Ten days later, her Pap smear is returned as "high-grade squamous intraepithelial lesion." Of the following options, the BEST course of action would be the performance of

(A) immediate wide-cuff hysterectomy

(B) repeated Pap smears at 3-month intervals

(C) fractional dilation and curettage (D&C)

(D) punch biopsy of anterior cervical lip

(E) colposcopy with biopsy

1343. The colposcope permits one to

(A) view the cervix at 1–4 power magnification

(B) see the entire transition zone in all patients

(C) choose the most suspicious areas on the cervical portio to biopsy

(D) treat invasive cancer with a biopsy

(E) make the diagnosis of cancer

1344. Leukoplakia refers to

(A) a microscopic lesion

(B) atrophy

(C) a cancer

(D) a white patch

(E) an ulcer

1345. A patient has a Pap smear that is read as "high-grade squamous intraepithelial lesion," followed by an inadequate colposcopic examination. Your next step should be

(A) fractional D&C

(B) simple hysterectomy, removing a large vaginal cuff

(C) cervical conization

(D) careful observation with repeat cytology at 6-month intervals

(E) colposcopic-directed biopsies from all suspicious areas of the cervix and endocervical curettage

1346. Conization of the cervix would be inappropriate in which of the following instances?

(A) when there is disparity between Pap smear and biopsy results

(B) when colposcopy is inadequate

(C) when microinvasion is diagnosed by biopsy

(D) when deeply invasive cancer is shown on a biopsy

(E) for treatment of biopsy-proven CIN III

1347. In treating CIN III, cryotherapy has a failure rate of about

(A) 1 to 5%

(B) 10 to 20%

(C) 25 to 30%

(D) 35 to 40%

(E) >40%

1348. Often, the first symptom of cervical cancer is

(A) leg pain

(B) pain with intercourse

(C) vaginal bleeding

(D) weight loss

(E) vulvar pruritus

1349. Most cervical cancers arise

(A) on the portio vaginalis

(B) at the internal os

(C) in the endocervix

(D) at the squamocolumnar junction

(E) at the exteral os

1350. What percentage of clinical stage I carcinomas of the cervix will have lymphatic spread?

(A) 0%

(B) 5%

(C) 15%

(D) 25%

(E) 40%

1351. Clinical staging of cervical carcinoma when correlated with findings at surgery has an accuracy of approximately

(A) 10%

(B) 25%

(C) 50%

(D) 75%

(E) 100%

1352. The factor most indicative of invasive cancer on colposcopic examination is

(A) white epithelium

(B) leukoplakia

(C) abnormal blood vessels

(D) punctation

(E) mosaic pattern

1353. If a non-healing ulcer is seen on the cervix, it is best evaluated by

(A) repeat examination

(B) Pap smear

(C) punch biopsy

(D) cone biopsy

(E) vaginal steroid cream

Questions 1354 and 1355

1354. A 43-year-old woman had a suspicious Pap smear and a normal pelvic examination. A colposcopically directed biopsy of a normal-appearing cervix revealed invasive carcinoma. The next step in the care of the patient should be

(A) metastatic evaluation

(B) conization

(C) radical hysterectomy

(D) radiation therapy

(E) both irradiation and radical hysterectomy

1355. The woman had a negative metastatic workup. Her clinical exam shows cancer growth shown in Figure 21–1. She is stage

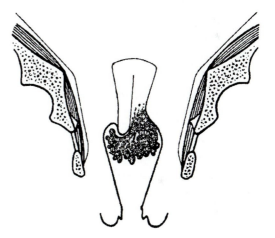

Figure 21–1.

(A) IA

(B) IB

(C) IIA

(D) IIB

(E) C

1356. The most common serious complication of radical hysterectomy is

(A) bowel obstruction

(B) illness from transfusion

(C) genitourinary fistula

(D) premature menopause

(E) intraoperative death

1357. Biopsy-proven carcinoma in situ of the uterine cervix, if otherwise untreated, will progress to invasive cancer in up to what percentage of patients?

(A) < 5%

(B) 30%

(C) 50%

(D) 70%

(E) > 90%

1358. The incidence of pelvic lymph node metastasis in stage I cervical squamous cell cancer (clinically confined to the cervix) is approximately

(A) < 1%

(B) 3 to 5%

(C) 15 to 20%

(D) 30 to 50%

(E) > 50%

1359. The majority of deaths from cervical carcinoma are due to

(A) local spread obstructing the ureters, causing renal failure

(B) brain metastasis with resultant cerebral hemorrhage

(C) hemorrhage into the pelvis from erosion of vessels by the tumor

(D) pulmonary failure secondary to metastatic disease filling the lungs

(E) bone metastasis causing crush injuries to the central nervous system

1360. The 5-year survival rate for all stages of invasive cervical cancer is approximately

(A) 15%

(B) 35%

(C) 50%

(D) 65%

(E) > 65%

1361. Extent of spread being equal, which of the following carcinomas of the cervix has the poorest prognosis?

(A) well-differentiated, keratinizing, large cell squamous carcinoma

(B) undifferentiated, large cell squamous carcinoma

(C) differentiated, small cell squamous carcinoma

(D) undifferentiated, small cell squamous carcinoma

(E) papillary adenocarcinoma

1362. A bulky, friable, papillary tumor mass growing from the cervix would be BEST termed

(A) exophytic

(B) endophytic

(C) nodular

(D) ulcerating

(E) edematous

1363. A 34-year-old woman is 16 weeks, pregnant and has a Pap smear suspicious for cancer. You advise her to

(A) have colposcopy with biopsy

(B) have colposcopy, but biopsy is too risky in pregnancy

(C) have a repeat Pap smear in 3 months

(D) undergo a termination of pregnancy and then undergo complete evaluation

(E) have cervical conization

1364. Vaginal intraepithelial neoplasia is most commonly found in which part of the vagina?

(A) the upper one third

(B) the mid-vagina

(C) the distal vagina

(D) at the hymenal ring

(E) the posterior fourchette

1365. The preferred treatment for stage I vaginal carcinoma confined to the upper one third of the lateral vagina in a 29-year-old woman would be

(A) intravaginal 5-FU

(B) upper vaginectomy

(C) simple hysterectomy and upper vaginectomy

(D) radical hysterectomy, pelvic lymphadenectomy, and partial vaginectomy

(E) anterior exenteration

DIRECTIONS (Questions 1366 through 1374): Each of the numbered items or incomplete statements in this section is followed by answers or by completions of the statement. Select the answers or completions that may apply.

1366. Which three of the following are true regarding cancer of the vulva?

(A) It is often associated with a long history of vulvar pruritus, discomfort, or a bloody discharge.

(B) It will often appear as a growth on the labia.

(C) Biopsy is necessary to make the diagnosis.

(D) The lesion is often curable by local excision.

(E) The peak incidence occurs at age 52.

1367. Management of a vaginal ulcer should include which four of the following?

(A) biopsy if it does not heal rapidly

(B) VDRL (Venereal Disease Research Laboratory)

(C) frequent observation

(D) referral to a psychiatrist to evaluate factitious etiologies

(E) discontinuation of tampons

1368. A 42-year-old presents with a history of postcoital spotting. Examination of the cervix reveals a raised/reddened area next to the os. This could represent which four of the following?

(A) carcinoma

(B) condyloma lata

(C) ectropion

(D) cervical polyp

(E) Nabothian cyst

1369. Reasons for cytology (Pap smears) to be unsatisfactory include which four of the following?

(A) extensive malignant necrosis

(B) poor sampling

(C) misreading

(D) cervical inflammation

(E) excessive bleeding

1370. The treatment of carcinoma of the cervix during pregnancy should depend on which three of the following?

(A) the desires of the oncologist

(B) the religious beliefs of the patient

(C) the trimester of the pregnancy

(D) the stage of the lesion

(E) the length of the cervix

1371. Which four of the following, of and by themselves, are indicative of a less favorable prognosis in cancer of the cervix?

(A) lymph node involvement

(B) increased size of primary tumor

(C) blood vessel or lymphatic space invasion

(D) low socioeconomic status of the patient

(E) underexpression of ras oncogene

1372. The therapy of a 26-year-old patient with microinvasive carcinoma of the cervix depends on which four of the following?

(A) depth of stromal invasion being < 3 mm

(B) no lymphatic space involvement

(C) desire to maintain reproductive capabilities

(D) small area of tumor involvement

(E) which other organs were involved with tumor

1373. A 42-year-old woman undergoes a radical hysterectomy and requires postop radiation. During the radiation therapy she returns complaining of watery vaginal discharge and recurrent urinary tract infections. Which four of the following might be reasonable evaluations?

(A) intravenous pyelogram (IVP)

(B) cystoscopy

(C) wet mount

(D) sigmoidoscopy

(E) inject diluted methylene blue in sterile water to the bladder with a catheter and examine the vagina

1374. A 31-year-old woman has multifocal VIN, grade II. Which four of the following therapies would be acceptable given current treatment patterns?

(A) simple vulvectomy

(B) wide local excision of the affected areas

(C) laser vaporization of the affected areas

(D) topical 5-FU applied to the vulva

(E) observation over time

Answers and Explanations

1317. (E) The etiologic agent for vulvar carcinoma is unknown. Vulvar diseases (squamous cell hyperplasia, previously known as hyperplastic dystrophy, sexually transmitted diseases, granulomatosis diseases) are all associated with an increased incidence of vulvar cancer, but none are considered the cause. Some authorities feel the etiologic agent may be viral in origin (HPV), while others feel it may be just a cofactor or an associated, not causative, finding. Some studies have shown about 50% of vulvar cancers are HPV positive.

1318. (E) Intraepithelial or in situ cancer implies a replacement of the full-thickness of the epithelial lining with undifferentiated abnormal cells. All of these lesions have been separated in the past but really are similar in terms of behavior, and are all treatable by local destruction when they are intraepithelial lesions. Invasion requires radical excision.

1319. (B) VIN can certainly recur, although it has a much longer transition time than CIN. Some VINs may regress spontaneously, but this is not guaranteed. VIN can be multifocal, and about 20% of patients with an initial biopsy of VIN III have been reported to have microinvasive cancer in the resected specimen. Steroid cream is the treatment of choice for pruritus from vulvar dystrophies, but this woman needs a vulvar exam and possible biopsy to rule out recurrence.

1320. (A) Paget's disease may be identified by the typical vacuolated large, pale, mucin-containing cells infiltrating the epidermis, often in a serpiginous fashion (Paget cells). About 15% of the time they have an associated adenocarcinoma. Most often, however, it represents an intraepithelial, not invasive, process.

1321. (B) Cancer of the vulva makes up about 5% of all gynecologic malignancies, and approximately 90% of vulvar cancer is squamous cell. Paget's disease is an intraepithelial lesion derived from an undifferentiated glandular cell. Extramammary Paget's disease is most often an intraepithelial lesion that may spread over the perineum. Adenocarcinoma probably arises from glandular structures of the vulva. Malignant melanoma can occur over any skin area but is relatively rare in the vulva (about 5% of cases).

1322. (B) At age 48, this lesion is probably a wart. However, it could be verrucous carcinoma, which is a locally invasive tumor that does not tend to metastasize via the lymphatics. Metastases are possible, however, and cannot be ruled out unless adequate surgery is performed. It may be HPV related. If any doubt exists, adequate biopsy should be done.

1323. (C) Pruritus is the presenting complaint in over one half of patients. Twenty percent are asymptomatic, and the remainder may have pain, bleeding, or a foul smell from tumor necrosis. Atrophy is not usually a complaint.

1324. (B) Although any of the options are possible, the most likely one is a varicosity due to the pampiniform plexus of veins found in the labia. Biopsy of a lesion such as this can lead to heavy bleeding. It is one of the few examples in which vulvar biopsy is detrimental.

1325. **(C)** The tumor could be of any size, but the positive nodes place the lesion in stage III. In the tumor, node, metastasis (TNM) staging, these would be N2 tumors. The TNM system seems to be more prognostic than the FIGO system.

1326. **(D)** In recent years a hemivulvectomy has been substituted for radical vulvectomy in many cases when tumor is isolated to one side of the vulva. Removing the ipsilateral groin and femoral lymph nodes is performed in the medically stable patient. Bilateral vulvectomy and lymph node dissection is still standard therapy for large tumors and tumors that impinge on the midline because vulvar lymphatics cross the midline. Deep pelvic nodes are excised only if the others are positive, and there is little salvage demonstrated by removing these deep pelvic lymph nodes.

1327. **(D)** If multiple inguinal nodes are positive, the cure rate drops to less than 15%, and if the deep nodes are involved, the cure rate is very low. This illustrates the importance of the lymphatic route of spread in this disease and the importance of extirpative surgery in treating the disease. Before radical surgery, almost no one survived this disease.

1328. **(D)** While all of the choices may be complications of radical vulvectomy, about 50% of the patients experience significant problems with wound healing. This is because of the large amount of tissue removed and the poor blood supply of the remaining tissues. Patients often spend 2 or more weeks in the hospital just for the postoperative care of their wounds. Leg edema is also common, and incontinence of urine is not unusual (likely due to resection of the distal third of the urethra), but neither are as frequent as wound problems.

1329. **(A)** The most common site of recurrence is the site of the primary surgical resection or the groin area where nodes were positive (if not previously resected). The tumor occurs centrally and seldom as distant metastases.

1330. **(D)** Pure basal cell tumors can be cured by wide excision. The other tumors are all treated as invasive carcinomas with radical surgery. Rhabdomyosarcomas are found in young patients, are extremely malignant, and, fortunately, are very rare.

1331. **(C)** Most vaginal cancer is asymptomatic and not visible to the unaided eye on routine examination nor palpable to the average examiner. Papanicolaou screening is the most common method for making the diagnosis. Advanced disease presents with bleeding, mass, foul-smelling discharge, and pain.

1332. **(E)** The only true vaginal carcinomas are those confined to the vagina. If cervix, vulva, or endometrium are involved, those organs are considered to be the source of the primary tumor. Vaginal cancers are rare, representing 1 to 2% of all gynecologic malignancies.

1333. **(C)** Vaginal clear cell or adenocarcinoma is quite rare, but it is increased in the offspring of women who took DES (incidence estimated at 0.14 to 1.4 per 1,000 exposed female fetuses).

1334. **(B)** Without the use of pre- or postoperative irradiation, the incidence of vaginal metastases from uterine adenocarcinoma is about 10%. Cervical cancer can also spread to the vagina and, when it does so, may change the staging of the disease. Remember, however, recurrence does not change initial staging.

1335. **(C)** This highly malignant tumor of the vagina is fortunately rare but must be thought of whenever vaginal bleeding or discharge occurs in a young female patient. A small scope or examination under anesthesia may be used for diagnostic purposes. Sarcoma botryoides, so called because of its sometimes grape-like gross appearance, is a highly malignant tumor.

1336. **(D)** Vaginal cancer staging criteria are similar to the criteria used in cervical cancer. Carcinoma of the vagina does not respond as well to treatment as carcinoma of the cervix.

1337. (E) Vaginal carcinoma is primarily squamous cell (80 to 90%) followed by adenocarcinoma (5%), melanoma (3%), and less frequent yet, verrucous and clear cell.

1338. (D) In this case, radiation therapy is the best choice. Surgery is unlikely to be able to remove all the tumor present. Chemotherapy is almost never curative for solid gynecologic tumors. Radiation will nonspecifically kill cells and preferentially kill the most rapidly growing cells, making it a valuable adjunct in the treatment of many malignancies.

1339. (C) Surgery is not a good choice because of the stage of the tumor and the frail condition of the patient. Chemotherapy alone does not do well with squamous cell cancer, and the combination of these therapies has unacceptable complication rates.

1340. (E) CIN is an asymptomatic disease generally found on Pap smear, with no findings present to the unaided eye. There are over 300,000 Pap smears per year in the United States with identified changes of CIN.

1341. (B) Though the exact etiology of CIN and cervical cancer is unknown, it has been known for more than 200 years that it is associated with the number of sexual partners, the incidence of many venereal diseases, and early age of first intercourse. HPV is a risk factor but is not considered a stand-alone etiologic factor; cigarette smoking also appears to be a cofactor. Genetics, obesity, and parity probably play little, if any, role.

1342. (E) The type and extent of the lesions must be determined before treatment. Most authorities would recommend a colposcopically directed cervical biopsy done by someone skilled in the technique for a smear suggestive of a high-grade (CIN II–III) intraepithelial lesion. If infection is suggested, appropriate examination, therapy, and reevaluation are also indicated.

1343. (C) The colposcope permits 6–40× power magnification and the addition of a bright light source. If one cannot see the entire cervical transition zone, the colposcopic examination is unsatisfactory, and other diagnostic methods must be used. One should have a tissue diagnosis before instituting treatment for invasive cancer. Colposcopy's greatest advantage is in allowing directed biopsies for diagnosis, not for making the diagnosis. Histologic confirmation is needed, and more than one biopsy should be taken if the suspicious area is large or more than one suspicious area is present.

1344. (D) Leukoplakia is a clinical term that describes the gross appearance of a lesion. These lesions show up as white prior to the application of acetic acid. It does not imply etiology or degree of abnormality.

1345. (E) Since the colposcopic examination is inadequate (cannot see the whole lesion), one must rule out invasive disease. The best way to do this is either by conization or by adequate colposcopically directed biopsy and endocervical curettage. Generally, biopsies are done prior to conization to rule out invasive cancer. Now, in-office LEEP (loop electrosurgical excision procedure) procedures can offer diagnosis and treatment and would also be an option.

1346. (D) If invasive cancer is diagnosed by the biopsy, you have all the necessary information. The next step is staging. One must always carefully examine a microinvasive lesion to rule out frank invasion, as the treatments are quite different. Patients with invasive cervical cancer are badly compromised by treatment for the lesser disease. If a possible invasive cancer cannot be adequately evaluated by colposcopic biopsy, a cone biopsy is indicated.

1347. (B) The best results are obtained with a double freeze in patients with CIN I and II and negative endocervical curettage specimens. However, in advanced abnormalities, the recurrence rate is high (10 to 20%), and follow-up must be meticulous. Follow-up examination may be made more difficult by the changes caused by the cryosurgery. For this reason, many clinicians use laser vaporization or LEEP to treat cervical dysplasia.

1348. **(C)** As vaginal bleeding may be due to many factors, one must be wary in attributing it to a less serious cause and thereby missing the underlying carcinoma. The cervix must always be inspected in these cases. Most bleeding will not be from carcinoma.

1349. **(D)** If the entire squamocolumnar junction is not seen on a colposcopic examination, that exam is inadequate. It is believed that abnormal change begins here because this is the site of metaplastic cells that are more capable of transformation.

1350. **(C)** Such lymphatic spread is often undetected during clinical staging of early cervical cancer. It may be the reason for the 10 to 15% 5-year mortality in stage I cervical cancer. Detection of the distant spread of tumors may require surgical sampling.

1351. **(B)** An identical diagnosis from two expert clinicians is only 89% accurate, and when clinical staging is compared with operative findings, the accuracy is much lower. Clinical overestimation occurs in about 20% and underestimation in about 50% of cases. Lymph node sampling at surgical exploration combined with quantification of tumor volume after removal are good indicators.

1352. **(C)** When any abnormality occurs, biopsy is indicated, as it may be more severe than expected. However, corkscrew or comma-shaped vessels are highly suspicious of malignancy. The key word here is suspicious—not diagnostic. Colposcopy does allow you to biopsy the most abnormal areas. Usually, more than one biopsy site is needed for adequate sampling.

1353. **(C)** Any unexplained lesion on the cervix that does not heal must be biopsied—the sooner the better. Treatment with creams does not replace adequate diagnosis. Do not forget to rule out syphilis and herpes as the cause of the ulcer.

1354. **(A)** This patient is already known to have invasive cancer. Proper staging and evaluation for surgery or irradiation is the next step. Surgery is done only on early lesions. Stages beyond IB or early IIA are treated with radiation.

1355. **(C)** Figure 21–2A depicts stage IB; Figure B stage IIA with carcinoma extending into the left vaginal vault; Figure C stage IIB with parametrium involved on both sides; Figure D stage IIIA; Figure E stage IIIB; and Figure F stage IVA.

1356. **(A)** The mortality rate for radical hysterectomy is less than 1%. Complications from transfusion are low at present. Urinary fistulization occurs in 1 to 2% of cases. Menopausal symptoms should not occur because the ovaries are not generally removed unless the patient is peri- or postmenopausal. Unrecognized and therefore unrepaired bowel injury is unlikely during hysterectomy of any kind. Late small bowel obstruction occurs 5% of the time and rises if postoperative radiation is used.

1357. **(B)** It is likely that about two thirds of the cases of carcinoma in situ will not progress to cervical cancer, even if not treated, but this also means that one third will, and a clinician cannot tell which patients will have progression and which will not. Therefore, carcinoma in situ is a serious lesion deserving complete removal both to rule out invasion and to avoid progression. Frequent follow-up is mandatory. Even with complete excision, this is a "field" type of disease, with multiple recurrences.

1358. **(C)** Some patients with no clinical evidence of metastatic spread will be shown to have positive nodes. These patients are at very high risk of persistent disease after treatment. It is for this reason that surgical staging of these malignancies has become popular. Stage II cancer has involvement of lymph nodes about 30% of the time, stage III about 60% of the time, and stage IV more than 75% of the time.

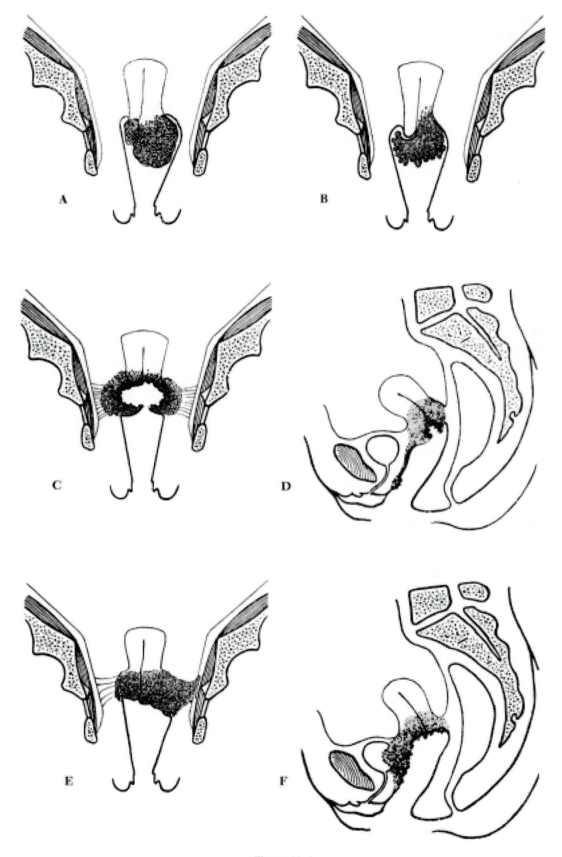

Figure 21–2.

1359. (A) Urinary or intestinal obstruction and simple wasting away (cachexia) cause the majority of deaths from cervical cancer. If the recurrence is totally central in the pelvis, exenteration may be indicated. With good selection, survival rates are fair.

1360. (E) This survival rate takes into account all stages of invasive cervical cancer and all modes of treatment. Obviously, the survival is greater in earlier stages. Adequate staging allows for the best treatment.

1361. (D) The greater the degree of undifferentiation (cellular ambivalence), the poorer the prognosis. Small cell carcinoma seems to have a more malignant course than large cell cancer. This, however, is not as constant a finding in the cervix as it is in the lung. Adenocarcinoma, stage for stage, has about the same prognosis as squamous cell carcinoma of the cervix.

1362. (A) Descriptive terms should mean the same thing to everyone using them. Exophytic lesions are seen and biopsied, while endophytic lesions may be quite large before they become visible. Exophytic lesions project outward from the cervix, like condylomata.

1363. (A) The pregnant patient with a suspicious Pap smear needs an evaluation (colposcopy and biopsy) to rule out invasive cancer. If CIN or carcinoma in situ is found, the patient can be observed and delivered at term, and then have a final evaluation and therapy 6 weeks postpartum. Cervical conization can be done in the second trimester if needed to rule out invasive cancer, but colposcopy and biopsy would be appropriate initial evaluation.

1364. (A) The majority of vaginal neoplasias are found in the upper one third of the vagina, probably related to the fact that this area at one time underwent metaplasia as a normal part of its maturation process.

1365. (D) An early stage of vaginal carcinoma in a young woman would be treated in a manner that would allow you to remove the lesion but preserve as much of her normal functions as possible. In this case, the cancer must be removed, but ovarian preservation and conservation of a functional vagina are the other great concern. The 5-FU would not cure an invasive cancer. The upper vaginectomy is also likely to fail because about 20% of the stage I patients will have pelvic lymph node metastases; therefore, the simple hysterectomy and vaginectomy will also fail in too high a percentage of patients. Radical hysterectomy with nodal extirpation and wide removal of the vagina will likely cure the cancer and preserve ovarian function, and a graft could be used to restore vaginal length, if necessary. Anterior exenteration (removal of all pelvic tissue in the anterior pelvis, including the bladder) is likely to be too much surgery.

1366. (A, B, C) Invasive vulvar cancer has a peak incidence in postmenopausal women over the age of 60. The peak incidence of carcinoma in situ (intraepithelial carcinoma) is about 10 years earlier. Women often have a history of long-standing vulvar irritation, vulvar dystrophy, or venereal disease. The most common lesion is found on the labium majus. Even with radical surgical excision, the overall cure rate is only about 65% in major centers.

1367. (A, B, C, E) As a general rule, any ulcer that does not heal completely in 2 weeks should be biopsied to rule out malignancy. Remember that a luetic chancre may heal, but the VDRL will become and remain positive. If present, the infection must be treated. Tampons are a common cause of vaginal ulcers. The patient does not need a psychiatric referral.

1368. (A, B, C, D) The purpose of this question is to reemphasize the point that a cervical lesion can be any number of abnormal findings, and the only way to be certain is to adequately sample the tissue by biopsy and microscopic evaluation. A Pap smear or colposcopic examination is not a substitute for evaluation of a gross cervical lesion. Biopsy is necessary. A Nabothian cyst is usually clear.

1369. (A, B, D, E) The most common cause of error is poor or inadequate sampling technique by the individual who obtains the smears. Pap smear errors can be decreased by improving the technique and obtaining repeat studies. Both the endocervical canal and squamo-columnar junction must be sampled. Misreading is not a cause of the smear being unsatisfactory, but may still yield erroneous information.

1370. (B, C, D) This question is designed to point out two things. The major medical concerns should be (1) the trimester of the pregnancy, and (2) the stage of the lesion involved. Patients in the first and early second trimester should not wait to begin treatment; the delay is too long. In the third trimester, treatment often can be postponed until a viable fetus can be delivered. Treatment with radiation versus surgery depends on the stage, size, and type (histologic differentiation) of the lesion involved. Treatment must be individualized, with decisions being made by an informed patient and a physician. Two commonly held fallacies—(1) cancer of the cervix grows more rapidly during pregnancy, and (2) delivery of an infant through a cancerous cervix spreads the disease—should be ignored; they do not appear to be true. The desires of the patient are also important and must be respected even though they might be contrary to current medical opinions. Neither the age of the patient nor the length of the cervix are important factors.

1371. (A, B, C, D) Physical characteristics of the tumor, such as a large volume or barrel shape, lymphatic and blood vessel invasion, and small cell type with undifferentiated histology, all indicate worse prognosis. Some non-tumor characteristics such as advanced patient age, poor general health, and low socioeconomic status also decrease survival. Overexpression of ras and cmyc oncogenes are also associated with a poor prognosis in cervical cancer. Treatment centers with less experienced caregivers also have lower survival rates in general.

1372. (A, B, C, D) A simple hysterectomy is generally felt to be adequate therapy for a patient whose microinvasive cervical carcinoma meets all the given criteria. Very few of these patients will have positive pelvic nodes. In a young woman wishing to preserve her reproductive function, a cone biopsy might be considered if all the above conditions were met, the patient fully understood the risks involved, and she would be reliable in her follow-up. Some gynecologic oncologists would disagree with this plan of management. Some prefer to define microinvasion as 1 mm or less of invasion for greatest patient safety. By definition, if the cervical cancer were microinvasive, no other organs would be affected.

1373. (A, B, C, E) A vesicovaginal fistula can occur after radiation therapy or hysterectomy (even a hysterectomy for benign disease). The classic symptoms are described in the case. Methylene blue–stained saline in the bladder can help make the diagnosis by visualizing blue dye in the vagina or by instilling the fluid in the bladder and placing a tampon in the vagina, which becomes stained. Cystoscopy can help in visualizing the lesion and assessing the size, location, and number of fistulas. An IVP is useful for diagnosing ureterovaginal fistula, which is a rarer complication but could present with watery vaginal discharge. A wet mount is useful for diagnosing vaginitis, which might occur, but the amount of discharge is likely to be much less with vaginitis than with a fistula. Sigmoidoscopy would not be helpful.

1374. (B, C, D, E) Though some might disagree as to "best" treatment, the lesion here is an intraepithelial one (corresponds to moderate dysplasia). The patient is a young woman, and her chance of ever developing vulvar carcinoma is low. A vulvectomy would be an unnecessarily deforming operation on her but would affect "cure," but all of the others are safe, even observation. Observation allows natural regression, which happens frequently.

CHAPTER 22

Gynecologic Oncology: Upper Genital Tract Malignancies
Questions

DIRECTIONS (Questions 1375 through 1466): Each of the numbered items or incomplete statements in this section is followed by answers or by completions of the statement. Select the ONE lettered answer or completion that is BEST in each case.

1375. A 44-year-old multiparous woman complains of abnormal vaginal bleeding of 5 months' duration. Pelvic examination demonstrates a small, anteverted uterus and a normal-appearing cervix. No adnexal masses are present. A serum pregnancy test is negative, and a cervical Papanicolaou smear is normal. Serum follicle-stimulating hormone (FSH), prolactin, and thyroid-stimulating hormone (TSH) levels are normal. The most efficient method to determine the etiology of the bleeding is

   (A) dilation and curettage (D&C)
   (B) endometrial biopsy
   (C) endometrial cytology
   (D) transvaginal sonography
   (E) hysteroscopy

1376. The most common symptom of endometrial hyperplasia is

   (A) vaginal discharge
   (B) vaginal bleeding
   (C) amenorrhea
   (D) pelvic pain
   (E) abdominal distention

1377. Which of the following statements regarding endometrial hyperplasia is TRUE?

   (A) Endometrial hyperplasia results from prolonged androgenic stimulation of the endometrium.
   (B) Endometrial hyperplasia is characterized by proliferation of glands but not stroma.
   (C) Endometrial hyperplasia rarely undergoes spontaneous regression.
   (D) Cytologic atypia is an important characteristic determining risk of progression to carcinoma.
   (E) The length of time required for endometrial hyperplasia to progress to carcinoma is less than 1 year.

1378. A 49-year-old woman experiences irregular vaginal bleeding of 3 months' duration. You perform an endometrial biopsy, which obtains copious tissue with a velvety, lobulated texture. The pathologist report shows proliferation of glandular and stromal elements with dilated endometrial glands. Cytologic atypia is absent. You advise the patient that

   (A) the presence of dilated endometrial glands is unusual
   (B) the histologic finding is called cystic atrophy
   (C) the tissue may be weakly premalignant
   (D) she requires a hysterectomy
   (E) no further therapy is needed

1379. A 48-year-old woman is referred to you for irregular vaginal bleeding of 6 months' duration. Her referring physician removed tissue protruding through the cervix 3 months ago. Microscopic examination of the tissue shows a mass with cystic hyperplasia and a central vascular channel surrounded on three sides by epithelium. The vaginal bleeding has continued. You advise that the

(A) risk of developing endometrial cancer is increased tenfold

(B) bleeding is from an endometrial polyp

(C) histology of the tissue may not reflect the source of the bleeding

(D) uterus should be probed with a forceps to remove more tissue

(E) patient should receive cyclic progestin therapy

1380. A 40-year-old nulligravida female pediatrician comes to see you for irregular vaginal bleeding of 1 year's duration. She has not been using birth control and had hoped to conceive. Endometrial biopsy revealed endometrial hyperplasia. She would like medical treatment and wants to know which factor is most important in determining premalignant potential. You advise that it is the

(A) age of the patient

(B) degree of cystic atrophy

(C) persistence of bleeding

(D) thickness of endometrial hyperplasia

(E) degree of cytologic atypia

1381. A 32-year-old woman with polycystic ovary syndrome (PCOS) has infertility of 1 year's duration. Her menses occur at irregular intervals, and basal body temperatures (BBTs) are monophasic. An endometrial biopsy shows endometrial hyperplasia with mild cytologic atypia. The most appropriate therapy is

(A) danazol

(B) megestrol acetate

(C) oral contraceptives (OCs)

(D) clomiphene citrate — *desires fertility*

(E) human menopausal gonadotropins (hMGs)

Questions 1382 and 1383

A 58-year-old woman on combined estrogen and progesterone hormone replacement has postmenopausal bleeding. You obtain a pelvic ultrasound, which shows an endometrial stripe thickness of 12 mm.

1382. Which of the following is true?

(A) If the endometrial stripe thickness had been less than 5 mm, you would have told the patient that no further evaluation was needed.

(B) An endometrial stripe thickness of 5 to 10 mm confers no risk of endometrial cancer.

(C) An endometrial stripe thickness of greater than 10 mm correlates with a 10 to 20% risk of hyperplasia or cancer.

(D) The endometrial stripe thickness in premenopausal women is interpreted similarly to the endometrial stripe thickness dimensions in postmenopausal women.

(E) Hysterectomy should be performed.

1383. The patient returns for testing. Office hysteroscopy shows thickened endometrium but no polyps or masses. Office endometrial biopsy results indicate grossly dilated glands with the classic "Swiss cheese" appearance and benign cellular architecture. There is no invasion or mitotic figures. The diagnosis is

(A) adenocanthoma

(B) complex atypical hyperplasia

(C) cystic endometrial hyperplasia

(D) clear cell adenocarcinoma

(E) squamous cell carcinoma of the endometrium

1384. An internist calls you for consultation regarding a 55-year-old postmenopausal woman with some vaginal spotting. On examination, a small, round, bright red mass was noted to protrude through the cervical os. It bled during the Pap smear. The Pap smear result was normal. The advice you give the internist is to

(A) recheck the mass in 6 months and refer if it enlarges

(B) refer the patient for probable polyp removal

(C) refer the patient for cone biopsy

(D) tell the patient not to worry since the Pap smear is negative

(E) tell the patient polyps are never cancerous and refer for removal

1385. A 44-year-old female biochemist has complex hyperplasia without atypia on endometrial biopsy. You prescribe 40 mg megestrol acetate daily. She inquires about the mechanism of action and regression rate. Which of the following explanations is TRUE?

(A) The regresion of endometrial hyperplasia takes at least 12 months.

(B) Progestins oppose estrogen action in endometrial tissue by reducing the amount of estrogen receptors.

(C) Hyperplastic endometrium has few progesterone receptors so a large dose of progestin is needed.

(D) If regression of endometrial hyperplasia occurs within 3 months, it will recur if she stops the medication.

(E) Progestins bind to progesterone receptors in the endometrium and convert the histology to proliferative endometrium.

1386. The most common uterine neoplasm is

(A) sarcoma

(B) adenocarcinoma

(C) adenomyosis

(D) choriocarcinoma

(E) leiomyoma

1387. The most common uterine malignancy is

(A) endometrial adenocarcinoma

(B) endometrial sarcoma

(C) leiomyosarcoma

(D) malignant mixed müllerian tumor

(E) endometrial stromal tumor

1388. Which of the following types of cancer is the leading cause of gynecologic/reproductive cancer death in women?

(A) cervical

(B) uterine

(C) ovarian

(D) breast

(E) vulva

1389. Which of the following 25-year-old patients is most likely to develop endometrial adenocarcinoma?

(A) a prostitute using OCs

(B) a married woman with PCOS

(C) a waitress with testicular feminization

(D) a high school gymnast with regular menses

(E) a physician with an intrauterine device (IUD)

1390. Endometrial adenocarcinoma is most often preceded by

(A) cystic hyperplasia

(B) endometrial hyperplasia

(C) endometrial hyperplasia with cytologic atypia

(D) Arias–Stella phenomenon

(E) microcystic glandular hyperplasia

1391. Endometrial carcinoma is most common in which of the following age groups?

(A) 10 to 25 years

(B) 25 to 30 years

(C) 30 to 40 years

(D) 40 to 50 years

(E) > 60 years

1392. A 69-year-old postmenopausal woman is being admitted for surgical treatment of endometrial cancer. She has no health insurance and would like to know which is the most important preoperative screening test to look for metastasis?

(A) chest x-ray

(B) hysterosalpingogram

(C) pelvic ultrasound

(D) intravenous pyelogram (IVP)

(E) barium enema

1393. A 58-year-old woman develops postmenopausal bleeding. An endometrial biopsy shows adenocarcinoma. She undergoes a total abdominal hysterectomy with pelvic lymph node sampling. The final pathology shows tumor extending from the uterus into the cervix but no other invasion (see Figure 22–1). Lymph nodes were negative for metastasis. The cancer is classified as stage

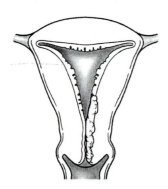

Figure 22–1.

(A) 0
(B) I
(C) II
(D) III
(E) IV

1394. Endometrial adenoacanthoma is BEST described as

(A) adenocarcinoma with benign squamous components
(B) adenocarcinoma with papillary formation
(C) squamous cell carcinoma with benign glandular components
(D) a mixture of malignant glandular and squamous components
(E) a mixture of benign glandular and squamous components

1395. Which of the following types of endometrial carcinoma has the BEST prognosis?

(A) adenosquamous carcinoma
(B) clear cell adenocarcinoma
(C) papillary serous carcinoma
(D) mucinous adenocarcinoma
(E) mixed carcinoma

1396. Most endometrial cancers are diagnosed as stage

(A) I
(B) II
(C) III
(D) IV
(E) recurrent

1397. An 80-year-old woman who has never taken estrogen develops a pink vaginal discharge. An endometrial biopsy shows adenocarcinoma of the endometrium. Papanicolaou smear is negative. Of the following, what is the most important prognostic indicator?

(A) body habitus
(B) level of CA-125
(C) nutritional status
(D) histologic type of tumor
(E) presence of peptide hormone receptors

Questions 1398 through 1401

A healthy 65-year-old woman is seen for postmenopausal bleeding. The pelvic examination is normal. A fractional D&C demonstrates adenocarcinoma of the endometrium. Histologically, endometrial glands are confluent without solid areas of tumor cells. The endocervical curettage shows normal endocervical cells. The cervical Pap smear and other preoperative investigations are normal.

1398. The grade of the endometrial tumor is

(A) well differentiated
(B) moderately well differentiated
(C) moderately differentiated
(D) poorly differentiated
(E) undifferentiated

1399. Which of the following statements regarding endometrial carcinoma in this patient is TRUE?

(A) Invasion of tumor through most of the myometrium will not be found.

(B) Invasion of tumor into pelvic lymph nodes will not occur.

(C) Steroid hormone receptors will not be present in tumor tissue.

(D) Radical hysterectomy and bilateral salpingo-oophorectomy is the primary treatment modality.

(E) Therapy depends on surgical and histologic evaluation of pelvic viscera, peritoneal cavity, and retroperitoneal lymph nodes.

1400. Exploratory laparotomy is negative for metastatic disease. The uterus is opened in the operating room and found to have tumor invasion into the myometrium. Histologic examination of the uterus confirms tumor invasion beyond the inner half of the myometrium. Peritoneal washings and pelvic and para-aortic nodes are negative for malignancy. You advise

(A) no further therapy

(B) radiation therapy

(C) hormonal therapy

(D) single-agent chemotherapy

(E) multiple-agent chemotherapy

1401. This patient underwent postoperative radiation. During radiation therapy she develops nausea, anorexia, diarrhea, and mild abdominal pain. The most likely diagnosis is

(A) radiation cystitis

(B) radiation enteritis

(C) radiation proctitis

(D) enterovaginal fistula

(E) vaginal ulceration

1402. Which of the following statements regarding steroid receptors in endometrial adenocarcinoma is TRUE?

(A) Steroid receptor levels in endometrial cancer are higher than in normal endometrium.

(B) Steroid receptor levels in endometrial cancer are lowest in well-differentiated tumors.

(C) The proportion of steroid receptor–positive tumors increases with advancing tumor stage.

(D) The presence of progesterone receptors in tumors predicts a response to progestin therapy.

(E) Steroid receptor status is not an important prognostic indicator of survival from endometrial carcinoma.

1403. Which of the following therapies is used in the treatment of stage IV endometrial cancer?

(A) surgery

(B) radiation therapy

(C) hormonal therapy

(D) multiagent chemotherapy

(E) all of the above

1404. A pulmonary nodule is discovered on the chest radiogram of a healthy 82-year-old woman. Four years ago, she was treated for endometrial adenocarcinoma. Excision of the nodule shows moderately differentiated endometrial adenocarcinoma–containing progesterone receptors. There is no other evidence of metastatic disease. You advise

(A) exploratory laparotomy

(B) lobectomy

(C) radiation therapy

(D) brachytherapy

(E) progestin therapy

1405. The most common uterine sarcoma is a(n)

(A) leiomyosarcoma

(B) endometrial stromal sarcoma

(C) endolymphatic stromal myosis

(D) malignant mixed müllerian tumor

(E) lymphoma

1406. Most uterine leiomyosarcomas are diagnosed by

   (A) sudden uterine enlargement
   (B) vaginal bleeding
   (C) pulmonary metastasis
   (D) histologic examination of excised myomas
   (E) pelvic pain

1407. A 55-year-old woman undergoes a total abdominal hysterectomy and bilateral salpingo-oophorectomy for a rapidly enlarging pelvic mass. A frozen section is sent, although the pathologist tells you he cannot distinguish leiomyosarcomas very well on frozen section. Nonetheless, the specimen looks very suspicious. You still have her abdomen open in the operating room. Which of the following statements is true?

   (A) Radical parametrectomy should be performed.
   (B) Lymphadenectomy should be performed.
   (C) Radiation to the pelvis has no effect on pelvic recurrence of sarcoma.
   (D) While radiation may be of benefit to prevent pelvic recurrence, if the sarcoma recurs, metastasis frequently occurs at distant sites.
   (E) Intraperitoneal radioactive phosphorus (^{32}P) should be considered for treatment.

1408. The incidence of sarcomatous degeneration in a uterine leiomyoma is

   (A) < 1%
   (B) 3%
   (C) 10%
   (D) 15%
   (E) 30%

1409. Treatment of uterine sarcomas is primarily by

   (A) surgery
   (B) radiation therapy
   (C) chemotherapy
   (D) hormonal therapy
   (E) chemohormonal therapy

Questions 1410 and 1411

A 49-year-old healthy woman experiences vaginal bleeding of 1 month's duration. Pelvic examination demonstrates an irregular uterus that is 12 gestational weeks' size. Six months ago, her physician was sure her pelvic examination was normal. A cervical Pap smear is normal. A D&C does not produce sufficient tissue for diagnosis. An abdominopelvic computed tomography (CT), IVP, blood chemistry and hematologic studies, and chest radiograph are normal. The patient does not request any further treatment, although another month passes and she is still bleeding.

1410. The most appropriate therapy is

   (A) observation
   (B) hysterectomy
   (C) radiation therapy
   (D) progestin therapy
   (E) chemotherapy

1411. The hysterectomy specimen shows a tumor with multiple rubbery wormlike outgrowths into the myometrium and periuterine vascular spaces. The tumor consists of cells with a spindle-like appearance resembling those of the uterine stroma. The tumor has 4 mitoses per 10 high-power fields. The diagnosis is

   (A) endometrial sarcoma
   (B) endometrial stromal nodule
   (C) endometrial stromal sarcoma (ESS)
   (D) uterine leiomyoma
   (E) intravenous leiomyomatosis

1412. Homologous malignant mixed müllerian tumors of the uterus consist of

   (A) carcinomatous epithelial elements and sarcomatous tissue foreign to the uterus
   (B) carcinomatous epithelial elements and sarcomatous tissue resembling normal uterine mesenchyme
   (C) benign epithelial elements and sarcomatous tissue resembling normal uterine mesenchyme
   (D) benign epithelial elements and sarcomatous tissue foreign to the uterus

(E) benign stromal elements and sarcomatous tissue resembling normal uterine mesenchyme

1413. A factor predisposing to the development of malignant mixed müllerian tumors is

(A) prenatal exposure to diethylstilbestrol (DES)
(B) exposure to mumps virus
(C) family history of ovarian cancer
(D) previous pelvic irradiation
(E) perineal use of talc

1414. Which of the following types of gynecologic cancer results in the greatest number of deaths?

(A) ovarian
(B) uterine
(C) cervical
(D) vaginal
(E) vulvar

1415. A 38-year-old nulliparous woman presents requesting a bilateral salpingo-oophorectomy. Her mother died of ovarian cancer at age 64, and her sister at age 48. There is no family history of other cancers. You advise her that her risk of developing ovarian cancer is

(A) 1 to 2%
(B) 5 to 7%
(C) 10 to 20%
(D) 30 to 40%
(E) > 50%

1416. The same patient gets on the Internet and returns asking about the hereditary types of epithelial ovarian cancer. Which statement is TRUE?

(A) A site-specific defect transmitting the trait for only ovarian carcinoma is common.
(B) A BrCA1 gene mutation increases her lifetime risk of ovarian cancer to 10%.
(C) Lynch type II cancer syndrome includes ovarian malignancy.

(D) Fifty percent of ovarian cancer is hereditary.

1417. Which of the following symptoms most commonly accompanies early ovarian carcinoma?

(A) pelvic pain
(B) bloating
(C) dysuria
(D) constipation
(E) none

1418. The cornerstone for detection of ovarian neoplasia is

(A) CA-125
(B) human chorionic gonadotropin (hCG)
(C) pelvic examination
(D) pelvic ultrasound
(E) alpha-fetoprotein

1419. The most important principle in the treatment of ovarian cancer is

(A) removal of all resectable disease
(B) examination of tumor cells cultured in vitro
(C) choice of chemotherapy
(D) calculation of radiation dose
(E) measurement of tumor hormone receptors

1420. The most important prognostic indicator of survival from advanced ovarian carcinoma is

(A) stage of disease
(B) grade of tumor differentiation
(C) nutritional status
(D) body mass index
(E) presence of sex steroid receptors

1421. The most widely used classification of ovarian neoplasia is based upon

(A) cell of origin
(B) hormonal activity
(C) degree of malignancy
(D) long-term prognosis
(E) severity of symptoms

1422. Ovarian neoplasms most commonly arise from

- (A) ovarian epithelium
- (B) ovarian stroma
- (C) ovarian germ cells
- (D) ovarian sex cords
- (E) metastatic disease

1423. Which of the following postmenopausal women is most protected from ovarian epithelial carcinoma?

- (A) a married woman using perineal talc powder
- (B) an unmarried woman with a history of breast cancer
- (C) a nun with a history of late menopause
- (D) a nulliparous woman with a history of regular menses
- (E) a multiparous woman who used OCPs and now is using postmenopausal estrogens

1424. Which of the following statements regarding ovarian epithelial carcinoma is TRUE?

- (A) The incidence of ovarian carcinoma increases with age until the seventh decade of life.
- (B) Elderly women are less likely than younger women to have disease diagnosed at an advanced stage.
- (C) Most women with ovarian cancer develop symptoms prior to dissemination of disease.
- (D) Seventy-five percent of all ovarian tumors in women over 50 years of age are malignant.
- (E) Twenty-five percent of all ovarian tumors in women between 20 and 40 years of age are malignant.

Questions 1425 and 1426

A 76-year-old woman has six courses of multiagent chemotherapy for her stage III, grade 3, ovarian epithelial carcinoma. She has no evidence of disease on examination and a normal CA-125. A second-look laparotomy is planned by surgeon A.

1425. Which of the following statements is TRUE?

- (A) There is a greater than 50% chance that there will be no pathologic evidence of disease.
- (B) She should not have a second look since she had advanced disease.
- (C) She has about a 50% chance of recurrence even if she had a negative second look.
- (D) Second-look laparotomy is not useful in evaluating chemotherapy response.
- (E) Further tumor debulking at second look does not improve survival.

1426. The patient decides to get a second opinion from surgeon B. Which of the following is appropriate?

- (A) observation
- (B) consolidation chemotherapy (giving different chemotherapy to continuously suppress possible recurrence)
- (C) second-look laparotomy
- (D) all of the above

1427. Calcific "sandlike" concretions associated with ovarian serous cystadenomas are called

- (A) papillomas
- (B) psammoma bodies
- (C) tubercles
- (D) giant cells
- (E) stones

1428. Which of the following ovarian epithelial tumors most commonly has external papillary excrescences?

- (A) mucinous cystadenomas
- (B) serous cystadenomas
- (C) dermoids
- (D) lutein cysts
- (E) Brenner tumors

1429. Brenner tumors tend to undergo which of the following types of transformation?

- (A) hemorrhagic
- (B) mucinous

(C) serous

(D) hyaline

(E) fibrous

Questions 1430 through 1432

A 35-year-old woman desiring fertility undergoes exploratory laparotomy for a 12-cm pelvic mass. At surgery, a large, lobulated, right ovarian mass is observed. It has a smooth external capsule and a bluish-gray appearance. The uterus, fallopian tubes, and left ovary appear normal. Abdominal exploration is negative for metastatic disease. A right salpingo-oophorectomy is performed. The tumor is opened intraoperatively and found to be divided by septa into lobules. Frozen section of the tumor shows a mucinous cystadenoma of low malignant potential.

1430. Which of the following statements regarding mucinous cystadenoma of low malignant potential is TRUE?

(A) Spread of the tumor outside the ovary occurs 30 to 40% of the time in the form of intraperitoneal growth of mucin-producing cells.

(B) It has a 30% incidence of bilaterality.

(C) It has a 5-year survival rate of 60%.

(D) It invades ovarian stroma.

(E) It may be mixed with invasive elements.

1431. Two days after surgery, you receive the pathology report of the ovarian tumor. It is a mucinous cystadenoma of low malignant potential mixed with well-differentiated carcinoma. The tumor has not invaded the ovarian capsule, lymphatics, or mesovarium. Omental and retroperitoneal lymph node biopsies and peritoneal washings are negative for tumor cells. You advise

(A) biopsy of the contralateral ovary

(B) removal of the uterus and contralateral adnexum

(C) postoperative chemotherapy

(D) postoperative radiation therapy

(E) no further therapy

1432. Suppose the final pathology report returns with the same findings as question 1431 except the tumor has invaded the ovarian capsule and lymphatics and omental biopsy and peritoneal washings are positive. You advise removal of the uterus and contralateral adnexa. You further advise

(A) postoperative chemotherapy

(B) she has a 74% 5-year survival rate

(C) observation

(D) no estrogen replacement therapy

(E) radiation

1433. A 54-year-old healthy woman comes for an annual examination. Her last menstrual period (LMP) was 4 years ago. The physical examination is normal. Pelvic examination shows vaginal atrophy and a small, mobile uterus. The right ovary is 2.5/4.5 cm in diameter. The left ovary is nonpalpable. Vaginal ultrasonography shows that the right ovary is similar in size to that of a premenopausal ovary. You advise that

(A) the ovaries of a postmenopausal woman are usually palpable

(B) the right ovary of a postmenopausal woman is usually palpable by right-handed examiners

(C) a palpable ovary in a postmenopausal woman is suspicious for malignancy

(D) the right ovary is still producing significant amounts of estrogen

(E) the vaginal ultrasound is an unnecessary diagnostic test

Questions 1434 through 1439

A 65-year-old woman has abdominal distention of 3 months' duration. Abdominal percussion causes a wavelike movement of fluid around a central tympanitic area. Pelvic examination shows a right adnexal mass. It is 8 cm in size, nodular, and fixed in the pelvis. The left ovary is nonpalpable. Blood chemistries, urinalysis, cervical Pap smear, mammography, and chest x-ray are normal. Stool guaiac examination and gastrointestinal studies are also normal. A serum CA-125 level is 250 U/mL (normal, < 35 U/mL).

1434. Which of the following statements regarding CA-125 is TRUE?

(A) It is a circulating antigenic marker for germ cell ovarian carcinoma.

(B) It is found in normal fetal and adult ovaries.

(C) It is secreted by mesothelial cells of the pleura, pericardium, and peritoneum.

(D) It is not useful in monitoring tumor progression.

(E) It is never elevated in the sera of women with benign diseases.

1435. The most likely diagnosis is

(A) gonadoblastoma

(B) Meigs' syndrome

(C) Krukenberg tumors

(D) serous cystadenocarcinoma

(E) endodermal sinus tumor

1436. Her surgical treatment should

(A) remove all gross disease if the risk of fatal complications is minimal

(B) avoid resection of bowel

(C) be done through a Pfannenstiel incision

(D) be done laparoscopically

(E) be done without a bowel preparation

1437. Exploratory laparotomy shows a tumor involving the right ovary. The left ovary appears normal. Several tumor implants are present on the peritoneal surfaces of small bowel and omentum. Biopsies of the peritoneal implants and ovarian tumor show moderately differentiated serous cystadenocarcinoma. There are no distant metastases, and the liver appears normal (see Figure 22–2). The stage of the tumor is

(A) 0

(B) I

(C) II

(D) III

(E) IV

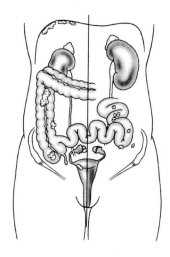

Figure 22–2.

1438. The immediate action after determining tumor stage is to

(A) terminate the operation

(B) remove the right ovary

(C) remove both ovaries

(D) remove uterus and both ovaries

(E) remove uterus, both ovaries, and all metastases

1439. The primary tumor and all metastases are surgically removed. You meet with the patient postoperatively to discuss her prognosis. You advise that

(A) the 5-year survival rate with no postoperative chemotherapy is about 70%

(B) the response to chemotherapy is related to the amount of residual disease after surgery

(C) older patients achieve results from postoperative chemotherapy superior to those of younger patients

(D) a second-look operation is performed in patients with incomplete response to chemotherapy

(E) few women thought to be free of disease after therapy have disease present at second-look operation

1440. Which of the following statements regarding pseudomyxoma peritonei is TRUE?

(A) The mean age of diagnosis is 70 years old.

(B) Chemotherapy is beneficial to survival.

(C) Radiation therapy is beneficial to survival.

(D) The appendix should be removed.

(E) The mortality rate is 10 to 20%.

1441. Which of the following ovarian tumors is the most common

(A) arrhenoblastoma

(B) granulosa cell tumor

(C) granulosa–thecal cell tumor

(D) endodermal sinus tumor

(E) mucinous cystadenoma

1442. What percentage of germ cell tumors in women under age 21 are malignant?

(A) 10%

(B) 30%

(C) 50%

(D) 70%

(E) 90%

1443. You are called to the operating room by the general surgeons at a local children's hospital. A 4-year-old girl with acute abdominal pain was thought to have appendicitis; instead, she has a large right ovary. The most likely diagnosis is

(A) germ cell tumor

(B) epithelial stromal tumor

(C) sex cord stromal tumor

(D) non-neoplastic follicle or theca–lutein cyst

(E) metastatic tumor

1444. An 18-year-old woman with a history of pelvic inflammatory disease (PID) undergoes a laparoscopic ovarian cystectomy for a 5-cm ovarian mass containing a tooth. The contents of the cyst spill during removal and contain thick sebaceous material and hair. Copious irrigation was used to remove this material. She is noted to have marked bowel adhesions in the pelvis, which require dissection to reach the ovarian cyst. Four days postoperatively she returns to the emergency de-

partment with a temperature of 101.1°F, abdominal pain, nausea, and vomiting. White blood cell count is 15.0. What is the most likely diagnosis?

(A) ileus

(B) narcotic-induced constipation

(C) chemical peritonitis

(D) influenza

(E) bowel perforation

1445. An 11-year-old girl presents with abdominal pain, and a right 5-cm solid ovarian mass is found. The alpha-fetoprotein level is elevated. You counsel the girl and parents that

(A) 70% of cases are stage I

(B) the tumor is common and accounts for half of all germ cell tumors

(C) bilateral salpingo-oophorectomy is indicated since bilateral tumors are common

(D) no surgery is indicated until after puberty

(E) if the tumor is stage I, no further therapy is needed

1446. Which of the following statements regarding germ cell tumors is TRUE?

(A) They are commonly seen during the fifth and sixth decades of life.

(B) They represent one half of all ovarian tumors.

(C) They occur only in the ovary.

(D) They are commonly malignant.

(E) They cause abdominal enlargement in children.

1447. The most common germ cell tumor is a(n)

(A) dysgerminoma

(B) endodermal sinus tumor

(C) embryonal carcinoma

(D) choriocarcinoma

(E) mature teratoma

1448. Rokitansky's protuberances

(A) stimulate vaginal development

(B) are solid projections within mature teratomas

(C) are required to diagnose a dysgerminoma

(D) produce alpha-fetoprotein

(E) produce hCG

1449. Which of the following statements regarding immature teratomas is TRUE?

(A) They are the most common malignant germ cell tumor.

(B) They are commonly bilateral.

(C) They produce alpha-fetoprotein.

(D) They commonly occur during the first two decades of life.

(E) They contain malignant squamous cell elements.

1450. A 56-year-old postmenopausal woman complains of paroxysmal flushing of the face and neck. Facial flushing is associated with colicky abdominal pain with diarrhea and shortness of breath. She has been told by her friends that she needs estrogen replacement therapy. Physical examination is normal. Pelvic examination demonstrates a 5-cm right adnexal mass. The most appropriate diagnostic test is

(A) a serum FSH

(B) a serum TSH

(C) serum thyroid function studies

(D) a urinary 5-hydroxyindole acetic acid

(E) urinary catecholamines

Questions 1451 and 1452

A 26-year-old nulliparous woman is seen in the emergency department for acute abdominal pain. Her vital signs are: blood pressure, 90/50; pulse, 120 bpm; and temperature, afebrile. Abdominal examination shows right lower quadrant tenderness with rebound. Pelvic examination demonstrates a painful 10-cm right adnexal mass. A serum pregnancy test is negative. A hematocrit is 24% (normal, 35 to 45%). Exploratory laparotomy confirms a he-

moperitoneum. A smooth right ovarian tumor is bleeding from its ruptured capsule. Inspection of the uterus, fallopian tubes, and left ovary is normal. A right salpingo-oophorectomy is performed. Frozen section of the tumor shows primitive germ cells with intervening connective tissue infiltrated by lymphocytes.

1451. The tumor is most likely a(n)

(A) dysgerminoma

(B) endodermal sinus tumor

(C) choriocarcinoma

(D) embryonal carcinoma

(E) mature teratoma

1452. Which of the following statements about the above tumor is TRUE?

(A) It occurs in women of all ages with equal frequency.

(B) It has a bilaterality rate of less than 1%.

(C) It is usually resistant to radiotherapy.

(D) It occurs in combination with other germ cell elements.

(E) It has a poor survival rate following unilateral adnexectomy for stage I disease.

1453. Schiller–Duvall bodies are found in which of the following germ cell tumors?

(A) endodermal sinus tumor

(B) polyembryoma

(C) mature teratoma

(D) immature teratoma

(E) dysgerminoma

1454. Which of the following neoplasms is classified as an embryonal ovarian tumor?

(A) endodermal sinus tumor

(B) polyembryoma

(C) dysgerminoma

(D) sarcoma

(E) serous cystadenoma

1455. Gonadoblastomas consist of

(A) stromal cells only

(B) mucin-producing cells and stromal cells

(C) germ cells and sex cord–stromal elements

(D) germ cells and germinal epithelium

(E) germinal epithelium and stromal cells

Questions 1456 through 1458

An 18-year-old woman with primary amenorrhea complains of a right inguinal mass. Physical examination demonstrates a normal-appearing female. Bilateral breast development is present. Axillary and pubic hair are sparse. The vulva appears normal, but the vagina ends in a blind pouch. The uterus is nonpalpable by rectal examination.

1456. The right inguinal mass is most likely a(n)

(A) lymph node

(B) gonad

(C) endometrioma

(D) cyst of Nuck's canal

(E) inguinal hernia

1457. Which of the following tumors is most likely to occur in the right inguinal mass?

(A) endodermal sinus tumor

(B) dysgerminoma

(C) choriocarcinoma

(D) gonadoblastoma

(E) Sertoli–Leydig cell tumor

1458. Malignant changes occur in what percentage of streak ovaries when a Y chromosome is present?

(A) 5%

(B) 25%

(C) 45%

(D) 65%

(E) 85%

1459. A 16-year-old phenotypic girl is seen for primary amenorrhea. Karyotyping shows 46,XY. In counseling, you advise gonadectomy

(A) when she is finished growing

(B) if the gonads are not in the normal location in the pelvis

(C) primarily because of the risk of malignancy

(D) primarily because there is no chance of pregnancy

(E) primarily because she will become virilized

1460. The patient in the preceding question has a gonadectomy. The pathology showed gonadoblastoma. At her 6-week postoperative check, she complains of feeling hot and getting flushed several times a day with no other symptoms. What is the most likely diagnosis?

(A) infection

(B) estrogen deficiency

(C) hyperthyroidism

(D) normal postoperative course

(E) carcinoid tumor

1461. A 5-year-old girl experiences early breast development. She is taller than her peers. Her mother has noticed blood at the girl's introitus. Serum gonadotropin levels are low and are unchanged after intravenous administration of gonadotropin-releasing hormone (GnRH). The most likely diagnosis is a(n)

(A) Sertoli–Leydig cell tumor

(B) granulosa cell tumor

(C) hilar cell tumor

(D) lipid tumor

(E) fibroma

1462. Granulosa cell tumors may be associated with

(A) endometrial hyperplasia

(B) congenital adrenal hyperplasia (CAH)

(C) Cushing syndrome

(D) PCOS

(E) dysgenetic gonads

1463. Reinke crystalloids are found in

(A) dysgerminomas

(B) granulosa cell tumors

(C) serous cystadenomas

(D) mature dermoids

(E) hilar cell (Leydig cell) tumors

1464. Metastatic tumors to the ovary rarely originate from the

(A) breast

(B) stomach

(C) large intestine

(D) uterus

(E) vagina

1465. A 75-year-old woman has bilateral, solid adnexal masses. Mammography is normal. Gastrointestinal studies show a stomach lesion suspicious for malignancy. The most likely diagnosis is

(A) Pick's adenoma

(B) Krukenberg tumor

(C) Brenner tumor

(D) struma ovarii

(E) carcinoid

1466. Which of the following statements is TRUE regarding ovarian leiomyomas?

(A) They account for 10% of benign ovarian neoplasms.

(B) They are usually vary large tumors.

(C) They are often malignant.

(D) They may arise from smooth muscle cells in the walls of blood vessels.

(E) Histologically, they appear different than leiomyomas of the uterus.

DIRECTIONS (Questions 1467 through 1470): Each of the numbered items or incomplete statements in this section is followed by answers or by completions of the statement. Select the answers or completions that may apply.

1467. Which four of the following conditions are likely to be associated with endometrial hyperplasia?

(A) hyperprolactinemia

(B) exogenous estrogen use

(C) granulosa–thecal cell tumor

(D) CAH

(E) PCOS

1468. Which four of the following factors are likely to adversely affect survival from stage I ovarian epithelial carcinoma?

(A) ascites

(B) tumor cell type

(C) tumor grade

(D) pelvic adhesions

(E) psammoma bodies

1469. Which four of the following tumors are likely to be hormonally active?

(A) Sertoli–Leydig cell tumor

(B) granulosa cell tumor

(C) hilar cell tumor

(D) fibroma

(E) thecoma

1470. Which four of the following neoplasms may cause androgen excess?

(A) nongestational choriocarcinoma

(B) embryonal carcinoma

(C) mixed germ cell tumor

(D) granulosa cell tumor

(E) gonadoblastoma

DIRECTIONS (Questions 1471 through 1489): Each set of items in this section consists of a list of lettered headings followed by several numbered words or phrases. For each numbered word or phrase, select the ONE lettered option that is most closely associated with it. Each lettered option may be selected once, more than once, or not at all.

Questions 1471 and 1472

Match the single BEST therapy for the case described.

(A) danazol

(B) progestin

(C) clomiphene citrate

(D) hysterectomy

(E) radical hysterectomy

(F) radiation

(G) no further treatment

1471. A 37-year-old female has a D&C for irregular bleeding. The pathology shows simple hyperplasia without atypia.

1472. A 48-year-old nulliparous female has a 20-year history of oligomenorrhea and hirsutism. She recently had an episode of menorrhagia. Office endometrial biopsy shows complex hyperplasia with severe atypia.

Questions 1473 through 1475

Match the rate of progression to endometrial cancer from the hyperplasia type.

  (A) 1 to 2%
  (B) 3 to 9%
  (C) 10 to 19%
  (D) 20 to 29%
  (E) 30 to 49%

1473. Complex hyperplasia

1474. A complex atypical hyperplasia

1475. Simple hyperplasia without atypia

Questions 1476 through 1479

  (A) serous tumor
  (B) mucinous tumor
  (C) endometrioid tumor
  (D) clear cell tumor
  (E) Brenner tumor

1476. The ovarian epithelial neoplasm with the lowest malignancy rate

1477. The ovarian epithelial neoplasm with the highest rate of bilaterality

1478. The ovarian epithelial neoplasm similar in histologic appearance to primary tubal carcinoma

Question 1479

  (A) epithelial cell
  (B) germ cell
  (C) sex cord–stromal cell
  (D) nonspecific mesenchyme

  (E) Krukenberg tumor
  (F) Brenner tumor

1479. Which of the above types of ovarian cancer is most likely to occur in a 65-year-old woman with a pelvic mass and malignant ascites? Mammography and gastrointestinal studies are normal.

Questions 1480 and 1481

  (A) radiation therapy
  (B) chemotherapy
  (C) both of the above
  (D) neither of the above

Which of the above therapies for ovarian cancer increases the risk of

1480. Bone marrow suppression?

1481. Bowel obstruction?

Questions 1482 through 1486

  (A) dysgerminoma
  (B) endodermal sinus tumor
  (C) choriocarcinoma
  (D) mature teratoma
  (E) struma ovarii
  (F) carcinoid
  (G) granulosa

Which of the above germ cell tumors is most likely to produce large amounts of

1482. Thyroxine

1483. Alpha-fetoprotein

1484. hCG

1485. Lactic dehydrogenase (LDH)

1486. Inhibin

Questions 1487 through 1489

A 25-year-old nulliparous woman has recently noticed rapid growth of facial hair. In the past 6 months, she has lost hair in the temporal regions and has noticed a deepening of her voice. Menstrual cycles occur at 28-day intervals. Irregular vaginal bleeding began 6 months ago. Physical examination shows temporal hair recession and coarse hair on the upper lip, chin, sternum, and lower abdomen. The breasts are small. Pelvic examination demonstrates clitoromegaly. Bimanual examination is difficult because of patient compliance. A pregnancy test is negative. Serum luteinizing hormone (LH) and FSH levels are 3 mIU/mL (normal, 3 to 28 mIU/mL) and 3 mIU/mL (normal, 2 to 17 mIU/mL). A serum testosterone value is 3.0 ng/mL (normal, < 0.8 ng/mL). Serum dehydroepiandrosterone sulfate (DHEAS) and 17-hydroxyprogesterone levels are normal.

(A) pituitary tumor

(B) PCOS

(C) stromal hyperthecosis

(D) Sertoli–Leydig cell tumor

(E) Krukenberg tumor

(F) lipid cell tumor

(G) granulosa cell tumor

(H) gynandroblastoma

With regard to this patient, which of the preceding conditions is most likely to be associated with

1487. 4-cm tumor composed of well-developed tubular structures separated by luteinized stroma

1488. 3-cm sex cord–stromal tumor consisting of both male and female cell types

1489. 2-cm tumor capable of producing glucocorticoids

Answers and Explanations

1375. (B) D&C has been the traditional method used to diagnose abnormalities of the endometrial lining. Dilation refers to opening of the cervix with a series of dilators to gain access to the intrauterine cavity: curettage refers to scraping of the uterine lining to obtain endometrial tissue. Unfortunately, pain accompanying cervical dilation usually requires that D&C be performed with paracervical or general anesthesia. D&C has been replaced by endometrial biopsy techniques performed as an office procedure. Endometrial biopsy has about a 90% accuracy in detecting endometrial hyperplasia and cancer. Techniques that obtain endometrial tissue are more accurate than those relying on endometrial cytology. Careful sampling of the intrauterine cavity by some method is mandatory, since some women with the histologic diagnosis of adenomatous hyperplasia have coexisting endometrial carcinoma. When an endometrial biopsy cannot be completed for technical reasons, a fractional D&C must be performed. Hysteroscopy is usually done at the same time as D&C to visualize and remove pathologic findings such as polyps or submucous fibroids. Transvaginal sonography is currently utilized in the evaluation of abnormal bleeding. When combined with injecting saline into the uterine cavity via the cervix (sonohysterography), abnormalities in the endometrial cavity such as submucous fibroids or polyps can be identified. However, no tissue is obtained for pathologic diagnosis. Also, an endocrinopathy causing anovulation is the most likely reason for the patient's irregular vaginal bleeding. Endometrial biopsy might prove this if proliferative endometrium is seen in the luteal phase of the menstrual cycle.

1376. (B) The most frequent symptoms of endometrial hyperplasia is abnormal vaginal bleeding. Fortunately, this usually occurs early and allows early detection.

1377. (D) Endometrial hyperplasia is characterized by proliferation of glandular and stromal elements with focal glandular crowding at the expense of stroma. It commonly undergoes spontaneous regression. Endometrial hyperplasia may be either simple or complex, depending on the extent of glandular crowding. Regardless of architectural pattern, cells lining the glands may exhibit varying degrees (mild to severe) of cytologic atypia, defined by nuclear enlargement, hyperchromasia, or irregularity in shape. Cytologic atypia is the most important morphologic characteristic of endometrial hyperplasia, which determines its risk of progression to invasive carcinoma. A new terminology to describe endometrial hyperplasias and their premalignant potential was adopted in 1988 by the International Society of Gynecologic Pathologists (ISGYP) (Table 22–1). Endometrial hyperplasia with severe cytologic atypia is also called carcinoma in situ because it represents a stage preceding stromal invasion in which abnormal cells are confined to the endometrial glands.

Table 22–1. Classifications of Endometrial Hyperplasias

Traditional	International Society of Gynecologic Pathologists
Cystic hyperplasia	Simple hyperplasia
Adenomatous hyperplasia	Complex hyperplasia (adenomatous hyperplasia without cytologic atypia)
Atypical adenomatous hyperplasia	Atypical hyperplasia (adenomatous hyperplasia with cytologic atypia)
Architectural atypia (mild, moderate, severe)	
Cytologic atypia (mild, moderate, severe)	

1378. (C) Endometrial hyperplasia causes the endometrium to thicken and acquire a velvety, lobulated texture with a yellowish appearance. Dilation of endometrial glands often occurs in a hyperplastic endometrium and is referred to as cystic hyperplasia (simple hyperplasia [ISGYP]), or "Swiss cheese hyperplasia." It is considered weakly premalignant because it progresses to endometrial carcinoma in less than 0.5% of women. The increased stromal thickness distinguishes cystic hyperplasia from inactive endometrium with cystic change (cystic atrophy). The latter normally occurs in postmenopausal women and is not a hyperplastic condition. Progestin administration to women with endometrial hyperplasia usually corrects the hyperplasia and the irregular vaginal bleeding.

1379. (C) Endometrial polyps arise as fingerlike endometrial projections and commonly occur under conditions of unopposed estrogen stimulation. They may be small in size (1 to 2 mm) or large enough to protrude through the cervix. Although frequently asymptomatic, abnormal bleeding is the most common symptom of an endometrial polyp. Pelvic pain may also occur if extrusion of the polyp through the cervix causes cervical dilation. Their histologic pattern consists of glandular and stromal elements and a central vascular channel surrounded on three sides by epithelium. Two thirds of endometrial polyps contain immature endometrium unresponsive to progesterone, occasionally associated with cystic hyperplasia. Endometrial polyps originate from functional endometrium undergoing cyclic histologic changes. Less than 1% of endometrial polyps are malignant. The risk of developing endometrial cancer in women with endometrial polyps increases twofold. Several endometrial polyps can occur together and may not be removed entirely by using a forceps at the time of D&C. Endometrial polyps frequently coexist with other endometrial pathology. It is important to separately examine polyps and endometrial lining to determine the source of irregular vaginal bleeding.

1380. (E) Patient age and degree of cytologic atypia are the most important factors in management planning of endometrial hyperplasia. Recent evidence suggests that the degree of cytologic atypia is the most important determinant of premalignant potential. One study found that 18% of women with endometrial hyperplasia developed endometrial carcinoma within 1 to 30 years of initial diagnosis. In women of childbearing age desiring fertility, endometrial hyperplasia with or without cytologic atypia may be treated with progestins (e.g., OCs, medroxyprogesterone acetate, megestrol acetate). An endometrial biopsy should be repeated in 3 to 6 months. If repeat endometrial sampling shows normal endometrium, progestins may be continued or the patient may be observed without hormone therapy for evidence of ovulation. Anovulatory patients interested in childbearing should be treated with ovulatory agents. Persistent symptomatology despite adequate therapy requires hysteroscopy combined with D&C to confirm adequacy of endometrial sampling and to identify coexisting uterine pathology. Perimenopausal women may be treated by progestins or hysterectomy, depending on severity of hyperplasia, desire for sterilization, or persistence of symptoms. Patients with moderate to severe atypical hyperplasia should consider hysterectomy. Individuals with lesser disease may receive progestin therapy but require hysterectomy if symptoms persist to eliminate the possibility of concomitant endometrial carcinoma or discover ovarian estrogen-producing tumors. Unless they are poor surgical candidates, most postmenopausal women with endometrial hyperplasia should consider hysterectomy with bilateral salpingo-oophorectomy, since uterine or ovarian disease may coexist.

1381. (D) This patient with PCOS is anovulatory, as confirmed by the absence of a biphasic shift in BBTs. Acyclic estrogen production unopposed by progesterone stimulates endometrial proliferation, increasing the risk of developing endometrial hyperplasia and carcinoma. In patients of reproductive age, OCs can be used if contraception is desired. Otherwise, progestins are prescribed. A biopsy should be repeated in 3 to 6 months. The most convenient method of ovulation induction in women with PCOS who desire pregnancy is clomiphene citrate. Intramuscular administration of hMGs is expensive and inconvenient and requires close monitoring.

1382. (C) An endometrial stripe of less than 5 mm in a postmenopausal woman confers no risk of cancer. A stripe of more than 10 mm correlates with a 10 to 20% risk of hyperplasia or cancer. The data on endometrial stripe thickness for premenopausal women is more difficult to interpret, but it appears that less than 12 mm confers little or no risk of cancer. A hysterectomy is not appropriate until a tissue diagnosis is obtained.

1383. (C) Cystic hyperplasia often occurs in a hyperplastic endometrium in menopausal or postmenopausal women. It will regress spontaneously in many cases. Complex atypical hyperplasia would show crowded glands although still architecturally ordered but with nuclear atypia. Adenocanthoma is atypical endometrioid adenocarcinoma with at least 10% of the tumor containing benign-appearing squamous metaplasia. Adenoacanthoma and clear cell and squamous cell carcinoma would all have malignant features on histology.

1384. (B) The mass the internist describes is likely to be a polyp. It could be endocervical or endometrial in origin, and the latter type can prolapse through the cervix. Adenomatous polyps may antedate endometrial hyperplasia, and abnormalities range from benign polyps to frank adenocarcinoma. The appropriate therapy is to remove the mass for pathologic evaluation. This can be done simply without performing a cone biopsy. Even with a negative Pap smear, the mass should be removed.

1385. (B) Progestins oppose estrogen action in endometrial tissue by decreasing the number of estrogen receptors and changing the lining to a secretory endometrium. Progesterone receptors are high in late proliferative and early secretory phases but even higher in endometrial hyperplastic states. The regression of endometrial hyperplasia often occurs within 3 months. There are some reports of disease being successfully controlled for more than 3 years, even after only 6 weeks of therapy. However, if an endocrinopathy (such as polycystic ovarian disease), obesity, estrogen-producing tumor, or other factor contributing to chronic endometrial exposure to estrogen still exists, the disease is likely to recur. Therapy with progestins can be continued long term.

1386. (E) A neoplasm is defined as abnormal tissue growth that persists and grows independently of its surrounding structures. The most common uterine neoplasms are benign leiomyomas. They are found anywhere in the uterus and may be pedunculated.

1387. (A) Uterine cancer is the most common gynecologic malignancy and represents the fourth most frequent malignancy in American women, following breast, colorectal, and lung cancer. The incidence of uterine cancer is two- and threefold that of cancer of the ovary and cervix. Endometrial adenocarcinoma is the most common uterine cancer. It varies in histologic type and degree of differentiation. Endometrial carcinoma usually develops after menopause (ages 50 to 59 years) as malignant glandular epithelium invades endometrial stroma. The remaining 5% of uterine malignancies are mostly sarcomas, derived from mesenchymal components of endometrial stroma, myometrium, or uterine connective tissue.

1388. (D) Breast cancer is the leading gynecologic cause of cancer death. It is also the primary cause of all deaths in women 40 to 44 years old. Approximately 1 in 9 (11%) American women develops breast carcinoma during her lifetime; 175,000 new cases are diagnosed annually, and about 44,000 women die of their disease each year. Endometrial carcinoma is the next most common gynecologic cancer, with 35,000 new cases per year in the

United States. Ovarian and cervical cancer occur less frequently than uterine cancer but are far more lethal. Approximately 12,000, 7,000, and 3,000 deaths occur annually from ovarian, cervical, and uterine cancers, respectively. Vulvar cancer is even less common.

1389. (B) Evidence suggests an association between endometrial cancer and prolonged endometrial exposure to estrogen unopposed by progesterone. Chronic anovulation accompanying PCOS and obesity increases the risk of developing endometrial carcinoma. During the 1970s, an increased frequency of endometrial cancer was also observed in postmenopausal women receiving exogenous estrogens without progestins.

1390. (C) Endometrial hyperplasia with cytologic atypia may progress to invasive carcinoma but usually is treatable by progesterone therapy, ovulatory agents, curettage, or hysterectomy. The rates at which simple, complex, simple atypical, and complex atypical hyperplasia progress to carcinoma are 1%, 3%, 8%, and 29%, respectively.

1391. (E) The median age of women with endometrial cancer is 60 years. The highest incidence of disease onset is in the sixth and seventh decades. Two to five percent of endometrial cancers occur before age 40, particularly in women with a history of chronic anovulation.

1392. (A) A chest radiograph should be performed because the lung is the main site of extrauterine spread from endometrial carcinoma (36% of cases). Once the diagnosis of endometrial cancer has been confirmed, further investigation for metastatic disease includes abdominopelvic computed tomography (CT scan), possibly IVP, liver function studies, bone and brain scans (if localized symptoms exist), and barium enema with sigmoidoscopy (if bowel symptoms occur). Preoperative evaluation also includes hematologic and renal studies, serum electrolytes, and a coagulation profile. A cervical Pap smear and endocervical curettage is performed to ex-

clude the presence of concomitant cervical pathology. Any cervical or vaginal lesions are biopsied. Pelvic ultrasound is helpful if an adnexal mass is suspected.

1393. (C) Adenocarcinoma of the endometrium with extension to the cervix is a stage II lesion (Table 22–2).

Table 22–2. Corpus Cancer Staging (Adopted 1988)

Stage	Characteristic
IA	Tumor limited to endometrium
IB	Invasion to < 1/2 myometrium
IC	Invasion to ≥ 1/2 myometrium
IIA	Endocervical glandular involvement only
IIB	Cervical stromal invasion
IIIA	Tumor invades serosa and/or adnexae, and/or positive peritoneal cytology
IIIB	Vaginal metastases
IIIC	Metastases to pelvic and/or para-aortic lymph nodes
IVA	Tumor invasion of bladder and/or bowel mucosa
IVB	Distant metastases including intra-abdominal and/or inguinal lymph node (See Figure 22–3.)

1394. (A) Endometrial adenoacanthoma refers to adenocarcinoma with benign squamous components. The squamous component results from metaplasia and should comprise more than 10% of the tumor. Adenoacanthoma comprises about 5% of endometrial carcinomas. The prognosis of adenoacanthoma is similar to that of adenocarcinoma of comparable differentiation. Adenoacanthoma should not be confused with adenosquamous carcinoma, in which both glandular and squamous components are malignant. Adenosquamous carcinoma has a poorer prognosis than either adenocarcinoma or adenoacanthoma.

1395. (D) About 75% of endometrial cancers are pure adenocarcinomas. Variants of adenocarcinoma with benign squamous elements (adenoacanthoma) or secretory cells (mucinous adenocarcinomas) have similar biological activities (Table 22–3). Adenocarcinomas containing malignant squamous epithelium (adenosquamous carcinoma), papillary structures (papillary serous adenocarcinoma), or polyhedral epithelial cells (clear cell carcinoma) carry a poorer prognosis.

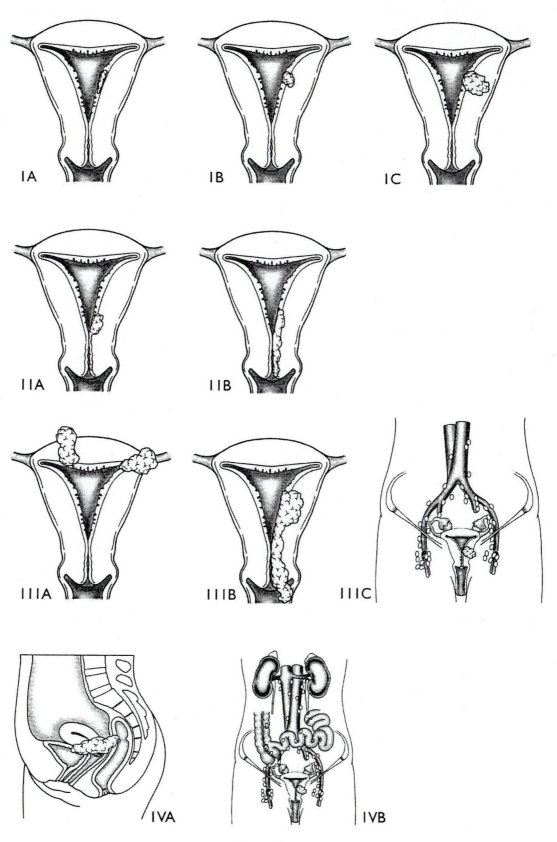

Figure 22–3.

Table 22–3. Endometrial Primary Adenocarcinomas

Typical endometrioid adenocarcinoma

    Adenocarcinoma (squamous metaplasia)

    Adenosquamous carcinoma (mixed adenocarcinoma and squamous cell carcinoma)

Papillary serous endometrial carcinoma

Clear cell adenocarcinoma

Mucinous adenocarcinoma

Adenosquamous carcinoma

Undifferentiated carcinoma

Mixed carcinoma

1396. **(A)** Seventy to seventy-five percent of endometrial cancers are diagnosed as stage I disease. Ten to fifteen percent of endometrial cancers are stage II at the time of diagnosis, while the remaining 10 to 15% are stages III and IV. The ability of women to seek medical advice at the onset of abnormal vaginal bleeding probably accounts for the early detection of disease.

1397. **(D)** Important prognostic indicators of survival from endometrial carcinoma include (1) stage of disease at the time of detection, (2) grade of tumor differentiation, (3) lymphatic/hematogenous spread, and (4) tumor type. Stage of disease is inversely correlated with 5-year survival rate (stage I, 86%; stage II, 66%; stage III, 44%; stage IV, 16%). In stage I disease, depth of myometrial invasion by tumor is an important prognostic factor. Tumor penetration beyond the middle half of the myometrium adversely affects survival and relapse rates. Malignant cells in peritoneal washings are found in 12 to 15% of women with early disease by clinical assessment and reduce the chance for survival. Other tumor indicators of poor prognosis are size (> 2 cm), absence of sex steroid receptors, and DNA ploidy. Many of these prognostic indicators are interrelated and occur together. Five-year survival rates range from 95% (in women with well-differentiated tumors that do not invade the myometrium) to 20% (in patients with poorly differentiated tumors that invade deeply into the myometrium). CA-125 is useful only when it is initially elevated, which occurs in 20% of clinical stage I or II patients with endometrial cancer.

1398. **(A)** Adenocarcinoma of the endometrium usually develops as proliferating glandular epithelium invades endometrial stroma. Malignant epithelial glands contain cells that are increased in size, are pseudostratified, and have enlarged nuclei with clumped nuclear chromatin. Crowding of glandular elements ("back-to-back glands") results from loss of stroma between these abnormal glands. The grade of the tumor is determined by the degree of abnormality of glandular architecture. Well-differentiated tumors (grade 1) have a glandular pattern similar to that of normal endometrium. Moderately (grade 2) and poorly differentiated (grade 3) carcinomas have glandular elements mixed with small or large amounts of solid areas of tumor. Tumor grade is one of the most sensitive indicators of prognosis. It correlates with depth of myometrial invasion. Poorly differentiated tumors of any size have a greater propensity for extrauterine spread than do well-differentiated tumors.

1399. **(E)** In women with stage I and II disease, exploratory laparotomy with total (not radical) abdominal hysterectomy and bilateral salpingo-oophorectomy treats early disease and determines extent of disease spread for planning of postoperative therapy. Peritoneal washings for malignant cells are obtained upon entering the abdomen. The uterus is opened in the operating room and examined for evidence of tumor invasion into the myometrium. Removal of pelvic and para-aortic nodes is also performed if tumor is found to be moderately or poorly differentiated, or if malignancy invades beyond the inner half of the myometrium. Bilateral salpingo-oophorectomy should be performed as 6 to 10% of patients with clinical stage I disease will have metastasis to the adnexa.

1400. **(B)** Treatment of early endometrial cancer depends on prognostic factors, pattern of disease spread, and probability of metastatic disease. The presence of extrauterine disease (nodal and/or adnexal metastases, malignant cells in peritoneal cytology) is associated with a high rate of disease recurrence. Generally, women with stage IA, grade 1 or 2 lesions are adequately treated with surgery alone since the risk of metastatic disease is low (4%). However, patients with stage I disease and poor prognostic factors (e.g., poorly differentiated tumor, tumor invasion beyond the inner half of the myometrium, nodal and/or adnexal metastases, malignant peritoneal cytology) and women with stage II disease involving the cervical stroma benefit from postoperative radiation therapy. Radiotherapy may be:

- External irradiation (external beam pelvic radiation)—reduces the risk of recurrent disease at the vaginal vault and pelvic wall. The radiation field may be extended to the para-aortic region in patients with nodal metastasis in this area.
- Brachytherapy (a form of radiation therapy in which the radioactive source is placed in close proximity to tumor)—reduces the risk of recurrent disease at the vaginal vault but not the pelvic wall. A common form of brachytherapy used in the treatment of endometrial cancer is intravaginal irradiation (radium, cesium, or cobalt).
- Intraperitoneal radioactive phosphorus (^{32}P)—advocated by some investigators for women with stage I disease in whom positive peritoneal washings for malignant cells are the only evidence of extrauterine disease. The use of radiation therapy is individualized to balance the risk of disease recurrence with the incidence of treatment side effects. The use of adjunctive hormones or cytotoxic agents to prevent systemic recurrence in high-risk patients with early disease is controversial.

1401. **(B)** Early and late complications from radiation therapy occur. Acute reactions, including cessation of mitotic activity and tissue edema with or without necrosis, may be associated with cystitis (hematuria, urgency, frequency), proctosigmoiditis (tenesmus, diarrhea, hematochezia), enteritis (nausea, vomiting, diarrhea, abdominal pain), and bone marrow suppression. Chronic reactions to radiation, occurring 6 to 24 months after completion of

radiation, include obliteration of small blood vessels, fibrosis, and reduced number of epithelial and parenchymal cells. Chronic reactions may be associated with enteropathy (proctosigmoiditis, ulceration, fistula, stenosis), vaginal vault necrosis and/or stenosis, and urologic injuries (cystitis, vesicovaginal fistula, uterovaginal fistula, ureteric stenosis).

1402. **(D)** Many endometrial adenocarcinomas contain estrogen and/or progesterone receptors. Steroid receptor levels in these tumors are generally lower than in normal endometrium. Steroid receptor status is a prognostic indicator of survival from endometrial carcinoma. Steroid receptor levels in endometrial cancer correlate with degree of tumor differentiation and are highest in well-differentiated tumors. The proportion of receptor-negative tumors increases with advancing tumor stage. Progestin therapy (medroxyprogesterone acetate, megestrol acetate) is more effective in treating recurrent or metastatic disease continuing progesterone receptors than receptor-negative tumors.

1403. **(E)** Treatment of women with stage III and IV disease may include surgery, radiation therapy, hormone therapy, and multiagent chemotherapy. Chemohormonal therapy is used to treat systemic disease. Overall, removal of the primary tumor is desirable in most situations, even with metastatic abdominal disease. Surgery is not curative but cytoreduction of tumor burden may improve the response to adjuvant therapy. Therapy must be individualized to suit the clinical condition of the patient.

1404. **(E)** Ninety percent of recurrences of endometrial adenocarcinoma occur within 5 years of the initial diagnosis. Half of the recurrences occur in the pelvis and vagina, while the most frequent sites of nonpelvic metastases are lung (17%), upper abdomen (10%), and bone (6%). One third of recurrent endometrial cancers have sex steroid receptors. High-dose progestin therapy (medroxyprogesterone acetate, megestrol acetate) with or without chemotherapy is often effective in controlling advanced or recurrent disease-containing progesterone receptors. The use of progestin combined with tamoxifen, an anti-estrogen, in these women is controversial but attractive since tamoxifen increases the progesterone receptor content of some tumors. Tumors without sex steroid receptors are usually treated with cytotoxic agents since their response to hormone therapy is poor. Some chemotherapeutic agents used singly and in combination for treatment of endometrial cancer include doxorubicin (adriamycin) and cisplatin. These are the most active agents. Other agents that might be used include paclitaxel and ifosfamide.

1405. **(A)** Uterine sarcomas consist of malignant mesenchymal (sarcomatous) components arising from endometrial stroma, myometrium, or uterine connective tissue. They comprise 2 to 6% of uterine cancers and are classified according to whether the sarcomatous element resembles tissue indigenous (homologous) or foreign (heterologous) to the uterus and exists alone (pure) or admixed with malignant epithelial (carcinomatous) tissue (Table 22–4). The most common types of uterine sarcoma in decreasing order of frequency are leiomyosarcoma (45%), malignant müllerian mixed tumor (40%), endometrial stromal tumors (10%), and other sarcomas (5%).

Table 22–4. Classification of Uterine Sarcoma

I. Pure sarcoma
    A. Homologous
        1. Leiomyosarcoma
        2. Endometrial stromal sarcoma
            a. Low-grade: endolymphatic stromal myosis
            b. High-grade: endometrial stromal sarcoma
    B. Heterologous
        1. Rhabdomyosarcoma
        2. Chondrosarcoma
        3. Osteosarcoma
        4. Liposarcoma
II. Malignant mixed müllerian tumors
    A. Homologous (carcinosarcoma): carcinoma + homologous sarcoma
    B. Heterologous: carcinoma + heterologous sarcoma
III. Other sarcomas

1406. **(D)** Although D&C occasionally diagnoses tumor extending into the uterine cavity, most leiomyosarcomas are discovered at the time of surgery for removal of a rapidly enlarging uterine tumor. The incidence of leiomyosarcoma found at the time of surgery in a patient presumed to have leiomyoma is between 0.2% and 0.7%. The possibility of leiomyosarcoma should be considered when rapid uterine growth occurs in older women. Almost 50% of women with leiomyosarcoma have extrauterine disease at the time of diagnosis so that 5-year survival is only 15%. Poor prognostic features include postmenopausal status, extrauterine disease, high mitotic count, and tumor arising de novo from myometrium rather than leiomyomata.

1407. **(D)** Radical hysterectomy and lymphadenectomy are not indicated since there does not appear to be orderly lymph node spread. Radiation has been reported to decrease local recurrence, but does not improve survival. Leiomyosarcoma does tend to spread hematogenously and chemotherapy offers fair results. In leiomyosarcoma, doxorubicin has significant activity with a response rate of about 25%. The overall 5-year survival rate is about 20%; for stage I and II leiomyosarcomas it is about 40%.

1408. **(A)** The incidence of sarcomatous degeneration in a uterine leiomyoma is less than 1%. The tumors usually originate from uterine myometrium but occasionally develop from preexisting leiomyomas. An important microscopic criterion for distinguishing leiomyosarcoma from leiomyoma is the number of mitoses present in tumor tissue (mitotic index):

- Greater than 10 mitoses per 10 high-power fields (hpf) is associated with frank malignancy (leiomyosarcoma).
- Between 5 and 10 mitoses per 10 hpf may be associated with malignant behavior, especially if atypia is seen.
- Less than 5 mitoses per 10 hpf and no atypia is associated with benign behavior (leiomyoma).

1409. (A) Uterine sarcomas discovered at an early stage (I and II) are treated by total abdominal hysterectomy and bilateral salpingo-oophorectomy. Postoperative irradiation decreases pelvic recurrences. Adjuvant chemotherapy may be attempted to prevent distant metastases. More advanced disease requires an aggressive, combined therapeutic approach consisting of surgery, radiotherapy, and chemotherapy. Commonly used chemotherapeutic agents include doxorubicin, ifosfamide, and paclitaxel. Etoposide, trimetrexate, and topotecan have no activity in leiomyosarcoma.

1410. (B) Total abdominal hysterectomy with bilateral salpingo-oophorectomy is advised when D&C fails to diagnose the source of bleeding in a perimenopausal woman with a rapidly enlarging uterus. Many sarcomas require a hysterectomy specimen to obtain adequate tissue for analysis.

1411. (C) Endometrial stromal tumors occur in perimenopausal women (ages 45 to 50) and consist of proliferating cells that resemble normal endometrial stroma. Based on differences in mitotic activity, vascular invasion, and prognosis, three types of endometrial stromal tumor exist:

1. Endometrial stromal nodule is a benign tumor that is cured by hysterectomy. Mitotic activity rarely exceeds 3 mitotic figures per 10 hpf.
2. Low-grade endometrial stromal sarcoma (ESS) is a low-grade malignancy capable of myometrial, vascular, and lymphatic invasion. Mitotic activity is usually less than 10 mitotic figures per 10 hpf. At laparotomy, tumors have multiple rubbery wormlike outgrowths into myometrium and pelvic blood vessels. One third of women with endometrial stromal sarcoma develop pelvic or abdominal recurrences, often years after initial diagnosis. Total abdominal hysterectomy with bilateral salpingo-oophorectomy is adequate for local disease. Incompletely resected or recurrent disease may respond to surgical resection, radiation therapy, or high-dose progesterone therapy.

3. High-grade ESS is a highly malignant neoplasm with mitotic rates greater than 10 mitotic figures per 10 hpf. One half of patients have metastatic disease to distant organs at the time of diagnosis, and few individuals survive beyond 3 years after initial surgery.

1412. (B) Malignant mixed müllerian tumors are derived from totipotential endometrial stromal cells that have the capacity for epithelial and stromal differentiation. They contain carcinomatous epithelial (glandular) elements and sarcomatous tissue resembling normal uterine mesenchyme (homologous or carcinosarcoma) or tissue foreign to the uterus (heterologous), such as cartilage bone or striated muscle.

1413. (D) Malignant mixed müllerian tumors develop from menopause (median age of patients, 62 years) as large, soft, polypoid masses filling the uterine cavity. One third of women with this disease have a history of previous pelvic irradiation for benign disease or cervical cancer. Malignant mixed müllerian tumors have a poor prognosis since up to 50% of patients have metastatic disease at the time of diagnosis.

1414. (A) Ovarian carcinoma is the second most common malignancy of the lower female genital tract. It occurs less frequently than endometrial cancer but more frequently than cervical cancer. Although representing only 25% of all gynecologic cancers, ovarian carcinoma is the most common cause of death resulting from female genital tract malignancy. It accounts for approximately 13,600 deaths annually. Lifetime risk is 1.4%

1415. (B) Her risk with two first-degree relatives having ovarian cancer is 5 to 7%. Given the poor prognosis with treatment of advanced ovarian cancer and no workable screening for early detection of disease, it is not unreasonable to consider bilateral oophorectomy. Bilateral oophorectomy can easily be accomplished as a day surgery with laparoscopic oophorectomy. However, if she desires childbearing, she may wish to delay surgical therapy until her family is complete. If she had known mutations of BRCAI or BRCAII, her risk would be even greater.

1416. **(C)** Lynch type II hereditary cancer syndrome includes nonpolyposis colorectal cancer and endometrial, breast, ovarian, and other gastrointestinal and genitourinary malignancies. The BrCA1 mutation increases her lifetime risk of up to 50% of developing ovarian cancer. Only 5 to 10% of ovarian cancer is hereditary.

1417. **(E)** Early ovarian cancer usually produces no symptoms. It may cause pelvic pain if the tumor undergoes torsion, rupture, or infection. Abdominal enlargement develops as the tumor grows beyond 15 cm in diameter. Invasion of pelvic viscera by malignancy leads to vague abdominal discomfort, urinary frequency (dysuria), or gastrointestinal disturbances. Irregular uterine bleeding may reflect uterine metastases or concomitant endometrial stimulation by endocrinologically active tumors. Other symptoms of ovarian malignancy include bloating, dyspepsia, weight loss, and shortness of breath (dyspnea) from pleural effusion. Symptoms of distant metastases to the skin, peripheral lymph nodes, lung, and brain are rare.

1418. **(C)** Most women with ovarian carcinoma have a palpable abdominal or pelvic mass. The pelvic examination remains the cornerstone for detection of ovarian neoplasia. The presence of a fixed, irregular, adnexal mass with cul-de-sac nodularity should be considered an ovarian carcinoma until proven otherwise. Unfortunately, no good screening test exists.

1419. **(A)** Exploratory laparotomy is the most important aspect of ovarian carcinoma management because it establishes the diagnosis, serves as effective therapy, and determines the extent of disease for planning of adjunctive therapy. The basic surgical tenet is to adequately stage the disease while removing primary tumor and all metastases (cytoreductive surgery).

1420. **(A)** Important prognostic indicators of survival from ovarian carcinoma include stage of the disease, age of the patient, and amount of residual tumor after surgery. The stage of ovarian malignancy is inversely correlated with the 5-year survival rate. Poorly differentiated (high-grade) tumors are commonly diagnosed in advanced stages, while well-differentiated (low-grade) tumors tend to be diagnosed in earlier stages. Grade is not incorporated into the FIGO classification of ovarian cancer. Grade is a useful prognostic indicator in early stage cancer, but this has not been proven in advanced stages. Older women are more likely than younger women to have advanced stage, poorly differentiated tumors. Moreover, women over age 50 have a worse prognosis than younger women after correction for tumor stage and grade. Individuals with residual tumor masses less than 2 to 3 cm in size after surgery have a longer length of survival than those with larger amounts of disease.

1421. **(A)** Ovarian neoplasms are classified according to their cell of origin: (1) coelomic epithelium (epithelial), (2) germ cells, (3) sex cord–stromal cells, (4) others: sarcoma, and (5) metastatic disease.

1422. **(A)** The percentage of ovarian neoplasms (benign and malignant) derived from epithelial cells, germ cells, and all other cell types is 65%, 25%, and 5 to 10%, respectively.

1423. **(E)** Ovulation appears to play a role in the pathogenesis of epithelial ovarian carcinoma. These tumors rarely develop in other mammals ovulating infrequently but occur commonly in fowl that ovulate regularly. Nulliparous women who are ovulatory and experience late menopause are at increased risk for developing ovarian cancer. Oral contraceptive use, pregnancy, and breast-feeding inhibit ovulation and protect against this disease. There are conflicting reports on other risk factors for developing ovarian cancer. Perineal use of talc powder (allowing an irritant to enter the peritoneal cavity via the reproductive tract), fat intake, and a history of mumps infection before menarche may be risk factors. Obesity and alcohol have also been weakly linked to ovarian cancer. The incidence of ovarian cancer is increased in affluent, industrialized countries such as the United States.

1424. **(A)** The incidence of ovarian carcinoma increases with age until the seventh decade of life. The malignancy rate of ovarian tumors in women between the ages of 20 and 40 and over age 50 is 10% and 50%, respectively. The mortality rate of ovarian cancer reflects the fact that most women with ovarian cancer have extensive disease by the time the symptoms appear. Elderly women are more likely to have their disease diagnosed at an advanced stage, contributing to a poorer prognosis compared to women with disease under age 65.

1425. **(C)** While the numbers vary between studies, probably 65% of patients with stage III disease and poorly differentiated tumors will have recurrence of disease despite appearing clinically free of disease. Only about 30% of patients with advanced disease (stages III and IV) will have no pathologic evidence of disease at second look. If disease is found at second-look laparotomy, tumor debulking does seem to improve survival in some studies. (Remember, having a second-look procedure implies there is no clinically detectable disease preoperatively.)

1426. **(D)** Second-look laparotomy is controversial today because 30 to 50% of patients with a negative second look experience recurrence.

1427. **(B)** Serous cystadenomas have a malignancy rate of 30%. Serous tumors, whether benign or malignant, tend to form calcific "sandlike" concretions, called psammoma bodies (from the Greek word *psammos*, meaning sand).

1428. **(B)** Serous tumors may have papillations, or excrescences, on their external or internal surfaces. Excrescences do not prove malignancy, so one should wait for histologic examination before deciding further surgical management.

1429. **(B)** One third of Brenner tumors are associated with mucinous elements. Brenner tumors are most likely to form mucinous cysts resembling mucinous cystadenomas.

1430. **(E)** About 20% of ovarian epithelial cancers are tumors of low malignant potential. The cells of these tumors do not invade ovarian stroma. Ovarian tumors of low malignant potential tend to occur in reproductive-age women and have an excellent prognosis regardless of stage (5-year survival rate, over 90%), although late recurrences are possible. A conservative surgical approach is advisable for early-stage disease in women desiring fertility. The most common types of "borderline" tumors are serous and mucinous, although other epithelial types also occur. Its external capsule is smoother and has a bluish-gray appearance; its interior is divided by septa into lobules. Each lobule contains clear viscid fluid produced by a single layer of columnar epithelium rich in mucin. The rate of bilaterality is 10 to 15%. Pseudomyxoma peritonei may also result from mucinous tumors of low malignant potential. Careful microscopic examination of these tumors is crucial to assure that invasive elements are not present.

1431. **(E)** Gynecologic surgeons recognize that intraoperative analysis of a large borderline tumor may fail to recognize small areas of invasive elements. It is important to conduct a thorough surgical staging to guard against the possibility that a borderline ovarian tumor harbors a malignant component. The standard operation for ovarian epithelial cancer (without gross disease beyond the ovary) is total abdominal hysterectomy, bilateral salpingo-oophorectomy, omentectomy, and complete surgical staging. Patients wishing to preserve fertility may undergo conservative surgery (e.g., unilateral salpingo-oophorectomy) under the following conditions:

- Tumor is confined to the ovary.
- Tumor is well differentiated without invasion of ovarian capsule, lymphatics, or mesovarium.

- Peritoneal washings are negative for tumor cells.
- Close surveillance is possible.
- Patient will consider excision of the contralateral ovary after childbearing is completed.

Biopsy of a normal-appearing contralateral ovary is not done because it is unlikely to uncover tumor and increases the risk of pelvic adhesions leading to infertility.

1432. (A) She now has a Stage III cancer with verified malignant extension to the omentum. Multiagent chemotherapy with paclitaxel (Taxol) plus carboplatin or cisplatin would be given after removal of the uterus and contralateral adnexa. Overall 5-year survival rates for patients with stage III epithelial ovarian cancer is 30%. She may do better since the tumor is well differentiated, she is younger, and she will have optional debulking. Hormone replacement therapy does not increase recurrence rate of ovarian cancer.

1433. (C) The ovaries of reproductive-age women are usually palpable, measuring about 1.5 × 2.5 × 4.0 cm in diameter. The postmenopausal ovary is usually nonpalpable because it decreases in size to 2.0 × 1.5 × 0.5 cm. Therefore, a palpable ovary in a woman beyond menopause always warrants dignostic studies to rule out the possibility of malignancy. Prior to the advent of diagnostic studies (e.g., tumor markers and vaginal ultrasonography), most postmenopausal women with a palpable ovary underwent exploratory laparotomy. It now appears that, in postmenopausal women, unilocular cysts less than 5 cm in diameter are usually benign. Ovarian masses that are solid, multiloculated, over 5 cm in diameter, or associated with elevated serum CA-125 levels should be removed. The decision to proceed with surgery depends on the patient's age, operative risk, serum CA-125 levels, and sonographic characteristics of the ovarian mass.

1434. (C) CA-125 is produced by normal tissue derived from coelomic epithelium, including the epithelial component of the müllerian system, and the mesothelial cells of the pleura, pericardium, and peritoneum. It is not found in normal fetal or adult ovaries. Although it is a circulating antigenic marker for epithelial ovarian carcinoma, serum CA-125 measurement for detection of pelvic malignancy is controversial. An elevated serum CA-125 level (> 35 U/mL) occurs in more than 80% of patients with nonmucinous epithelial ovarian carcinomas but also accompanies other malignancies and benign diseases, including pregnancy, endometriosis, fibroids, pelvic inflammatory disease, hepatocellular disease, chronic peritonitis, and carcinomas of the endometrium, fallopian tube, endocervix, pancreas, colon, breast, and lung. Evaluation of a pelvic mass should not be based solely on a serum CA-125 but should also depend on history, pelvic examination, and ultrasound. A serum CA-125 level greater than 200 U/mL in any individual suggests the presence of an ovarian malignancy. An elevated CA-125 at the time of surgery is useful to monitor tumor progression and to follow the clinical response of the patient to therapy.

1435. (D) A 65-year-old woman with ascites and a fixed pelvic mass is most likely to have ovarian epithelial cancer. Preoperative studies are used to exclude other etiologies for a pelvic mass. Mammography is used to detect primary mammary cancer with metastases to the ovary. Stool guaiac examination, sigmoidoscopy, and intestinal tract imaging are useful for detecting gastrointestinal cancers in patients with appropriate symptoms. A chest x-ray will detect pulmonary disease and/or pleural effusions. Cervical Pap smear and endometrial biopsy (if necessary) eliminate cervical and endometrial disease. An IVP is useful if the patient is symptomatic for genitourinary disease. It will detect ureteral obstruction and will also show pelvic calcifications suggestive of benign or malignant disease. Laboratory tests including a complete blood count, blood chemistries, and urinalysis are also helpful. Ultrasonography and/or a CT scan of the abdomen and pelvis will also be of assistance.

1436. (A) Although further studies are required to improve long-term survival, several statements can be made about the current treatment of ovarian epithelial cancer. The most important principle in ovarian cancer therapy is removal of all gross disease if the risk of fatal complications is minimal. A midline incision should be used and bowel may be removed if necessary. Areas of risk for metastases in the peritoneal cavity and retroperitoneal lymph nodes also should be sampled since 10 to 20% of women with apparent stage I disease have para-aortic nodal metastases. Other treatment may include the following:

- Postoperative ^{32}P may be used in low-stage tumors (IC) in which there is a risk of intraperitoneal tumor spread without residual disease.
- Postoperative external radiation is used when primary tumor is limited to the pelvis and gross disease is removed at the time of surgery. To date, comparative survival and complication rates between whole abdomen radiation and multidrug chemotherapy have yet to be published.
- First-line multiagent chemotherapy with paclitaxel plus a plantinum compound (carboplatin or cisplatin) is used for patients with stage IA to IB, grade 3 (some oncologists treat grade 2), stage II to IV, or with residual disease after initial tumor removal.

1437. (D) The stage of ovarian cancer is determined by physical examination, roentgenologic studies, surgical findings, histologic analysis of tumor, pelvic organs, omentum, and biopsies of suspicious areas, and cytology examination of peritoneal fluid. At surgery, careful inspection of the pelvic viscera, peritoneal serosa, gastrointestinal tract, omentum, liver, diaphragm, retroperitoneal nodes, pancreas, and biliary structures is mandatory. Peritoneal fluid should be collected for cytologic examination. Omentectomy is performed because the omentum is a common site for metastases. Lymph node sampling is recommended, and palpable nodes should be excised in all but obviously advanced cases. The staging system for ovar-

ian carcinoma, as defined by the International Federation of Gynecology and Obstetrics (FIGO), is based on the following:

- *Stage I*—growth limited to the ovaries but can include malignant cells in the peritoneal cavity, ovarian surface excrescences, capsule rupture, or involvement of both ovaries
- *Stage II*—growth involving one or both ovaries with pelvic extension to the uterus, tubes, or other pelvic structures
- *Stage III*—abdominal metastases and their size, positive retroperitoneal lymph nodes, or extension to small bowel or omentum
- *Stage IV*—distant metastases, including liver metastases or malignant pleural effusion   (See Figure 22–4.)

1438. (E) In postmenopausal women, both adnexa and the uterus are removed to eliminate the risks of having occult disease or another primary cancer in the opposite ovary. Patients with advanced disease whose residual tumor nodules are less than 1.5 cm in diameter after cytoreduction have the best chance for survival. In a reproductive-age woman desiring fertility, a salpingo-oophorectomy may be considered for unilateral, well-differentiated tumor without evidence of metastatic disease.

1439. (B) Despite the benefit of cytoreductive surgery, the 3-year survival rate of patients with stage III ovarian cancer without residual disease after cytoreduction is only 30%. Therefore, combination chemotherapy (e.g., cisplatinum and paclitaxel) is commonly given after cytoreductive surgery. The use of combination chemotherapy for the treatment of high-stage disease appears to provide superior survival rates compared to single-agent chemotherapy. The response to chemotherapy is related to the amount of residual disease after surgery. Younger patients achieve results from postoperative therapy superior to those of older patients. The response to chemotherapy usually occurs within 6 months. If the patient with a stage III cancer appears to have a complete response to chemotherapy (by physical examination and

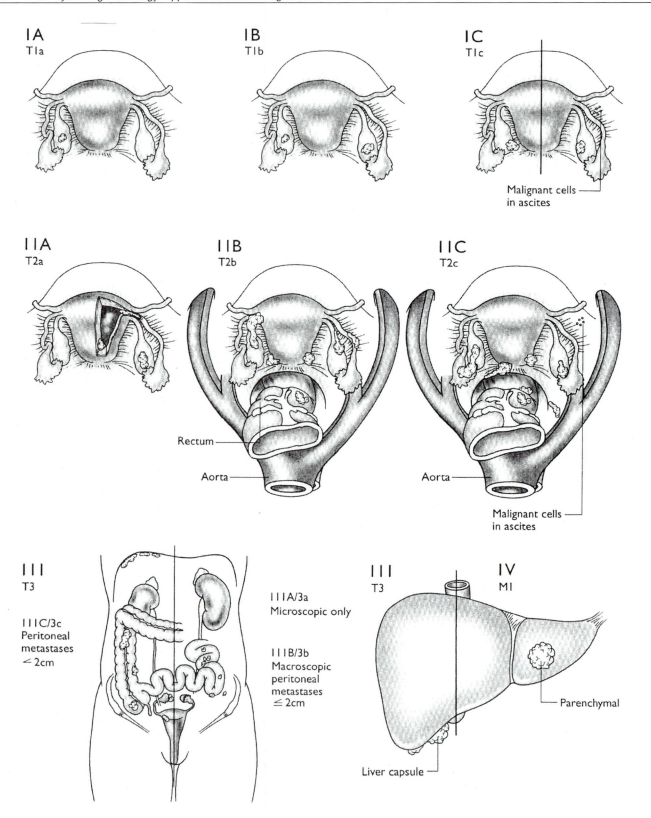

IA
T1a

IB
T1b

IC
T1c

Malignant cells in ascites

IIA
T2a

IIB
T2b

Rectum

Aorta

IIC
T2c

Aorta

Malignant cells in ascites

III
T3

IIIC/3c
Peritoneal metastases ≤ 2cm

IIIA/3a
Microscopic only

IIIB/3b
Macroscopic peritoneal metastases ≤ 2cm

III
T3

IV
M1

Parenchymal

Liver capsule

Figure 22–4.

diagnostic testing), a second-look operation is sometimes performed. Under this condition, about one half of women thought to be free of cancer have disease present at second-look operation.

1440. (D) The mean age of diagnosis is 41 years for mucinous borderline tumors of the intestinal type, which is similar to the age distribution for all borderline tumors. The value of post-operative radiation and chemotherapy is controversial and there is no firm evidence that it prolongs survival. The appendix should always be removed because microscopic evidence of similar disease is almost always present, suggesting that the ovarian tumors may be metastatic from the appendix. The majority of patients with pseudomyxoma peritonei will eventually die of their disease.

1441. (E) As a group, ovarian epithelial tumors are the most common ovarian neoplasms. Germ cell tumors are the second most common group of ovarian tumors.

1442. (B) Germ cell tumors are believed to originate from primitive germ cells that differentiate toward developmental tissues of either embryonic (e.g., ectoderm, mesoderm, endoderm) or extraembryonic (e.g., yolk sac, trophoblast) origin. They are the most common neoplasms in women under age 30 (representing 60% of ovarian neoplasms in infants and children). About one third of germ cell tumors found in women under age 21 are malignant. The incidence of malignancy in germ cell tumors increases to 84% in girls younger than 10 years of age. Germ cell tumors are the main cause of ovarian malignancy in young women but account for only 3% of all ovarian malignancies.

1443. (D) Pediatric ovarian malignancies are rare (1.7/100,000 per year) so only 36 to 64% of cases are identified before surgery. The most common incorrect diagnosis is acute appendicitis since the most common presenting symptom is abdominal pain. Germ cell tumors represent 70% of ovarian neoplasms in children. However, when reviewing any ovarian enlargement, 67% of masses are be-nign and are frequently non-neoplastic follicles or theca lutein cysts.

1444. (E) Bowel perforation is a well-recognized complication of laparoscopy and injuries are not always recognized at the time of surgery. Most patients present with postoperative symptoms within 10 days. The diagnosis is not always clear. While ileus and severe obstipation from narcotics give similar symptoms, the marked fever and elevated white blood cell count argue for bowel perforation. Similarly, although chemical peritonitis has been reported with dermoids, bowel perforation is more likely given the clinical scenario.

1445. (A) The likely diagnosis is endodermal sinus tumor given the elevated alpha-fetoprotein. The majority of cases are stage I and bilaterality is rare so unilateral adnexectomy is appropriate. However, simple surgical therapy results in frequent recurrences so chemotherapy is also indicated. The majority of stage I patients survive with modern chemotherapy. This tumor accounts for about 10% of malignant germ-cell tumors. Almost all cases have elevated alpha-fetoprotein levels, and it is a useful marker for following these tumors clinically.

1446. (E) Germ cell tumors represent one quarter of all ovarian tumors and occur anatomically anywhere along the migration route of primordial germ cells from the yolk sac to the genital ridge. Germ cell tumors are commonly unilateral and are usually seen during the second and third decades of life. Most germ cell tumors are benign and represent mature teratomas. Five percent of germ cell tumors are malignant and occur predominantly in prepubertal girls. Abdominal enlargement is the most common sign of a malignant germ cell tumor in children.

1447. (E) The mature teratoma, or dermoid cyst, is the most common germ cell tumor and accounts for 25% of all ovarian neoplasms. Dysgerminomas are the most common malignant germ cell tumors and account for 1 to 2% of ovarian cancers.

1448. (B) Bone fragments, teeth, and gastrointestinal mucosa are often located adjacent to projections within mature teratomas, referred to as Rokitansky's protuberances. These protuberances are the sites from which mature teratomas are thought to undergo malignant transformation.

1449. (D) Immature teratomas contain embryonal (immature) tissue, resembling that normally found in the human embryo. Tumor grade is based on the maturity of the ectodermal neural tissue. Hair is present in 40% of tumors, and calcified bone is usually grossly evident. Immature teratomas are the second most common malignant germ cell tumor (the first being dysgerminoma). Seventy-five percent of these tumors are discovered during the first two decades of life. Survival varies from 81 to 30% for grades 1 to 3. Bilaterality is rare, although 5% of immature teratomas are associated with a mature teratoma in the contralateral ovary. Stage I, grade 1 disease may be treated by unilateral salpingo-oophorectomy, but adjuvant chemotherapy is required for higher grades or more advanced stages. Pure immature teratomas do not produce alpha-fetoprotein or hCG.

1450. (D) Highly specialized teratomas include carcinoid and struma ovarii. Primary ovarian carcinoid originates from gastrointestinal or respiratory epithelium within a teratoma. It is diagnosed by finding an elevation in the amount of urinary 5-hydroxyindoleacetic acid. One third of cases produce the carcinoid syndrome (paroxysmal flushing of the face and neck, colicky abdominal pain with diarrhea, and asthma-like respiratory distress). Although the tumor is usually benign and treated by simple excision, malignant transformation is possible.

1451. (A) Dysgerminoma is the most common malignant germ cell tumor of the ovary. Histologically, dysgerminoma are composed of primordial germ cells and intervening connective tissue infiltrated by lymphocytes. The tumors are usually smooth, rounded, and thinly encapsulated. Rupture of the capsule may lead to intra-abdominal hemorrhage.

1452. (D) Dysgerminoma occurs primarily in women under age 30. It has the highest rate of bilaterality (10 to 15%) of all malignant germ cell tumors. The 5-year survival rate following unilateral salpingo-oophorectomy for tumor confined to one ovary is more than 90%. Survival rates drop to about 60% when disease extends beyond the ovary. Dysgerminoma is sensitive to chemotherapy and radiotherapy. Other germ-cell tumors (e.g., teratoma, gonadoblastoma) may coexist with dysgerminomas and may worsen the prognosis.

1453. (A) Endodermal sinus tumors have several histologic patterns. The most notable pattern consists of scattered tubules lined by a single layer of cuboidal cells, a loose stroma, and a papillary structure containing a central blood vessel (Schiller–Duvall body).

1454. (B) Embryonal carcinoma is one of the most malignant ovarian cancers and originates from undifferentiated primordial germ cells. Histologically, primitive pleomorphic cells, with vacuolated cytoplasm and vesicular nuclei, form glandlike spaces. Clusters of syncytiotrophoblast-like and mononuclear cells produce hCG and alpha-fetoprotein. More than half of patients with this tumor have hormonal abnormalities, including hirsutism, virilization, irregular uterine bleeding, and sexual precocity. Survival for patients with stage I embryonal carcinoma has increased above 50% with the use of adjuvant combination chemotherapy. Polyembryoma is a rare, highly malignant, germ cell neoplasm composed of numerous embryoid bodies, which have the structural appearance of normal embryos. The polyembryoma probably represents the most immature stage of development of the fetus (i.e., that immediately following the blastocyst). It is one of the most undifferentiated of lesions and its prognosis is very poor.

1455. (C) Gonadoblastomas are generally benign tumors consisting of primordial germ cells and sex cord–stromal elements resembling granulosa or Sertoli tumor. Leydig cells and luteinized cells also may be present.

1456. (B) Physical examination strongly suggests testicular feminization, a disorder in males due to defective androgen action. The uterus is absent and the vagina ends blindly, causing amenorrhea. The testes are located in the pelvis or within an inguinal hernia and contain immature seminiferous tubules.

1457. (D) Gonadoblastoma is the most common neoplasm associated with dysgenetic gonads. Eighty percent of patients with this tumor are phenotypic women, most of whom are virilized and have a Y chromosome. Adolescent patients with gonadoblastoma may experience delayed puberty due to primary gonadal failure. Many of these tumors are small and contain calcifications. Bilaterality occurs in at least half of the patients. Fifty percent of gonadoblastomas contain malignant germ cell elements, predominantly dysgerminoma, which reduce the chance for survival. Bilateral salpingo-oophorectomy is usually performed in patients with dysgenetic gonads containing a gonadoblastoma because malignant germ cell elements may be present and bilaterality is common. Gonadectomy is usually delayed until after puberty in patients with testicular feminization to allow hormone-dependent pubertal changes.

1458. (B) The presence of a Y chromosome in an individual with dysgenetic gonads carries a 25% chance of developing a germ cell tumor (e.g., gonadoblastoma, dysgerminoma, endodermal sinus tumor, choriocarcinoma). Most of these malignant changes occur after puberty and before the age of 30.

1459. (C) Gonadectomy is indicated at the time the abnormality is detected because of the risk of malignancy. These patients can develop gonadoblastoma or malignant germ cell tumors (primarily dysgerminoma). Gonadectomy is indicated regardless of the location of the gonad. These abnormal gonads are almost always useless for fertility and many will become virilized, but the primary reason for removal is the cancer risk.

1460. (B) While gonadoblastomas frequently cause virilization secondary to androgen excess,

they also can produce estrogen. Hot flashes have been reported postoperatively.

1461. (B) The serum gonadotropin response to exogenous GnRH differentiates children with true sexual precocity from those with pseudoprecocious puberty. Granulosa cell tumors occur in all ages and juvenile granulosa cell tumors commonly induce pseudosexual precocity. The tumors are predominantly unilateral, solid tumors containing granulosa-like cells with longitudinal nuclear grooving (coffee bean appearance). They vary in amounts of thecomatous stromal matrix. Cystic tumor elements containing serous fluid or clotted blood may rupture, leading to hemoperitoneum.

1462. (A) Granulosa cell tumors in postmenopausal women may cause vaginal bleeding due to endometrial hyperplasia or carcinoma. Granulosa cell tumors in reproductive-age women may disrupt ovulation.

1463. (E) Cytoplasmic inclusions, called Reinke crystalloids, are a characteristic feature of testicular interstitial cells. Reinke crystalloids also are found in hilar cell (Leydig cell) tumors and are pathognomonic if present.

1464. (E) Metastatic tumors to the ovary usually originate in the breast, gastrointestinal tract, or uterus. They account for 4 to 8% of ovarian carcinomas. Lymphatic channels are probably the most important route of ovarian metastasis. Other means of cancer spread to the ovaries include direct extension, intraperitoneal dissemination, metastasis via the lumen of the fallopian tube, and hematogenous metastasis.

1465. (B) One type of metastatic ovarian tumor is the Krukenberg tumor. It is characterized histologically by nests of mucin-filled cells with a "signet ring" appearance in a cellular stroma. Krukenberg tumors form large, bilateral masses, containing gelatinous necrosis and hemorrhage. They usually arise in the gastrointestinal tract, primarily the stomach. The next most frequent primary site of origin is the large intestine. These tumors occasionally arise from the breast and other mucus-producing organs, such as the appendix and urinary bladder.

1466. **(D)** Nonspecific mesenchymal tumors of the ovary arise from ovarian-supporting structures that are common to most organs. These unusual tumors may be benign or malignant. They include hemangiomas, leiomyomas, sarcomas, and lymphomas. More than 50 cases of ovarian leiomyoma have been reported in adults, accounting for possibly almost 1% of benign ovarian neoplasms. Many reported cases have been small tumors.

1467. **(B, C, D, E)** Most endometrial hyperplasia results from persistent estrogen stimulation unopposed by progesterone. Endometrial hyperplasia frequently develops immediately after menarche and shortly before menopause when anovulatory cycles associated with persistent estrogen stimulation are common. Conditions predisposing to development of endometrial hyperplasia are: chronic anovulation with serum estrogen levels unopposed by progesterone (PCOS, obesity, congenital adrenal hyperplasia); estrogen-producing tumors (granulosa–thecal cell tumors, ovarian thecomas); and exogenous estrogen administration. Hyperprolactinemia inhibits hypothalamic GnRH activity and usually causes amenorrhea, due to low circulating estrogen levels.

1468. **(A, B, C, D)** Tumor grade is a major determinant of prognosis when survival is examined for each stage of disease. Tumor cell type also affects prognosis (e.g., serous tumors have a worse prognosis than mucinous, endometrioid, and clear-cell tumors). Serous tumors tend to be more poorly differentiated and identified at a higher stage than other tumors. Other factors adversely affecting survival from stage I ovarian epithelial carcinoma include pelvic adhesions and ascitic fluid (> 250 mL). Women with well-differentiated tumors confined to the ovary do not require further treatment after surgery. Individuals with poorly differentiated stage I disease and stage II disease usually receive postoperative adjuvant therapy (e.g., radiotherapy or

chemotherapy). Psammoma bodies have no prognostic significance in gynecologic cancer.

1469. **(A, B, C, E)** Fibromas and thecomas are benign tumors derived from stromal mesenchyme. They can occur at any age but are most common in peri- and postmenopausal women. The tumors are solid, irregular, and mobile, ranging in size from small to several thousand grams. The fibroma is the most common benign solid ovarian tumor. It does not produce hormones but can be associated with Meigs' syndrome. The thecoma is almost always unilateral, and is composed of endocrinologically active stromal cells bearing a resemblance to lipid-laden thecal cells. Its yellow appearance on cross-section is due to the presence of steroid-producing cells. Granulosa cell tumors produce estrogen; hilar cell and Sertoli–Leydig tumors produce androgens.

1470. **(A, B, C, E)** Gonadal tumors may produce androgens directly (gonadoblastoma) or indirectly through the secretion of chorionic gonadotropin (e.g., nongestational choriocarcinoma, embryonal carcinoma, and mixed germ cell tumor).

1471. **(B)** Only a few cases (about 2%) of simple hyperplasia without atypia will progress to carcinoma and the progression is slow. The D&C alone often removes the hyperplasia. Progestin is a standard treatment. Appropriate follow-up includes repeat endometrial sampling in 6 months to assure resolution of the process. A hysterectomy is not indicated unless bleeding problems persist despite hormonal treatment or the disease progresses to hyperplasia with atypia.

1472. **(D)** Severe atypical hyperplasia may progress to endometrial carcinoma so hysterectomy is warranted. In severe atypia, about 25% develop carcinoma, 25% regress, and 50% persist. She is likely to have PCOS, causing anovulation and prolonged estrogen exposure.

1473. **(B)** Three to five percent of patients with complex hyperplasia will ultimately develop endometrial cancer. The precise mechanism of progression to carcinoma is unknown.

1474. (D) Probably 21 to 29% of women with atypia in the hyperplasia will progress to a malignant cancer. This is why hysterectomy is offered when childbearing is completed.

1475. (A) Simple hyperplasia without atypia rarely progresses to endometrial cancer.

1476. (E) Less than 5% of Brenner tumors are malignant. The malignancy rates for mucinous and serous tumors are 15% and 30%, respectively. Almost all endometrioid and clear cell tumors are malignant.

1477. (A) The risk of bilaterality is an important issue in the treatment of ovarian tumors. Malignant tumors have a higher rate of bilaterality than benign tumors. The bilaterality rates of ovarian epithelial neoplasms are, in decreasing order of frequency: serous cystadenocarcinoma (33 to 66%), mucinous cystadenocarcinoma (10 to 20%), endometrioid carcinoma (13 to 30%), and Brenner tumor (6%).

1478. (A) Serous ovarian tumors have an appearance similar to that of tubal epithelium. Ovarian and tubal tumors also may contain papillae or papillary structures. Ovarian disease metastatic to the fallopian tube is diagnosed when the tubal mucosa is intact and malignant cells are present in the subepithelial lymphatics. Some patients have small ovaries (< 4 cm in diameter) and widespread serous carcinoma in the abdomen, referred to as papillary serous carcinoma of the peritoneum. Occasionally the primary site of papillary serous carcinoma is difficult to determine.

1479. (A) Eighty-five to 90% of malignant ovarian neoplasms are derived from coelomic epithelium. These malignancies are uncommon prior to age 40. More than one half of epithelial ovarian cancers occur in women beyond the age of 50. Malignant ascites is defined as accumulation of serous fluid containing cancerous cells within the abdominal cavity. It

may develop with intraperitoneal spread of tumor. Ascites is often attributed to simple weight gain by women who notice tightening of their abdominal clothing. It may be associated with malignant pleural effusion, defined as the accumulation of fluid containing cancerous cells within the pleural cavity.

1480. (C) Bone marrow suppression may accompany chemotherapy or radiation therapy. It is common when abdominopelvic radiation follows chemotherapy.

1481. (A) Radiation-induced bowel obstruction can lead to a surgical emergency. In addition, intestinal injuries commonly occur when surgery is performed after abdominopelvic radiation. Adhesions resulting from intestinal injury may cause symptoms of bowel obstruction (e.g., postprandial crampy abdominal pain, vomiting, anorexia), which are similar to those of recurrent disease.

1482. (E) Struma ovarii refers to a teratoma in which thyroid tissue represents more than half of the tumor. One quarter of these tumors are associated with clinical hyperthyroidism.

1483. (B) Alpha-fetoprotein is produced by endodermal sinus tumors. It can be detected in the serum of patients with primary and recurrent disease. The prognosis for patients with endodermal sinus tumor has improved markedly with the recent use of multidrug chemotherapy (stage I, 80%; stage II, 60%; stage III, 30% survival).

1484. (C) Choriocarcinoma may develop from a germ cell (nongestational) or a pregnancy (gestational) arising in the ovary or elsewhere in the genital tract. All of these tumors produce hCG and contain sheets of cytotrophoblastic and syncytiotrophoblastic tissue. Nongestational choriocarcinoma is less responsive than gestational choriocarcinoma to chemotherapy. The prognosis of patients with nongestational choriocarcinoma is poor.

1485. (A) Pure dysgerminomas occasionally produce large amounts of lactic dehydrogenase.

They do not secrete significant amounts of alpha-fetoprotein or hCG.

1486. (G) Inhibin is produced by granulosa cell tumor and may be used as a serum marker for this tumor.

1487. (D) Sertoli–Leydig cell tumors (arrhenoblastoma, androblastoma) are rare tumors composed of Sertoli cells within a stromal matrix of Leydig cells. They occur most commonly as unilateral tumors in women between the ages of 11 and 45. These tumors have a low malignant potential with biologic behavior depending on degree of differentiation (e.g., well-differentiated tumors have a benign biologic behavior). Most Sertoli–Leydig cell tumors produce large amounts of testosterone, causing circulating testosterone levels to exceed 2.0 ng/mL (normal female, < 0.8 ng/mL). Progressive masculinization may occur and is characterized by temporal balding, voice deepening, and clitoromegaly. Conservative salpingo-oophorectomy is justified in young women with disease limited to one ovary. Patients with extraovarian metastasis and/or differentiated tumors require multidrug chemotherapy.

1488. (H) Gynandroblastoma refers to a neoplasm in which both Sertoli–Leydig and granulosa–thecal elements are present in significant proportions. These tumors may produce androgens or estrogens and also have low malignant potential.

1489. (F) Lipid (lipoid) cell tumors are a heterogeneous group of stromal neoplasms having in common an endocrine-type histologic appearance with lipid-containing cells. Malignancy occurs in some lipid cell tumors and is associated with tumors greater than 7 cm in diameter, nuclear atypia, and the presence of mitotic figures. Lipid-cell tumors include the following:

- *Hilar cell (Leydig cell) tumors*—small (usually < 5 cm), unilateral neoplasms found within the hilar region of the ovary; this tumor is usually benign.
- *Adrenal-like tumors*—generally benign tumors with a histologic appearance similar to that of an adrenocortical adenoma.
- *Indeterminant lipid cell tumors*—neoplasms that cannot be categorized into the above groups.

Breast Cancer
Questions

1490. Which of the following is the greatest risk factor for the development of breast cancer?

(A) delayed childbearing
(B) a family history of breast cancer
(C) increased dietary fat intake
(D) smoking
(E) atypical epithelial hyperplasia

1491. Which of the following is most likely to detect early breast cancer?

(A) bloody discharge from the nipple
(B) a palpable mass on self-examination
(C) a palpable mass on annual examination at the caregiver's office
(D) mammographic abnormalities
(E) a mobile tender cyst

1492. Which of the following is the most likely to be a late finding in a patient with breast cancer?

(A) greenish-gray discharge
(B) drooping of the breasts
(C) darkening of the areola
(D) asymmetry of the breast size
(E) skin or nipple retraction

1493. Which of the following statements regarding breast cancer is TRUE?

(A) It is the most common malignancy in women.
(B) It is the most common cause of death from malignancy in women.
(C) The median age of women with breast cancer is about 40.
(D) In the United States, breast cancer is more common in Caucasian populations.
(E) Most patients with breast cancer can be identified by risk factors.

1494. The most common site for breast cancer to occur within the breast is the

(A) upper outer quadrant
(B) upper inner quadrant
(C) lower outer quadrant
(D) lower inner quadrant
(E) under the nipple

1495. The diagnostic accuracy of cytology of a nipple discharge or fluid from breast cyst aspiration

(A) has generally been shown to be of little benefit
(B) has an extremely high false-positive rate
(C) is diagnostically correct about 75% of the time
(D) is accurate nearly 100% of the time in diagnosing breast cancer

1496. A patient is deciding whether or not she will have a mammogram and asks you about the advantages and disadvantages of the procedure. You can correctly tell her

(A) mammography can be performed with a radiation exposure of 1 rad

(B) mammography can be used to evaluate suspicious breast masses and save women from biopsy in many cases

(C) mammography and physical examination are equally effective in the diagnosis of all types of breast cancer

(D) mammographic screening of new populations for breast cancer will identify about 1 cancer for every 1,000 women screened

(E) mammography is a much more effective technique for diagnosing breast cancer than is breast ultrasound

1497. A woman asks you what the advantages of mammography are. You can correctly tell her

(A) it can detect some breast cancers as early as 2 years before they would reach a palpable size

(B) it can detect all cancers greater than 1 cm in diameter

(C) it can effectively screen all women after age 30

(D) it is an equally effective screening technique in both premenopausal and postmenopausal women

(E) it can be decreased to every 3 years in women over the age of 70 because their risk of breast cancer is decreased compared to the 50 to 70 age group

1498. In the BI-RADs (American College of Radiology Breast Imaging, Reporting and Data System) terminology, the designation zero means

(A) normal mammogram

(B) benign lesion

(C) probably benign lesion

(D) suspicious for malignancy

(E) needs additional evaluation

1499. Ultrasound of the breast is most useful to diagnose

(A) fibroid adenomas

(B) invasive cancer

(C) in situ carcinoma

(D) interductal papillomas

(E) benign cysts

1500. How many years of growth does the average breast cancer require to reach a diameter of 1 cm?

(A) 1.5

(B) 2

(C) 4

(D) 6

(E) 10

1501. Clinical breast examination discovers approximately what percentage of breast cancers that are missed by mammography

(A) < 1%

(B) 5 to 8%

(C) 15 to 20%

(D) 25 to 28%

(E) > 33%

1502. Breast self-examination in reproductive-age women is best performed

(A) at the onset of menses

(B) just after menses

(C) at midcycle

(D) just before the onset of menses

(E) monthly at any time during the cycle

1503. A 25-year-old G2P2 healthy woman's mother developed breast cancer at age 52. The patient's sister was diagnosed with breast cancer at age 30. Both her mother and sister are living. She wants to know if there are any tests she should get to help her evaluate her risks of getting breast cancer. You can correctly explain to her that in her case

(A) decreased T-cell levels cause a decline in protective antibodies, which results in an increased risk of breast cancer

(B) HER-2/Reu gene overexpression is associated with later development of breast cancer

(C) BRCA1 and BRCA2 mutations may predict increased risk of breast cancer

(D) decreased B cells can cause increased risk of breast cancer because of decreased cell-mediated immunity

(E) CA-125 is a good prognostic marker for breast cancer

1504. The most common pathologic type of breast malignancy is

(A) lobular in situ

(B) ductal in situ

(C) Paget's

(D) infiltrating lobular carcinoma

(E) infiltrating ductal carcinoma

1505. The major importance of estrogen receptor status in breast cancers is that

(A) if a tumor lacks estrogen receptors, it is generally more amenable to treatment

(B) tumors with estrogen and/or progesterone receptors generally do not require adjuvant chemotherapy

(C) antiestrogen therapy (such as tamoxifen) may improve survival in patients with a positive receptor status

(D) diethylstilbestrol (DES) may be given as a curative agent in many of these patients

1506. A 59-year-old woman presents with a 3-cm, irregular, mobile mass in the upper outer quadrant of her breast. Her right axilla has two palpable, very small, rubbery, mobile lymph nodes. If the primary mass is malignant, her stage would most likely be

(A) 0

(B) I

(C) II

(D) III

(E) IV

1507. A woman is operated on for stage II breast cancer with a lumpectomy and axillary node dissection on the involved side. Three lymph nodes are positive for breast cancer. Which of the following statements can you correctly tell her regarding her prognosis?

(A) Her chance of 5-year survival should be about 85%.

(B) Her chance of 10-year survival is nearly the same as her 5-year survival rate.

(C) Breast cancer with 0 to 3 positive axillary nodes gives a 50% chance of survival at 5 years.

(D) She has greater than a 70% chance of dying from her breast cancer.

(E) She should be cured of her cancer.

1508. During counseling of a patient with stage I breast cancer prior to surgery, she asks what the chances are of finding cancer in her axillary lymph nodes during the surgery. There are no clinically palpable nodes present on her preoperative examination. You answer that

(A) there is nearly a 0% chance

(B) the chance is about 10%

(C) the chances are about 30%

(D) the chances are greater than 50%

(E) most women have some degree of lymph node involvement in any breast cancer

1509. A procedure designed to prevent many of the surgical complications of axillary lymph node dissection, which has very good positive and negative predictive values for detecting lymph node metastasis, is

(A) magnetic resonance imaging (MRI)

(B) fine-needle biopsy

(C) sentinel node mapping

(D) HER-2/neu detection

(E) clinical palpations

1510. Involvement of supraclavicular lymph nodes with breast cancer usually indicates

(A) the same prognosis as axillary lymph node involvement

(B) a slightly better prognosis than axillary lymph node involvement

(C) a slightly worse prognosis than axillary lymph node involvement

(D) a very poor prognosis

1511. An 88-year-old woman complains of itching of the nipple on her left breast over the past 2 months. On examination, you see excoriation and superficial ulceration of the nipple area. How should you counsel this patient?

(A) She most likely has eczema of the breast and should be treated with corticosteroids.

(B) This is a common finding in postmenopausal women. If her mammogram is negative, topical estrogen therapy or oral estrogen therapy is indicated.

(C) Wearing gloves to bed will usually stop the scratch–itch cycle and resolve the problem. A small bandage over the area at night may also accomplish this task.

(D) This presentation is nearly pathognomonic for breast cancer in a woman this age. A mammogram should be performed to confirm the diagnosis.

(E) The woman may have Paget's disease of the breast. The eroded area should be biopsied.

1512. A 46-year-old woman has an irregular, firm, 2-cm mass on breast examination. Her axillary examination is normal. On clinical grounds, you are very suspicious of a cancer. She asks you, "What are the chances that this will be benign?" You tell her that the chances that it is benign are

(A) nearly 0%

(B) about 15%

(C) about 30%

(D) about 50%

(E) > 70%

1513. You are counseling a patient about biopsying a lesion found in her breast. You can correctly tell her that

(A) a needle biopsy has been proven to be as good as open biopsy in nearly all cases

(B) needle biopsy has little or no role in the evaluation of breast masses

(C) needle biopsy can be falsely negative in 15 to 20% of cases

(D) open breast biopsy should remove an entire breast lobule surrounding the mass

(E) general anesthesia is necessary to do an adequate breast biopsy in most cases

1514. A 61-year-old woman has a clinically suspicious, relatively superficial breast mass. Her ipsilateral axilla is normal. A biopsy is recommended. She asks how the biopsy should be done. Of the following, the best option is

(A) to do her biopsy in the office today

(B) a lumpectomy and axillary dissection or mastectomy in your ambulatory surgery center as indicated after gross inspection of the specimen

(C) an outpatient biopsy in the ambulatory surgery center and await the final pathology reports before proceeding with any further evaluation or treatment

(D) doing the biopsy in the hospital and proceeding with axillary dissection or mastectomy depending on the pathologist's frozen section report

1515. Excluding recurrence of the cancer, the most common complication following the treatment of breast cancer is

(A) edema of the ipsilateral arm

(B) complications from breast reconstruction

(C) development of leukemia from adjuvant chemotherapy

(D) permanent alopecia

(E) agranulocytosis

1516. Which of the following is the most effective method to prevent breast cancer in a high-risk patient?

(A) bilateral oophorectomy

(B) tamoxifen

(C) bilateral mastectomy

(D) avoid weight gain

(E) have first term birth before age 20

1517. A 68-year-old woman consults with you because she has discovered a single firm nodule in the upper outer quadant of her left breast. Examination reveals a discrete nodule with no skin edema, no enlargement of lymph nodes, no retraction, no redness, and no pain. The immediate course of action should include

(A) needle aspiration of the nodule

(B) repeat examination in 2 weeks

(C) radiation therapy

(D) biopsy of the lesion

1518. Which of the following statements is TRUE of breast cancer during pregnancy?

(A) Pregnancy greatly accelerates the growth of breast cancer because of its elevated hormone levels.

(B) Treatment of breast cancer should be withheld during pregnancy or lactation.

(C) Breast cancer in pregnancy is rare, with an incidence of about 1 per 100,000 pregnancies.

(D) Because of pregnancy, the diagnosis of breast cancer is often delayed, but stage-for-stage prognosis is the same with prompt treatment.

(E) Axillary metastases are less common in pregnant than in nonpregnant patients at the time when breast cancer is diagnosed.

DIRECTIONS (Questions 1519 and 1520): Each set of the numbered items or incomplete statements in this section is followed by answers or by completions of the statement. Select the answers or completions that may apply.

1519. Which four of the following are in the differential diagnosis of a breast mass?

(A) mammary dysplasia (fibrocystic changes of the breast)

(B) microglandular hyperplasia secondary to oral contraceptives (OCs)

(C) fibroadenoma

(D) intraductal papilloma

(E) fat necrosis

1520. Which two of the following will improve the detection of malignant cells in axillary nodes by 10 to 30% above routine cytology in patients with breast cancer?

(A) immunohistochemical staining for cytokeratin

(B) palpation

(C) HER-2/neu detection

(D) sentinel node mapping

(E) serial sectioning

DIRECTIONS (Questions 1521 through 1525): Each set of matching questions in this section consists of a list of lettered headings followed by several numbered items. For each numbered item, select the ONE lettered option that is most closely associated with it. Each lettered option may be selected once, more than once, or not at all. Match the type of mastectomy operation with its appropriate descriptor.

Questions 1521 through 1525

(A) extended radical mastectomy

(B) modified radical mastectomy

(C) radical mastectomy

(D) segmental mastectomy

(E) simple mastectomy

1521. Includes en bloc removal of the breast, pectoral muscles, and axillary nodes

1522. Includes removal of the entire breast, but leaves the axillary nodes intact

1523. Includes removal of the internal mammary nodes

1524. Includes en bloc removal of the breast, with underlying pectoralis major fascia and axillary lymph nodes

1525. Includes excision of a quadrant of the breast or lumpectomy

Answers and Explanations

1490. (E) Delayed childbearing, non-breast-feeding, high-fat diet, a positive family history, late menopause, early menarche, and mammary dysplasia are all risk factors in the development of breast cancer. Of the options listed, atypical epithelial hyperplasia is the greatest risk factor. Smoking is not proven to increase the risk of breast cancer.

1491. (D) While most breast cancer is found by the patient during self-examination, the earliest detectable lesions are most likely to be discovered using screening mammography in an asymptomatic, postmenopausal population.

1492. (E) Late findings in breast cancer include skin or nipple retraction, axillary adenopathy, sudden breast enlargement, redness, edema, chest wall pain, and fixation of a mass to the chest wall. Greenish-gray discharge is most often just ductal epithelial breakdown. Drooping of the breasts is a phenomenon of aging. Darkening of the areola is a progesterone effect most often seen in pregnancy. Most women have slightly asymmetric breast development, but this should be a lifelong condition. Skin or nipple retraction suggests interference with normal breast architecture, which occurs with malignancy.

1493. (D) Breast cancer is a disease that affects more than 1 of every 10 women if they live into their 80s. It is most common in postmenopausal white women who are nulliparous. Though some families have a strong genetic predisposition for breast cancer, 90 to 95% of women with the disease will have no first-degree relative with the disease and only about 20 to 25% have any identifiable risk factors. The survival after treatment in the early stages is high, but falls rapidly as the stage at diagnosis increases. The most common cancer in women is of the skin, and the cancer causing the greatest number of deaths is of the lung. Sixty is the median and mean age of women diagnosed with breast cancer.

1494. (A) The presenting complaint of about 70% of women with breast cancer is a painless lump. About 90% of these masses will be discovered by the patient herself. Breast cancer is usually slow growing. By the time a mass is palpable (1 to 2 cm), it may have been present 8 years! Nearly one half of breast cancers will occur in the upper outer quadrant and another 25% under the nipple and areola.

1495. (A) Cytology of nipple discharge and breast cyst aspirate is seldom diagnostic. It also has a high false-negative rate. Most experienced evaluators do not send the fluid for cytologic examination routinely unless the fluid is bloody. The fluid can be checked for blood by microscopy or guaiac. If it is bloody, further evaluation may be indicated. Negative results of such evaluation, however, cannot be considered reassuring.

1496. (E) Mammography is an excellent screening procedure in appropriate patients (postmenopausal and premenopausal patients with risk factors). The radiation is very low (approximately 0.1 rad with new equipment) and can be considered noncarcinogenic. It can detect nonpalpable breast cancer very accurately. When combined with physical examination in screening programs for new populations, a diagnosis rate for breast cancer as high as 6 per 1,000 is attained. About 80% of affected women diagnosed by mammogram have negative axillary lymph nodes, compared to 45% of those diagnosed by physical examination alone. However, mammography is not as good in diagnosing medullary carcinoma of the breast, and it has been reported that as high as 40% of some types of cancer can be diagnosed by palpation but do not show on mammography. While mammography is certainly indicated to aid in the diagnosis of a suspicious breast mass, the mass itself needs to be removed. Mammography is not a substitute for biopsy. Mammography is a much more effective technique than ultrasonography in detecting cancer, but ultrasound is useful to distinguish cystic from solid masses in the breast.

1497. **(A)** Many breast cancers may take 8 to 10 years to reach a palpable size. Mammograms may detect them several years before they become palpable. On the other hand, many breast cancers can be palpated that are not seen on mammograms. The clinical examination and mammography are complementary. While there are differences of opinion regarding when mammogram screening should begin and how often it should be performed in premenopausal women, there is agreement that all postmenopausal women should have annual mammographic screening, and the American College of Obstetricians and Gynecologists (ACOG) now recommends that women should be offered annual mammograms at age 40. There are groups of high-risk patients, such as those shown to be at genetic risk, who should begin screening in their 30s. Mammographic lesions are more difficult to detect in young women than lesions in postmenopausal women because the density of young women's breast tissue is greater. Their breast parenchyma has not yet been replaced by less dense fat. Women over 50 should definitely have yearly mammograms. Screening should not be stopped at age 70. Unlike many other cancers, the longer

a woman lives, the more likely she is to get breast cancer.

1498. **(E)** BI-RAD was devised to make mammographic terminology more standardized and to reduce confusion. Zero means more evaluation is needed, such as repeat mammogram film or ultrasound. One is a normal mammogram. Two is a benign lesion. For both of these, yearly screening is recommended. Three is a probably benign lesion, which demands a shorter follow-up. There is a low (< 2%) chance of malignancy. Four and five are suspicious or highly suspicious of malignancy, usually demanding biopsy.

1499. **(E)** Ultrasound helps most in distinguishing whether a mass detected on mammogram is cystic or solid. If the mass is cystic with a thin lining and no excretions, it can be safely aspirated, as it is almost always benign.

1500. **(D)** Although a few breast carcinomas grow very rapidly, most grow slowly and give time for screening to pick them up early enough for treatment to be highly efficacious. Women who do routine breast self-exam find lesions at approximately 2 cm in size.

1501. **(C)** Clinical breast exams can discover between 15 and 20% of breast cancers that are not detected by mammography. The examination will detect more masses if it is done systematically by both inspecting and palpating the breasts and taking 3 to 5 minutes to accomplish.

1502. **(B)** Breast self-examination is generally recommended for all women over the age of 20. Beginning at this age helps women get used to doing a normal examination and establish a routine, and provides them with a valuable cost-free disease prevention technique. Examining during the luteal phase of the cycle increases the probability of finding breast cysts and other changes in the parenchyma that are hormonally influenced. These changes can make the examination confusing in the menstrual-age patient. Examination is best performed just after menses when the breast is usually in its most quiescent state.

1503. (C) The BRCA1 gene is located on chromosome 17. It is a suppressor gene, and if a patient has a mutation, the risk of breast cancer in her lifetime is quite high, with small subsets of patients having an 80 to 85% risk during their lifetime. BRCA2, which is located on chromosome 13, also results in a similar increased breast cancer risk. As both members of this patient's family with breast cancer are alive, they can be checked for a BRCA1 or 2 gene mutation. If one is found, the patient can be evaluated for a similar mutation. Women with either BRCA1 or 2 mutations are at increased risk for ovarian cancer as well. These women should utilize recognized screening procedures to help detect cancer at an early stage. HER-2/neu is associated with decreased prognosis of known breast cancer but has not been of use as a screening diagnostic test. Neither T- nor B-cell levels are breast cancer screening tests. T cells are associated with cell-mediated immunity and B cells with antibody production. CA-125 has been found helpful to follow ovarian cancer, but has not been helpful for screening. It is not helpful for screening for breast cancer.

1504. (E) Lobular carcinoma in situ comprises approximately 2% of breast cancer, while 8% of breast cancer is invasive lobular. Ductal carcinoma in situ comprises approximately 10%, and infiltrating ductal carcinoma comprises 65% of breast cancer. Other types are less common.

1505. (C) Generally, patients with positive hormone status are more amenable to hormonal therapy (80% responders when metastatic disease is present). Chemotherapy is of benefit even in the estrogen/progesterone receptor–positive tumor. Tamoxifen is effective as an adjuvant to surgery or radiation, especially in receptor-positive patients. Chemotherapy is a benefit in both estrogen/progesterone receptor–positive and -negative tumors. DES was once given to induce receptors, but it is no longer administered.

1506. (C) A stage I tumor is less than 2 cm in diameter. Stage II tumors are less than 5 cm in di-

ameter and without any suspicious nodes. In this case, the nodes found are small and rubbery, and not suspicious for metastic disease. Stage III disease demonstrates tumor greater than 5 cm in diameter or tumor of any size with invasion of skin or attached to the chest wall. Supraclavicular nodes must be negative, and there should be no sign of distant metastases. Stage IV disease shows evidence of distant metastases (Table 23–1).

Table 23-1. Clinical and Histologic Staging of Breast Carcinoma and Relation to Survival

Clinical Staging (American Joint Committee)	Crude 5-Year Survival (%)
Stage I	85
Tumor < 2 cm in diameter	
Nodes, if present, not felt to contain metastases	
Without distant metastases	
Stage II	66
Tumor < 5 cm in diameter	
Nodes, if palpable, not fixed	
Without distant metastases	
Stage III	41
Tumor > 5 cm or—	
Tumor any size with invasion of skin or attached to chest wall	
Nodes in supraclavicular area	
Without distant metastases	
Stage IV	10
With distant metastases	

1507. (C) The histologic findings of lymph node dissection are extremely important in prognosis of early-stage breast cancers. Stage II breast cancer should have about a 66% survival rate at 5 years (stage I—85%, stage III—41%, stage IV—10%), but lymph node involvement can greatly alter prognosis. Unlike most other cancers, breast cancer survival at 5-year survival does not equate with cure. A patient with one positive lymph node has a 5-year chance of survival of about 60% and a 10-year chance of about 40%. A patient with more than four axillary lymph nodes positive for cancer has a 32% chance of survival at 5 years but only a 13% chance at 10 years. The survival rate appears to be increasing (see Table 23–2).

Table 23–2. Clinical and Histologic Staging of Breast Carcinoma and Relation to Survival

	Crude Survival (%)	
Histologic Staging	5 Years	10 Years
All patients	63	46
Negative axillary lymph nodes	78	65
Positive axillary lymph nodes	46	25
1–3 positive axillary lymph nodes	62	38
>4 positive axillary lymph nodes	32	13

1508. (C) Studies show that about 30% of patients who have clinically negative axillary nodes actually have spread of their breast cancer to these nodes. When the experienced clinician thinks nodes are involved at the time of surgery, cancer is found about 85% of the time.

1509. (C) The routine removal of all lymph nodes in the axilla creates a high incidence of chronic lymphedema. A method of injecting radioactive tracers and dye in the area of the tumor allows the lymph nodes that drain that tumor to be identified and removed without doing a complete axillary disection unless those nodes are positive.

1510. (D) Usually, no supraclavicular nodes are found to be involved. When they are, the cancer should be considered to be metastatic and stage III. Other ominous findings include suspicious infraclavicular lymph nodes and/or edema of the ipsilateral arm (see Table 23–1).

1511. (E) Paget's carcinoma of the breast is uncommon. It classically presents as itching and an erosion. Biopsy of the erosion makes the diagnosis. There may be no palpable mass, and the mammogram is unlikely to help in making the diagnosis. There are two learning points here: (1) breast pruritus is an uncommon complaint, and (2) a physical finding suggestive of tissue destruction merits biopsy.

1512. (C) About 30% of lesions thought to be cancerous prior to biopsy are benign, and about 15% (roughly one in seven) thought to be benign are cancerous. This emphasizes the need for biopsy for an accurate diagnosis.

1513. (C) Needle biopsies are excellent at making a diagnosis in most cases but have been reported to have false-negative rates as high as 20%. A negative biopsy, therefore, may have to be followed with an open biopsy in some patients. Open breast biopsies can usually be done as outpatient procedures with local anesthetic. In most cases, there is no need to remove more than the lump with a small margin of normal tissue surrounding it.

1514. (C) The first two options are unacceptable. Many patients will not have cancer on their biopsy, even when an experienced surgeon predicts it will be. These patients should be well informed about their problem, its diagnostic course, and possible outcomes; but they do not need to be unnecessarily frightened or subjected to uncertainties, such as "What will I find when I wake up?" For these reasons, the National Cancer Institute recommends a two-step approach. First, the patient is educated about the need for biopsy and the procedure of biopsy. After the biopsy, final reports are obtained and discussed so that she has time to consider treatment options, including reconstructive surgery. She should make a decision based on all the facts. Different patients have different needs, and evaluation regimens might have to be modified in some cases. The delay of the two-step regimen has not been shown to adversely effect prognosis for breast cancer.

1515. (A) Following either local excision of tumor plus radiotherapy or radical surgery, there is a 10 to 30% incidence of chronic edema of the ipsilateral arm. Breast reconstruction or implants seldom cause problems for the patient, despite what our media would have us believe. Still, most women choose not to have reconstructive surgery. Alopecia and leukocytopenia are almost always transient. Leukemia is a rare complication of combination chemotherapy, occurring most often with alkylating agents.

1516. (C) Bilateral mastectomy is the most effective means of preventing breast cancer in high-risk patients with up to 91% prevention. Bilateral oophorectomy may prevent 70%. First term birth before age 20 provides up to 50% prevention. Tamoxifen will prevent approximately 50%, and avoiding weight gain is the best lifestyle modification, which also includes the avoidance of smoking and drinking alcohol.

1517. (D) Any breast nodule in a postmenopausal woman should be biopsied immediately. Aspiration may be indicated for cystic masses during the menstrual years but has no place in this age group. Therapy, of course, is dependent on the pathology. If you do not perform radical breast surgery, immediate referral for biopsy and further care is indicated.

1518. (D) The diagnosis of breast cancer may be delayed during pregnancy because of the other changes in breast architecture and a lowered index of suspicion, but stage-for-stage prognosis is the same. Treatment can be carried out at any stage of pregnancy and by any technique in most cases. While not common, the incidence of breast cancer is about 10 to 30 per 100,000 pregnancies. By the time breast cancer is diagnosed and treated, about two thirds of pregnant patients have axillary metastases.

1519. (A, C, D, E) OCs may cause microglandular hyperplasia in the cervix but have no such effect on the breast. Fibrocystic changes and fibroadenomas are common conditions of the breast. Intraductal papillomas and fat necrosis are less common but may cause a mass. Mammary dysplasia or fibrocystic change (formerly called fibrocystic disease of the breast) is not a disease. Such changes are normal findings and are not felt to be precursors to cancer. Intraductal papilloma is a common cause of bloody discharge from the nipple. Fat necrosis most often results from injury to the breast and produces an indurated area.

1520. (A, E) Many women will have negative nodes at initial surgery, but 30 to 40% who do not appear to have grossly positive nodes have metastasis discovered during histologic examination. By addition of immunohistochemical staining for cytokeratin and serially sectioning the axillary nodes, 10 to 30% of women who were initially thought to have negative nodes by routine histologic evaluation will be found to have positive nodes.

1521–1525. (1521-C, 1522-E, 1523-A, 1524-B, 1525-D) Simple mastectomy removes the breast only, leaving the muscle, its fascia, and the axillary nodes. Lumpectomy removes only the mass and a small amount of surrounding normal tissue. Quadrantectomy is an extended lumpectomy and is also called segmental mastectomy. The radical mastectomy removes the breast, the pectoral muscles, and the axillary nodes en bloc. It was the standard operation on the breast for cure from the early 1900s through the early 1980s. In addition, the extended radical mastectomy removes the internal mammary nodes. The modified radical mastectomy removes the breast, with underlying pectoralis major fascia and axillary lymph nodes en bloc, but spares the pectoralis muscle.

CHAPTER 24

Gynecologic Oncology: Chemotherapy and Radiation Therapy in the Treatment of Malignancies of the Female Genital Tract

Questions

DIRECTIONS (Questions 1526 through 1545): Each of the numbered items or incomplete statements in this section is followed by answers or by completions of the statement. Select the ONE lettered answer or completion that is BEST in each case.

1526. The basic idea behind gynecologic chemotherapy is to exploit the fact that

(A) tumor cells and nontumor cells are different enough so that tumor cells might be able to be selectively killed

(B) all gynecologic malignancies have estrogen and progesterone receptors

(C) tumor cells can be made necrotic by destroying their oxygen-carrying capacity

(D) all of the above

1527. Tumors grow exponentially due to

(A) rapid proliferation

(B) Gompertzian growth

(C) rapid doubling time

(D) disruption in the regulation of programmed cell death (apoptosis)

1528. The mitotic index is the

(A) best indicator of a cell's dividing capacity

(B) fraction of cells in a steady-state condition

(C) way to determine the cell type of an actively dividing cell

(D) measure of estrogen effect in superficial cells in the female genital tract

1529. Growth fraction refers to the

(A) percentage of cells in the S phase at a particular time

(B) use of tritiated thymidine to produce measurable curves

(C) overall proportion of proliferating cells in a tumor

(D) rate at which a recurring tumor will grow

1530. The stem cell theory states that

(A) all malignant change begins in the primitive cells of the hematopoietic system

(B) malignancies are actually formed at the time of embryonic development and lie dormant until activated

(C) any cell has the capability to become malignant under the influence of releaser cells called "stems"

(D) only certain undifferentiated cells (stem cells) are able to divide to reproduce a tissue

(E) malignancy results from a disruption of a major organ system—by background radiation, constant irritation, or other mechanism

1531. The cell kill hypothesis is the fundamental principle behind the use of chemotherapeutic agents. It states that

(A) agents that are not tumoricidal (kill tumor cells) cannot be used alone in the treatment of malignancy

(B) chemotherapeutic agents will kill fewer cells with each subsequent course

(C) the proportion of cells killed is constant, despite the amount of therapeutic agent administered

(D) chemotherapy kills a constant proportion, not number of cells

(E) the relative sensitivity of cells to a given therapeutic agent must be tested before use or cells may not be killed (sensitivity testing)

1532. Which of the following statements regarding a malignancy is TRUE?

(A) As a tumor increases in size, the doubling time becomes much shorter.

(B) Death occurs with a tumor burden of about 10^{12} cells.

(C) A course of chemotherapy generally kills all but a few cells, and the tumor regrows from these few stem cells.

(D) Chemotherapy is scheduled such that every session will catch the tumor cells at their most vulnerable point and maximize tissue effect.

(E) A chemotherapeutic agent is considered curative when after a course only 10^4 cells remain.

1533. A 35-year-old female with stage IIB squamous cell carcinoma of the cervix will receive radiation. Regarding reproductive changes, you advise that

(A) ovaries are radioresistant

(B) fertility can be maintained

(C) radiation will likely result in endometrial ablation

(D) younger patients are more susceptible to radiation-induced castration

(E) there is no change in vaginal function

1534. As a tumor grows, host defenses seem to

(A) become less and less

(B) be unaffected

(C) become hyperactive

(D) be variably affected (stronger T-cell immunity, less B-cell immunity)

(E) none of the above

1535. As a general rule, drugs used in multiagent chemotherapeutic regimes must be

(A) effective as individual agents if they are to be effective together

(B) less effective than large-dose single agents, but also less toxic

(C) used in smaller doses to prevent tumor resistance

(D) most effective on slow-growing tumors

1536. During treatment with chemotherapy, an accepted definition of tumor response is

(A) complete response (CR) with no measurable tumor clinically over 6 months

(B) partial response (PR) with at least a 25% decrease in lesion size

(C) stable disease (SD) with no new lesions over 4 weeks

(D) progressive disease (PD) with at least a 75% increase in the lesion size

1537. Radiation medicine most typically involves the therapeutic manipulation of

(A) ionizing radiation

(B) nuclear energy

(C) nonionizing radiation

(D) beta radiation

(E) alpha radiation

1538. Radiant energy produces biologic change most commonly by

(A) inducing the growth of new, normal tissue

(B) damaging the DNA of target tissues

(C) producing heat that causes tissue dessication

(D) eliminating hydroxyl radicals (free radicals) from tissue

(E) all of the above

1539. The biologic effect of a course of radiation depends on

(A) total dose

(B) fractional design

(C) total treatment time

(D) field size

(E) all of the above

1540. Dosimetry means

(A) giving a uniform dose throughout the treatment field

(B) giving the largest tolerable dose of radiation to any given tissue

(C) the measure of the amount of radiation absorbed by the patient in any given area

(D) the size of the radiation source

(E) none of the above

1541. Previously, radiation therapy produced severe injuries to skin and external structures. Today, little skin injury is produced because

(A) far less radiation is administered

(B) radiation can now be administered from many more angles with precise movement of the patient to many delivery ports

(C) radiation sources today accelerate particles much faster and with less scatter, thus penetrating deeply and quickly and avoiding the skin

(D) radiation sources do not come in direct contact with the body because shielding is used

(E) pure uranium is used today instead of radium or cobalt

1542. The inverse square law states that

(A) the intensity of radiation delivered is inversely proportional to the square of the distance from the source

(B) radiation dosage delivered to a tumor when squared is inversely proportional to patient survival

(C) the square of the distance across a radiation field is inversely proportional to the total dosage of radiation that can be delivered to the lowest isodose zone

(D) the size of a delivery port (field) is inversely proportional to the field most distant to it within the treatment area

(E) the less dynamic your radiation therapist is, the more likely you are to be cured

1543. Regarding choriocarcinoma, which of the following statements is TRUE?

(A) It is generally effectively treated only with surgery.

(B) Chemotherapy has allowed a salvage rate for this disease of about 25%.

(C) Up to 90% of patients with choriocarcinoma can achieve a normal life expectancy.

(D) Choriocarcinoma is 100% curable in all cases with combination chemotherapy.

1544. A 46-year-old obese woman smokes two packs of cigarettes a day. She had a radical hysterectomy with a para-aortic and pelvic lymphadenectomy for stage IB squamous cell carcinoma of the cervix. At surgery she was found to have dense pelvic small bowel adhesions from a prior ruptured appendix and appendectomy. Lymph nodes were positive for cancer cells. In discussing postoperative radiation, you counsel her that she has an increased rate of radiation-related complication because of

(A) obesity

(B) excision of lymph nodes

(C) decreased bowel motility from adhesions

(D) age

(E) stage of the cancer

1545. A 43-year-old woman has stage III epithelial ovarian carcinoma. She had surgical debulking and has received five courses of carboplatin and paclitaxel. She is now due for her sixth course. She comes to clinic complaining of fatigue and myalgias. She has a temperature of 101.3°F. On examination, you find no obvious source of the fever. White blood cell (WBC) count is 1,000/mm³ (normal 4,500–11,000/mm³). Your next course of action is to

(A) send home and instruct to check temperature twice a day

(B) give a broad-spectrum antibiotic as outpatient

(C) admit to hospital and observe

(D) admit to hospital and start antibiotics

(E) admit to hospital and give sixth course of chemotherapy

DIRECTIONS (Questions 1546 through 1549): Each of the numbered items or incomplete statements in this section is followed by answers or by completions of the statement. Select the answers or completions that may apply.

1546. Which four of the following statements regarding the principles of clinical chemotherapy are TRUE?

(A) The chief aim of therapy is to achieve maximum cell kill with minimum toxicity.

(B) A steep dose–response curve for most drugs indicates that the highest tolerable dose producing an acceptable level of reversible toxicity should be used in treatment of susceptible tumors.

(C) In general, a therapeutic concentration of cell cycle–specific drugs is obtained by a 5-day course.

(D) Low-dose intermittent therapy has been most successful against tumors with a large growth fraction.

(E) Chronic therapy is feasible if toxicity is negligible.

1547. Toxic chemotherapeutic drugs may be used in which four of the following ways?

(A) in conjunction with surgery

(B) in conjunction with irradiation

(C) as a single treatment modality

(D) for palliation

(E) for cancer prevention

1548. Classes of drugs used in gynecologic cancer chemotherapy include which four of the following?

(A) alkylating agents

(B) antibiotics

(C) antimetabolites

(D) hormones

(E) antitussives

1549. Which three of the following statements regarding radiotherapy are TRUE?

(A) There is significant correlation between tumor responsiveness to irradiation and radiocurability.

(B) The standard daily dosage of radiation is about 400 to 500 rads.

(C) A course of pelvic radiotherapy will last 5 to 6 weeks to deliver the appropriate amount of radiation.

(D) Calculation of radiation dose to the pelvis is traditionally done as dosages to two theoretical points called A and B.

(E) A given dose of radiation kills a constant fraction of tumor cells.

DIRECTIONS (Questions 1550 through 1565): Each set of items in this section consists of a list of lettered headings followed by several numbered words or phrases. For each numbered word or phrase, select the ONE lettered option that is most closely associated with it. Each lettered option may be selected once, more than once, or not at all.

Questions 1550 through 1557

Match the class of chemotherapeutic agents with the most appropriate descriptor.

(A) alkylating agents

(B) antimetabolites

(C) antibiotics

(D) hormones

(E) none of the above

1550. Inhibit synthesis of DNA

1551. Act directly by arresting mitosis

1552. Disrupt DNA by binding of an alkyl group

1553. Act on more highly differentiated endometrial tumors

1554. Chlorambucil

1555. Dactinomycin

1556. Fluorouracil

1557. Ifosfamide

Questions 1558 through 1561

Match each chemotherapeutic agent with the most appropriate clinical description.

(A) carboplatin

(B) cyclophosphamide

(C) methotrexate

(D) paclitaxel

(E) mesna

(F) vinblastine

(G) doxorubicin

1558. A 60-year-old woman with stage III papillary serous ovarian cancer received standard surgical debulking treatment. She is on her third cycle of chemotherapy with typical agents for ovarian cancer. It is 3 weeks after her chemotherapy injection and her gums are bleeding and she has a nosebleed that will not stop. A platelet count is $10,000/mm^3$ (normal 150,000 to 400,000/mm^3).

1559. The patient in question 1558 is also receiving a second typical chemotherapeutic agent for ovarian cancer. The standard prophylactic medications were not ordered and her second cycle of chemotherapy was given. Ten minutes after the dose she develops dyspnea with bronchospasm, urticaria, and hypotension. You call for emergency equipment.

1560. A 53-year-old woman with advanced epithelial ovarian cancer is receiving an alkylating agent. Despite receiving 2 liters of normal saline with her chemotherapy, 4 days later she returns with gross hematuria. A platelet count is $110,000/mm^3$ (normal 150,000 to 400,000/mm^3).

1561. The patient in question 1560 returns for her next course of chemotherapy. You wish to continue the same regimen so you administer a chemoprotective agent to inactivate the bladder toxic metabolite.

Questions 1562 through 1565

(A) ovarian cancer

(B) vulvar cancer

(C) endometrial cancer

(D) cervical cancer

1562. The cornerstone of treatment is surgical, but adjuvant radiation therapy may be given pre- or postoperatively, depending on the grade of the tumor and depth of tumor invasion.

1563. The problem in this disease relates to the large field of radiation needed to treat it in most cases. A tumoricidal dose would cause serious bowel complications.

1564. Surgery is reserved for only early invasive lesions, and radiotherapy is the cornerstone of therapy for lesions stage IIB and greater.

1565. Tissues are so intolerant of radiotherapy that it is generally used only in cases with extremely large tumors prior to surgical debulking.

Answers and Explanations

1526. (A) Chemotherapy for gynecologic malignancies makes use of differences between normal and tumor cells in order to kill the tumor cells. All gynecologic malignancies do not have estrogen and progesterone receptors. Tumor cells die better when they are well oxygenated, not when they are deprived of oxygen (ask any radiotherapist).

1527. (D) Tumors grow exponentially because of disruption in the regulation of programmed cell death (apoptosis), not because of rapid proliferation. Gompertzian growth is the concept that as the tumor grows larger, the rate of growth slows.

1528. (B) A knowledge of the terminology of cell kinetics is helpful in understanding the dynamics of tumor cells. Some cells divide more slowly than others and will arrest in different stages of cell cycle. Cell division is halted with a vinca alkaloid and all the cells are counted. The number of cells in the process of division per 1,000 cells counted gives the mitotic index.

1529. (C) Growth fraction is the overall proportion of proliferating tumor cells in any given tumor. The percentage of S-phase cells in the cycle is another estimate of tumor growth. Growth fraction is not used clinically to treat recurrence.

1530. (D) The stem cell theory states that only certain undifferentiated cells (stem cells) are able to divide to reproduce a tissue. The remainder of the cells are well differentiated (specialized) and cannot undergo this change. Tumors are thought to arise from an individual stem cell. Malignant cells are thought to escape the normal regulation of cells in some as yet undetermined fashion.

1531. (D) The cell kill hypothesis states that the effect of cancer chemotherapy on cell populations is to kill a constant proportion of the cells present, not a constant number. The percentage of cells killed and therefore indirectly the number of cells killed in one cycle is dependent on the dose of the chemotherapeutic agent given.

1532. (B) This number (10^{12}) of tumor cells is only 1 to 2 orders of magnitude less than the total of number of cells in the body. As a tumor grows, its doubling time usually slows. Chemotherapy kills about 90% of cells as its maximum effect; 100% would have to be killed for the chemotherapy to be curative. Chemotherapy is spaced so that a large percentage of tumor cells will be killed but so that normal cells have time to recover between the courses, or else the patient might not survive the treatment, let alone the disease.

1533. (C) Ovaries are very radiosensitive organs. Radiation-induced castration can occur with doses as low as 500 rads (or less) in women over 40. Younger women are more resistant to radiation effects on the ovaries, but at doses of 1,000 to 1,500 rads, virtually all women will become postmenopausal from ovarian failure. The typical dose for cervical cancer is in the range of 6,000 to 6,500 rads, so she will lose her reproductive capacity, because of both ovarian failure and endometrial ablation. She will also have loss of vaginal elasticity. Vaginal stenosis can be a major problem if not addressed early.

1534. (A) Not only does the host's immune system seem to lose its abilities to fight off disease, but this effect is compounded by the fact that most chemotherapy drugs also suppress the immune system. Drugs like bacillus Calmette–Guérin (bCG) and *Corynebacterium parvum* have been used to try to increase host immunocompetence to overcome these problems.

1535. (A) In multiagent chemotherapy, each drug should be effective against the tumor. If each is not, effect is less. Toxicity at comparable dosage is no different than in single-agent therapy, and each drug must be monitored for its own side effects. Multiagent chemotherapy is used in the same general doses as if the agents were used alone. Generally, the faster growing a tumor is, the more susceptible it is to chemotherapeutic agents.

1536. (C) Stable disease encompasses anything from steady-state response less than partial response (see below) to progression less than progressive disease, lasting at least 4 weeks with no new lesions appearing. One should read articles carefully to ascertain the criteria used to determine significant responses to therapy. Complete response is complete disappearance of all clinical evidence of tumor determined by two evaluations at least 4 weeks apart. A partial response is a greater than 50% decrease in lesion size and no new lesions appearing. Progressive disease is an increase of at least 50% in lesion size or new lesions. Also remember, response does not necessarily correlate with survival in cancer treatment.

1537. (A) Ionizing radiation may be classified as electromagnetic (gamma ray, x-rays, photons) or particulate (electrons). Ionizing radiation is most commonly used in radiation medicine. Alpha, beta, and nonionizing radiation are not generally used in cancer therapy. While ionizing radiation is a form of nuclear energy, it is generally not considered in this way in the context of medical care. Beta emitters in the form 32P are sometimes used in the treatment of minimal-volume ovarian cancer.

1538. (B) Radiant energy is a nonspecific killer that destroys the DNA of cells that get in its path whether the cells are normal or abnormal. It is hoped that normal cells recover better than diseased ones. It does not burn cells. It creates free radicals.

1539. (E) To be effective, a radiation dose must be tumoricidal. The total dose of radiation delivered is important for tumor control and preservation of normal tissue. If a low dose is used so that no normal tissue is damaged, control of the tumor is unlikely. The opposite is true as well—if a large radiation dose is delivered to kill the tumor completely, unacceptably high damage to normal tissue may occur. Fractionation is dividing radiation treatments into small doses per session to shrink the rapidly dividing tumor cells but allow time for repair of normal cells. The energy of radiation absorbed depends on the size of the field being radiated. Large fields contain more scattered radiation and lead to a larger dose at a given depth.

1540. (C) Dosimetry is the measurement of the amount of radiation absorbed by the patient. It is measured in rads (1 centigray), gray (100 rads), or milligram hours (which are hard to convert to rads). Measuring the doses in a radiation field produces isodose curves (Figure 24–1) that allow exact measures of the radiation delivered.

1541. (C) The use of the linear accelerator produces very high energy with very little scatter. Radiation can penetrate deeply into tissue with very little surface damage. We could also use many delivery ports.

1542. (A) The inverse square law states that the intensity of radiation delivered to an area is inversely proportional to the square of the distance that area is from the source. An

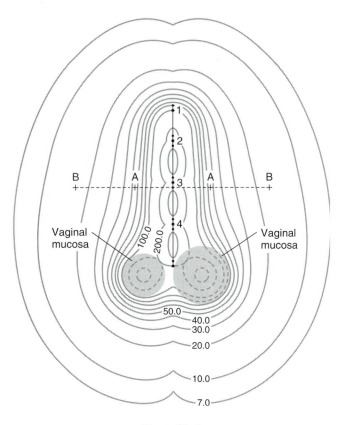

Figure 24–1.

important application of this law is that the rapid fall-off of energy from the source does not permit delivering cancericidal doses at the margins of a field without causing significant damage throughout the field. On the flip side, a higher dose of radiation may be delivered to the tumor site, with rapid fall off of the dose sparing surrounding normal tissue.

1543. (C) Choriocarcinoma used to be almost universally fatal. It can now be cured in nearly 100% of cases when it is not metastatic and in 90% of all cases. Surgery to evacuate the uterus is still used, but it is not the most effective mainstay of treatment.

1544. (C) After previous surgery where marked adhesions were found, it is likely that adhesions will reform and lead to bowel being fixed in place. These fixed loops of bowel will receive a higher-than-normal dose of radiation. There may also be decreased vascularity after surgery, which can make the bowel

more susceptible to radiation damage. Other factors that may increase the risk of radiation injury include concomitant chemotherapy, superimposed infection, presence of malnutrition, and use of tobacco. She should be advised to stop smoking.

1545. (D) Chemotherapy commonly induces neutropenia, which puts patients at risk for serious infections including bacteremia. Often, fever is the only complaint of patients with neutropenia and bacteremia. These infections can progress rapidly. The diagnosis is made by blood culture, chest x-ray, and urine culture. Any febrile, neutropenic patient should be admitted and placed on two antibiotics, although some investigators recommend single-antibiotic therapy with agents like imipenem. Giving the sixth course of chemotherapy is contraindicated with the current neutropenia and should be delayed. Granulocyte colony stimulating factors (GCSFs) may decrease the duration of neutropenia.

1546. (A, B, C, E) High-dose intermittent therapy is most successful. All the other statements are true.

1547. (A, B, C, D) Chemotherapy may be curative for solid tumors. It is the initial treatment of choice for trophoblastic disease. Otherwise, in gynecologic malignancy, tumor burden is reduced prior to its use, either with radiation or surgery. In some cancers, especially ovarian carcinoma, the patient may be made more comfortable and have less ascites through the use of such agents, even though the chance for cure is minimal. Some nontoxic drugs (e.g., tamoxifen) may be used for prevention.

1548. (A, B, C, D) These are the major categories of drugs used along with plant alkaloids and antiestrogens. You should know the general method of action of each basic type. Plant alkaloids are effective in arresting mitosis. Currently, the most active agents in gynecologic malignancy are platinum variants, paclitaxel, and antiestrogens. Antitussives are used to suppress coughs.

1549. (C, D, E) There is no significant correlation between the responsiveness of a tumor to irradiation and radiocurability. A tumor may be radiosensitive but not curable (lymphoma) or radioresistant but curable (adenocarcinoma of the cervix). A given dose of radiation kills a constant fraction of tumor cells. The standard daily dosage of radiation is 180 to 200 rads over 5 to 6 weeks and given 5 days out of 7, which often leads to excessive tissue damage. Whole pelvis radiation is followed with isodose curves, but points A and B are traditional indicators of therapy. Point A is an imaginary point, 2 cm lateral to the endocervical canal and 2 cm above the lateral vaginal fornix. Point B is 5 cm lateral to the endocervical canal in the same transverse plane as point A. The dose to point A, theoretically, is the dose to the parametrial tissue, and the dose to point B is the dose to the pelvic sidewall.

1550. (B) By competing in the metabolic process, the antimetabolites inhibit the formation of DNA and RNA. They work on the basis of cancer cells being the most rapid to divide (see Figure 24–2).

1551. (E) Vinblastine and vincristine are alkaloids that act by arresting mitosis, as does colchicine. The vinca alkaloids inhibit the assembly of the microtubules. Colchicine is used for arresting cell mitosis for chromosomal analysis, not chemotherapy.

1552. (A) A cross-linkage is destroyed, preventing RNA formation. Melphalan and cyclophosphamide are common examples.

1553. (D) A good example of hormonal action is the effect on well-differentiated carcinoma of the endometrium by progesterone. The more differentiated cells may cease their proliferation and eventually become atrophic. Pulmonary metastases often respond well.

1554. (A) Chlorambucil is an alkylating agent that may be given orally.

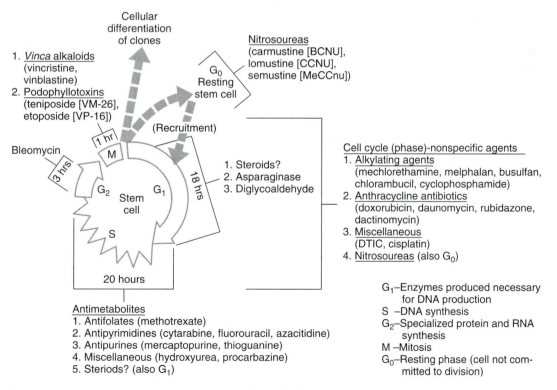

Figure 24–2.

1555. (C) Actinomycin D is another name for this antibiotic used in chemotherapy. It intercalates DNA and inhibits DNA transcription and RNA translation. It is gastrointestinal (GI) toxic and limited in the total amount that can be used. Alopecia and mouth ulcers can be severe. It has proven active in treatment of germ cell tumors of the ovary and of gestational trophoblastic disease.

1556. (B) The name itself should give a clue as to this compound's competitive status with needed metabolites. It is a well-tolerated drug, used most often in the treatment of colon cancer. However, it is also used as a radiation sensitizer in cervical cancer, recurrent ovarian cancer, and vaginal dysplasia (5% cream).

1557. (A) Ifosfamide is an alkylating agent used for first-line treatment for advanced or recurrent cervical cancer and some gynecologic sarcomas or for second-line treatment for advanced ovarian cancer.

1558. (A) Carboplatin is a typical platinum-based agent used for advanced ovarian cancer of epithelial origin. It appears to cause DNA lesions intracellularly by intercalating DNA. Carboplatin toxicities differ slightly from cisplatin. The most frequent dose-limiting complication of carboplatin is bone marrow suppression, particularly thrombocytopenia. The platelet nadir occurs 3 weeks after dosing. Nephrotoxicity is less common than with cisplatin.

1559. (D) Paclitaxel (Taxol) is an important addition to the chemotherapy drugs for advanced ovarian cancer. It is derived from the needles and bark of the Western Yew tree. Prior to giving standard premedication with dexamethasone, diphenhydramine, and cimetidine (or equivalents), major hypersensitivity reactions occurred in 25 to 39% of women. With premedication, the reaction occurs less than 2% of the time. It usually occurs after the first or second dose of paclitaxel. Other toxicities include myelosuppression (mostly neutropenia) and neurotoxicity.

1560. (B) A cyclophosphamide metabolite, acrolein, can alkylate bladder mucosa and cause hemorrhagic cystitis. For that reason, patients are often prehydrated and instructed to drink eight glasses of fluid daily during the 2 days after cyclophosphamide dosing. Sterile hemorrhagic cystitis can occur any time after dosing for up to several weeks. Her platelet count is sufficiently high, so you would not expect thrombocytopenia to be the cause of her hematuria.

1561. (E) Mesna is a sulfhydryl-containing compound that can neutralize the cyclophosphamide and ifosfamide metabolite acrolein. Administration of mesna does not decrease antitumor activity.

1562. (C) In endometrial cancer, the cornerstone of treatment is surgical, but adjuvant radiation therapy may be given pre- or postoperatively, depending on the grade of the tumor and the depth of tumor invasion.

1563. (A) In ovarian cancer, the problem of treating with radiation is related to the large field needed to treat the disease in most cases. A tumoricidal dose would cause intolerable serious bowel complications. The complications to bowel, such as enteritis, proctitis, fistulization, perforation, and obstruction, would be so high from tumoricidal doses that patients could not survive the treatment. These complications occasionally occur despite the most cautious and well-thought-out treatment with the latest techniques and information.

1564. (D) In cervical cancer therapy, radical hysterectomy is reserved for only early invasive lesions (IB–IIA), and radiotherapy is the cornerstone of therapy for lesions stage IIB and greater.

1565. (B) Vulvar tissues are intolerant of radiotherapy, which is generally used only in cases with extremely large tumors prior to surgery. If the tumor can be radiated and the remainder of the vulva spared, some degrees of success may be experienced.

CHAPTER 25

Infectious Diseases in Obstetrics and Gynecology
Questions

DIRECTIONS (Questions 1566 through 1599): Each of the numbered items or incomplete statements in this section is followed by answers or by completions of the statement. Select the ONE lettered answer or completion that is BEST in each case.

1566. A 23-year-old woman at 29 weeks' gestation ruptures her amniotic membranes. She is admitted to the hospital and 3 days later she is found to have a temperature of 101.1°F, a white blood count (WBC) of 15,000, fetal tachycardia, and mild tenderness over her lower abdomen. What is the most likely diagnosis for this patient?

(A) intra-amniotic infection

(B) lower urinary tract infection

(C) pyelonephritis

(D) genital herpes

(E) cytomegalovirus

1567. Three weeks after delivery, a 29-year-old primipara, who is breast-feeding twin girls, presents to the clinic complaining of a tender right breast mass. On physical examination, you find a 5-cm fluctuant, swollen, reddened mass in her right breast that is exquisitely tender to the touch. Axillary lymph nodes on the ipsilateral side are enlarged and tender. Which of the following statements regarding this patient is TRUE?

(A) This mass requires a breast biopsy.

(B) These findings are consistent with an inflammatory carcinoma of the breast, as well as puerperal mastitis.

(C) The causative organism is most likely *Escherichia coli* secondary to contamination from the infants' stools.

(D) She should continue to breast-feed on the other side, and this mass is likely to subside spontaneously if she just manually expresses the involved breast.

(E) The mass should be incised and drained and antibiotics given to the mother; the infants need no therapy.

1568. Two weeks after the birth of her infant, a new mother brings the child in to see you. The child's eyes are edematous, with conjunctival erythema and a mucopurulent discharge. Your evaluation and treatment should include

(A) a pelvic examination (using a small scope) of the infant

(B) a pelvic examination of the mother and a swab of the maternal cervix for evaluation

(C) anaerobic cultures of the infant's and mother's eyes

(D) immunoglobulin M (IgM) titers of the infant

(E) penicillin VK for both the mother and infant

1569. Three days after an elective termination of pregnancy, a 29-year-old woman presents to the emergency department with a history of mild abdominal pain and fever, a physical examination showing pelvic tenderness, and a purulent cervical discharge. A Gram stain of the cervical discharge shows gram-negative intracellular diplococci. Which of the following statements is TRUE?

(A) Gonorrhea is the likely diagnosis.

(B) These findings are most consistent with a chlamydial infection.

(C) A careful search for a chancre or ulcer-like lesion should be made.

(D) The Gram stain is pathognomonic and no culture is needed.

(E) You should provide no treatment until culture results return.

1570. Which of the following is TRUE regarding congenital syphilis?

(A) Adequate maternal treatment before 16 weeks' gestation prevents congenital syphilis.

(B) The Jarisch–Herxheimer reaction refers to the reddish burrows made under the skin that are pathognomonic of syphilis.

(C) Recommended treatment for maternal syphilis is 10 to 14 days of oral tetracycline.

(D) The Venereal Disease Research Laboratory test (VDRL) is a more specific but less sensitive test for syphilis than the fluorescent treponemal antibody absorption test (FTA-ABS).

(E) Fetal and neonatal IgM testing can readily identify syphilis in the infant at risk.

1571. A woman has a stillborn infant covered with a petechial rash. Which of the following infections would be most likely?

(A) herpes zoster

(B) herpes simplex

(C) *Listeria monocytogenes*

(D) human papillomavirus (HPV)

(E) chronic active hepatitis

1572. Regarding immunization during pregnancy, which of the following vaccines would be the safest to receive during pregnancy?

(A) mumps

(B) polio

(C) rabies

(D) rubella

(E) rubeola

1573. A seropositive HIV-infected mother comes to your clinic at 9 weeks' gestation. She wants to know about her risks in pregnancy. Which of the following statements is TRUE?

(A) Without treatment, the chance of transmission to the infant is nearly 100%.

(B) Because of their known teratogenicity, protease inhibitors are contraindicated in pregnancy.

(C) A tuberculin skin test should be done as a routine part of prenatal care.

(D) Breast-feeding is safe for the infant and should be encouraged.

(E) Pregnancy predisposes the gravida to change from seropositivity to developing the AIDS-related complex of problems.

1574. Herpes simplex virus (HSV) infection in pregnancy is associated with

(A) a nearly 50% neonatal mortality rate in untreated infected infants

(B) a nearly 100% transmission rate in infants born to mothers with active infection at the time of delivery

(C) a nearly 0% transmission rate to infants of mothers treated with zidovudine (AZT) during pregnancy

(D) a higher risk of neonatal infection in women with recurrent infection compared to women with primary infection

(E) a nearly 50% reduction in vertical transmission of HSV-2 if the mother has pre-existing antibody to HSV-1

1575. An infant, seemingly well when born, demonstrates microcephaly, chorioretinitis, deafness, and delayed development later in life. Which of the following is the most likely cause?

   (A) herpes hominis type 2 virus acquired at the time of delivery

   (B) cytomegalovirus (CMV) infection during pregnancy

   (C) vitamin K deficiency in the newborn

   (D) late-onset group B streptococcal infection

   (E) parvovirus infection

1576. A 19-year-old woman who has never had chickenpox has just been exposed to the disease (about 36 hours ago) at 16 weeks' gestation. She presents to your office, and you correctly tell her that

   (A) varicella-zoster, the causative virus, is not very contagious and infection is unlikely

   (B) varicella-zoster has been shown to have little or no effect during pregnancy; nothing needs to be done

   (C) though she may get chickenpox and be at increased risk for related pneumonia, fetal effects of this illness would be nil

   (D) the pregnancy now has about a 25 to 30% chance of major anomalies, and she should consider termination

   (E) the administration of varicella-zoster immune globulin should attenuate the maternal effects of varicella infection (VZIG)

1577. A 27-year-old gravida you have been following throughout her pregnancy presents at 22 weeks' gestation not feeling well. She complains of fever, cough, a runny nose, conjunctivitis, and on examination has white spots surrounded by a halo of erythema on her buccal mucosa and an erythematous maculopapular rash on her abdomen. You tell her that

   (A) this disease will be teratogenic

   (B) she should be immediately vaccinated

   (C) she has measles (rubeola), but the chance of its affecting her baby are small

   (D) stillbirth is a 50% likelihood

   (E) she has pneumonia

1578. Mumps in pregnancy is associated with

   (A) increased fetal wastage

   (B) limb reduction defects

   (C) maternal pneumonia

   (D) no major complications

   (E) congenital deafness

1579. Rubella in pregnancy is associated with

   (A) severe fetal congenital malformations and pregnancy wastage

   (B) increased maternal mortality

   (C) a rapidly declining incidence

   (D) the maternal development of type 2 diabetes

   (E) all of the above

1580. A 24-year-old primigravida at 36 weeks' gestation is exposed to chickenpox. She has no history of varicella. You recommend

   (A) the varicella vaccine within 48 hours of exposure

   (B) immediate administration of VZIG and acyclovir

   (C) intravenous acyclovir and the varicella vaccine within 96 hours

   (D) immediate serologic testing for varicella, and if negative, administration of VZIG

   (E) VZIG within 96 hours

1581. Of the following individuals, who would theoretically be at highest demographic risk for toxoplasmosis infection during pregnancy?

   (A) country–western singer

   (B) medical technologist

   (C) plumber

   (D) cat breeder

   (E) kitchen worker in Los Angeles

1582. A 22-year-old medical missionary is 16 weeks' pregnant and headed for a mission in an area of West Africa that is endemic for malaria. She consults you about her risks from malaria in pregnancy. The most appropriate thing to tell her is that

(A) her risks can be made considerably less by taking malarial prophylaxis

(B) antimalarial prophylaxis is dangerous for the fetus

(C) both her risk and the fetal risk from malaria can be lessened by chloroquine prophylaxis

(D) only quinine is safe for malarial prophylaxis during pregnancy

(E) primigravid women are relatively immune to malaria because of the tremendous increase in, and the suppressive effect of, progesterone on *Plasmodium falciparum*

1583. A 25-year-old sexually active woman complains of a "fishy" smelling gray-white vaginal discharge. You examine this on wet mount and see epithelial cells with clusters of bacteria obscuring their borders. The vaginal pH is 5.5. Which of the statements below is TRUE regarding her infection?

(A) Her male sex partner is likely symptomatic.

(B) It has been implicated in preterm birth in pregnant women.

(C) Regular douching would have prevented her infection.

(D) Culture is recommended to confirm the diagnosis.

(E) The treatment of choice is penicillin.

1584. Which of the following statements regarding the sequelae of chronic salpingitis is TRUE?

(A) Teenagers may be more likely to develop upper genital tract disease than women in their late 20s.

(B) Despite geographic location or ethnic background, the rates of gonorrheal infection are nearly the same across all U.S. population subsets.

(C) Chronic salpingitis from a chlamydial infection is much more likely to be associated with extensive tubal damage than is that from gonorrheal organisms or anaerobes.

(D) The recovery of anaerobic organisms in chronic pelvic inflammatory disease (PID) with an abscess portends an especially bad prognosis for the infected woman.

(E) The bacteria and viral particles involved are smaller than the pores in a latex condom; therefore, passage of these pathogens is almost guaranteed.

1585. A 39-year-old woman presents complaining of severe, low abdominal–pelvic pain that began the day after her menses ended. She has noticed some increase in vaginal discharge. Her social history shows she and her late husband had been medical missionaries their entire lives. He was her only sexual partner, and since his death 1 year ago, she has not had intercourse. Physical examination shows a temperature of 99.6°F. She is on the examining table on her side, doubled over, and clutching her abdomen with both arms. She has abdominal tenderness with mild rebound (right greater than left), cervical motion tenderness (greatest on rectal examination), and mild tenderness in the area of the right adnexa with no masses felt. Gram stain of her cervix shows a "few WBCs"; WBC is 10,400 (normal 3,600 to 10,000), and an erythrocyte sedimentation rate of 47 mm/hr (normal 0 to 25). A urine pregnancy test is negative. The next logical step in evaluation of this patient would be to

(A) admit her to the hospital with presumed PID, begin parenteral antibiotics, and wait 24 to 48 hours to assess her progress

(B) perform culdocentesis

(C) perform a pelvic ultrasound

(D) order a computed tomography (CT) scan of the abdomen and pelvis

(E) take her to the operating room for diagnostic laparoscopy

1586. A 45-year-old Laotian woman is visiting her daughter. She comes to your office complaining of frequent intermenstrual bleeding for years. You examine her and feel that her pelvis is "firmly fixed," with little mobility of the organs. You perform an endometrial biopsy. The pathology report returns stating that "frequent giant cells, caseous necrosis, and granuloma formation" are seen. Which of the following is TRUE?

(A) She should be tested for syphilis.

(B) A formal dilation and curettage (D&C) is required with these findings suggestive of malignancy.

(C) Testing for tuberculosis, with culture of an endometrial aspirate, and chest x-ray is indicated.

(D) Fungal cultures of the endometrium are indicated.

(E) Treatment of this condition will require major pelvic surgery.

1587. Which of the following statements is TRUE regarding intrauterine device (IUD)-associated infections?

(A) *Actinomyces* on a Pap smear is pathognomonic of infection.

(B) All IUDs are associated with about the same incidence of infection.

(C) An IUD in place during pregnancy increases the risk of spontaneous abortion.

(D) Antibiotics should be given for 2 weeks after every IUD insertion.

(E) Only the sexually promiscuous user will have an increased incidence of PID from the IUD.

1588. A 43-year-old woman has had a history of frequency, urgency, and dysuria for the past 8 years. She has had five negative urine cultures and urinalyses in the last year. Cystoscopy 1 month ago showed a normal bladder and reddened urethra. An intravenous pyelogram (IVP) is normal. The most likely diagnosis is

(A) the patient is surreptitiously using antibiotics to mask her laboratory results

(B) tuberculous urethritis

(C) vulvar vestibulitis syndrome

(D) urethral syndrome

(E) urethral gonorrhea

1589. A 51-year-old woman presents complaining of dysuria, dyspareunia, frequency of urination, dribbling of urine from the urethra when she stands after voiding, and a painful swelling under her urethra. Which of the following is the most likely diagnosis?

(A) simple cystitis

(B) urethral syndrome

(C) infection of the Skene's glands

(D) infected urethral diverticulum

(E) urethral carcinoma

1590. On the evening after a vaginal hysterectomy, a patient develops a temperature of 100.4°C. You are called to evaluate her. Which of the following do you consider most likely prior to examining the patient?

(A) She probably has a urinary tract infection (UTI).

(B) Ureteral obstruction is likely.

(C) Her fever may be factitious.

(D) She may be having an allergic reaction to her medications.

(E) The temperature elevation is most likely unrelated to a surgical infection.

1591. The same patient continues to have fever in the 102° to 104°F range over the next few days. A pelvic examination is repeated and a midline, tender mass about 8 cm in diameter is noted over the vaginal cuff. What should be your next step?

(A) Obtain an erythrocyte sedimentation rate (ESR) and WBC, and change the antibiotics.

(B) Get an infectious disease consult.

(C) Send a vaginal culture to assess the coverage of your antibiotics.

(D) Open the vaginal cuff in the midline.

(E) Aspirate the vaginal cuff for culture.

1592. For which of the following procedures would prophylactic antibiotics be appropriate?

(A) amniocentesis

(B) laparoscopy

(C) tubal sterilization

(D) vaginal hysterectomy

(E) episiotomy repair

1593. The term *pelvic cellulitis* refers to

(A) an infection secondary to gonorrhea

(B) a mixed anaerobic infection

(C) redness in the groin and upper thighs

(D) soft tissue infections, generally of the contiguous retroperitoneal space above the vaginal apex

(E) an infected collection of blood

1594. Bacterial vaginosis in pregnancy has been associated with which of the following complications?

(A) intrauterine growth restriction and neonatal immunodeficiency

(B) preterm premature rupture of the membranes, neonatal jaundice, and ocular infection in the neonate

(C) preterm premature rupture of the membranes, preterm labor, and chorioamnionitis

(D) preterm labor, chorioamnionitis, and ocular infection in the neonate

(E) intrauterine growth restriction, preterm premature rupture of the membranes, and neonatal jaundice

1595. A 35-year-old woman undergoes a cesarean section after a failed induction for past dates. Three days after surgery, she develops a high spiking fever. Ampicillin and gentamicin are administered. Complete physical examination shows no abnormality except a tender uterus. Blood, urine, and sputum cultures are negative. On the fifth day after surgery, a hectic (spiking) fever is still present. The antibiotics are changed to ampicillin, genta-

micin, and clindamycin in high dosage. Forty-eight hours later, the fever persists, and examination shows a tender uterus. A chest x-ray is normal. Pelvic CT is consistent with parametrial thrombosed vessels but no abscess. Which of the following is the next best step in managing this patient?

(A) Reoperate to find the source of the fever.

(B) Anticoagulate the patient with heparin.

(C) Get an infectious disease consult.

(D) Discontinue all antibiotic medication and reculture the patient.

(E) Change antibiotics again.

1596. A 34-year-old woman (gravida 2, para 1) is at 13 weeks' gestation by last menstrual period (LMP) with a desired pregnancy. She presents to the emergency department very anxious with a 10-hour history of low abdominal cramping and vaginal bleeding. Her temperature is 102.2°F, and her uterus is markedly tender on bimanual examination. Ultrasound shows an intrauterine pregnancy with a crown–rump length consistent with her LMP and fetal cardiac activity present. Her cervix is dilated 1 cm. Her WBC is 26,000. The best management for her is to

(A) place a cervical cerclage immediately after administering antibiotics

(B) administer antibiotics and expectantly manage her

(C) evacuate her uterus after administering antibiotics

(D) administer antibiotics, and if she does not spontaneously abort after 24 hours of observation, place a cervical cerclage

(E) place her on bed rest and administer both a tocolytic and antibiotics

1597. On the seventh day after abdominal hysterectomy, a morbidly obese patient stands to go to the bathroom and spontaneously passes "a large amount (more than a liter) of serosanguinous fluid" from her abdominal wound. This sign most likely indicates that

(A) she has a wound dehiscence

(B) a wound hematoma has spontaneously drained

(C) a medical student should stay in the room to see if there is more drainage from the wound

(D) you will need to remove the skin staples fron the wound, as they are likely causing an allergic reaction

(E) there is a urinary tract draining spontaneously through the patient's wound

Questions 1598 and 1599

A 22-year-old primigravida learns she is HIV positive with a high viral load at 10 weeks' gestation.

1598. In counseling her on initiating multiagent active antiretroviral therapy, you explain that

(A) the transmission rate without therapy is approximately 80%

(B) the drugs are not likely to have significant effects on her immune system; they are used exclusively to reduce the risk of perinatal transmission

(C) the regimen should routinely be discontinued following delivery

(D) the full effects of multiagent therapy on the fetus are not well delineated

(E) antiretroviral drug therapy is less effective during pregnancy

1599. At 36 weeks' gestation, despite multiagent therapy, her viral load is greater than 1,000 copies per milliliter. In discussing the potential benefit of scheduled cesarean section, you explain that

(A) most perinatal transmission occurs as a result of hematogenous dissemination early in pregnancy

(B) there is no evidence that scheduled cesarean section reduces perinatal transmission rates in women on antiretroviral therapy

(C) scheduled cesarean section may decrease her risk of transmitting HIV to her infant

(D) compared with HIV-negative women undergoing cesarean section, her risk of endometritis is 10-fold higher

(E) cesarean section, if performed after the initiation of labor or rupture of membranes, poses a greater risk of HIV transmission than does uncomplicated vaginal birth

Questions 1600 through 1602

An asymptomatic 24-year-old African-American woman with sickle cell trait is found on routine prenatal screening at 14 weeks' gestation to have symptomatic bacteriuria (10^5 colonies/mL).

1600. Her risk of developing pyelonephritis if untreated is

(A) 5 to 10%

(B) 20 to 30%

(C) 40 to 50%

(D) 60 to 70%

(E) 90 to 100%

1601. The most likely organism to be cultured is

(A) group B streptococcus

(B) *Klebsiella pneumoniae*

(C) *Chlamydia trachomatis*

(D) *Proteus* species

(E) *Escherichia coli*

1602. An appropriate choice of antibiotic therapy for this patient pending culture results is

(A) ampicillin

(B) tetracycline

(C) ciprofloxacin

(D) nitrofurantoin

(E) metronidazole

DIRECTIONS (Questions 1603 through 1609): Each of the numbered items or incomplete statements in this section is followed by answers or completions of the statement. Select the answers or completions that may apply.

1603. Which four of the following are associated with toxic shock syndrome?

(A) a woman colonized with *Staphylococcus aureus*

(B) an organism producing an associated toxin

(C) an abrasion or trauma site to provide a portal of entry into the systemic circulation

(D) facultative anaerobic organisms

(E) shock and multisystem organ failure

1604. Which three of the following statements regarding viral influenza during pregnancy are TRUE?

(A) The most common serious complication of influenza during pregnancy is pneumonia.

(B) Amantadine should be used to treat most pregnant women with influenza during the third trimester because of the potential adverse sequelae in pregnancy and the fetus.

(C) Viral influenza is associated with an increased risk of maternal mortality.

(D) There is concern about teratogenicity of the influenza vaccine if used in the first trimester.

(E) Women who are at high risk for influenza complications because of other diseases, such as diabetes or heart disease, should be vaccinated against influenza.

1605. Regarding acute salpingitis or acute PID, which two of the following statements are TRUE?

(A) Acute PID is usually polymicrobial in etiology.

(B) PID is an ascending infection, with organisms gaining access to the abdominal cavity through the vagina, cervix, uter-

ine corpus, and finally through the fallopian tube.

(C) The longer an infection incubates, the more likely gonorrheal organisms are to be cultured from the cervix or fallopian tubes of the patient.

(D) There is a good correlation (> 80%) between organisms cultured from the cervix and those cultured from the tube at the time of laparoscopy.

(E) Women who use oral contraceptives (OCs) are at higher risk for developing acute PID.

1606. Which three of the following statements regarding lower UTI (cystitis) are TRUE?

(A) The most common symptoms of lower UTI are frequency, urgency, and dysuria.

(B) Incontinence is not a symptom associated with UTI.

(C) One in five women will develop UTI in her lifetime.

(D) Cystitis is often associated with greater than 10^5 bacteria per milliliter of urine.

(E) *Streptococcus faecalis* is the most common organism recovered from the urine of young healthy women with cystitis.

1607. Which three of the following statements regarding postoperative wound infection are TRUE?

(A) In treatment, antibiotics are more important than drainage.

(B) The patient's systemic resistance is important in preventing postoperative wound infections.

(C) Obesity may increase the incidence of wound infection.

(D) Corticosteroids may suppress the inflammatory phase of the wound healing process.

(E) The first symptoms of wound infection usually begin between the second and fourth postoperative days.

1608. Necrotizing fasciitis is a particularly virulent, rapidly progressing soft tissue infection.

Which two of the following are other characteristics of this infection?

(A) It is easily diagnosed based on clinical findings.
(B) Treatment requires wide debridement of all necrotic tissue up to bleeding margins.
(C) Antibiotics are not needed for treatment.
(D) Obese patients are more susceptible.
(E) Patients do not generally appear toxic.

1609. A woman delivers and 48 hours later is noted to have a fever of 101.3°F, uterine tenderness, low abdominal pain, and leukocytosis. You obtain cultures from the uterine cavity by cleansing the cervix with povidone–iodine and inserting a sterile cotton-tipped swab into the endometrial cavity and inoculating a culture medium for aerobic and anaerobic bacteria. Of the following, which four would your laboratory be most likely to report?

(A) group B streptococcus
(B) enterococcus
(C) *Escherichia coli*
(D) *Chlamydia trachomatis*
(E) *Bacteroides* species

DIRECTIONS (Questions 1610 through 1627): Each set of items in this section consists of a list of lettered headings followed by several numbered words or phrases. For each numbered word or phrase, select the ONE lettered option that is most closely associated with it. Each lettered option may be selected once, more than once, or not at all.

Questions 1610 through 1616

Match the type of infection with the most appropriate descriptor.

(A) candidal vaginal infections
(B) *Trichomonas*
(C) bacterial vaginosis
(D) atrophic vaginitis
(E) mucopurulent cervicitis
(F) foreign body

1610. Most common type of vaginitis with a high pH in the sexually active mature patient.

1611. In cases of treatment failure, combined oral and intravenous therapy with metronidazole may be indicated.

1612. The patient complains of a white, curdy discharge and vaginal burning and itching; on examination, the copious discharge is confirmed. The vaginal pH is 3.0.

1613. Associated most commonly with chlamydia or gonorrhea.

1614. Diagnosis may require vaginoscopy.

1615. The treatment should include intravaginal estrogen therapy.

1616. The most likely causative organism also has a high associated incidence of upper genital tract infection.

Questions 1617 through 1627

Match the choices with the most closely associated descriptor.

(A) uncomplicated anogenital gonorrhea
(B) disseminated gonococcal infection
(C) syphilis
(D) chancroid
(E) lymphogranuloma venereum
(F) donovanosis
(G) pediculosis pubis
(H) scabies
(I) molluscum contagiosum
(J) genital herpes infection
(K) HPV infection
(L) genital mycoplasma

1617. Diagnosis is made from culture on Thayer–Martin or Transgrow media.

1618. An asymptomatic disease on the vulvar skin, spread by close contact; it can be found as a disseminated disease in children that is not necessarily spread by sexual contact.

1619. The causative organism for genital condyloma, it is an etiologic agent, cofactor, or enhancer for the development of most intraepithelial neoplasias of the genital tract.

1620. A 44-year-old schoolteacher returns from a vacation in Haiti where she had unprotected intercourse with a native Haitian about 3 weeks previously; she now has a painless vulvar ulcer.

1621. A 48-year-old Nigerian woman presents with vesicular and pustular lesions with ulceration of the vulvar areas. She also has painful elevated inguinal nodes.

1622. One of the most infectious of all sexually transmitted diseases (STDs); characteristic lesions are found at the base of hair follicles.

1623. One week after her first intercourse, an 18-year-old college student presents to your office with intense, constant itching in the area of her pubic hair; on examination, you think you see red "moles" that are moving.

1624. A patient reports having had intercourse with a new sexual partner about 8 days ago and now complains of general malaise and fever, vulvar pain, pruritus, and vaginal discharge; genital examination shows tender inguinal lymphadenopathy and vesicles and ulcers on the labia majora bilaterally.

1625. A 41-year-old woman returns from a job on a Caribbean cruise ship. She had several new sexual partners during the 3-week cruise. A few days before coming to see you, she noticed the growth of an asymptomatic vulvar nodule. The skin ulcerated over the nodule, and she now has a beefy-red ulcer. She thinks additional nodules may be developing. The ulcer is painless, and there are no associated groin lesions or enlarged lymph nodes.

1626. Caused by *Hemophilus ducreyi*, the disease is characterized by a painful ulcer, most commonly of the vaginal vestibule.

1627. Frequently isolated from the cervix and vagina, its role as a cervical pathogen is unclear.

Answers and Explanations

1566. (A) The diagnosis of intra-amniotic infection (also called chorioamnionitis) is often one of exclusion. The most common physical findings are fever, maternal/fetal tachycardia, uterine tenderness, foul-smelling vaginal discharge, and preterm labor. The most common causative organisms are bacteria and probably most often are polymicrobial. The primary treatment is delivery and secondarily initiation of antibiotic therapy. The most common neonatal sequela is pneumonia. For this reason, it is becoming a more common practice to initiate penicillin or ampicillin in cases of premature rupture of membranes that are managed conservatively to protect from group B streptococci.

1567. (E) This is a classic presentation of puerperal mastitis with a localized breast abscess. Inflammatory breast carcinoma generally involves the entire breast. The most common causative organism is *Staphylococcus aureus* from the infants' normal mouth flora. The abscess needs to be drained and a staph-resistant antibiotic given to the mother (unlikely to affect the babies). Authorities differ, but most feel the mother may continue to breast-feed if she can tolerate the discomfort; also, twins might get very hungry sharing the same breast.

1568. (B) The infant is very likely to have a *Chlamydia trachomatis* conjunctivitis from passage through the birth canal of the infected mother. It causes conjunctivitis 1 to 2 weeks after delivery in the infant and may be an indolent organism that causes pelvic infection in the mother. The diagnosis is made from immunologic enzyme assay in most cases.

The mother can be treated with a tetracycline or preferably with erythromycin if she is breast feeding. The infant should be treated with oral erythromycin and/or sulfa ointment to the eyes. Tetracycline can stain the infant's permanent teeth.

1569. (A) While not pathognomonic, the finding of gram-negative intracellular diplococci combined with the history of intrauterine instrumentation, the likelihood of gonorrhea is nearly 100%. A syphilitic lesion should be sought on all patients with venereal disease, but it is not a high-prevalence STD in most settings. Given the likelihood of gonorrhea as the causative organism, the patient and all recent partners should be treated.

1570. (A) The incidence of syphilis has been increasing in recent years in the United States. It is a treponemal infection and before 18 weeks' gestation these organisms seldom affect the fetus. Maternal treatment would consist of penicillin in most cases and never tetracycline because of its adverse fetal effects. Due to prior transplacental transport, erythromycin is not effective therapy in the pregnant woman. For this reason, pencillin (after desensitization) is used even in penicillin-allergic patients. The FTA-ABS is the most specific and sensitive test to diagnose syphilis, but the VDRL is simpler and less expensive. Fetal IgG testing will identify syphilis, but there is no early IgM response. The Jarisch–Herxheimer reaction refers to the febrile reaction many people have after the treatment of syphilis, perhaps related to toxin release as penicillin destroys the spirochetes.

1571. (C) Listeriosis is characterized by abortion, stillbirth, septicemia, and encephalitis. It has a characteristic rash in infants that is often described as petechial or granulomatous in appearance and is a good candidate for the stillbirth. It causes overwhelming sepsis in infants much like group B streptococcus. Maternal septicemia is also common. It is unusual for listeriosis to cause repetitive pregnancy loss.

1572. (B) Polio vaccine is generally a vaccine made from a killed virus and, therefore, safe to receive during pregnancy. Mumps, rabies, rubella, and rubeola are live virus vaccines and, therefore, not generally felt to be as safe in pregnancy. Other killed virus vaccines include hepatitis B and influenza vaccines. Killed bacterial vaccines include pertussis, typhoid, typhus, cholera, meningococcus, and rickettsia. Toxoids include diphtheria and tetanus. Killed bacteria vaccines and toxoids are also thought to be safe during pregnancy.

1573. (C) The predisposition of HIV-infected patients to developing tuberculosis, pneumocystic pneumonia, CMV, and candidiasis has led to recommendations that prenatal patients be screened with tuberculin skin tests, receive a chest x-ray, and be tested for other opportunistic infections. The actual management of prenatal and intrapartum care does not differ all that much from routine pregnancy with the exception that CD4 counts are followed. The use of highly active antiretroviral therapy, including protease inhibitors, has been shown to decrease the risk of vertical transmission. While they have not been shown to be teratogenic, the long-term effects of many of these newer drugs are unknown. In countries where bottle-feeding of these infants is possible, it is most likely a safer alternative than breast-feeding.

1574. (A) Genital herpes is usually symptomatic in mothers when infants are overtly infected. Genital lesions can usually be found. Transmission rates to infants are probably about 30% in mothers who have primary outbreak late in pregnancy and only 3% when maternal infections are recurrent. Transmission is associated

with high neonatal mortality rates, nearly 50% among nontreated infants. Preexisting antibody to HSV-2 but not to HSV-1 reduces the risk of vertical transmission of HSV-2. Acyclovir has been demonstrated to be effective in diminishing the rate of recurrent genital herpes outbreaks, but AZT (zidovudine) is not used in the treatment of genital herpes.

1575. (B) CMV is an asymptomatic maternal infection passed to the infant during gestation. Virus can be isolated from any body fluid. Nearly all of the infected infants will be asymptomatic at birth, but 5 to 15% will develop the central nervous system manifestations during early childhood. Vitamin K deficiency causes neonatal coagulopathy. Late onset group B streptococcal infection is typically manifested by bacteremia, meningitis, and pneumonia. In utero infection with parvovirus is a cause of fetal hydrops. Infection in young children is generally associated with fever, malaise, adenopathy, and a characteristic rash.

1576. (E) Varicella-zoster is a highly contagious virus that causes chickenpox. It is a more severe disease in adults than children and has been reported to cause pneumonia in 10% of infected pregnant women. About 10% of fetuses can become infected in utero when the gravida is exposed in early pregnancy. Severe congenital malformation of the limbs, chorioretinitis, and cerebral cortical atrophy are possible as a result of exposure. The administration of VZIG within 96 hours of exposure will attenuate most infections. Before administering VZIG, maternal serum can be tested to see if the patient is immune.

1577. (C) This is a classic presentation of measles (rubeola), especially the pathognomonic (Koplik) spots. It seldom has an effect in midgestation. Vaccination is not indicated during pregnancy, and if you already have the infection, vaccination is of no value. Some authorities would recommend passive immunity.

1578. (D) Mumps show no evidence of fetal damage when compared to the general noninfected population. Congenital mumps is extremely rare.

1579. (A) Congenital rubella is teratogenic and often fatal to the fetus or neonate. It is seldom dangerous to the gravida but has been increasing in frequency in recent years. Vaccination is the key to prevention and should be performed shortly after pregnancy or when adequate contraception is being used. While vaccination during pregnancy is not recommended, it has not been shown to cause any excess morbidity in mother or child.

1580. (D) Primary infection with the varicella-zoster virus causes chickenpox, which has an attack rate of 90% in seronegative individuals. Fortunately, over three quarters of adults are immune from prior symptomatic or asymptomatic infection. Therefore, the best course of action is to determine whether this patient is immune. If so, nothing more need be done. If not, then administration of VZIG within 96 hours of exposure is recommended to attenuate varicella infection. The varicella vaccine, a live, attenuated vaccine, is not recommended for pregnant women and would not be effective in preventing infection after exposure has already occurred. Finally, intravenous acyclovir is recommended for the treatment of varicella pneumonia, which has been found to lower the mortality rate in pregnancy from 35 to 15%.

1581. (D) Those who eat raw meat and those who handle cat feces (litter box cleaners) are at greatest risk for toxoplasmosis infection during pregnancy. The cat breeder is at greatest risk. The rate of primary infection in pregnancy is low (about 1:1,000) and only 10% of those infected will have serious neonatal sequelae. Women who desire to be tested for this disease will show appropriate immune IgG titers that can be measured before pregnancy. During pregnancy, the most appropriate test is to follow titers to see if a dramatic rise can be demonstrated. A patient with a household pet is highly unlikely to be exposed to toxoplasmosis and so screening is *not* typically offered. These women may opt to not be responsible for cleaning the litter box if they are concerned.

1582. (C) Malarial prophylaxis is important during pregnancy when the gravida is at a great risk of infection. Chloroquine, quinidine, and mefloquine are safe for mother and fetus. These drugs inhibit maternal infection and the passing of the infection transplacentally to the fetus. Primigravid women seem to be more susceptible to infection, not less. Progesterone does not have a suppressive effect on the parasite that is transmitted by the mosquito vector.

1583. (B) The infection described is bacterial vaginosis, which results from an overgrowth of many anaerobic bacteria. It has been associated with preterm birth, and oral, rather than topical, therapy is preferred in pregnancy. The treatment of choice is metronidazole; clindamycin and amoxicillin/clavulanic acid are also effective. Douching is not a recommended practice because it can disturb the natural flora (i.e., lower the concentration of lactobacillus), which can make women more prone to vaginal infections. The male partner is not symptomatic and does not generally require treatment.

1584. (A) Teenagers are less immunocompetent toward gonorrheal antigens and are less able to form antibodies to this bacteria than are older women. Unfortunately, it is also demographically a disease of young women (75% are under 25), non-Caucasian women, and economically disadvantaged women. One in eight sexually active adolescent women will develop acute PID. One in four who develop a lower tract infection will develop salpingitis. Abscesses, nearly 100% of which contain anaerobes, probably do not spontaneously reinfect but are more likely reinfected by a new organism. Foam and condoms may be the best protection for the high-risk woman for two reasons: (1) foam (active ingredient: nonoxynol-9) is highly bactericidal and (2) latex pores are 1,000 times smaller than even viral particles and provide an excellent barrier against infection.

1585. (E) While this woman meets the standard criteria for PID on the basis of clinical criteria, her history is disparate with this diagnosis. Admitting and treating for a disease she is unlikely to have "in order to see how things go" is poor medicine. Culdocentesis is reasonable, but if you find pus, it will not tell where the pus comes from. Neither a pelvic ultrasound nor CT is likely to make the diagnosis and may postpone what is needed, although U.S. physicians are getting better at diagnosing appendicitis. Diagnostic laparoscopy is most apt to determine the source of this woman's problem and should be used in cases in which the diagnosis is unclear. In this case, it was appendicitis.

1586. **(C)** Tuberculosis of the female genital tract is found in Asia, Latin America, and the Middle East as a cause of infertility and PID. The diagnosis can be established by biopsy in the secretory phase of the cycle. Treatment consists of 24 months of combination antituberculous drugs. Surgery is reserved for those who fail medical therapy.

1587. **(C)** Insertion of an IUD increases the risk of genital tract infection. Some IUDs have much higher infection rates, but they are no longer marketed in the United States. The highest risk of infection is within 2 months after insertion, but prophylactic antibiotics do not decrease the risk of infection. The IUD increases the chance of spontaneous abortion when left in place during intrauterine pregnancy. If the string is visible, the IUD should be removed from the pregnant patient.

1588. **(D)** Urethral syndrome has the same symptoms as cystitis. Its etiology is unknown, and the only physical findings may be tenderness of the urethra and redness of the urethra on urethroscopic examination. While tuberculosis and gonorrhea may give you sterile cultures (because a special medium is needed) with urethral infection, both do produce a pyuria, which is not present in this patient. Antibiotics should make the symptoms better and not mask a diagnosis of simple cystitis.

1589. **(D)** This patient has the classic triad of symptoms for urethral diverticulum: dysuria, dyspareunia, and dribbling of urine after voiding. The tender suburethral mass is the most common physical finding. The mass needs to be excised as a source of chronic infection.

1590. **(E)** Seventy-five percent of women may show some elevation of temperature during the evening after having had surgery, more so after vaginal than abdominal hysterectomy. Only one fifth of postoperative fevers are related to infection. UTI is the most common cause of true infection in any patient who has been catheterized at the time of surgery. It is not the most common cause of an isolated temperature elevation. Ureteral obstruction, factitious fevers, and febrile allergic reactions are uncommon. Postsurgical atelectasis is by far the most common cause.

1591. **(D)** This history, combined with the finding of a tender mass, gives you the diagnosis of pelvic abscess. Abscesses need to be opened and drained. Opening the vaginal cuff is easy, and material for culture usually comes flowing out. This alone will lead to cure in 12 to 36 hours in most cases.

1592. **(D)** There has been no benefit shown from antibiotic prophylaxis for minor procedures unless the patient is immunocompromised or is at high risk for infecting an abnormal heart valve. Prophylactic use of antibiotics has been shown to be of benefit in both abdominal and vaginal hysterectomies. Interestingly, a single dose of almost any antibiotic about 30 minutes before the operation shows the same positive effect as multiple doses continued after surgery.

1593. **(D)** This term is used to refer to postsurgical infection of the soft tissue above the vaginal apex. It may describe a mild or severe infection caused by aerobic or anaerobic organisms. The diagnosis is made from these criteria: a fever, excessive postoperative tenderness at the cuff site, and induration of the cuff. It is generally treated by antibiotic administration.

1594. **(C)** Bacterial vaginosis has been associated with preterm labor, preterm premature rupture of the membranes, and chorioamnionitis as well as puerperal endometritis. A number of infections (e.g., CMV, toxoplasmosis, rubella) have been implicated in intrauterine growth restriction, but bacterial vaginosis has not. Neonatal ophthalmic infection can be caused by both *Chlamydia trachomatis* and *Neisseria gonorrhoeae*. While jaundice has resulted from sepsis, bacterial vaginosis per se has not been implicated as a direct cause.

1595. **(B)** In this case, the patient has all the classic findings of septic pelvic thrombophlebitis, especially a spiking (hectic) fever. She has had an adequate trial of a broad-spectrum antibiotic followed by combination broad-spectrum antibiotics without success. It is thought that tiny, inflamed clots need to be anticoagulated while waiting for resolution.

1596. **(C)** This woman is undergoing a septic abortion, a potentially fatal condition if not treated promptly and appropriately. The fetus is not salvageable. After adequate blood levels of broad-spectrum antibiotics are achieved, her uterus must be promptly evacuated.

1597. **(A)** Passage of a large amount of serosanguinous fluid through the wound on postoperative days 5 to 8 indicates that this wound has dehisced (deep fascial layers are no longer intact). Rather than the fascia just separating, there is more likely a tear of the fascia. About 50% of the time the wound is also infected. The wound must be explored, and in most cases the patient will have to be taken back to the operating room, debrided, and closed again with internal or external retention sutures.

1598. **(D)** Most studies show that the average risk of perinatal HIV transmission is 20 to 30%. The rate is higher with high maternal viral loads, but probably not as high as 80%. The goal of multiagent antiretroviral therapy is to decrease the risk of perinatal transmission and improve the course of the disease. Once initiated, the therapy may be continued beyond pregnancy; this decision is dependent on the health status of the mother. Since many of the drugs are relatively new, the full effects of the drugs on the fetus are still unknown. There is no evidence that these agents are less effective in pregnancy, and there is little data on disease progression in pregnancy.

1599. **(C)** While hematogenous dissemination may occur, evidence suggests that most vertical transmission may occur intrapartum. The added benefit of cesarean section in lowering perinatal transmission for women on highly active antiretroviral therapy with undetectable viral loads is questionable. Given that this women still has a viral load greater than 1,000 copies per milliliter, however, cesarean section will likely be of benefit. The most important risk factor for postpartum endometritis is cesarean section. Women with HIV have a higher risk of this complication, but this risk is not as high as 10-fold over that of HIV-negative women. While cesarean section does not pose a greater risk of perinatal transmission than vaginal delivery, the data indicate no reduction in transmisison rate if it is performed after the onset of labor or rupture of membranes.

1600. **(B)** The prevalence of asymptomatic bacteriuria in pregnancy is 5 to 10 percent, and all pregnant women should have urine cultures at their first prenatal visit to detect this. Treatment reduces the risk of acute cystitis and pyelonephritis. Approximately 20 to 30% of women with untreated lower urinary tract infection will develop pyelonephritis. Pyelonephritis in pregnancy can result in preterm labor, septic shock, and adult respiratory distress syndrome.

1601. **(E)** *E. coli* is the most frequent organism identified on urine culture, responsible for 80 to 90% of initial infections. Other common organisms include *Staphylococcus, Saprophyticus, Klebsiella pneumoniae, Proteus* species, and enterococci.

1602. **(D)** In recent years, 20 to 30% of *E. coli* strains have developed resistance to ampicillin, so this is not a good choice unless sensitivity tests are known. Tetracycline and ciprofloxacin are contraindicated in pregnancy because of their teratogenic effects. Metronidazole is effective against anaerobes that are a cause of pelvic infection but are not common uropathogens. Nitrofurantoin is the best choice. It has activity against most gram-negative aerobic bacilli and its cost is relatively low.

1603. **(A, B, C, E)** This is one of the few pelvic infections in which anaerobes are not blamed. Toxic shock syndrome is produced by the toxin produced by a subspecies of *S. aureus*. The abrasive lesions caused by tampons, contraceptive sponges, and diaphragms have all been implicated. Antibiotic therapy is of no proven value in treatment of the initial episode, but may prevent recurrence. The goal is to provide multisystem (mainly ventilation, vascular, and renal) supportive therapy until the patient is able to clear the toxin.

1604. **(A, C, E)** Influenza in pregnancy is generally treated symptomatically, and amantadine is not routinely used. However, amantadine can reduce the severity of symptoms if given within the first 48 hours. It is reserved for nonimmunized women at high risk for influenza complications. The influenza vaccine has not been found to be teratogenic. There is an increased risk of maternal mortality associated with influenza pandemics.

1605. **(A, B)** The clinical behavior of acute pelvic infection has been reinvestigated in recent years, and traditional wisdom has been found to be lacking. It would appear that gonorrhea and chlamydia still play a major role in the etiology of PID, but the process includes a polymicrobial infection that inoculates the cervix and ascends the genital tract to the abdominal cavity. The longer the process exists, the less likely the practitioner is to culture gonorrhea or chlamydia (or both 25 to 40% of the time) from the cervix or the fallopian tubes. This makes cervical cultures much less useful than previously thought and explains why a person with classic symptoms and physical findings often does not have the expected positive cultures. Although women using OCs are more likely to harbor *Chlamydia* in their cervices, they are at lower risk of developing PID. This may be related to the thickened cervical mucus preventing access of organisms to the upper genital tract.

1606. **(A, C, D)** A UTI most commonly presents with symptoms of frequency, urgency, and dysuria. Twenty percent of the female population will suffer a UTI in their lifetime. It may lead to temporary incontinence, and a culture should be done on all women who have this complaint. While a clean-catch specimen culturing greater than 100,000 colonies per milliliter was considered to be diagnostic, many physicians treat infection with lower (100) bacterial counts if the woman is symptomatic. *E. coli* is the most common cause of UTI.

1607. **(B, C, D)** Wound infections usually occur or manifest themselves between the fifth and tenth postoperative days. With the practice of early discharge after surgery, many wound infections may not be recognized in hospital. Factors such as age, obesity, chronic illness, immunosuppression, and overall health and nutrition certainly affect wound healing. Opening, draining, cleaning, and debridement of the wound are the best care that can be given. Antibiotics are rarely needed.

1608. **(B, D)** Necrotizing fasciitis is a life-threatening surgical emergency. Prompt aggressive debridement must be performed to remove the necrotic tissue involving the subcutaneous tissue and fascia. The initial presentation may be consistent with cellulitis, but the patient generally appears toxic with signs of sepsis. Surgical explorations are required to rule necrotizing fasciitis in such suspicious cases. Broad-spectrum antibiotics are necessary for treatment. Patients with diabetes, malnutrition, obesity, and poor tissue perfusion are more suspectible.

1609. **(A, B, C, E)** *C. trachomatis* is the least likely organism to be found for two reasons: (1) Anaerobic bacteria may be present in more than 50% of puerperal infections and include peptostreptococci, peptococci, and *Bacteroides* species. The most common aerobic bacteria as pathogens are the aerobic bacteria group B, D, and A streptococcus and *E. coli*. Polymicrobial infections may also have *Gardnerella vaginalis*. The role of *Chlamydia* is somewhat uncertain, but it may be associated with a late (2 to 6 days after delivery) endometritis. (2) *Chlamydia* is difficult to culture and requires special media. It is more commonly found using rapid antigen detection tests. Culturing for "routine" aerobes and anaerobes will not isolate *Chlamydia*.

1610–1616. (1610-C, 1611-B, 1612-A, 1613-E, 1614-F, 1615-D, 1616-E) Vulvovaginitis and mucopurulent cervicitis are the two most common symptoms of infections in the lower genital tract. Vaginitis is more common, affecting nearly every woman at some time in her life. Bacterial vaginosis (previously called *Gardnerella* vaginitis) is the most common cause of vaginitis with a pH greater than 4.7. Laboratory evaluation of vaginitis includes taking a pH of the vaginal secretions and looking at wet mounts of the secretions diluted respectively with normal saline and potassium hydroxide (KOH). *Candida* does not change the normal pH of the vagina (3 to 4.5). *Trichomonas* and bacterial vaginosis are treated with metronidazole, but *Trichomonas* may be resistant to standard doses and require both oral and intravenous therapy in some cases. Children also are susceptible to the same types of vaginal infections but must also be considered as having foreign bodies (the most common one being toilet paper) as a common cause. Because of the small vagina in children, a small diameter scope might have to be used to make the diagnosis and perhaps used for removal of the foreign body (vaginoscopy). Elderly women may also suffer from vaginitis symptoms because of the vaginal atrophy induced by lack of estrogen. Replacement therapy with estrogen will generally alleviate this problem. Finally, it must be remembered that not all discharge from the vagina is from vaginal infection. Cervicitis from gonorrhea, *Chlamydia*, herpes simplex, and flat condyloma can cause excessive discharge. Whenever discharge from the cervix is seen, STDs must be strongly suspected, and the caregiver must realize that the patient is at great risk of infection in the upper genital tract (Figure 25–1).

1617. (A) Uncomplicated anogenital gonorrhea is most often asymptomatic in women. The most common symptom when present would be vaginal discharge followed by dysuria and/or anogenital itching. Diagnosis is made by culture onto a selective media such as Thayer–Martin or Transgrow media. Patients with gonorrhea may have a 20 to 40% chance of also being infected with *Chlamydia*.

1618. (I) Molluscum contagiosum is a viral disease. Women are generally asymptomatic other than for the unpleasant appearance of the lesions on the vulvar skin. The disease is spread by close contact but is not very contagious, despite what the name implies. It may be a disseminated disease in children that is not necessarily spread by sexual contact. The incubation period is weeks to months. Characteristic small nodules or firm vesicles with a waxy appearance and some with umbilicated centers are present. Either the gross appearance or biopsy is diagnostic. They are treated by simple debridement.

1619. (K) HPV is the causative organism for genital condyloma acuminata (not condyloma latum, which is associated with syphilis). HPV also may be the etiologic agent (or cofactor or enhancer) for the development of most intraepithelial neoplasias of the genital tract.

1620. (C) Primary syphilis is associated with painless genital ulcers (chancre) on the labia, vulva, vagina, cervix, anus, lips, or nipples. The lesion appears 10 to 90 days after the initial infection. The chancre lasts 1 to 5 weeks and will resolve without treatment; the infective organism remains, however. The disease is treated with penicillin, erythromycin, or tetracycline. Haiti is endemic for syphilis.

1621. (E) In lymphogranuloma venereum, the causative organism is *C. trachomatis*. Transmission is venereal, with men affected six times more frequently than women. It presents as vesicular and pustular lesions with ulceration of the inguinal and vulvar areas. The characteristic exquisitely painful in-

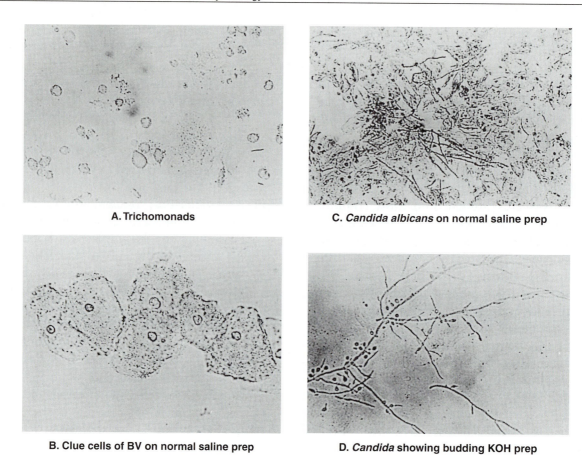

A. Trichomonads

C. *Candida albicans* on normal saline prep

B. Clue cells of BV on normal saline prep

D. *Candida* showing budding KOH prep

Figure 25–1. Vaginitis.
(Reproduced, with permission, from DeCherney AH, Nathan L. *Current Obstetric and Gynecologic Diagnosis & Treatment*, 9th ed. New York: McGraw-Hill, 2003.)

guinal lesion is called a bubo. Late complications include rectal strictures. The disease is treated with doxycycline, tetracycline, erythromycin, or sulfa drugs.

1622. **(G)** Pediculosis pubis is an infestation by the crab louse, *Phthirius pubis,* and is generally confined to the hairy areas of the vulva but occasionally may be found in the eyelashes. It may be the most infectious of all STDs. Characteristic lesions are found at the base of hair follicles; colposcopy is an excellent way to see these lesions.

1623. **(H)** Scabies is caused by *Sarcoptes scabiei,* a parasite with a red appearance resulting from blood consumption. They may be found anywhere on the body. Both pediculosis pubis and scabies are treatable with 5% permethrin (Nix) or lindane (Kwell) shampoo or cream.

1624. **(J)** Genital herpes can produce systemic symptoms, including general malaise and fever, in women during the primary infection. Symptoms of vulvar pain, pruritus, and discharge peak between days 7 and 11 of the primary infection. The patient has severe symptoms for 14 days in these cases. However the primary infection may be relatively asymptomatic and they are unrecognized in half of early cases. Severity of symptoms necessitates hospitalization for approximately 5 to 10% of women with known primary infection. Notorious as a recurring disease, genital herpes may be prophylactically treated with acyclovir.

1625. **(F)** This is a classic presentation of donovanosis (granuloma inguinale), caused by *Calymmatobacterium granulomatis.* It is an STD (in most cases) that incubates in 1 to 12 weeks. It is transmitted to 10 to 50% of partners during intercourse. It presents as coalescing, ulcerating nodules that may not be painful unless secondarily infected. It is usually diagnosed by its clinical manifestations. The pathognomonic Donovan bodies are dark-staining (with silver stain) bacteria found in the cytoplasm of the infected cells. It is generally treated with tetracycline.

1626. **(D)** Chancroid is an STD that is very uncommon in the United States. It is predominantly a male disease (10:1). It is caused by *H. ducreyi,* a very contagious, gram-negative rod. The disease cannot penetrate normal skin, so there must be an area of trauma where it enters. Lesions may be solitary or multiple and begin as a papule that later ulcerates. Lymph nodes are involved about half of the time. The diagnosis is made from a combination of Gram stain, culture, and biopsy. Tetracycline, cephalosporins, penicillins, and sulfa drugs have all been used successfully for treatment.

1627. **(L)** Genital mycoplasmas include *Mycoplasma hominis* and *Ureaplasma urealyticum.* It is doubtful whether these organisms can cause mucopurulent cervicitis, and it is also doubtful that they cause any genital tract damage. They are often cultured and treated in infertility patients. Little useful information about their pathogenicity exists.

CHAPTER 26

Special Topics in Gynecology: Pediatric and Adolescent Gynecology, Sexual Abuse, Medical Ethics, and Medical–Legal Considerations
Questions

1628. Which of the following patients is most likely to have an acidic vaginal pH?

(A) 2-day-old girl

(B) 4-year-old girl

(C) 16-year-old adolescent with vaginal trichomoniasis

(D) 21-year-old woman with vaginal bleeding

(E) 65-year-old postmenopausal woman

1629. Which of the following conditions is the most likely cause of vulvovaginal symptoms in children?

(A) foreign body

(B) lichen sclerosis

(C) physiologic leukorrhea

(D) trauma

(E) nonspecific

1630. The most common symptom of urethral prolapse in the prepubertal, unestrogenized girl is

(A) dysuria

(B) urinary frequency

(C) urinary retention

(D) painless genital bleeding

(E) hematuria

1631. Premature thelarche differs from true precocious puberty in that premature thelarche is associated with

(A) pubic hair development

(B) axillary hair development

(C) spontaneous ovulations

(D) voice changes

(E) isolated breast development

1632. Puberty marks the transition period between childhood and sexual maturity. Which of the following signs occurs initially in preadolescent girls?

(A) axillary hair growth

(B) breast development

(C) menarche

(D) peak growth spurt

(E) pubic hair growth

1633. A 16-year-old girl is seen in the emergency department for evaluation of nausea and vomiting. Her vital signs are: blood pressure, 80/40; pulse, 130 bpm; and temperature, 102.2°F. Physical examination shows conjunctivitis, oropharyngeal hyperemia, and a sunburn-like macular rash over the face, proximal extremities, and trunk. Palpation of the extremities elicits muscle tenderness. Pelvic examination is normal, and a bloody tampon is present in the vagina. The most likely diagnosis is

(A) erysipelas
(B) syphilis
(C) Kawasaki disease
(D) toxic shock syndrome (TSS)
(E) human immunodeficiency virus (HIV)

1634. A 14-year-old girl has a chronic cough with copious expectoration. A biopsy of the respiratory mucosa shows ciliated epithelium devoid of dynein arms. Which of the following conditions is most likely to occur in later life?

(A) abnormal vaginal bleeding
(B) infertility
(C) pelvic pain
(D) urinary incontinence
(E) chronic diarrhea

1635. The percentage of sexually abused children who know their assailant is

(A) 15%
(B) 35%
(C) 55%
(D) 75%
(E) 95%

1636. The most commonly reported form of incest is

(A) father–daughter
(B) father–son
(C) stepfather–daughter
(D) mother–son
(E) brother–sister

1637. The appropriate "emergency contraception" for a sexual assault patient who is found to be at risk for pregnancy is

(A) irrigation of the vagina with normal saline at the time of vaginal examination
(B) combination low-dose oral contraceptive (OC) agent in standard single-dose therapy for the next 30 days
(C) an injection of Depo-Provera at the time of the visit
(D) two tablets of a low-dose OC at the time the victim is seen and 12 hours later
(E) two tablets of a high-dose OC at the time the victim is seen and 12 hours later

1638. When childhood sexual assault is suspected within the past 72 hours, the next action of the physician should be to

(A) perform a complete physical examination
(B) bring family members together for an interview
(C) report the incident to Child Protective Services
(D) contact mental health workers
(E) notify the police

1639. Which of the following is a legal but not a medical responsibility of the physician caring for an alleged sexual assault victim?

(A) offering postcoital hormonal prophylaxis to prevent pregnancy
(B) providing counseling and emotional support
(C) obtaining a complete gynecologic history
(D) obtaining informed consent from patient
(E) collecting samples of hair and vaginal secretions, and microscopic evaluation of motile sperm

1640. Which of the following legal theories describes the failure of a physician to disclose the risks of a procedure?

(A) breach of duty
(B) intentional tort

(C) abandonment

(D) informed consent

(E) lack of diligence

1641. The physician witness should

(A) interrupt the interrogating attorney when necessary

(B) interpret the meaning of a document prepared by another person

(C) use medical language as much as possible

(D) not defer to another physician or author as an authoritative expert

(E) depersonalize the plaintiff

1642. Professional liability insurance that protects against claims made during the policy period, regardless of when the suit is filed, is a(n)

(A) claims-made policy

(B) occurrence policy

(C) tail policy

(D) nose policy

(E) none of the above

DIRECTIONS (Question 1643): Each of the numbered items or incomplete statements in this section is followed by answers or by completions of the statement. Select the answers or completions that may apply.

1643. Which four of the following are torts?

(A) personal injury

(B) automobile accident

(C) slip and fall

(D) professional liability claim

(E) assault

DIRECTIONS (Questions 1644 through 1650): Each set of items in this section consists of a list of lettered headings followed by several numbered words or phrases. For each numbered word or phrase, select the ONE lettered option that is most closely associated with it. Each lettered option may be selected once, more than once, or not at all.

Questions 1644 through 1646

(A) *Escherichia coli*

(B) *Staphylococcus aureus*

(C) *Streptococcus pyogenes*

(D) *Candida albicans*

(E) *Gardnerella vaginalis*

(F) *Chlamydia trachomatis*

(G) *Enterobius vermicularis*

(H) none of the above

Which of the above organisms is most likely to cause childhood vaginitis associated with

1644. Previous respiratory infection

1645. Small red papules and an erythematous vulva

1646. Perianal pruritus and excoriations

Questions 1647 and 1648

A 39-year-old multiparous woman is infertile after acute salpingitis. A salpingoplasty has been unsuccessful and the patient requires in vitro fertilization (IVF). She has three children from a previous marriage and desires another child with her new husband. The husband is ambivalent about her wishes to conceive. He believes that they do not have the financial resources to care for another child. The couple has enough money to pay for a single IVF attempt.

(A) Parenthood refers to the emotional capacity for loving a child.

(B) Parenthood refers to the ability of providing for a child's well-being.

(C) both of the above

(D) neither of the above

Which of the above statements best agrees with the decision to

1647. Recommend in vitro fertilization

1648. Recommend no therapy at this time

Questions 1649 and 1650

A 39-year-old woman, after using fertility drugs to induce ovulation, has a quadruplet pregnancy. You advise the patient and her husband that, without intervention, she probably faces preterm labor, which risks the survival of all the pregnancies. Selective termination of at least one fetus may improve the chance of survival for the remaining fetuses. The couple returns 1 week later and wants to schedule the procedure.

(A) The parents have an absolute right in deciding what type of care will be given to affect pregnancy outcome.

(B) The parents should bear full responsibility for the decision because they will live with its consequences.

(C) The parents have the responsibility to protect the well-being of all the fetuses.

(D) more than one of the above

Which of the above statements BEST supports the decision to

1649. Perform selective termination

1650. Not perform selective termination

Answers and Explanations

1628. (A) Hormone-sensitive tissues in the female infant are affected for several weeks by the estrogen-rich milieu of pregnancy. The vagina responds to maternal estrogens by developing a thick, glycogen-rich epithelium that favors the growth of *Lactobacillus* (Doderlein's bacilli). *Lactobacillus* and other bacteria acquired during passage through the birth canal metabolize glycogen to lactic acid, producing an acidic vaginal pH between 3.7 and 6.3. As circulating estrogen levels decline during childhood, the vaginal pH increases to 6.8 to 7.2. The vaginal pH of reproductive-age women is 4.0 to 5.0, while that of postmenopausal women is more basic due to the decline in serum estrogen levels. The acid–base status of the vagina is an important factor in diagnosing vaginitis. A vaginal pH greater than 4.5 is found with bacterial vaginosis, trichomoniasis, or blood in the vagina.

1629. (E) Nonspecific vulvovaginitis (NSV) accounts for 25 to 75% of vulvovaginal symptoms in children. The predominant vaginal organism cultured in NSV is *Escherichia coli.* Although vaginal colonization with *E. coli* occurs in asymptomatic girls, half of 3- to 10-year-old girls with NSV have this organism present in the vagina.

1630. (D) Girls with urethral prolapse typically experience painless genital bleeding. This symptom can be precipitated by straining or constipation. Urinary frequency and retention can also be seen occasionally. Dysuria and hematuria occurs only with significant irritation and inflammation. Conservative management with estrogen cream and sitz

baths is appropriate with surgical intervention only in extreme cases.

1631. (E) Premature thelarche is the spontaneous development of breast tissue as an isolated event without other pubertal changes. Premature onset of puberty involves spontaneous ovulation, increases in estradiol levels, and the development of breast tissue.

1632. (B) Pubertal changes are marked by various stages of sexual and somatic development. Breast development or thelarche is the first sign of puberty in the female, usually occurring between the ages of 9 and 11 years. Breast development is complete within 3.5 years after onset. Adrenarche is the onset of sexual hair growth. Pubic hair growth occurs between ages 11 and 12 years, while axillary hair growth occurs later. Menarche is the final stage of puberty and occurs after 12 years of age.

1633. (D) TSS has an incidence of about 6.2 per 100,000 menstruating women annually. It was originally associated with one brand of super-absorbent tampon (Rely) but continues to occur (albeit with lower frequency) after removal of the blamed tampon from the market in 1980. TSS occurs occasionally with the use of diaphragms, vaginal sponges, cervical caps, and postoperative wound infections. Symptoms of TSS occur during menstruation and include sudden high fever, flulike symptoms (sore throat, headache, diarrhea), erythroderma, signs of multisystemic failure, and hypotension. TSS is usually associated with vaginal strains of *Staphylococcus aureus* producing an exfoliative exotoxin (TSST-1). Adolescent females are at greatest risk for TSS because they have not yet developed an immunity against TSST-1. Treatment of TSS includes aggressive supportive therapy (e.g., hydration, transfusion, replacement of coagulation factors, use of vasoactive agents) and antistaphylococcal antibiotic therapy. Mechanical ventilation and hemodialysis may be required to treat adult respiratory distress syndrome and renal failure. Risk for recurrence of TSS is 30% and may be reduced by intermittent use of tampons during menses or by not using tampons.

1634. (B) Immobile cilia syndrome, or Kartagener's syndrome, refers to the congenital absence of dynein arms in ciliated epithelium. Abnormalities of microtubular structure may coexist. Patients with Kartagener's syndrome suffer from chronic cough, sinusitis, bronchiectasis, and airway obstruction. The diagnosis is usually made by microscopic examination of the respiratory mucosa. Immobile cilia may coexist in the fallopian tube epithelium and may increase the risk of infertility in some individuals.

1635. (D) About 75% of sexually abused children know their assailant. At least one half of these cases involve another family member.

1636. (A) Incest refers to a sexual relationship between people who are related and cannot legally marry. The most commonly reported form of incest involves the father and his own daughter (75% of reported cases). Brother–sister incest may actually be the most common form of incest but is not reported often. A sexual relationship between a stepfather and child or between a mother's boyfriend and child is called "functional parent incest" because the individuals are not related.

1637. (E) High-dose OCs such as Ovral should be given in double dosage at the time of the evaluation and 12 hours later. This form of emergency contraception can be effective up to 72 hours after unprotected intercourse. A pregnancy test should be performed at the next visit if indicated. Alternatively, low-dose OCs can be substituted in quadruple dosage at the time of evaluation and 12 hours later. Use of an antiemetic at the time of administration will reduce the side effect of nausea experienced with high estrogen doses such as these treatments. Depo-Provera is not appropriate treatment in preventing pregnancy nor is standard dosing of OCs.

1638. (A) Any child in whom sexual assault is suspected within the past 72 hours should be examined immediately to document physical findings corroborating the assault. Since the child of an incestuous relationship may not disclose the full history in the presence of the involved family member, the parents and child should be interviewed separately. When sexual assault is suspected weeks to months earlier, the child can be examined after the interviewing process is completed.

1639. (E) It is important to distinguish legal from medical responsibilities in the care of an alleged sexual assault victim. The collection of hair and vaginal secretions for the microscopic evaluation of motile sperm and semen is a legal responsibility to provide evidence to the authorities for the sake of documentation. All of the other answers provided represent medical responsibilities to the patient.

1640. (D) The doctrine of informed consent states that a patient suffering an unfavorable result from a procedure may seek recovery for failure of the physician to properly disclose the risks of the procedure. Recovery is not sought for medical negligence or fault. To avoid lawsuits claiming lack of informed consent, the physician should provide complete, understandable information regarding treatment, document informed discussions about the treatment, and personally obtain written consent from the patient after answering any questions. If the risk of a treatment has a 1% incidence of occurrence, it must be disclosed along with alternative treatments.

1641. (D) The physician witness should not defer to another physician or author as an authoritative expert. If so, opposing counsel may seek the physician witness to accept a statement from that individual as inviolate. Such statements rarely apply to the circumstances under review and may be made in improper context. A medical writing may be acknowledged by the physician witness but should not supersede the witness's testimony.

1642. (B) An occurrence policy protects against claims made during the policy period, regardless of when the suit is filed. This form of insurance is expensive for obstetric coverage. A claims-made policy protects against claims made during the life of the policy. It does not provide coverage if the policy is discontinued and the physician is subsequently sued for an event occurring when the policy was in effect. (For such coverage, an additional tail policy can be purchased when the claims-made policy is discontinued.)

1643. (A, B, C, D) A tort is an act causing harm to another person or his or her property for which the injured party seeks monetary compensation. All personal injury claims (e.g., automobile accidents, slip and falls, medical professional liability claims) are types of tort.

1644. (C) Childhood vaginitis may be caused by respiratory pathogens (*Streptococcus pyogenes* [group A streptococcus], *Streptococcus pneumoniae, Neisseria meningitidis*). These bacteria should be suspected when childhood vaginitis follows a respiratory infection in the child or another family member.

1645. (D) Vaginitis due to *Candida albicans* causes a thick, cheesy, pruritic discharge. The vulva may be reddened and covered by red satellite papules. Fissures on the posterior fourchette are common. Predisposing factors for *C. albicans* are diabetes mellitus, antibiotic use, corticosteroid therapy, obesity, diaper use, and tight-fitting clothing.

1646. (G) Children complaining of perianal pruritus and excoriations should be screened for pinworm (*Enterobius vermicularis*) infestation. Cellophane tape is placed on the perineum in the morning. The tape is removed later and examined microscopically for eggs. Occasionally perineal inspection at night will show adult worms.

1647. (A) The ethical dilemma for an infertile couple requesting fertility is whether successful therapy enhances or debases the meaning of parenthood. Attempts at pregnancy may be ethical if the nature of parenthood is enhanced but may be unethical if becoming a parent degrades the parenthood role. The ethical value judgments in this case reflect differences in the meaning of parenthood. Assisted reproductive technology (ART) may be appropriate for this couple if parenthood refers to the emotional capacity of loving a child.

1648. (B) If parenthood refers to the ability of providing for a child's well-being, the financial resources of the couple may enter the decision-making process. For example, the husband is already ambivalent about his wife's decision to attempt IVF, and any further financial difficulty may adversely affect the marriage. Delaying assisted reproductive technology (until the couple can provide for a child's well-being) may be appropriate but encourages selective use of health care by those who can afford it. This issue raises another ethical dilemma.

1649. (D) Human menopausal gonadotropin therapy is associated with a 10% twin pregnancy rate and a 1% chance of having a higher number of conceptuses. Obstetric outcomes of multifetal gestations (e.g., triplets or more) are poorer than those of singleton or twin pregnancies. Without intervention, pregnant women with quadruplets face a significant chance of preterm delivery associated with prolonged hospitalization, pregnancy-induced hypertension, polyhydramnios, anemia, and postpartum hemorrhage. Premature birth may cause neonatal death and serious mental or physical handicaps. Abortion of all fetuses is usually not an option because conception was achieved at great psychological and economic cost and may not occur again. The ethical dilemma is whether to reduce the number of fetuses to increase the probability of survival for some of them. People who believe that the main concern in pregnancy is the well-being of the woman and that selective termination in multifetal gestation is permissible to avoid harm to her and the remaining fetuses will make ethical value judgments supporting use of selective termination. Under these conditions, parents have an absolute right in deciding what care will be given to affect pregnancy outcome. They bear full responsibility for the decision because they will live with its consequences.

1650. **(C)** An alternative ethical value judgment regarding the use of selective termination believes that any act to deliberately destroy human fetal life should be morally condemned. Parents with this opinion have the moral responsibility to protect the well-being of all fetuses. This ethical position places little significance to the unwantedness of a pregnancy and may view selective termination as a precedent to euthanasia.

CHAPTER 27

Primary Health Care for Women
Questions

DIRECTIONS (Questions 1651 through 1675): Each of the numbered items or incomplete statements in this section is followed by answers or by completions of the statement. Select the ONE lettered answer or completion that is BEST in each case.

1651. A 46-year-old patient has her serum cholesterol tested in your lab, and it is 280 mg/dL. Which of the following statements regarding this finding would be accurate to tell her?

(A) The pizza she had for lunch the previous day probably is responsible for the elevation.

(B) Further evaluation will be needed.

(C) She needs to see an internist immediately.

(D) Elevated serum cholesterol is the most significant risk factor in the development of ischemic cardiac disease.

(E) Unless there is a family history of cardiac disease, she is less likely to develop heart problems than the rest of the population.

1652. A 70-year-old woman who is in good health comes to your office for the first time. Her only disease prevention issue is that she smokes. While discussing this with her, you should tell her that

(A) at 70, smoking is up to her, and she is certainly mature enough to make her own decisions

(B) if she got to be 70 and smokes, it is probably good for her

(C) assure her that 70 is too old to be worrying about quitting smoking

(D) inform her that her life expectancy may be 15 to 20 more years or longer, and that if she would like to try to quit smoking, you will assist her

(E) 25% of people will die of cancer, and the greatest risk factor we know of for developing cancer is smoking

1653. The most important feature of mammography is that it

(A) provides the caregiver with a medical–legal safety screen

(B) leads to a reduction in mortality in breast cancer in women aged 50 to 64

(C) essentially misses no cancer

(D) can detect lesions as small as 1 mm

(E) allays fears in women

1654. Exercise may

(A) help to control weight

(B) reduce blood pressure

(C) improve glucose tolerance

(D) prevent coronary artery disease

(E) all of the above

Questions 1655 through 1659

A 43-year-old woman is 5 feet 4 inches tall (163 cm) and weighs 176 lbs (80 kg).

1655. Her body mass index (BMI) is

(A) 26

(B) 28

(C) 30

(D) 32

(E) 34

1656. She would like to weigh 125 to 130 pounds. She asks, "How many calories do you think I am eating a day?" You respond

(A) 1,000
(B) 1,800
(C) 2,600
(D) 3,000
(E) 3,500

1657. She then asks, "How many calories would I have to cut out each day to lose 1 pound per week?" You answer

(A) 100
(B) 500
(C) 900
(D) 1,300
(E) 1,800

1658. She asks, "How would it be most reasonable to change my diet to lose this amount?" You tell her to

(A) eliminate dietary fat
(B) decrease protein content
(C) decrease carbohydrate content
(D) decrease amount of water intake, and less calories will be retained
(E) decrease overall food intake with the greatest decrease being fats

1659. You also encourage her to exercise. Given her current status, which of the following is the best initial form of exercise for her to maximize the calories burned per week?

(A) bicycling
(B) jogging/running
(C) swimming
(D) tennis
(E) walking

1660. As part of a premarital examination, a 24-year-old teacher would like a measles vaccination because she is nonimmune. She asks, "Do I need to avoid pregnancy after getting this vaccination?" You answer

(A) no, it is a killed vaccine and unnecessary
(B) no, it is a form of passive immunization and therefore noninfective
(C) yes, for 6 weeks
(D) yes, for 12 weeks because it is a live, attenuated vaccine
(E) yes, and if pregnancy is attained before 1 year, abortion is recommended

1661. A woman who has been splenectomized as a result of a car accident wonders if there is any special immunization she should have as a result. You answer

(A) measles
(B) mumps
(C) pertussis
(D) pneumococcus
(E) meningococcus

1662. A county sheriff, who works within the confines of the jail, asks if she should receive a tetanus injection; her last was 3 years ago. You answer

(A) yes, yearly
(B) yes, every 3 years
(C) no, only once every 10 years
(D) only if she has been injured in the last 6 months
(E) no, once in a lifetime is enough

1663. A patient presents to you with excruciating pain, and you confirm the diagnosis of a kidney stone. You would like to provide the greatest amount of pain relief possible until the stone can be treated or passes. Of the following narcotics, which has the greatest analgesic potency (administered parenterally) when compared to morphine?

(A) codeine
(B) oxycodone
(C) methadone
(D) meperidine
(E) hydromorphone

1664. A 77-year-old woman comes to see you with her daughter. The mother has recently moved in with the daughter because it is difficult for her to care for herself completely. At night the mother seems to become confused, does not know where she is, and cannot recognize her daughter. This is

(A) a normal variant of aging and should be accepted

(B) an indication that the mother needs to be restrained at night for fear of hurting herself

(C) an indication of possible early dementia or organic brain syndrome, needing further evaluation

(D) expected to resolve completely as the mother becomes more aware of her new surroundings

(E) controllable by administration of sleep medication early in the evening

1665. A 19-year-old patient comes in for an annual refill of her birth control pills. For the past 6 years her family physician has treated her for nodular cystic acne with what the patient feels are poor results. Which of the following would you recommend?

(A) topical benzoyl peroxide

(B) systemic tetracycline

(C) topical clindamycin

(D) stopping her oral contraceptives (OCs)

(E) isotretinoin

1666. A 23-year-old Native American woman recently discharged from the Air Force presents with a severe cough of several weeks' duration. She has been working as a nurse's aide for 2 years in a pulmonary ward in the Philippines. She thinks she may have tuberculosis (TB) since she knows she has been exposed. The most reliable way to make the diagnosis would be with

(A) chest x-ray

(B) Gram stain of her sputum

(C) culture of her sputum

(D) bronchial washings for cytology

(E) tuberculin skin test

1667. A woman and her husband are planning a trip to Mexico for their 25th anniversary. She has heard about "traveler's diarrhea" and wonders what advice you can give her. You tell her

(A) not to worry about it; very few people ever get it

(B) she will get it no matter what she does, and it will subside quickly on its own

(C) to be sure to drink plenty of water, not to eat uncooked meat or vegetables, and she will likely be fine

(D) to take oral clindamycin before they get to Mexico and all during their stay

(E) to take trimethoprim–sulfa tablets along and begin them at the first signs of diarrhea

1668. A 39-year-old woman comes in complaining that every night just after going to bed she awakens with a severe, substernal burning that is relieved when she drinks a glass of milk. She is allergic to codeine and has a known gallstone. Physical examination shows she is 5 feet 4 inches tall and weighs 209 pounds. Her general examination is normal. There is no abdominal tenderness. Her stool is guaiac-negative. She would like to know what to do for long-term relief. You advise

(A) weight loss and no eating within 3 hours of bedtime

(B) an upper gastrointestinal x-ray series

(C) cholecystectomy

(D) antacids before bedtime

(E) histamine blockers

1669. A 44-year-old multigravid patient comes to your office with two complaints. She has difficulty having bowel movements. They occur about twice weekly and are associated with significant straining. She has also noticed a painful mass at the anus and some bright red blood on her toilet paper. On examination you see a bluish lump about 2 cm across at the anus, a mild rectocele, and a normal digital rectal examination. A stool specimen is guaiac-negative. You advise her

(A) to have a colonoscopy

(B) that a biopsy of the mass is necessary

(C) to use hydrocortisone suppositories for the discomfort

(D) to drink 8 to 10 glasses of water each day, increase the amount of fiber in her diet, and soak the area in a tub of warm water twice daily

(E) to see a colorectal surgeon

1670. A 27-year-old woman has just begun a new job as an administrative assistant after working for years as an account representative at another bank. Over the last few weeks, she has developed a chronic, bilateral, nonpulsatile headache that begins every afternoon. Her 79-year-old aunt has recently died of a cerebral aneurysm, and she had a cousin who she believes died of a "brain tumor." Her neurologic examination is within normal limits. What do you tell her about the origin of her headaches?

(A) She needs to see a neurologist.

(B) She needs to see a psychiatrist.

(C) It is a common migraine headache, and she will need further evaluation.

(D) Given her family history, an angiogram is indicated.

(E) The headaches are most likely stress-related and can be managed without further testing.

1671. A 48-year-old patient (gravida 2, para 2) presents for an annual exam. She has had a tubal ligation for contraception. She reports her menses occur every 25 to 28 days and are "normal." Her history and examination, including stool guaiac and skin, are unremarkable other than she appears somewhat pale on examination. Which of the following laboratory results should prompt an evaluation for a cause other than simply iron deficiency from menstrual loss?

(A) hemoglobin < 11.5 g/dL

(B) increased total iron-binding capacity (TIBC)

(C) microcytic hypochromic cells on peripheral smear

(D) normal indices on an automatic analysis of peripheral smear

(E) normal to high reticulocyte count once corrected for the anemia

1672. A 19-year-old woman (gravida 0, para 0) presents for her annual sports physical. She is 5 feet 10 inches tall and weighs 110 lbs. She states she has been this weight for "a while" and attributes it to being the star forward for her nationally ranked college soccer team. She does note her last menses was more than 3 months ago. Her urine human chorionic gonadotropin (hCG) is negative. Which of the following findings would be inconsistent that her presentation is due to athletic involvement and instead raise the concern of an anorexic disorder?

(A) increased exercise tolerance

(B) increased physical activity

(C) lanugo hair

(D) low body weight

(E) resting bradycardia and hypotension

1673. A 14-year-old patient presents complaining of knee pain that has been increasing over the past few months. Since she is the goalie for the high school soccer team, you suspect patellofemoral dysfunction. Which of the following would DECREASE a postpubertal girl's risk for this problem?

(A) increased angle from knee to pelvic girdle

(B) tight vastus medialis obliquus musculature

(C) tight vastus lateralis musculature

(D) shallow trochlear groove configuration

1674. A 38-year-old woman presents with the complaints of symmetric polyarthritis, especially in the hands and wrists, marked morning stiffness that lasts for up to an hour, and nodules over her elbows. These complaints have been present and increasing over the past 3 to 4 months. Of the following differential list, which is the most likely diagnosis?

(A) ankylosing spondylitis
(B) gout
(C) osteoarthritis
(D) Reiter syndrome
(E) rheumatoid arthritis

1675. A patient asks what she can do to minimize her risks of developing skin cancer. You inform her that

(A) application of sunscreen is best just before sun exposure
(B) high altitudes are less dangerous for sun exposure dermal injury
(C) one will get sun damage on overcast days
(D) tanning booths use a form of ultraviolet (UV) radiation that is safer than sun exposure
(E) she should use a sunblocker with a sun protection factor (SPF) rating of 8 or less

DIRECTIONS (Questions 1676 through 1685): Each of the numbered items or incomplete statements in this section is followed by answers or by completions of the statement. Select the answers or completions that may apply.

1676. Which three of the following routine yearly health care screening tests is appropriate in an apparently healthy 55-year-old woman?

(A) hematocrit
(B) mammography
(C) Pap smear
(D) serum creatinine
(E) urine dipstick for glucose and protein

1677. A 59-year-old woman complains that she is not sleeping at night. Of the following, which four would be appropriate steps for her primary care physican after hearing this complaint?

(A) asking her why she feels she has a difficult time sleeping
(B) assessing the stresses and recent changes in her life
(C) inquiring about her dietary intake of caffeine
(D) obtaining a detailed history of her sleeping habits
(E) prescribing a sleeping medication

1678. Which four of the following are advantages of estrogen replacement therapy (ERT) in the postmenopausal woman?

(A) improved sleep in many women
(B) increased high-density lipoprotein (HDL)
(C) prevention of breast cancer
(D) prevention of genital atrophy
(E) retardation of bone loss

1679. Which four of the following would be considered part of primary health care?

(A) genetic counseling
(B) performing a general history and physical examination
(C) providing contraceptive teaching
(D) screening blood pressure
(E) trying to foster healthy behavior in the patient

1680. A 20-year-old female college student gives a history of having five different sexual partners in the past 2 years. Your job as her health care provider should be to do which two of the following?

(A) call her parents/guardian
(B) offer testing for gonorrhea, chlamydia, syphilis, and human immunodeficiency virus (HIV)
(C) provide contraception information
(D) tell her she is promiscuous and that she should stop sexual activity until she is more serious about her relationships with others
(E) try to convince her to get counseling

1681. Which three of the following are TRUE statements regarding cancer of the colon?

(A) Adenocarcinoma of the colon is the most common cancer in women in the United States.

(B) Physical examination will detect most cancers of the colon, providing a rectal examination is done.

(C) Screening with stool guaiac tests should be performed annually in women over age 50.

(D) Sigmoidoscopy should be performed every 3 to 5 years in women over the age of 50.

(E) There is often a hereditary component to colon cancer.

1682. When prescribing medication for a patient, which four of the following should be major concerns for the practitioner?

(A) always inquiring about patient allergies and adverse reactions

(B) choosing the least expensive drug available

(C) considering the metabolism, route of excretion, and adverse effects, as well as the indication

(D) individualizing doses based on patient's age, size, health status, and problem

(E) prescribing as few drugs as possible

1683. A 52-year-old patient with a strong family history of breast cancer presents to discuss hormone replacement. She is very hesitant to use estrogen due to recent articles in the paper. She requests a dexa-scan to evaluate her risk for osteoporosis. The scan reveals that osteoporosis is already present. Which four of the following are secondary causes for the finding of osteoporosis?

(A) chronic use of heparin

(B) chronic use of glucocorticoids

(C) hyperprolactinemia

(D) hypothyroidism

(E) subtotal gastrectomy

1684. The previous patient is not found to have any secondary cause for her osteoporosis. You feel it is due to her surgical castration 10 years ago without estrogen supplementation. Which four of the following interventions that may be used to increase bone mass have been shown to decrease the incidence of fractures?

(A) biphosphonates

(B) calcitonin

(C) calcium

(D) estrogen

(E) sodium fluoride

1685. During her annual examination, a patient states that she is very concerned about developing skin cancer due to a strong family history. You instruct her in the components of a skin exam, which involves evaluating a lesion for which two of the following are danger signs for melanoma?

(A) asymmetry

(B) raised surface

(C) consistency of color

(D) diameter > 6 mm

(E) smooth border

DIRECTIONS (Questions 1686 through 1699): Each set of items in this section consists of a list of lettered headings followed by several numbered words or phrases. For each numbered word or phrase, select the ONE lettered option that is most closely associated with it. Each lettered option may be selected once, more than once, or not at all.

Questions 1686 through 1689

(A) androgenic alopecia

(B) alopecia areata

(C) syphilitic alopecia

(D) systemic lupus-related alopecia

(E) telogen effluvium

(F) traumatic alopecia

1686. A patient presents with acute hair loss in patches. Inspection of the patches shows complete hair loss without signs of inflammation and without scarring. Hair can be easily plucked at the edge of these patches.

1687. A patient complains of thinning of her hair on her crown over the past months. She reports her mother had a similar problem.

1688. A patient presents 3 months' postpartum complaining that she is going bald. She describes large amounts of hair in her brush each morning and her hairdresser says her hair is thinner.

1689. A patient presents complaining of temporal balding. She is African-American and has worn her hair in plaited braids for years.

Questions 1690 through 1693

Choose the best diagnosis for each patient presentation.

    (A) drug rash

    (B) erythema multiforme

    (C) Lyme disease

    (D) measles

    (E) pityriasis rosea

    (F) rubella

    (G) varicella

1690. A 24-year-old woman presents with a generalized eruption of small oval lesions that are aligned along skin lines. She denies any constitutional symptoms. She did note a single larger lesion a few days prior to the generalized rash.

1691. A 22-year-old schoolteacher presents complaining of a rash that started as a bull's-eye pattern that rapidly enlarged. She had a flu-like illness prior to the rash. Although she hikes often, she denies any tick bites.

1692. A 19-year-old woman presents with vesicular pustular pruritic lesions on an erythematous base. The rash followed a high temperature. The rash started in the hairline and has rapidly spread to the entire body.

1693. An 18-year-old college student from Vietnam presents with the complaint of a macu-lopapular rash that started on her face and rapidly spread. The rash followed a day of malaise, fever, headache, and conjunctivitis. Lymphadenopathy is evident in the postauricular and suboccipital nodes.

Questions 1694 through 1696

Of the following causes for mortality in women, which is the primary cause for each of the age groups?

    (A) accidents

    (B) cancer

    (C) cerebral vascular disease

    (D) chronic obstructive lung disease

    (E) heart disease

    (F) HIV infection

    (G) homicide

    (H) suicide

1694. Women aged 15 to 34

1695. Women aged 35 to 54

1696. Women aged 55 to 74

Questions 1697 through 1699

    (A) degenerative disease

    (B) disk disease

    (C) nerve root pain

    (D) ankylosing spondylitis

    (E) referred pain from pelvic viscera

1697. A 65-year-old patient presents with complaints of back pain that is worse after exercise or at the end of the day.

1698. A 30-year-old patient complains of back pain that is worse in the morning. Her examination reveals decreased range of motion of the spine and tenderness over the sacroiliac joints. There is a loss of lordosis.

1699. A 45-year-old woman presents complaining of back pain that radiates down her legs and is accompanied by numbness, paresthesia, and some weakness. The pain is increased with normal activities and improved with rest.

Answers and Explanations

1651. (B) A serum cholesterol of 280 mg/dL is well outside the normal range. Cholesterol as a risk factor may be greatly overemphasized, but further evaluation is needed. You will need to fractionate it to determine her levels of low-density lipoprotein (LDL) and high-density lipoprotein (HDL). You will need to assess any other cardiac risk factors, such as a positive family history, 30% or more over ideal weight, smoking, exercise level, blood pressure, dietary intake, and other medical conditions (diabetes, hypothyroidism, hyper-uricemia, etc.).

1652. (D) Smoking is associated with heart disease, chronic respiratory disease, and multiple cancers (head, neck, lung, and cervix). While no one lives forever, a 70-year-old woman could easily live to be 90. Wouldn't you help a 20-year-old live to age 40? Offer this woman smoking cessation therapy; she may be more interested than one might think.

1653. (B) Mammography is the most common method of detecting asymptomatic malignant disease in the breast, the second most prevalent of cancers in women. It can be wrong and seldom finds cancer of less than 0.5 cm. It may create as much anxiety as it solves. Although there has been some recent controversy, most organizations still recommend regular mammograms for women once they reach age 40.

1654. (E) Exercise can help to control weight, reduce blood pressure, improve glucose tolerance, and prevent coronary artery disease. Twenty to thirty minutes of aerobic exercise three times weekly may be enough. A goal of exercise is to reach and maintain a specific heart rate over a minimum time period. The calculation of the target heart rate is (220 − age) × (60 to 80%).

1655. (C) The calculation for BMI is weight (in kilos) divided by height (in meters) squared. A BMI of more than 29.9 is considered obese. A BMI of 25.0 to 29.9 is overweight. By this definition 55% of the American population is overweight or obese.

1656. (C) The formula for basal metabolic rate in women (kcal/M^2/hr) = 655 + (9.6 × W) + (1.8 × H) − (4.7 × A), or in her case = 655 + (9.6 × 80) + (1.8 × 163) − (4.7 × 43). (W = weight in kg, H = height in cm, A = age in years.) This is the Harris–Benedict equation and can be done without nomograms. In this case, it works out to about 1,500 kcal/day; then figuring in 1,200 kcal per day for light to moderate work, she takes in about 2,600 to 2,800 kcal/day. Another way to figure it is to assume a person uses 30 to 35 kcal per day per kg to maintain weight. So 80 kg × 33 kcal/kg = about 2,650.

1657. (B) This is a very simple calculation. A negative calorie balance of 3,500 kcal is required to lose 1 pound. So 3,500 kcal/pound divided by 7 means 500 kcal less per day loses about 1 pound per week.

1658. (E) Fat has 9 kcal/g; carbohydrate and protein each have about 4 kcal/g. Eliminating all fat is unpalatable and impossible. Decreasing overall intake with proportionately less fat is better than trying to eliminate something altogether. In fact, with the new commercially available fat-free products, it is possible to be fat free and still gain weight. This is because many of these food products use corn syrup instead of oil so the caloric intake is still similar. The key to sustained weight loss is moderation, especially of fat intake.

1659. (E) Although bicycling or swimming will use up 200 cal/hr and tennis and jogging even more, it is difficult for an overweight person who has not been exercising to do these activities for more than a few minutes. However, walking (at 150 cal/hr) is more consistent with their abilities. Thus, the patient will typically be more successful at walking for 30 or more minutes per session and do it three or four times per week. As their conditioning improves, they can change to more demanding activities if they prefer.

1660. (D) Measles is a live, attenuated vaccine. It is given as a single SQ dose. It is recommended for all persons born after 1956 who are non-immune. Pregnancy is recommended to be avoided for 3 months.

1661. (D) Pneumococcus vaccine is given as a single dose of purified capsular polysaccharide to people over 2 years of age who are at increased risk of infection with pneumococcus. Splenectomy, chronic cardiovascular disease or pulmonary disease (excluding asthma), metabolic or hepatic disease, or immunocompromised state (e.g., HIV) increases that risk.

1662. (C) Tetanus is generally given as a toxoid to those over 7 years of age and only once every 10 years unless there is an *acute* severe puncture or penetrating wound. One way to help individuals remember is to synchronize the doses to the decades of their birth. In other words, when a patient turns 30, 40, 50, and so on, he or she should receive a booster.

1663. (E) The relative potency of a parenteral dose of the listed medications would be (most potent to least potent): hydromorphone > oxy-

codone = methadone > meperidine > codeine in a ratio of 6:1:1:0.15:0.10, respectively. For pain as intense as a kidney stone and a sure diagnosis, maximum pain relief is indicated.

1664. (C) This is referred to as "sundowning." Confusion in the late afternoon or early evening is the key symptom. It can be associated with dementia, organic brain syndrome, unfamiliar environments, and aging. In this case, the fact that the mother does not recognize her daughter is most worrisome and would lead you to pursue a more detailed cause than simply aging. It may improve over time, but it may well need to be treated. Restraints (physical or chemical) are not the answer. More specific therapy can be recommended.

1665. (E) Isotretinoin is a vitamin A derivative that is indicated for just this problem. You should be certain that other therapies (especially A, B, and C) have been tried and failed, failing because of ineffectiveness rather than non-compliance. The patient should also be informed of the need to continue effective contraception when using this medication because of its known teratogenicity. Also, OCs will often help in the improvement of the acne.

1666. (C) The most reliable form of diagnosis would be culture, but it is also very slow. Presumptive evidence can be gleaned from chest x-ray findings or staining the sputum for acid-fast bacilli. Skin testing can cause an extreme reaction in patients with active tuberculosis and should be avoided in a patient in whom there is a high index of suspicion for active TB. Cultures are important to rule out a resistant form of TB. In this case, a culture, chest x-ray, and Gram stain of her sputum should all be taken, and if any indicate infection, treatment should be started.

1667. (E) Traveler's diarrhea results from the ingestion of contaminated water or food, so advising large water consumption or consumption of uncooked but washed raw foods is poor advice. The disease is common, and most physicians will recommend either prophylaxis or treatment immediately with the onset of symptoms. Trimethoprim–sulfa or ciprofloxacin is the best choice. The diarrhea without treatment can last for a long time. Clindamycin is a poor choice because it not only provides poor coverage, but in its oral form may be associated with colitis.

1668. **(A)** Most likely, she has simple reflux esophagitis. An upper gastrointestinal series would lend little to the resolution of this problem. Milk calms it, but in the long run probably exacerbates the problem. Antacids at the bedside or chronic administration of histamine blockers could treat the discomfort. However, the real problem is increased intra-abdominal pressure, probably related to her weight and to overeating, especially before bedtime. A gallstone would be associated with a different type of pain and would be unlikely to resolve as a result of the ingestion of milk. The surgical removal of asymptomatic gallstones is debatable.

1669. **(D)** This is a simple case of hemorrhoids brought on or exacerbated by constipation. Adding fluids and bulk-forming agents, and providing relief with sitz baths, astringents, or topical anti-inflammatory creams should help. Referral is unnecessary at this point, and biopsy is one of the biggest mistakes you will ever make in the office setting. Bright red blood per rectum on the toilet paper is unlikely to be a malignancy, and colonoscopy should be reserved for persistent or changing symptoms.

1670. **(E)** The history given is classic for stress-related headache. Her family history is unlikely to contribute in this instance. There is little that is hereditary in either case. Reducing her stress, small doses of analgesic, and patient education about stress-related headaches are most appropriate. The only other suggestion may be to have an eye examination to determine if corrective lens are indicated. Otherwise, referral would be inappropriate at this time.

1671. **(E)** The most common cause of anemia in a premenopausal–perimenopausal patient is iron deficiency. The other choices are all consistent with iron deficiency and support the conservative approach of iron supplementation unless the history would imply a source other than menses for the loss. An elevated reticulocyte count would imply that there are adequate iron stores, and there is another source such as hemolysis for the anemia.

1672. **(C)** The diagnosis of anorexia is very important since this can become life threatening. A patient may be embarrassed by her problem or not see it as a problem and provide the physician with a number of "explanations" for her body mass. Conversely, as more women become involved in sports, the lean build may reflect this athletic involvement and not an eating disorder (see Table 27–1). Although increased exercise tolerance is mainly associated with the athletic individual, the findings other than the lanugo hair are common in both groups.

1673. **(B)** As more women become involved in sports at a competitive level, physicians are seeing more knee injuries. The exact reason for this is unclear but is partially due to the wider pelvic girdle, which causes more lateral placement of the proximal attachments of the anterior thigh muscles. This, along with a common finding of an asymmetry in the strength of the knee muscles with more strength evident laterally, encourages the patella to track abnormally with resultant patellofemoral irritation and pain. Activities that involve repetitive hyperextension (such as punting a soccer ball) will often precipitate this problem. Muscle strengthening exercises, appropriate bracing or taping, and modification of activity are all part of the therapy.

1674. **(E)** This is classic for rheumatoid arthritis. It is two to three times more common in women. The etiology is unknown. Occasionally, the arthritis may begin in a more asymmetric fashion but will generally become more symmetric as it progresses. Unlike osteoarthritis, this is a systemic disease, hence

Table 27–1. Characteristics of Anorectics and Athletes

	Anorectics	Athletes
Distinguishing features	Aimless physical activity	Purposeful training
	Poor or decreasing exercise performance	Increased exercise tolerance
	Poor muscle development	Strong muscular development
	Flawed body image	Accurate body image
	Body fat below normal level	Body fat level within defined normal range
	Electrolyte abnormalities if abusing laxatives or diuretics	Increased plasma volume
	Cold intolerance	Increased 2 extraction from blood
	Dry skin	Efficient energy metabolism
	Cardiac arrhythmias	Increased high-density lipoprotein-2
	Lanugo hair	
	Leukocyte dysfunction	
Shared features	Dietary faddism	
	Controlled caloric consumption	
	Specific carbohydrate avoidance	
	Low body weight	
	Resting bradycardia and hypotension	
	Increased physical activity	
	Amenorrhea or oligomenorrhea	
	Anemia (sometimes)	

Reproduced, with permission, from McSherry JA. The diagnostic challenge of anorexia nervosa. *Am Fam Physician* 1988;29:144.

the nodules. Although osteoarthritis of the hip occurs at the same rate in men as women, women are more likely to have problems with knees and hands. Factors that predispose to osteoarthritis are prior injury or stresses to the affected joint. Ankylosing spondylitis and Reiter syndrome are spondyloarthropathies and tend to be more central in their location (e.g., vertebral and sacroiliac joints). Gout involves isolated joints that are swollen, warm, erythematous, and markedly tender.

1675. **(C)** The recommendation is to use sun protection factor (SPF) 32 sunscreens and apply approximately 2 hours prior to sun exposure to allow skin absorption. The damage is from the UV lightwaves, which are present on cloudy days and are at high intensity at higher altitudes due to the thinner atmosphere. The UV lights in tanning booths are just as bad as natural sunlight and perhaps worse since one does not get hot and hence may increase time of exposure and the amount of skin exposed.

1676. **(B, C, E)** In most instances the Pap smear, mammography, and dipstick urinalysis are done as a routine part of yearly health care screening. Serum creatinine would generally be reserved for only those patients with suspected renal disease, and hematocrit if indicated by previous history or other finding.

1677. **(A, B, C, D)** There are many causes for poor sleep: depression, use of stimulants, worry, and others. Finding out why the patient is not sleeping is more important than simply giving her a medication to sleep. Ask about all the sleep-related issues that you can in order to treat the cause and not the symptom.

1678. **(A, B, D, E)** ERT may increase breast cancer risks slightly if it affects breast cancer at all. It should be noted that obesity is a much greater risk factor than ERT for the development of breast cancer. When combined with a progestin, it reduces the chance of endometrial carcinoma over that of the general population. It stops bone loss, improves lipid profile, stops hot flushes (thus promoting sleep) and prevents atrophy of the vagina and urethra. Many women will take estrogen therapy for at least a short period during menopause. The debate now concerns how long a woman should consider estrogen use.

1679. (B, C, D, E) Primary health care includes those things that contribute to the ongoing health maintenance of an individual: routine screening for symptoms, physical findings, basic laboratory analysis, and providing ongoing health care needs. Genetic counseling is a specialized service that cannot be provided by all primary caregivers and may involve referral in most cases. However, a brief genetic screening history at initial intake of a new patient for risk patterns is becoming a more standard element of care, especially for women considering a pregnancy.

1680. (B, C) While the more paternal among us may consider choices A, D, and E, none of these things are truly our job. Making the patient aware of the need for contraception if she does not wish to become pregnant is part of our responsibility, even when not specifically requested. Offering sexually transmitted disease (STD) testing is also a routine part of health maintenance, as would be informing her that she is at increased risk of acquiring an STD if she continues having multiple partners. Also, consider hepatitis B immunization if she has not completed the series.

1681. (C, D, E) Most colon cancer lesions cannot be felt on rectal examination, but every annual examination after the age of 50 should also include a rectal examination. Colon cancer comprises 15% of all cancers in women. The most common organ to have cancer is breast followed by the lungs and then the colon. There is a hereditary component to colon cancer, so her positive family history may indicate a need to initiate screening sooner.

1682. (A, C, D, E) The prescribing of medication means that you do what is necessary to pick the right medication in the correct dosage to treat the disease process identified. The past medical history will need to be reviewed for allergies, adverse reactions, and previous successes or failure. Though you might not believe it in these times of saving money, cost should not be the primary concern in determining the need for an indicated medicine. This does not mean most expensive is best. It

does mean that an ineffective drug is not good for your patient, regardless of cost savings. Probably the best cost savings can be obtained by picking a generic form of a known reliable drug.

1683. (A, B, C, E) In a patient with documented osteoporosis, especially so close to menopause, other causes for osteoporosis need to be considered. All of these can cause increased calcium loss except for hypothyroidism. It is hyperthyroidism that is more of a problem. Obviously, if a secondary cause is found, it should be treated directly and not just assumed that estrogen replacement will manage the problem. In this woman, tamoxifen may be a consideration since it may protect from breast cancer and still offer some bone protection. However, there are increased risks of endometrial cancer and thromboembolic problems.

1684. (A, B, C, D) All except fluoride have been shown to decrease fractures. Although sodium fluoride increases osteoblastic activity and increases bone density in the spine, it does not increase the density in other sites of trabecular bone. Despite the increased density, studies show an increase in nonvertebral fractures and no decrease in vertebral fractures with the use of fluoride.

1685. (A, D) When evaluating a skin lesion for potential malignant risks, one should look for the ABCD of melanoma: A is for asymmetry of the lesion; a benign lesion is very symmetrical. B is for border, which should be smooth and distinct. C is for color; blackness is not as much of a problem as is a variation of coloring within a malignant lesion. The diameter should be smaller than the diameter of the eraser on a No. 2 pencil. If larger, it is suspicious for melanoma.

1686. (B) The hairs that are plucked will often show a clubbed hair root. Usually there is spontaneous regrowth of hair in 2 to 6 months. Due to the spontaneous recovery, it is hard to know what the best therapy is. The cause is unknown.

1687. (A) This is similar to the form of alopecia in men as they get older. This condition is genetic, with onset in reproductive-age women. A biopsy may be helpful in diagnosis, and topical minoxidil will help some patients.

1688. (E) This is the loss of resting hairs. Pregnancy and other stresses appear to cause a synchronization of hair follicles so a larger portion enter telogen at the same time and then are shed at once. This is usually time limited, and the hair regrows within 6 months.

1689. (F) The constant tension placed on a hair follicle can cause permanent damage and scarring, resulting in permanent hair loss in the affected areas. Some of the current hair styles, especially among blacks, are predisposed to this complication.

1690. (E) This is classic pityriasis rosea with the herald patch. If one looks at the back, the rash will line up with the skin in a diagonal Christmas-tree look. This rash is self-limiting and is probably viral in origin.

1691. (C) This is likely to be early Lyme disease despite the lack of a history of a tick bite. Laboratory confirmation is difficult as many of the serologic assays are not reliable. Since early Lyme disease is easily treated with prolonged tetracycline or amoxicillin with probenecid, it is often wise to treat if one suspects the diagnosis.

1692. (G) This is classic varicella. In a healthy adult, treatment is symptomatic, with careful monitoring for the development of varicella pneumonia. Acyclovir has no place in the treatment of an uncomplicated case of varicella.

1693. (F) This is classic rubella. This is not commonly seen in the United States due to mandatory immunization of schoolchildren but still occurs occasionally. Since this has grave implications for a fetus, it is important to make the diagnosis and then to assure that the patient is not pregnant and that she does not expose other pregnant women.

1694. (A) Over 25% of deaths in the 15 to 34 age group are related to accidents. The next most frequent cause is cancer, which accounts for about 15%. Homicide and suicide are third and fourth.

1695. (B) Forty percent of deaths in the 35 to 54 age group are related to cancer. The second most common cause is heart disease, accounting for 15%. Accidents and cerebrovascular accidents follow as third and fourth.

1696. (B) Cancer is the number 1 killer in women aged 55 to 74, with heart disease second and chronic obstructive lung disease third.

1697. (A) This is typical of degenerative disease. It occurs in older patients and is worse at the end of the day.

1698. (D) There may also be a decrease in chest expansion. Aortic stenosis and uveitis can be seen in some patients. There is a strong association with HLA-B27.

1699. (C) Anything that stretches the nerve, such as bending, will increase the pain. Sciatica is a form of nerve root pain. If clear muscle weakness is demonstrated, active intervention may be indicated and a referral to an orthopedist may be wise. Otherwise, conservative therapy with anti-inflammatory medications, analgesics, and muscle relaxants is the first-line therapy.

CHAPTER 28

Practice Test
Questions

DIRECTIONS (Questions 1 through 115): Each of the numbered items or incomplete statements in this section is followed by answers or by completions of the statement. Select the ONE lettered answer or completion that is BEST in each case.

1. A patient wishes you to explain the concept of cervical intraepithelial neoplasia (CIN) III, which has been diagnosed from her cervical biopsy after a low-grade squamous intraepithelial lesion (LGSIL) was found on a Pap smear. You can correctly tell her CIN III

   (A) is an invasive cancer
   (B) includes carcinoma in situ (CIS)
   (C) requires no further treatment
   (D) is due to a bacterial infection
   (E) corresponds to the LGSIL shown on her prior Pap smear

2. The major histocompatibility complex (MHC) in human beings is located on which chromosome?

   (A) 1
   (B) 6
   (C) 13
   (D) 16
   (E) 21

3. With respect to genetics, linkage means that the

   (A) spindles have formed in the equatorial plate
   (B) pairing of homologous chromosomes has occurred
   (C) centromere is acrosomic
   (D) involved genes have crossed over
   (E) involved gene loci lie near one another on the same chromosome

4. Which of the following alleles has no detectable product?

   (A) A of the ABO blood group
   (B) B of the ABO blood group
   (C) O of the ABO blood group
   (D) D of the Rh group
   (E) K of the Kell blood group

5. Which of the following is most likely to be the best donor for a kidney transplant patient?

   (A) father
   (B) mother
   (C) grandfather
   (D) aunt
   (E) brother

6. A 22-year-old patient is involved in a skiing accident with head injuries. Six months after her apparent recovery she has not had a menstrual cycle. She also complains of hot flushes. Her luteinizing hormone (LH), follicle-stimulating hormone (FSH), and estradiol levels are all very low. This implies an injury to the

   (A) periventricular nucleus
   (B) supraoptic nucleus
   (C) suprachiasmatic nucleus
   (D) arcuate nucleus
   (E) paraventricular nucleus

7. Which of the following hormones is a single chain peptide?

   (A) thyroid-stimulating hormone (TSH)
   (B) LH
   (C) adrenocorticotropic hormone (ACTH)
   (D) FSH
   (E) human chorionic gonadotropin (hCG)

8. A male infant is born with hypertension and hypokalemia. One suspects an absence of 17-alpha hydroxylase. This can be verified if there is an elevation of

   (A) 17-alpha hydroxyprogesterone
   (B) androstenedione
   (C) testosterone
   (D) deoxycorticosterone
   (E) cortisone

9. The synthesis of a progesterone-like product that was biologically active after oral ingestion was critical to the effectiveness of oral contraceptive (OC) pills. These 19-nortestosterones are so named because they

   (A) have a northern orientation in a magnetic field
   (B) are minus a methyl group
   (C) are neither estrogen nor androgen
   (D) are precursors to testosterone
   (E) none of the above

10. A ubiquitous 20-carbon fatty acid with a variety of biologic effects is

    (A) progesterone
    (B) dopamine
    (C) ACTH
    (D) FSH
    (E) prostaglandin (PG)

11. The fetal gonad is critical to the phenotypic sexual development of the fetus. Which of the following statements best describes the function of the fetal gonad?

    (A) Estrogen produced by the fetal ovary induces female internal genitalia development.
    (B) Müllerian inhibitory factor produced by the fetal testis induces regression of female external genitalia.
    (C) Testosterone produced by the fetal testis induces male internal genital development.
    (D) Dihydrotestosterone produced by the fetal testis induces male external genitalia development.

12. Precocious puberty has a number of physical and psychological consequences. However, one of the steroid effects is not reversible or correctable and has major long-term implications. For this reason, which of the following steroid effects would be the prime consideration in management of female precocious puberty?

    (A) epiphyseal closure
    (B) hair growth
    (C) genital development
    (D) breast tissue development
    (E) fat redistribution

13. The absence of 17-alpha hydroxylase is associated with

    (A) hypergonadotropic hypogonadism
    (B) hypogonadotropic hypogonadism
    (C) true precocious puberty
    (D) pseudo-precocious puberty
    (E) normal puberty

14. Growth in most follicles is usually followed by

    (A) ovulation
    (B) cyst formation
    (C) atresia
    (D) arrest
    (E) regression

15. Which of the following physical findings should prompt an evaluation of a pathologic process in a menopausal woman?

    (A) atrophic vaginal mucosa
    (B) clitoromegaly
    (C) small labia minora
    (D) amenorrhea

16. The darkening of the vaginal mucosa that occurs early in gestation is called

   (A) Hegar's sign

   (B) Chadwick's sign

   (C) Braxton Hicks contractions

   (D) Von Fernwald's sign

   (E) Cullen's sign

17. Which of the following situations generally applies to the uterus during pregnancy?

   (A) rotates to the right because of the sacral promontory

   (B) exhibits no rotation

   (C) rotates to the right because of the rectosigmoid

   (D) rotates to the left because of the sacral promontory

   (E) rotates to the left because of the sigmoid colon

18. The symptom of excessive salivation that may occur during pregnancy is called

   (A) deglutition

   (B) pruritus

   (C) emesis

   (D) eructation

   (E) ptyalism

19. A lowered hemoglobin during normal pregnancy is a physiologic finding. It is due mainly to

   (A) low iron stores

   (B) blood lost to the placenta and fetus

   (C) increased plasma volume

   (D) increased cardiac output resulting in greater red cell destruction

   (E) decreased reticulocytosis

20. The average woman can expect to retain as much as 7 L of water during a normal gestation. Factors that play a role in this retention include

   (A) decreased venous pressure in the lower fourth of the body

   (B) increased plasma oncotic pressure

   (C) increased capillary permeability

   (D) marked increase (> 50 g) in the maternal exchangeable sodium

   (E) a physiologic cardiac failure resulting in edema, fluid retention, and enlargement of the heart

21. Maternal serum prolactin levels in pregnancy are highest

   (A) at the end of gestation just before delivery of the infant

   (B) just after delivery of the infant

   (C) as the placenta is released

   (D) the third to fourth day postpartum

   (E) during breast-feeding

22. Normally, the pregnant woman hyperventilates. This is compensated by

   (A) increased tidal volume

   (B) respiratory alkalosis

   (C) decreased P_{CO_2} of the blood

   (D) decreased plasma bicarbonate

   (E) decreased serum pH

23. Immediately after spontaneous rupture of membranes there is moderate vaginal bleeding and the development of fetal distress. Concern is raised about a fetal hemorrhage from a vasa previa. It is critical to act quickly because the normal fetal blood volume compared to fetal weight near term is approximately

   (A) 15 mL/kg

   (B) 50 mL/kg

   (C) 80 mL/kg

   (D) 100 mL/kg

   (E) 150 mL/kg

24. A cytomegalovirus (CMV) infection may cause an acute fetal hemolysis. If a fetal intrauterine transfusion becomes indicated, which of the following blood products is best to use?

   (A) AB-positive donor red blood cells

   (B) O-negative maternal whole blood

   (C) AB-negative paternal plasma

   (D) O-positive donor red blood cells

   (E) O-negative donor red blood cells

25. A patient presents at 30 weeks' gestation in labor that cannot be stopped. Lung maturity is unlikely. Fetal lung surfactant production may be increased by a number of factors. Which of the following is proven clinically useful?

(A) estrogen

(B) prolactin

(C) thyroxine

(D) glucocorticosteroids

(E) alpha-fetoprotein

26. The only class of hormones relevant to the embryogenesis of the external genitalia is

(A) androgens

(B) estrogens

(C) cortisol

(D) hCG

(E) progesterone

27. Of the following laboratory studies, which would be done routinely in a pregnant patient?

(A) electrolytes

(B) urinary estriol

(C) serum glutamic-oxaloacetic transaminase (SGOT)

(D) VDRL (Venereal Disease Research Laboratory)

(E) fluorescent treponemal antibody absorption (FTA-ABS)

28. Asked about the fetal safety of a category B drug when taken by a pregnant woman, you respond that a drug in this category has

(A) proven risks that outweigh its benefits

(B) fetal risk, but the benefits far outweigh the risks

(C) no adequate studies showing adverse effects in animals, but there are no human data

(D) animal studies showing no fetal risks, or if there are risks, they are not shown in well-controlled human studies

29. An Rh-negative pregnant woman at 18 weeks' gestation was found to have a titer of 1:32 anti-Lewis antibodies and no other evidence of sensitization to red-cell antigens. You should

(A) perform a repeat blood test at 4 weeks to see if the titer increases

(B) advise termination of pregnancy

(C) plan serial amniocentesis, starting at 24 to 26 weeks

(D) plan exchange transfusion as soon as fetal viability is assured

(E) plan to give D-immunoglobulin at 28 weeks' gestation

30. When counseling a patient regarding fetal abnormalities during prenatal care, the greatest advantage of chorionic villus sampling (CVS) over amniocentesis is

(A) the ability to provide results sooner

(B) the ability to perform enzyme studies

(C) a decreased fetal risk

(D) obtaining far superior cellular sample

(E) a lack of maternal cell contamination

31. When performing clinical pelvimetry in a gynecoid pelvis, the diagonal conjugate should be at least

(A) 7.5 cm

(B) 9.5 cm

(C) 11.5 cm

(D) 13.5 cm

(E) 15.5 cm

32. A 26-year-old primigravida at her first prenatal visit reports that she is in excellent health and refuses the prenatal vitamins you prescribe. Your dietary review indicates that she does follow a nutritious, well-balanced diet. Nonetheless, you explain that the only nutrient for which requirements during pregnancy could not be met by diet alone is

(A) vitamin C

(B) calcium

(C) iron

(D) zinc

(E) vitamin D

33. You are called to the bedside of a laboring patient who has just received an injection in her epidural. She has become panicked. She cannot breathe and begins to convulse. Your first step in treating a severe systemic reaction to this local anesthetic agent is

   (A) oxygen administration
   (B) IV fluids
   (C) stopping convulsions
   (D) supporting blood pressure
   (E) clearing the airway

34. The greatest amount of blood would normally be lost in which of the following procedures?

   (A) a vaginal delivery of a normal-term infant
   (B) an uncomplicated cesarean section of a single fetus at term
   (C) an uncomplicated vaginal delivery of twins at term
   (D) an uncomplicated cesarean section of twins at term
   (E) an elective dilation and curettage (D&C) done in the nonpregnant state

35. The implantation of a placenta in which there is a defect in the fibrinoid layer at the implantation site, allowing the placental villi to invade and penetrate into but not through the myometrium, is called

   (A) placenta accreta
   (B) placenta increta
   (C) placenta percreta
   (D) placental infarct
   (E) placenta previa

36. You are checking a term patient in labor. The examination of the fetal presentation feels unusual. Which of the following would be incompatible with a spontaneous delivery?

   (A) occiput posterior
   (B) mentum posterior
   (C) brow asynclitic
   (D) occiput transverse
   (E) sacrum posterior

37. Ritodrine is a beta-adrenergic receptor stimulator that is used to arrest preterm labor. Which of the following is a major maternal risk associated with its use?

   (A) hypertension
   (B) decreased plasma glucose
   (C) decreased serum potassium
   (D) cardiac arrhythmias
   (E) asthma

38. You are taking care of a 29-year-old primigravida who is having a postpartum hemorrhage. The placenta delivered spontaneously, intact. Labor was 9¾ hours and was unremarkable. There are no obvious lacerations. You are becoming concerned about coagulopathy. The most readily available test for blood clotting defects during labor and delivery is

   (A) prothrombin time
   (B) serum fibrinogen
   (C) fibrin split products
   (D) observance of a tube of whole blood
   (E) platelet count

39. In the presence of a complete longitudinal vaginal septum

   (A) delivery is usually difficult
   (B) the uterus is less likely to be abnormal
   (C) conception is nearly impossible
   (D) there is an above-average incidence of urinary tract abnormalities
   (E) prophylactic cesarean delivery is indicated

40. The hemostatic mechanism most important in combating postpartum hemorrhage is

   (A) increased blood clotting factors in pregnancy
   (B) contraction of interlacing uterine muscle bundles
   (C) markedly decreased blood pressure in the uterine venules
   (D) intramyometrial vascular coagulation due to vasoconstriction
   (E) enhanced platelet aggregation during pregnancy

41. A 32-year-old white woman (gravida 4, para 3) at 38 weeks' gestation by good dates presents in your office with painless moderate vaginal bleeding (soaking two pads) after an otherwise uneventful gestation. The bleeding presently has ceased and no uterine contractions are present; the fetal heart tones (FHTs) are 140. You should

    (A) perform a complete pelvic examination
    (B) reassure the patient and send her home to await spontaneous labor
    (C) admit the patient to the hospital the following morning for induction of labor
    (D) perform an ultrasound
    (E) perform an immediate cesarean section

42. As part of the hospital quality assurance program, the incidence of maternal morbidity is tracked. Infectious maternal (puerperal) morbidity is defined as

    (A) any fever after pregnancy
    (B) a temperature over 100.4°F during the first 24 hours after delivery
    (C) a temperature over 100.4°F in any two 24-hour periods of the 10 days immediately after delivery
    (D) a temperature over 102.2°F in any two 24-hour periods
    (E) a temperature over 100°F in any two 24-hour periods

43. A patient has an uncomplicated vaginal delivery of a 3500-g infant. The placenta delivers spontaneously in 15 minutes. Forty-five minutes after this delivery, you are notified by a nurse that the patient has an unusual amount of bleeding but that vital signs are stable. You should

    (A) order Pitocin IV
    (B) type and crossmatch two units of blood
    (C) reassure the nurse and wait
    (D) have the nurse call you back in 1 hour if bleeding persists
    (E) examine the patient

44. A 3-day postpartum patient developed a temperature of 104°F and a tender uterus with a foul-smelling discharge. Of the following organisms, the most likely offender is

    (A) *Escherichia coli*
    (B) *Bacteroides*
    (C) beta-streptococcus
    (D) gonococcus
    (E) *Staphylococcus*

45. A patient wishes to breast-feed. With which of the following active infections in the immediate postpartum period would it still be acceptable for a woman to breast-feed?

    (A) genital herpes
    (B) hepatitis B
    (C) HIV
    (D) varicella
    (E) CMV

46. Which of the following is normally found in the immediate postpartum period after a normal delivery?

    (A) leukopenia
    (B) large drop in hematocrit
    (C) elevated erythrocyte sedimentation rate (ESR)
    (D) retention of fluid
    (E) rapid fall in plasma fibrinogen

47. Once respirations are established, which of the following is the most important aspect of immediate care of the newborn?

    (A) drying the skin
    (B) warming the infant
    (C) placing identification bands
    (D) doing a brief physical examination
    (E) measuring the hematocrit

48. The most common cause of newborn jaundice (icterus neonatorum) is

    (A) indirect bilirubin
    (B) direct bilirubin

(C) lack of carotene production in the new-born liver

(D) meconium obstruction of the newborn digestive system

(E) bottle-feeding

49. A newborn is noted to have a darkened swelling of the scalp that does not cross the midline. This is most likely a

(A) caput succedaneum

(B) subdural hemorrhage

(C) cephalhematoma

(D) subarachnoid hemorrhage

(E) tentorial tear

50. After delivery, paralysis is noted on one side of the face in a newborn. This is most often associated with

(A) pressure on the trigeminal nerve during delivery

(B) neonatal sepsis

(C) facial swelling

(D) forceps-induced nerve injury

(E) abnormalities of the central nervous system (CNS)

51. A male infant is born with prominent epicanthal folds, a flattened nose, skin that appears "loose," and large, low-set ears. The baby does not spontaneously breathe, and you intubate the child and find it almost impossible to ventilate. Which of the following is the most likely diagnosis?

(A) postmaturity syndrome

(B) normal pressure hydrocephalus

(C) renal agenesis

(D) pyloric stenosis

(E) diaphragmatic hernia

52. A couple returns to your clinic after initial evaluation of their infertility condition. Semen analysis revealed 35 million sperm/mL, 50% motility, and 50% normal forms. Hysterosalpingogram demonstrated a normal endometrial cavity with unilateral proximal tubal obstruction. The female patient has regular menstrual cycles with appropriate basal body temperature (BBT) rise indicating a 14-day luteal phase. A serum progesterone level was 15.2 ng/mL. A diagnostic laparoscopy showed no adhesions or endometriosis, with bilateral free spill of dye from her tubes. What is the most appropriate diagnosis in this case?

(A) tubal factor infertility

(B) luteal-phase deficiency

(C) male factor infertility

(D) oligo-ovulation

(E) unexplained infertility

53. A 27-year-old woman with regular menstrual cycles presents to your clinic with her husband. Their previous studies included a normal hysterosalpingogram, normal semen analysis, and normal serum progesterone level. At the time of her visit, she is on cycle day 10 with intercourse 6 hours prior to this office visit. You perform a postcoital test, finding clear, scant mucus with minimal ferning pattern. Two nonmotile sperm are seen per high-power field (HPF). What is the most likely reason for this result?

(A) poor timing of the postcoital

(B) sperm antibody

(C) cervical factor

(D) progesterone dominance

(E) endocervicitis

54. The most common chromosomal abnormality found in tissue from first-trimester spontaneous abortions is

(A) autosomal trisomy

(B) sex-chromosome monosomy

(C) sex-chromosome polysomy

(D) triploidy

(E) tetraploidy

55. A 31-year-old patient comes to your clinic with irregular menstrual cycles and infertility of 2 years' duration. After evaluation you determine that clomiphene citrate would be the appropriate mode of therapy. Which of the following statements should be explained to the patient?

(A) There is an increased risk of fetal anomalies if pregnancy results.

(B) Approximately 25% of patients will respond by ovulating with this medication.

(C) The risk of multiple pregnancy is 7%.

(D) Ovulation usually occurs 3 weeks after the last day of clomiphene citrate ingestion.

(E) The risk of severe ovarian hyperstimulation syndrome is 25%.

56. Estrogen synthesis during pregnancy depends on the

(A) placenta only

(B) fetus only

(C) placenta and fetus

(D) placenta and mother

(E) placenta, fetus, and mother

57. A 22-year-old woman experiences amenorrhea of 6 months' duration. Physical examination demonstrates normal breast development and normal pelvic organs. There is no hirsutism or galactorrhea. Serum TSH and prolactin levels are normal. A serum pregnancy test is negative. The next course of action would be to

(A) administer progesterone

(B) administer estrogen followed by progesterone

(C) measure circulating estrogen levels

(D) measure circulating testosterone levels

(E) obtain radiologic evaluation of the sella turcica

58. A couple is using "natural family planning" for contraception. Shown is the basal temperature graph made by the couple the previous month (Figure 28–1). Which letter most closely identifies when unprotected intercourse may most safely resume?

(A) A

(B) B

(C) C

(D) D

(E) E

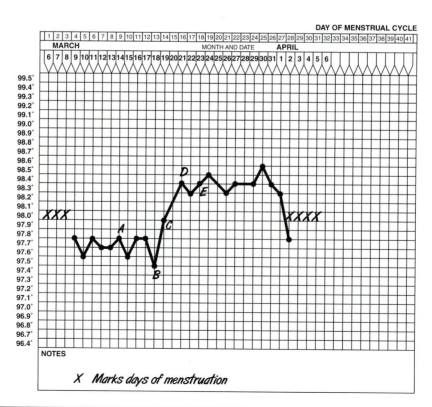

Figure 28–1.

59. A 33-year-old woman cannot feel the string of her intrauterine device (IUD). Her last menstrual period was 1 week ago. A serum pregnancy test is negative. The BEST immediate action is to

(A) obtain an abdominal radiogram
(B) probe the cervical canal gently to pull down the string
(C) obtain a pelvic ultrasound
(D) perform a hysterosalpingogram
(E) insert another IUD to replace the lost one

60. The most common side effect of low-dose OCs is

(A) breakthrough bleeding
(B) dysmenorrhea
(C) nausea
(D) mastalgia
(E) chloasma

61. A 35-year-old woman complains of irregular vaginal bleeding and abdominal pain. Her last menstrual period (LMP) was 8 weeks ago. A laparoscopic tubal fulguration was performed 2 years ago for permanent sterilization. She wants to know if her symptoms are related to the previous surgical sterilization. You advise her that a postoperative complication of female sterilization is

(A) dysmenorrhea
(B) anovulation
(C) irregular bleeding
(D) ovarian cyst formation
(E) ectopic pregnancy

62. A 32-year-old woman has an intrauterine fetal demise at 35 weeks' gestation. Which of the following pregnancy termination methods is associated with the highest rate of complications?

(A) intravenous oxytocin
(B) intravenous PG
(C) intravaginal PG
(D) intramuscular PG
(E) dilation and evacuation (D&E)

63. A 58-year-old woman consults you for vulvar pruritus. On pelvic examination, you note thin, atrophic skin with whitish coloration over the entire vulva. Of the following diagnoses, which would be most likely?

(A) vulvar carcinoma
(B) vulvar intraepithelial neoplasia
(C) hyperkeratosis
(D) atrophic vulvitis
(E) lichen sclerosis

64. A 53-year-old woman who has not menstruated for 1 year is started on cyclic hormonal replacement therapy. She has scant vaginal bleeding of 2 days' duration as she starts her second cycle of replacement. She is healthy, body mass index (BMI) 21, normal blood pressure, and used OCs until age 42. The next step in the management of her bleeding, if she refuses an endometrial sampling, is to

(A) begin a menstrual (bleeding) calendar
(B) take a Pap smear, including vaginal pool sampling
(C) insist on an endometrial sample
(D) perform colposcopy
(E) perform a transvaginal ultrasonography for endometrial thickness

65. Currently, the most effective treatment for primary dysmenorrhea in a woman who does not desire contraception is

(A) depo-medroxyprogesterone acetate
(B) birth control pills
(C) gonadotropin-releasing hormone (GnRH) agonist
(D) estrogen supplement in the luteal phase
(E) PG synthetase inhibitors

66. Endometriosis treated with prolonged estrogen and progesterone combination therapy exhibits which of the following histologic characteristics?

(A) marked edema
(B) atrophy
(C) glandular hypertrophy
(D) inflammatory infiltrate
(E) cyclic changes

67. The major symptom of adenomyosis is

(A) irregular uterine enlargement

(B) menorrhagia and dysmenorrhea

(C) urinary frequency

(D) menstrual irregularity and infertility

(E) uterine tenderness

68. A 35-year-old complains of increasing dysmenorrhea and pelvic pain. She has not become pregnant despite 3 years of unprotected intercourse. Her pelvic examination demonstrates tenderness and nodularity over her uterosacral ligaments and a 4-cm right ovarian cyst. What is her most likely diagnosis?

(A) adenomyosis

(B) pelvic congestion syndrome

(C) ectopic pregnancy

(D) endometriosis

(E) chronic pelvic inflammatory disease (PID)

69. An 80-year-old woman returns to your office 1 year after a surgical repair for genital prolapse. You performed a vaginal hysterectomy and anterior and posterior colporrhaphy. A few months ago she was hospitalized with pneumonia. She now complains of a large bulge protruding out her vagina. On examination, you diagnose a vaginal vault prolapse. Which of the following statements is TRUE?

(A) Prolapse must be repaired surgically in order to relieve symptoms.

(B) Fourth-degree vaginal prolapse cannot be adequately repaired by surgery in at least one half of cases.

(C) Prolapse of any female genital organ is likely to be accompanied by prolapse of one or more of the other genital organs at the time of diagnosis.

(D) The greatest risk factor for developing genital prolapse is a prior hysterectomy.

(E) Nulliparous patients are not reported to have genital prolapse.

70. A 65-year-old woman (gravida 3, para 3) is being counseled regarding the risks of having

a Burch operation for stress incontinence. She has had a prior hysterectomy. On examination, she has a second-degree cystocele. Urodynamic testing confirmed genuine stress incontinence. Which statement is TRUE?

(A) The incontinence operation will fail 25 to 30% of the time.

(B) Immediate postoperative urinary retention is the most common complication after continence surgery.

(C) The risk of ureteral injury is 10%.

(D) The risk of later developing an enterocele and/or rectocele is less than 5%.

(E) The failure rate is higher because of the prior hysterectomy.

71. A vigorous 79-year-old woman with worsening urinary incontinence over the past year comes to see you. The leakage seems to be without warning. Frequent small volumes leak at a time. It is interfering with her exercise program. She denies neurologic symptoms, stress incontinence symptoms, or voiding problems. She is on insulin for diabetes. Physical examination reveals normal neurologic and pelvic findings. A postvoid residual urine was 240 mL. Urodynamic testing shows uninhibited detrusor contractions with leakage. She generated a low-level detrusor contraction with voiding but has incomplete bladder emptying with residuals around 200 mL. Her bladder capacity is 350 mL. How will you achieve better bladder emptying with the fewest risks?

(A) teach her clean intermittent self-catheterization (CISC)

(B) place a Foley catheter

(C) start her on anticholinergic-type medication

(D) start her on PG inhibitor medication

(E) offer her a urinary diversion

72. A 1-year-old girl has an abdominal mass. Rectal examination demonstrates a mass extending into the right pelvis. The cervix is not palpable. Abdominal sonography shows that the uterus and vagina are absent. Both ovaries appear normal. The origin of the mass is most likely

(A) gastrointestinal (GI)

(B) renal

(C) musculoskeletal

(D) hepatic

(E) pancreatic

73. A 6-cm nontender, mobile, right adnexal mass is present in a 19-year-old woman. One year ago, while using OCs, she was hospitalized for left leg deep vein thrombophlebitis. Transvaginal sonography shows a 4-cm unilocular smooth ovarian cyst without internal excrescences. A serum pregnancy test is negative. You advise

(A) observation

(B) OCs

(C) estrogen therapy

(D) laparoscopy

(E) laparotomy

74. A 17-year-old girl experiences sudden right lower abdominal pain. Her LMP was 7 weeks ago. She has severe nausea and breast tenderness. Vital signs are: blood pressure, 120/80 mm Hg; pulse, 80 bpm; and afebrile. Abdominal examination is unremarkable. Pelvic examination shows blood in the vagina and a normal-appearing cervix. The uterus is slightly enlarged. A tender 4-cm right adnexal mass is present. The most appropriate diagnostic test is a(n)

(A) hematocrit

(B) white blood count (WBC)

(C) ESR

(D) serum hCG determination

(E) transvaginal sonogram

75. A 75-year-old woman presents with a 7-cm adnexal mass. Approximately what percentage of such masses in postmenopausal women are malignant?

(A) 10%

(B) 30%

(C) 50%

(D) 70%

(E) 90%

76. A 23-year-old woman asks about her recent biopsy diagnosis of vulvar intraepithelial neoplasia. You can correctly tell her that it commonly

(A) progresses to invasive cancer within a few years

(B) is a multicentric lesion

(C) arises from a glandular component in the skin

(D) exhibits nearly the same findings in each case—a raised, hard, white lesion

(E) can be cured with improved vulvar hygiene

77. A 69-year-old women presents with a 2-cm firm nodule in the right labium majus without signs of inflammation. Which of the following is the most appropriate course of action?

(A) excisional biopsy

(B) reassurance

(C) hot packs

(D) triple sulfa and cortisone cream

(E) simple vulvectomy

78. While viewing a cervical biopsy, squamous cell atypia is noted. It extends from the basal layer to a little more than one half the thickness of the epithelium. Beyond that level, maturation is evident. There is no invasion of stroma. This biopsy shows

(A) adenocarcinoma

(B) microglandular hyperplasia

(C) moderate dysplasia (CIN II)

(D) CIS

(E) invasive squamous cell carcinoma

79. The diagnosis of carcinoma of the cervix, International Federation of Gynecology and Obstetrics (FIGO) stage III, is assigned when

    (A) the carcinoma has infiltrated the bladder base
    (B) the carcinoma involves the distal vaginal mucosa
    (C) the carcinoma has extended into the parametria, but not to the pelvic side wall
    (D) x-ray reveals tumor
    (E) adenocarcinoma is present

80. A 57-year-old woman has been on unopposed estrogen for 7 years as she is intolerant of progestins. You have counseled her that

    (A) the risk ratio for developing endometrial cancer is between 3 and 8
    (B) the cumulative risk of developing endometrial cancer after 10 years is 20%
    (C) if she develops endometrial cancer while on estrogen, the 5-year survival rate is 50%
    (D) obesity is a risk factor among estrogen users
    (E) the biologic and clinical characteristics of endometrial cancer in estrogen users and nonusers is similar

81. A 62-year-old obese woman on unopposed estrogen develops abnormal vaginal bleeding. Her cervical Pap smear is normal. She is best evaluated by which of the following procedures?

    (A) transvaginal sonography
    (B) cervical conization
    (C) endometrial biopsy
    (D) endometrial cytology
    (E) colposcopy and cervical biopsy

82. Uterine sarcoma is most likely to occur in a

    (A) 10-year-old girl with recent onset vaginal bleeding
    (B) 9-year-old girl with a rapidly enlarging pelvic mass
    (C) 55-year-old woman with a rapidly enlarging uterus

    (D) 40-year-old woman with a slowly enlarging uterus
    (E) 25-year-old woman with a rapidly enlarging uterus

83. The most common site of metastases from ovarian carcinoma is

    (A) contralateral ovary
    (B) uterus
    (C) peritoneum
    (D) liver
    (E) lung

84. Which of the following sequelae is most likely to result from a ruptured mucinous cystadenoma?

    (A) pulmonary metastases
    (B) cerebral metastases
    (C) liver metastases
    (D) pseudomyxoma peritonei
    (E) ureteral obstruction

85. A woman has a hormonally active ovarian neoplasm. It is most likely to be

    (A) an epithelial tumor
    (B) a germ cell tumor
    (C) a sex cord–stromal tumor
    (D) a lipid cell tumor
    (E) a gonadoblastoma

86. A 45-year-old woman has an ovarian epithelial neoplasm. It is most likely to be a(n)

    (A) serous tumor
    (B) mucinous tumor
    (C) endometrioid tumor
    (D) clear cell tumor
    (E) Brenner tumor

87. Which of the therapies for ovarian cancer increases the risk of leukemia?

    (A) radiation therapy
    (B) chemotherapy
    (C) both of the above
    (D) neither of the above

88. A 56-year-old woman has gradual virilization. Which of the following conditions is most likely to be associated with her 5-cm left ovarian mass, which is found to contain nests of luteinized thecal cells within the stroma?

    (A) pituitary tumor
    (B) polycystic ovarian syndrome (PCOS)
    (C) stromal hyperthecosis
    (D) Sertoli–Leydig cell tumor
    (E) Krukenberg tumor

89. Which of the following findings would be the most suspicious for breast carcinoma?

    (A) diffuse nodularity in both breasts
    (B) a single cyst in the lower inner quadrant of the left breast
    (C) a single nodule in the upper outer quadrant of the right breast
    (D) multiple cystic masses in both breasts
    (E) a lump in the breast that appears just before menses

90. Which of the following statements regarding the treatment of breast cancer is TRUE?

    (A) Radical mastectomy has a higher local recurrence rate than modified radical or simple mastectomy.
    (B) The addition of radiotherapy increases the incidence of local recurrence after surgery.
    (C) The removal of axillary lymph nodes improves survival from breast cancer.
    (D) Radiation alone achieves local control of breast cancer in about 85% of cases.
    (E) Both pre- and postmenopausal women with positive lymph nodes and either receptor-positive or receptor-negative lymph nodes should be treated with adjuvant combination chemotherapy.

91. Doubling time is the time

    (A) required for the number of cells in a tumor to increase their number by a factor of two

    (B) needed for the volume of tumor cells to increase by a factor of two
    (C) needed by a proliferating cell to progress completely through the cell cycle to produce a daughter cell
    (D) that elapses before clinical recurrence

92. Which of the following is of greatest concern in treating cancer of the cervix? Delivering a dose of medication that will kill the tumor but will not

    (A) harm small bowel
    (B) induce sarcoma of the uterus
    (C) destroy the bladder or rectum
    (D) cause infection or necrosis
    (E) destroy surrounding pelvic muscles

93. A 27-year-old nurse in good health comes in and wonders when would be the best time of the year for her to get her flu shot. You correctly answer

    (A) spring
    (B) summer
    (C) fall
    (D) winter
    (E) at age 27, you advise against it

94. A 39-year-old woman comes into your office for a routine yearly examination. Her blood pressure is 150/110. You should first

    (A) take her blood pressure several more times with her as relaxed as possible
    (B) start a calcium channel blocker
    (C) start a diuretic
    (D) start a beta blocker
    (E) make a note to recheck her in 6 months

95. A 21-year-old college student presents to the student health clinic with complaints of increasing nervousness, fatigue, weight loss, and palpitations. She is a premedical student with a stressful academic load. She reports normal monthly menses. Her examination is remarkable for a documented 10-pound weight loss since her last clinic visit 6 months ago, warm skin, no goiter, and tachycardia without a murmur or click. The next step in her evaluation or therapy is to

    (A) schedule an echocardiogram to rule out mitral valve prolapse
    (B) initiate antianxiety medications
    (C) provide psychiatric/psychological referral for stress management
    (D) perform thyroid scan
    (E) measure TSH levels

96. When making a lower midline abdominal incision, would you find the lower border of the posterior rectus fascia (sheath) at the

    (A) insertion of the rectus muscles
    (B) same position as the lower end of the anterior rectus sheath
    (C) arcuate line (linea semicircularis)
    (D) area approximately 2 to 3 cm above the pubic symphysis

97. Classification of a living female patient's bony pelvis into one of the four major groups of Caldwell and Moloy

    (A) depends on the midplane configuration of the pelvis
    (B) depends on the inlet configuration of the pelvis
    (C) does not help to prognosticate the case of delivery
    (D) requires x-ray pelvimetry

98. A woman's medical record stated that she had a red birthmark on her pudenda. From this you could localize the birthmark to her

    (A) mons pubis
    (B) vulva
    (C) labia

    (D) external genitalia
    (E) none of the above

99. The portio vaginalis of the cervix is that part which

    (A) extends cephalad from the vagina
    (B) protrudes into the vagina
    (C) forms an internal isthmus or os
    (D) is normally covered with endocervical epithelium

100. The ovaries have which of the following characteristics?

    (A) They normally remain constant in size throughout a woman's lifetime.
    (B) They are supported by the round ligaments.
    (C) They secrete hormones and store germ cells.
    (D) They lie in the ovarian fossa of the false pelvis, overlying the external iliac vessels.

101. The nerve supply to the vulva is primarily from the

    (A) pudendal nerve
    (B) obturator nerve
    (C) ilioinguinal nerve
    (D) genitofemoral nerve
    (E) femoral nerve

102. The nerve supply to the uterus is characterized by

    (A) motor fibers leaving the spinal cord below the sensory fibers
    (B) being under voluntary control
    (C) being transmitted to the uterus via the cervical ganglion of Frankenhauser
    (D) having good point discrimination

103. Which of the following is a branch of the anterior division of the internal iliac artery?

    (A) pudenal artery
    (B) superior hemorrhoidal artery
    (C) superior gluteal artery

(D) ovarian artery

(E) iliolumbar artery

104. The second meiotic division of the oocyte with the release of a polar body is normally completed

(A) at the stage of the primary follicle

(B) at the stage of the graafian follicle

(C) in the peritoneal cavity

(D) in the uterus at the time of implantation

(E) after the sperm penetrates the secondary oocyte

105. An unregistered obstetric patient with no prenatal care comes in and delivers after a tumultuous labor. About 20 hours after delivery, her infant develops septic shock, pneumonia, and a positive Gram stain is obtained from the infant's blood. The clinical picture in this infant is most consistent with

(A) maternal syphilis

(B) group A streptococcal infection

(C) neonatal gonorrhea

(D) group B steptococcal infection

(E) infant cytomegalovirus

106. You are caring for a pregnant woman who is a recent immigrant from southeast Asia and are concerned about tuberculosis (TB). Which of the following statements is TRUE regarding TB in pregnancy?

(A) Skin tests have an unusually high false-positive rate in pregnancy.

(B) Two-drug antituberculous therapy in pregnancy is contraindicated.

(C) The best single drug for therapy of TB in pregnancy is streptomycin.

(D) If a patient is treated adequately during pregnancy, TB generally has no deleterious effect on mother or child.

(E) All southeast Asian immigrants should have a chest x-ray in pregnancy.

107. A 37-year-old hemodialysis technician is seen at 31 weeks' gestation. She has a temperature of 100.4°F and a blood pressure of 118/72. She complains of general malaise, myalgia, anorexia, nausea, and vomiting. On physical examination, her liver is slightly enlarged and tender. Her urine protein and bilirubin are elevated on the urine dipstick test. Your plan of action would be to

(A) have her come back in a week to repeat her blood pressure and urine dipstick test

(B) perform a roll-over test to rule out preeclampsia

(C) admit the patient to the hospital, begin intravenous antibiotic therapy, and administer high-dose steroids

(D) order an ultrasound of the gallbladder

(E) order a serum SGOT, SGPT (ALT), and alkaline phosphatase

108. Diagnostic laparoscopy is performed in a 19-year-old woman to determine the presence or absence of PID. The woman is a known alcoholic and intravenous drug user. The laparoscopic procedure shows copious pus and a left-sided infectious, tubo-ovarian complex. In examining the right upper quadrant of her abdomen with the laparoscope, you see an inflamed-appearing liver capsule with "violin string" adhesion from the surface of the liver to the parietal peritoneum of the overlying anterior abdominal wall and to the diaphragm. Which of the following is most likely to be her problem?

(A) The diagnosis is hepatitis B.

(B) Cholecystitis is present.

(C) Perihepatitis secondary to the pelvic infection.

(D) Liver abscess has secondarily infected her reproductive tract, simulating PID.

109. On the seventh day after abdominal hysterectomy, a morbidly obese patient stands to go to the bathroom and spontaneously passes "a large amount (more than a liter) of serosanguinous fluid" from her abdominal wound. The most appropriate consideration is that

(A) she has a wound dehiscence
(B) a wound hematoma has spontaneously drained
(C) a medical student should stay in the room to see if there is more drainage from the wound
(D) you will need to remove the skin staples from the wound, as they are likely causing an allergic reaction
(E) there is a urinary tract injury draining spontaneously through the patient's wound

110. A 2-year-old girl is brought in for evaluation of vaginal bleeding. Physical examination shows grape-like lesions protruding from the vaginal introitus. The most likely diagnosis is

(A) urethral prolapse
(B) condyloma acuminata
(C) sarcoma botryoides
(D) vaginal polyps
(E) hymenal tags

111. When an alert woman with normal vital signs is evaluated in an emergency department for sexual assault, which of the following should be performed first?

(A) physical examination
(B) report to authorities
(C) counseling
(D) baseline serologic testing for sexually transmitted diseases (STDs)
(E) informed consent

Questions 112 through 115

A 31-year-old woman (gravida 6, para 1, abortus 0, prematures 5) comes to you at 10 weeks' gestation with the history of having had progressively earlier deliveries, all without painful contractions. Her first child was born at 34 weeks' and survived, the next delivered at 26 weeks', the next two at 22 weeks', and the last one at 20 weeks'. No congenital abnormalities were found. On examination, her uterus is 10- to 12-week size, FHTs are present with Doppler, and the cervix is soft, three quarters effaced, and 2 cm dilated.

112. With this information, your first diagnosis is intrauterine gestation and

(A) genetic disease
(B) progesterone lack
(C) fibroid uterus
(D) premature labor
(E) incompetent cervical os

113. Which of the following would constitute the most efficacious therapy?

(A) bed rest
(B) progesterone injections 250 mg weekly
(C) McDonald procedure
(D) Lash procedure
(E) pessary until 24 weeks

114. During later delivery of a 9½-lb infant, the mother sustained a third-degree perineal laceration with involvement of the rectal mucosa. You should

(A) repair the defect with through-and-through sutures
(B) pack the defect open for secondary closure
(C) repair the anal sphincter and perineal muscles only
(D) leave the tear to heal primarily by itself, because of contamination
(E) repair the defect in layers

115. Having utilized the proper mode of therapy for a fourth-degree laceration, you can expect early satisfactory results in about what percentage of the cases?

(A) 90 to 95%
(B) 70 to 75%
(C) 50 to 55%
(D) 30 to 35%
(E) 10 to 15%

DIRECTIONS (Questions 116 through 131): Each of the numbered items or incomplete statements in this section is followed by answers or by completions of the statement. Select the answers or completions that may apply.

116. When describing fetal abnormalities, which three of the following are considered to be a general classification of genetic disorders?

(A) single gene defects

(B) chromosome disorders

(C) multifactorial inheritance

(D) environmental teratogenesis

117. A 21-year-old woman with no prenatal care presents to labor and delivery. She gives the date of her LMP and states that her pregnancy has been uncomplicated. Her estimated date of conception (EDC), calculated by Nägele's rule, places her at 43 weeks' gestation. Which four of the following are most likely to describe her pregnancy?

(A) postterm

(B) a normal variation

(C) an uncertain date of LMP

(D) an anencephalic fetus

(E) twins

118. A 31-year-old woman (gravida 4, para 3) is at 6 cm with a suspicious fetal heart tracing. You perform fetal scalp sampling. Which two of the following fetal scalp pH results should cause you to consider cesarean delivery?

(A) 7.30

(B) 7.22

(C) 7.18

(D) 7.15

(E) 7.25

119. Helpful maneuvers in managing shoulder dystocia include which two of the following?

(A) internal podalic version

(B) fundal pressure

(C) Ritgen maneuver

(D) McRoberts maneuver

(E) Wood's screw maneuver

120. Three fetal complications of vacuum extraction include

(A) subgaleal hemorrhage

(B) cephalhematoma

(C) fetal rib fractures

(D) facial lacerations

(E) fetal retinal hemorrhage

121. Which four of the following are indications for measuring a serum prolactin level in your gynecologic patient?

(A) galactorrhea

(B) enlarged sella turcica

(C) amenorrhea

(D) oligomenorrhea

(E) pregnancy

122. Which four of the following statements regarding breast-feeding are true?

(A) Serum prolactin levels in breast-feeding women remain elevated for at least 6 months postpartum.

(B) Serum prolactin levels in non-breast-feeding women decline to normal by the fifth postpartum week.

(C) Prolactin secretion during suckling stimulates casein production.

(D) Oxytocin secretion during suckling stimulates milk letdown.

(E) GnRH secretion during suckling stimulates gonadotropin secretion.

123. A patient (gravida 0) has galactorrhea (nongestational lactation). This may result from which four of the following?

(A) pituitary adenoma

(B) hypothyroidism

(C) renal failure

(D) intrapartum hemorrhage

(E) bronchogenic carcinoma

124. A female pseudohermaphrodite may have which four of the following conditions?

(A) androgen-secreting maternal tumor
(B) 20-22 desmolase deficiency
(C) 3-beta hydroxysteroid dehydrogenase deficiency
(D) 21-hydroxylase deficiency
(E) 11-beta hydroxylase deficiency

125. Which four of the following are routine health-screening activities in a 45-year-old woman?

(A) urine dipstick for glucose
(B) mammogram every 1 to 2 years
(C) Pap smear yearly
(D) serum creatinine yearly
(E) serum cholesterol every 5 years

126. During an annual examination, you determine that your patient is depressed. You offer her one of the newer antidepressant medications but warn her that anticholinergic effects are common. These would include which four of the following?

(A) blurred vision
(B) confusion
(C) diarrhea
(D) dry mouth
(E) urinary hesitance

127. Which four of the following factors are most likely to predispose to toxic shock syndrome (TSS)?

(A) tampon absorbency
(B) method of tampon use
(C) neutral vaginal pH
(D) high vaginal oxygen content
(E) coital frequency

128. A medical professional liability claim must prove which four of the following elements of negligence?

(A) duty
(B) breach of duty
(C) causation
(D) intention
(E) damage

129. Synonyms for, or types of, CIN include which four of the following?

(A) cervical dysplasia
(B) CIS
(C) high-grade squamous intraepithelial lesion (HGSIL)
(D) LGSIL
(E) metaplasia

130. Important principles(s) of radiotherapy include which four of the following?

(A) repair of sublethal injury
(B) repopulation
(C) reoxygenation
(D) radiation-induced synchrony
(E) selective regeneration of T and B cells

131. Necrotizing fasciitis is a particularly virulent, rapidly progressing soft tissue infection. Two other characteristics of this infection are

(A) it is easily diagnosed based on clinical findings
(B) treatment requires wide debridement of all necrotic tissue up to bleeding margins
(C) antibiotics are not needed for treatment
(D) obese patients are more susceptible
(E) patients do not generally appear toxic

DIRECTIONS (Questions 132 through 134): Each set of items in this section consists of a list of lettered headings followed by several numbered words or phrases. For each numbered word or phrase, select the ONE lettered option that is most closely associated with it. Each lettered option may be selected once, more than once, or not at all. Match the following complications with the clinical scenario.

Questions 132 through 134

(A) bowel perforation
(B) erosion of the urethra
(C) foreign body granulomatous response

(D) osteitis pubis

(E) osteomyelitis

(F) retropubic abscess

(G) retropubic space hematoma

(H) urinary tract infection (UTI)

132. A 42-year-old woman is 6 weeks' postoperative from a Marshall–Marchetti–Krantz (MMK) procedure for stress incontinence. She complains of suprapubic pain and burning with walking and standing. She is voiding fine and denies fever or vaginal discharge. On examination, she has tenderness over the pubic symphysis and limitation of abduction. WBC is 9,500. Microscopic urine evaluation shows no pyuria.

133. A 60-year-old woman had a Mersiline pubovaginal sling placed for recurrent stress incontinence after a prior MMK. She has had prior pelvic radiation for cervical cancer. For what serious complication does this procedure put her at risk?

134. A 42-year-old woman had a Stamey operation for stress incontinence. She had had a prior abdominal hysterectomy. A suprapubic catheter was placed in the operating room. Four days postoperatively she calls your office to report fever, lower abdominal pain, and chills. She has had no bowel movement. She comes to the office and appears quite toxic. She has generalized abdominal tenderness and rebound. What is the most likely diagnosis?

Answers and Explanations

1. **(B)** CIN III includes severe dysplasia and CIS. It is not invasive and therefore is not cancer. If it is not treated appropriately, however, approximately 30% will progress to invasive cancer. We do not know what causes CIN III, but it is not due to bacterial infection. It is more severe than one would predict from the prior LGSIL found on her Pap smear. If her Pap smear had been an HGSIL, the Pap smear and the biopsy would be better correlated.

2. **(B)** The MHC in human beings is designated histocompatibility locus antigen (HLA) (human lymphocyte A) and contains at least four major loci. Matching of HLA and ABO types is important in organ transplantation. The major histocompatibility antigens are on the short arm of chromosome 6.

3. **(E)** Linked genes are apt to be transmitted together rather than independently; this characteristic may be used to estimate where a certain gene is located. Genes on the same chromosome with a small measurable distance between them are said to be linked.

4. **(C)** Persons with O negative blood are called universal donors. O-type blood may have factors that can cause reactions to other factors in other blood group systems; however, they lack A or B antigens.

5. **(E)** Siblings have one chance in four of being the same HLA haplotype. Parents or more distant relatives are unlikely to have both haplotypes (each with four HLA-determinant loci), the same as those of the child.

6. **(D)** The principal hypothalamic locus for GnRH secretion is the arcuate nucleus. Lesions in this area cause gonadal atrophy and amenorrhea. Cell bodies for dopamine synthesis are found in the arcuate and periventricular nuclei. Separate cells in the paraventricular and supraoptic nuclei make vasopressin and oxytocin.

7. **(C)** ACTH is a single-chain peptide (39 amino acids in length) formed from the precursor molecule proopiomelanocortin. LH, FSH, hCG, and TSH are composed of two peptide subunits (alpha and beta), containing carbohydrate sidechains (glycoprotein hormones). The alpha subunit is common to all of these glycoproteins. The beta subunit is unique to each hormone, and determines its specificity. Carbohydrate attachment to protein hormone subunits (glycosylation) affects hormone-receptor activation and diminishes the metabolic clearance of hormone from the circulation. LH contains fewer carbohydrate sidechains (oligosaccharides) than FSH and, therefore, has a shorter circulating half-life (1 hour) than FSH (4 hours).

8. **(D)** Although the pathway from pregnenolone to aldosterone would function, there would be no cortisol production. Without cortisol negative feedback on the pituitary, ACTH secretion increases, causing adrenal hyperplasia in an attempt to maintain cortisol production. In the absence of sex steroid production, gonadotropin secretion also increases.

9. **(B)** Prefixes are used in steroid nomenclature to modify steroid names. The prefix *nor-* denotes elimination of a methyl group at carbon 19.

10. **(E)** Prostaglandins, which are 20-carbon fatty acids, are used for both induction of labor and abortion. They also play a role in the mediation of pain, as in dysmenorrhea. Recent evidence suggests a role for PGs in follicle rupture and luteolysis.

11. **(C)** The fetal ovary is not essential for female reproductive tract development. The fetal testis is essential for female reproductive tract regression and male reproductive tract development. Müllerian inhibitory factor induces müllerian duct regression. Testosterone induces the mesonephric system to undergo male internal genitalia development. (The mesonephric tubules contacting the rete testis cords form the ductuli efferentes of the testis, while the mesonephric duct elongates into the principal male genital duct, forming the epididymis, ductus deferens, seminal vesicles, and ejaculatory duct.) Target tissues (e.g., urogenital sinus and external genital anlagen) are capable of utilizing the enzyme, 4-alpha-reductase, to convert circulating testosterone to a more potent androgen, dihydrotestosterone (DHT). DHT production in target tissues is responsible for male external genitalia development.

12. **(A)** The major problem in children with idiopathic precocious puberty is that increased circulating sex steroid levels induce accelerated childhood bone growth but premature epiphyseal closure. Affected individuals are taller than peers as children but short in stature as adults. A radiogram of the wrist is the easiest test to confirm changes in bone composition induced by sex steroids. GnRH analogues have been used in children with true sexual precocity to suppress the hypothalamus and delay epiphyseal closure.

13. **(A)** In the absence of 17-hydroxylase, circulating levels of cortisol and sex steroids are low. Without negative feedback of cortisol and sex steroids, ACTH and gonadotropin levels are elevated. The resulting increase in circulating gonadotropin levels accompanying absence of gonadal sex steroids is referred to as hypergonadotropic hypogonadism. This rare cause of congenital adrenal hyperplasia causes delayed puberty and is associated with hypertension due to accumulation of mineralocorticoids (e.g., deoxycorticosterone).

14. **(C)** Of the many follicles present at birth, only about 400 follicles ever mature and extrude on ovum. Most that start to develop become atretic. No new follicles are formed after birth. Usually, only one follicle ovulates during each cycle.

15. **(B)** Estrogen deficiency causes atrophy of estrogen-dependent tissue. Consequently, postmenopausal women commonly develop amenorrhea, vaginal stenosis, atrophic vaginal mucosa, and small labia minora. Clitoromegaly accompanies high circulating androgen levels and raises the real possibility of an androgen-producing tumor.

16. **(B)** During pregnancy the vaginal mucosa appears purplish-red, which results from hyperemia. This is called Chadwick's sign. At times the softness of the cervical isthmus will mislead uninitiated examiners to conclude that there is a small uterus (really just the cervix) and a large globular pelvic mass (really the pregnant fundus). This is Hegar's sign. Braxton Hicks contractions are rhythmic nonprogressive uterine contractions prior to actual labor. Von Fernwald's sign is irregular softening of the uterine fundus over the placental implantation site. Cullen's sign is ecchymosis of the periumbilical area secondary to retroperitoneal bleeding.

17. **(C)** The rotation usually occurs to the right and is thought to be due to the presence of the rectosigmoid on the left. Rotation should be determined prior to performing C-section. A pelvic mass on the right, such as transplanted kidney, will result in levorotation.

18. **(E)** The saliva may be related to nausea. The symptom may be helped by atropine. It will spontaneously regress after pregnancy.

19. **(C)** Though the total amount of hemoglobin increases in pregnancy, the plasma volume increases to a greater extent and the hemoglobin and hematocrit both fall. Blood volume increases by 45%, while hematocrit, in total, increases by only 33%. Adequate iron supplementation will decrease this disparity.

20. **(C)** Some dependent edema is normal during pregnancy and can be alleviated by instructing the patient to rest on her side and to wear fitted, graded, pressure elastic support hose without constricting bands. The heart, however, remains an effective pump. The decreased plasma oncotic pressure and increased capillary permeability help to exacerbate this edema.

21. **(A)** Prolactin levels are highest in the weeks just before the birth of the baby. Prolactin shows a marked increase throughout pregnancy. Lactation is initiated by prolactin and allowed to occur when estrogen levels decrease in the postpartum period. Estrogen causes inhibition of lactation in the breast. Whether nursing or not, prolactin will return to normal in the weeks after delivery.

22. **(D)** Compensation of a lowered P_{CO_2} is affected by metabolic reduction of bicarbonate. The pH change is minimal. Pulmonary function is not impaired by pregnancy. Changes are physiologically compensated.

23. **(C)** The blood volume for the fetus and placenta is approximately 125 mg/kg of fetal weight. Approximately 45 mL/kg are retained in the placenta at delivery, leaving approximately 80 mL/kg for the newborn infant. The fetal blood volume can potentially be raised or lowered by various cord-handling techniques at delivery.

24. **(E)** Fetal cells need to be protected and a fetal immune cell response avoided; therefore, the least antigenic blood should be used. Fresh cells allow for the longest possible life span. The cells should be packed so that many can be given in a small volume to avoid fetal cardiac compromise. Since plasma will not correct anemia, it would be a poor choice.

25. **(D)** The exact relationship these varying compounds have in promoting lipoprotein synthesis and surfactant production is unclear, but some evidence exists supporting roles for each of the compounds listed. Perhaps some complex interaction of all of them is needed. One of the few widely used clinical techniques to promote the development of fetal lung maturity is the maternal administration of glucocorticoids. There is appreciable evidence supporting the administration of glucocorticosteroids in large amounts to the mother at certain critical times during gestation to effect an increased rate of maturation in the fetal lungs when preterm delivery is anticipated.

26. **(A)** Androgens are the only hormones relevant to the embryogenesis of the external genitalia. In the absence of androgens, female external genitalia will form. The active androgen is dihydrotestosterone (DHT).

27. **(D)** A VDRL should be obtained to rule out lues. If the patient has syphilis, she can be treated before the spirochete crosses the placenta, and before the fetal immune system is active, thereby eliminating the possibility of congenital syphilis. When treated before 18 weeks, the fetal prognosis is very good.

28. **(D)** The Food and Drug Administration has established categories for medications with regard to the drug's fetal effect. For category B drugs, animal studies show no fetal risk and there are no human studies or there have been adverse effects in animals, but human studies have shown no risks. Category A has no fetal risk in human studies. In category C, there may be adverse effects in animals, but there is no available human data. Category D drugs have fetal risk, but the benefits may outweigh risks. Category X has proven significant fetal risks.

29. (E) The Lewis antigen is not associated with fetal hydropic disease; therefore, one should not plan termination of pregnancy, serial amniocentesis, or any invasive procedure because of this finding. On the other hand, the patient is Rh-negative and should receive a dose of 300 µg of D-immunoglobulin, if she is not immunized, at 28 to 32 weeks and within 3 days after delivery if the infant is proved to be Rh-positive. This is done routinely to prevent sensitization from an Rh-positive infant.

30. (A) The greatest advantage to CVS is that fetal cells can be obtained at an earlier stage of gestation and, because of their rapid division, obviate the need for cell culture, thereby allowing earlier results. A disadvantage is that fetuses with chromosomal abnormalities, which would spontaneously abort if one waited a slightly longer time, may be present. One can perform enzyme studies on cells after either CVS or amniocentesis, so that in itself is not a specific benefit of the CVS. CVS is associated with a slightly increased fetal risk when compared to amniocentesis. The cell sample is good, but, because of maternal contamination, the possibility exsists of fetal and maternal chromosomes being confused. CVS also requires a greater learning time for the clinician to perform it adequately.

31. (C) The diagonal conjugate is the distance from the pubic arch to the sacrum promontory and should be at least 11.5 cm. By subtracting approximately 1.5 cm, you will have a good approximation of the obstetric conjugate. The intertuberous distance should be approximately 8 cm. The angle of the pubic rami should be approximately 85 to 90 degrees. The sacrum should be hollow and deep. The midpelvis is difficult to measure clinically, and x-ray or computed tomography (CT) exams have been used in special situations. A thorough clinical examination of the bony pelvis allows one to predict the ease or difficulty of delivering a normal-sized infant.

32. (C) Although the need for many nutrients increases during pregnancy and lactation, the Institute of Medicine concluded that iron was the only known nutrient for which requirements during pregnancy could not be met by diet alone.

33. (E) All the procedures must be done, but none will be of any avail if the airway is not clear. A clear airway is the first priority in any emergency, for without availability of oxygen, the patient will die in a few minutes regardless of what else is done.

34. (D) Both cesarean section and twin gestations increase the loss of blood at delivery, everything else being equal. Both overdistention and transabdominal delivery are predisposing factors to hemorrhage.

35. (B) When the placenta is firmly attached to *and invades* the myometrium, it is a placenta increta if it has *not* penetrated the entire depth of the myometrium and placenta percreta if it has. These defects in placental site attachment occur most commonly after previous cesarean section or curettage or with women of high parity. They are dangerous because hemorrhage may occur antepartum, intrapartum, and/or postpartum. This is particularly true if it is in the lower uterine segment, where thin myometrium does not allow adequate compression of the enlarged, ruptured blood vessels after an attempt is made to deliver the placenta.

36. (B) A face presentation with mentum posterior presents a large cephalic diameter to the pelvis and does not allow extension as a normal mechanism of labor. To deliver the head, rotation to mentum anterior must occur to allow extension. Often, the rotation will be spontaneous.

37. (D) Cardiac arrhythmias and pulmonary edema are serious side effects of beta-adrenergic stimulation. Pulmonary edema usually occurs only with concomitant infection or corticosteroids. Plasma glucose increases and blood pressure usually decreases. Hypokalemia is seldom a major problem. Beta-mimetic agents are used to treat asthma.

38. **(D)** Drawing blood and observing for clotting retraction and stability can be done every 10 to 15 minutes while waiting for other, more precise parameters. A serum fibrinogen will always be zero, as, by definition, serum has already been clotted. Split products may be found in serum.

39. **(D)** Remember the common association of genital and urinary malformations. A longitudinal vaginal septum does not usually constitute a barrier to either conception or delivery. If the uterus is deformed, implantation may be compromised.

40. **(B)** The tamponade effect of the myometrium is remarkable. Patients on heparin therapy whose blood does not clot do not bleed unusually at delivery if the uterus contracts well and no lacerations are present. Uterine atony can be a serious problem.

41. **(D)** The diagnosis that must be ruled out immediately is placenta previa. Ultrasound should be used to confirm the diagnosis. Pelvic examination for the purpose of diagnosis is contraindicated without a double setup. The fetus is mature enough to be delivered now if a placenta is found.

42. **(C)** This diagnosis requires that the temperature be 100°F or higher on two of the first 10 days postpartum. Temperatures are to be taken orally at least three times per day. Temperatures during the first 24 hours after delivery are not included.

43. **(E)** The most common cause of bleeding during the hour after delivery is uterine atony, especially if a proper postpartum examination of the cervix and vaginal canal has been done to help rule out lacerations. However, the excess bleeding necessitates rapid assessment to rule out other factors. If they are ruled out and massage causes the bleeding to cease, you can maintain uterine tone and continue observation. If bleeding persists, ex-

amination under anesthesia (EUA) and D&C may be done to rule out retained secundae or uterine tears not visible from below.

44. **(B)** *E. coli* may be a more common infecting agent, but it does not have a foul odor. Anerobic bacteria such as *Bacteroides* and anaerobic *Streptococcus* both produce a foul odor. *Bacteroides* is a frequent cause of postoperative pelvic abscess.

45. **(A)** Nursing is contraindicated in industrialized countries with availability of good alternative sources of formula, when the mother has active CMV, chronic active hepatitis B, or HIV. If the mother has an active outbreak of varicella at delivery, she should avoid contact with the infant until the vesicles are gone, which includes breast-feeding. As long as there are no herpetic lesions on the breast, nursing is acceptable with the mother observing good handwashing technique.

46. **(C)** The plasma fibrinogen remains high for several days and as a result the ESR remains moderately elevated as well. The hematocrit should remain stable unless there was excessive blood loss. Diuresis should occur, rather than fluid retention.

47. **(A)** The immediate care of the newborn is directed toward the same concepts as the critical care of any patient—make sure the patient is breathing and the airway is clear. Once this has been accomplished, attention must be directed to protecting the infant from the hazards of heat loss. Since the infant is naked and wet and will lose heat to the atmosphere, predisposing to metabolic problems, it should be dried and warmed. The most effective way to accomplish this end is vigorous and immediate drying of the newborn. A quick physical examination is indicated but is not an immediate priority. Hematocrit is indicated only if anemia or blood dyscrasia is suspected, and then only after the newborn has been stabilized.

48. **(A)** The infant's liver does not have adequate enzyme systems to conjugate the bilirubin

load. Mild jaundice often occurs because unconjugated bilirubin is poorly excreted. It can be photoabsorbed with great therapeutic results by light, even simple sunlight.

49. **(C)** A cephalhematoma lies beneath the periosteum in the subperiosteal space and, therefore, is limited by the midline periosteal attachment to the skull. Subdural hemorrhage, subarachnoid hemorrhage, and tentorial tears result in bleeding directly into the CNS.

50. **(D)** Facial paralysis may occur after either spontaneous (one third of cases) or forceps delivery (two thirds of cases) by pressure at the stylomastoid foramen. It is most often transient and rapidly clears within a few days after delivery.

51. **(C)** Renal agenesis (Potter syndrome) occurs about 1 in 4,000 births. It is more frequent in male infants. Prenatally, a low amniotic fluid volume is seen (because there is no urine made). The constellation of findings described in the problem are found in addition to the lack of kidneys. One third of infants with this syndrome are stillborn; the others die within 48 hours of life.

52. **(E)** *Unexplained infertility* is a term used to define couples who have completed their entire infertility workup with no clear etiology for their infertility problem. In this case, although the hysterosalpingogram demonstrated unilateral proximal obstruction, the diagnostic laparoscopy demonstrated patent tubes bilaterally. It is important to note that the laparoscopy is necessary for the workup to exclude endometriosis or pelvic adhesions. The semen analysis is normal with excellent concentration, motility, and morphology. Luteal-phase deficiency is unlikely given the normal-length luteal phase and serum progesterone level (> 10 ng/mL).

53. **(A)** This test may be abnormal due to poor timing, particularly if the patient has a prolonged follicular phase. Sperm antibodies may be present if the patient's partner has a

history of a vasovasostomy. Although intrauterine insemination would be the appropriate treatment for cervical factors, documentation of mucus abnormalities is an important first step. Progesterone would cause a thick, sticky mucus. Clear mucus is not likely to be present in endocervicitis.

54. **(A)** Autosomal trisomy is the most common chromosomal abnormality associated with first-trimester spontaneous abortion. X monosomy is the next most common chromosomal abnormality. Triploidy commonly accompanies hydropic placental degeneration. Tetraploidy and sex chromosome polysomy are rare causes of first-trimester spontaneous abortion.

55. **(C)** Clomiphene citrate is typically utilized as a first-line agent in the treatment of anovulation in patients. The course of therapy usually involves clomiphene citrate for 5 days, with ovulation usually occurring in 7 days after the last tablet has been ingested. It is quite successful, causing ovulation in 75 to 80% of all patients with a multiple pregnancy rate of 7%. There is no increased risk of congenital anomalies in clomiphene citrate–induced pregnancies. Severe ovarian hyperstimulation syndrome occurs rarely in patients treated with clomiphene citrate.

56. **(E)** The placenta is an incomplete steroid-producing organ, depending on precursors from the maternal and fetal circulations. The placenta readily converts maternal circulating cholesterol to pregnenolone and progesterone but cannot further metabolize these steroids to estrogen because it lacks 17-alpha hydroxylase. Therefore, circulating androgens of fetal and maternal origin are used by the placenta as substrate for estrogen production. This functional interdependence of fetus, mother, and placenta is referred to as the fetoplacental–maternal unit.

57. **(A)** Secondary amenorrhea refers to absence of menses for 6 months or a duration of three of the previous menstrual cycle lengths. Although the distinction between primary and

secondary amenorrhea tends to identify groups of individuals with different disorders (e.g., abnormal gonadal development occurs in 30 to 40% of women with primary amenorrhea but occurs less frequently in women with secondary amenorrhea), the diagnostic approach to primary and secondary amenorrhea is similar. After obtaining a history regarding sexual activity, contraception, use of medication associated with amenorrhea, stress, exercise, weight change, and instrumentation of the uterus (e.g., induced abortion), a serum hCG level should be obtained to exclude pregnancy. Serum prolactin and TSH should also be measured because abnormalities of prolactin secretion and thyroid function disrupt ovulation. The next step is to determine whether menstruation occurs 2 to 7 days after progesterone administration (progesterone challenge). The ability of progesterone to induce menstruation (positive response) requires a circulating E_2 value about 40 pg/mL and an endometrium responsive to estrogen. Individuals with a positive response to progesterone challenge have a functional hypothalamo–pituitary–gonadal axis and do not have an anatomic abnormality of the hypothalamus or pituitary.

58. **(E)** Based on the duration that the ovum may be fertilized, most authorities would recommend that 24 to 36 hours elapse after ovulation before unprotected intercourse may be resumed. In the temperature graph shown, the most likely day of ovulation is that identified by letter B. Given that the ovum may be fertilized for 24 to 36 hours after ovulation, the earliest possible time for the resumption of unprotected intercourse could be at the time labeled D. This date may be established in retrospect, but for the couple using the temperature graph in a prospective manner, with the uncertainties of establishing the ovulation as occurring at B and not C and the possibility that the temperature elevation found at D may represent normal temperature variation, it is safest to not resume unprotected intercourse until the point identified as E.

59. **(B)** The IUD string may retract into the cervical canal so that it is not palpable. It may also become displaced because of pregnancy, malposition, expulsion, and perforation. The latter complication accompanies about 1:1000 IUD insertions and occurs more frequently with insertions performed postpartum when uterine involution is incomplete. The IUD string can often be found by gently probing the cervical canal. If cervical probing is unsuccessful, further studies, including colposcopy with an endocervical speculum, pelvic ultrasound, abdominal radiography, or hysteroscopy may be necessary.

60. **(A)** The most common side effect associated with OC use is breakthrough bleeding. It usually occurs during the first one or two cycles and resolves spontaneously. Another common problem is amenorrhea. Persistent breakthrough bleeding and amenorrhea commonly reflect an atrophic endometrium and may be corrected by using a pill with a higher estrogen or lower progestin content. Other side effects include nausea, fluid retention (and perhaps weight gain), mood change, headache, breast tenderness (mastalgia), and a brownish discoloration of the face, particularly the forehead and cheeks (chloasma). Nausea usually remits spontaneously but also may decrease by taking pills with food or at bedtime. Generally, these side effects are minimal with "low-dose pills." OCs decrease prostaglandin levels in menstrual fluid and lessen dysmenorrhea.

61. **(E)** Excessive tubal destruction during female sterilization can create a small cornual fistula between the uterine and peritoneal cavities. This complication occurs most commonly when the tube is fulgurated near its uterine insertion rather than at its midportion. Spermatozoa migrating through the fistula can enter the fimbriated end of the tube. If fertilization occurs, 50% of the resulting pregnancies are ectopic. The remaining intrauterine pregnancies probably result from spontaneous tubal recannulation, failure of mechanical devices, and incomplete tissue damage by electrocoagulation. Although

pelvic pain and menstrual abnormalities after tubal ligation have been called the "post-tubal ligation syndrome," there is no evidence that female sterilization increases the risk of dysmenorrhea, anovulation, irregular bleeding, or ovarian cyst formation.

62. **(E)** Second-trimester pregnancy termination may be accomplished by either surgical evacuation of the uterus or induction of labor. D&E is a surgical procedure in which the cervix is dilated and the intrauterine contents are removed with a forceps and blunt curet. Unlike the evacuation of the uterus employed with early (first-trimester) terminations, evacuating the contents of a pregnancy at 25 weeks is associated with a much increased risk of perforation, sepsis, and retained products (incomplete removal). Labor may be induced by parenteral, vaginal, or intra-amniotic administration of prostaglandins. Intravenous oxytocin administration is less effective in inducing labor, although it is frequently used in conjunction with prostaglandin therapy.

63. **(E)** This is a description of lichen sclerosis, a common problem in postmenopausal women. It has been shown to exhibit increased metabolic activity. It must be followed closely and biopsied if other abnormal areas appear. Experience using the topical corticosteroid clobetasol proprionate ointment has shown improved results over previously recommended testosterone and progesterone ointment. About 25% of patients with lichen sclerosis will have associated areas of squamous cell hyperplasia and up to 5% will be associated with intraepithelial neoplasia. Lichen sclerosis should not be confused with the changes found in atrophic (postmenopausal) vulvitis. In atrophic vulvitis, the tissues are thinned and shiny, but lack the whitish coloration found in lichen sclerosis.

64. **(E)** Endometrial carcinoma must be ruled out in a postmenopausal woman who bleeds from the vagina, even if the bleeding is of short duration. Once a woman this age has gone for 12 consecutive months without menstrual bleeding, she is considered menopausal. An office biopsy or curettage is recommended. However, if the woman refuses a sampling, a transvaginal sonogram may be a reasonable alternative since she is at low risk for endometrial cancer (she is not obese, was on OCs until age 40, is not hypertensive, and is recently menopausal; she also bled after a progesterone withdrawal). An endometrial stripe of ≤5 mm on ultrasound is very unlikely to be associated with a premalignant or malignant process.

65. **(E)** The PG synthetase inhibitors (NSAIDs) decrease the formation of PGF_2-alpha in the endometrium. They have side effects similar to aspirin but are very effective. Most dysmenorrhea can be treated successfully with these medications.

66. **(B)** The usage of combined estrogen and progesterone eliminates hormonal cycling and gradually produces atrophy of the ectopic endometrial glands. This atrophy is the desired treatment effect. Antiestrogens, gonadotropin analogues, and androgens will produce similar suppressive results.

67. **(B)** The classic history is that of progressive dysmenorrhea and increased bleeding with periods in a 38- to 48-year-old multiparous woman. Clinical findings include a diffusely enlarged uterus often associated with tenderness (a sign, not a symptom). Unfortunately, the diagnosis can be confirmed only by hysteroscopic biopsy or hysterectomy. It is thought that up to 60% of women in this age group may have adenomyosis, and most are asymptomatic.

68. **(D)** Endometriosis affects 10 to 20% of reproductive-age women and is the most common reason for hospitalization in reproductive-age women. The classic symptoms are increasingly severe dysmenorrhea, pelvic pain, and infertility. It is diagnosed by direct visualization and biopsy. Ectopic endometrial glands surrounded by endometrial stroma should be seen. It can be treated either by surgical extirpation or hormonal suppression of the ectopic endometrial glands.

69. **(C)** The greatest risk factor for prolapse is multiparity, followed by aging. Prolapse surgery is not the only means to relieve symptoms. A properly fitted pessary can be comfortable and relieve symptoms, although, as mentioned earlier, retention of a pessary can be difficult with severe prolapse. Mild degrees of prolapse can be treated with Kegel exercises (cystocele/incontinence), bowel regimens (rectocele), rest (enterocele), or mechanical devices to hold the organs in place (pessary). Even severe prolapse has excellent surgical results—but only when all defects are repaired together, and this is the point of this question. Multiple defects occur simultaneously and must be repaired simultaneously to get the best result possible. While completely accurate incidence data is not available, it is estimated that 1 to 2% of nulliparous women suffer from genital prolapse.

70. **(B)** The Burch operation has a quoted success rate of 85 to 95%. The risk of ureteral injury is 0.1 to 1.5%. The risk of permanent urinary retention is fortunately rare, but altered voiding habits are not uncommon (slower stream of urine), as immediate postoperative urinary retention is reported to occur 16 to 25% of the time following a Burch procedure. The risk of later enterocele and/or rectocele is 15 to 20%.

71. **(A)** She has detrusor hyperreflexia with impaired contractility probably due to a neurologic etiology and/or a diabetic neuropathy. Most patients with good hand dexterity can easily master CISC with few risks. Long-term continuous drainage with a Foley has a much higher complication rate with infection, stones, contracted bladder, discomfort, and urethral dilation. While both medications might help the leakage, they can both worsen the voiding dysfunction. Once CISC is mastered, medications can be added if needed.

72. **(B)** Forty percent of abdominal masses in children under the age of 2 years are renal in origin. An ectopic pelvic kidney occurs in up to 15% of girls without a uterus or vagina. The pelvic kidney may be palpable abdominally or rectally.

73. **(A)** A functional ovarian cyst is the most common pelvic mass in menstruating reproductive-age women. It is usually nontender, mobile, and less than 8 cm in diameter. A unilocular smooth ovarian cyst without internal excrescences is usually a functional cyst. Functional ovarian cysts commonly regress spontaneously over 1 to 2 months and also may be suppressed with OCs. With a history of thrombophlebitis when taking OCs, observation is the safest for this patient. OCs for the purpose of cyst suppression are generally not recommended for cysts greater than 8 cm because the chance of neoplasia is too great.

74. **(D)** A painful adnexal mass in an amenorrheic, reproductive-age woman is suspicious of an ectopic pregnancy (implantation of an embryo outside the uterine cavity). One to two percent of all pregnancies are ectopically located, most of which occur in the fallopian tube (tubal pregnancy) as a consequence of chronic salpingitis. Hemorrhage at the implantation site causes a painful adnexal mass due to tubal distention. A serum pregnancy test should be performed in all reproductive-age women with pelvic pain, amenorrhea, and irregular vaginal bleeding. Sonography may be helpful in determining the location of the pregnancy.

75. **(B)** Approximately 30% of adnexal masses detected in women older than age 50 are malignant. In women under age 30, approximately 90% of ovarian masses are benign. The probability of an adnexal mass being malignant is important to remember when planning therapy for your patient.

76. **(B)** Vulvar intraepithelial neoplasia is an epidermal lesion, confined solely to the superficial skin. It is often multicentric in young women and actually very rarely progresses to invasive cancer (1 to 4%). It is known for being protean in appearance (raised, flat, verrucous, white, red, black, brown). It may spontaneously regress, especially after a pregnancy, and though good hygiene is recommended, it is not a cornerstone of present accepted therapy.

77. (A) Any solid tumor of the vulva in a women of this age should be biopsied without delay. It will most often be benign. An excisional biopsy may be curative, and most important, you will find any cancer present.

78. (C) Cellular atypia extending less than the full thickness of the squamous cervical epithelium justifies the diagnosis of dysplasia, in this case, probably a moderate dysplasia. More recent terms for classifying the degrees of atypia are CIN grades I, II, and III; the grades depend largely on the distance the atypical cells extend through the epithelium. The treatment techniques and outcomes are very similar no matter what the grade of the CIN.

79. (B) The criteria for staging of carcinoma of the cervix should be memorized (see Table 28–1). Once performed, the clinical stage remains the same, even if subsequent events prove that the tumor was either more or less extensive than thought at the time of the initial staging. Staging is mainly by clinical examination and the few tests used for staging are readily available.

80. (A) The excess risk for developing endometrial cancer is between 3 and 8. The cumulative risk after 10 years is 3.6% compared to 0.8% in nonusers. The 5-year survival rate is over 90% as cancers associated with estrogen use tend to be diagnosed in early stages with well-differentiated tumors and low rates of myometrial invasion and metastasis. This represents different biologic/clinical behavior than cancers developing in nonusers. Obesity is a significant risk factor in nonusers of estrogen but not in estrogen users.

Table 28–1. International Classification of Cancer of the Cervix (FIGO, 1994)

Stage	Description
Preinvasive Carcinoma	
Stage 0	Carcinoma in situ, intraepithelial carcinoma.
Invasive Carcinoma	
Stage I	Strictly confined to the cervix. Extension to corpus should be disregarded.
IA	Preclinical carcinomas of the cervix (those diagnosed only by microscopy).
IA1	Measured microscopic stromal invasion no greater than 3-mm deep and 7-mm wide.
IA2	Microscopic lesions larger than IA1. The upper limit of the measurement should not show a depth of invasion of > 5 mm from the base of the epithelium, either surface or glandular, and the horizontal spread must not exceed 7 mm.
IB	Lesions confined to the cervix of greater dimensions than stage IA2 lesions, whether seen clinically or not.
Stage II	Carcinoma extends beyond the cervix but has not extended onto the pelvic wall. The carcinoma involves the vagina, but not the lower third.
IIA	No obvious parametrial involvement.
IIB	Obvious parametrial involvement.
Stage III	Carcinoma has extended onto the pelvic wall. On rectal examination, there is no cancer-free space between the tumor and the pelvic wall. The tumor involves the lower third of the vagina. All cases with hydronephrosis or nonfunctioning kidney unless known to be due to another cause.
IIIA	No extension onto the pelvic wall, but involvement of the lower third of vagina.
IIIB	Extension onto the pelvic wall and/or hydronephrosis or nonfunctioning kidney due to tumor.
Stage IV	Carcinoma extended beyond the true pelvis or clinically involving the mucosa of the bladder or rectum.
IVA	Spread of growth to adjacent organs (that is, rectum or bladder with positive biopsy from these organs).
IVB	Spread of growth to distant organs.

81. (C) Endometrial biopsy allows a histologic evaluation of the endometrial lining in a patient who has several risk factors for endometrial cancer, including her age, obesity, and unopposed ERT. The sampling done by the biopsy must be complete. Transvaginal sonography is playing an increasing role in evaluating postmenopausal bleeding. An endometrial stripe thickness of less than 5 mm indicates a very small chance of endometrial cancer. However, no tissue is obtained for diagnosis.

82. (C) Sarcomas can occur at any age but are most common after age 40. Most women with uterine sarcoma experience symptoms of short-term duration, including abdominal pain (from a rapidly enlarging uterus), vaginal discharge, and/or vaginal bleeding. Based on similar patterns of disease spread, staging of uterine sarcoma uses the same system as that for endometrial carcinoma. Sarcomas tend to disseminate systemically by hematogenous spread so that they are often diagnosed at an advanced stage and associated with a poor prognosis (25% overall 5-year survival rate). Tumor also may extend by lymphatic channels and contiguous spread. Distant metastases commonly occur in the liver, abdomen, brain, and lung.

83. **(C)** Ovarian cancer usually spreads along the peritoneal surfaces of pelvic and abdominal viscera, including the undersurface of the diaphragm. Sites of metastases from ovarian carcinoma, in decreasing order of frequency, are peritoneum (85%), omentum (70%), contralateral ovary (70%), liver (35%), lung (25%), uterus (20%), vagina (15%), and bone (15%). Malnutrition and death usually occur when malignancy invades beyond pelvic structures and spreads along the peritoneal serosa and surface of the bowel, leading to intestinal obstruction. Lymphatic dissemination, particularly to para-aortic nodes, also occurs. Hematogenous metastases and spread of disease to liver and lungs are less common.

84. **(D)** Pseudomyxoma peritonei refers to massive intra-abdominal accumulation of gelatinous material from rupture of mucinous tumors or appendiceal mucoceles. The material is histologically benign but can cause intestinal obstruction. Mucinous cystadenomas are often large tumors (up to 15 to 30 cm in diameter) and are associated with a lower rate of malignancy (15%) than serous cystadenomas.

85. **(C)** Sex cord–stromal tumors originate from cells derived from sex cords and/or specialized gonadal stroma. They account for 6% of ovarian neoplasms. Many sex cord–stromal tumors are hormonally active and have cells of mixed origin (granulosa and thecal cells; Sertoli and Leydig cells). These tumors occur at any age but most commonly develop in reproductive-age and postmenopausal women.

86. **(A)** Serous tumors are the most frequent ovarian epithelial tumors. They represent 20 to 50% of ovarian neoplasms and 35 to 40% of ovarian malignancies.

87. **(B)** Administration of alkylating agents (e.g., melphalan, chlorambucil, cyclophosphamide) increases the risk of developing leukemia. The risk is time dependent, increasing from 29% to 10% after 4 years and 8 years of treatment. The use of cis-platinum and doxorubicin may also be associated with an increased risk of leukemia, which is not seen after radiation therapy.

88. **(C)** Stromal hyperthecosis is a benign ovarian disorder in which nests of luteinized stromal cells are present within the gonadal stroma. Circulating androgen levels may be markedly elevated, mimicking those accompanying an ovarian tumor. Virilization occurs gradually over several years, and gross ovarian morphology is similar to that of polycystic ovaries.

89. **(C)** A single, firm nodule is statistically more worrisome than multiple nodules, and cancer is most common in the upper outer quadrant. Any firm lump in a postmenopausal woman's breast must be biopsied or aspirated, and a mammogram should also be done both to evaluate the lump and to rule out other suspicious areas in both breasts.

90. **(E)** Radiation alone achieves local control of tumor in breast cancer only about 50% of the time. The National Surgical Adjuvant Breast Project showed that disease-free survival rates for patients treated with partial mastectomy, axillary dissection, and postoperative radiotherapy were the same as patients treated with modified radical mastectomy. Therefore, removal of the local tumor with radiation is used to control the disease, and axillary dissection aids in adjuvant therapy selection and predicting prognosis. Radical

mastectomy decreases local recurrence but does not prevent the growth of metastic lesions already in other sites.

Chemotherapy is used as an adjuvant therapy in patients with curable breast cancer and positive axillary nodes in the hope that it will destroy microscopic occult metastases. Cyclophosphamide, methotrexate, and fluorouracil are given monthly for 6 months after treatment and seems to be of value in premenopausal women with positive axillary nodes. Response is less in postmenopausal women or those with positive axillary nodes. Tamoxifen has been shown to be of benefit in both pre- and postmenopausal women with breast cancer and is being tested as a prophylactic agent for breast cancer.

91. **(A)** Doubling time is the time a tumor cell population needs to double in cell number, not volume.

92. **(C)** Bladder and bowel are the greatest concerns in the radiation treatment of cervical cancer. The dosage to kill tumor is very close to the dosage that will seriously harm these organs. Small bowel is generally far enough from the field so that it survives. Pelvic mucles are very radioresistant. Radiation seldom induces infection.

93. **(C)** Influenza vaccine is a multivalent agent in most cases, given SQ or IM, usually in the fall (at the beginning of the flu season). It is an annual vaccination for those at risk of serious complications and also for medical care personnel. Because she is in a high-risk occupation, she should take it in spite of her age.

94. **(A)** Multiple measures of blood pressure with the patient as relaxed as possible are the best initial evaluation. This can be done in your office, by a nurse at work, by a first-aid technician, or at many paramedic stations (including fire stations), who offer this service without charge. A thorough physical examination to assess any end-organ damage needs to be done. Only when hypertension has been established and an evaluation done should you start any kind of medication.

95. **(E)** Although these changes could represent an anxiety- or stress-related disorder, those are diagnoses of exclusion. Women are at increased risk for thyroid dysfunction, including hyperthyroidism. Even without a clinical goiter, this patient may be hyperthyroid. A very low TSH and an elevated thyroxine (T_4) will make the diagnosis. A thyroid scan may become part of the workup but is not the initial screening test. If the thyroid workup is negative, an evaluation for mitral valve prolapse with a good cardiac examination or echocardiogram, or even an evaluation for dysautonomia if postural blood pressure changes are present, may be warranted.

96. **(C)** The rectus sheath serves to both support and control the rectus muscles. The posterior rectus fascia (sheath) ends at the arcuate line (also called the semicircular line, linea semicircularis, line of Douglas) midway between the umbilicus and pubic symphysis. The rectus muscles are attached mainly to the anterior rectus sheath.

97. **(B)** The characteristics of each of the four major pelvic inlet configurations should be well known. The pelvic inlet can be classified clinically and helps predict ease of delivery. Clinically, these pelvic types often appear in mixed form (i.e., the forepelvis is one type and the posterior pelvis is another). The types are not necessarily exclusive.

98. **(D)** *Pudenda, vulva,* and *external genitalia* are used as synonymous terms, referring to the external genital organs. They describe the area from the mons veneris anteriorly to the rectum posteriorly, bounded laterally by the labia majora and minora. In addition to these organs, the vulva includes the clitoris, vaginal vestibule, and associated glandular openings, the distal urethra, and the perineal body. Therefore, the birthmark could be on any of these structures.

99. **(B)** The portio or portio vaginalis is that part of the cervix that extends into the vaginal canal. It is normally covered with squamous epithelium, and the external os is located at its distal end.

100. **(C)** The ovary has hormonally active stroma and follicles. The germ cells are also stored here prior to ovulation. These are the two primary functions of the ovaries. The ovary can vary normally in size from the post-menopausal patient, measuring 1 cm × 1 cm × 0.5 × 3 cm × 2 cm in the reproductive-age patient with multicystic ovaries. The ovary lies in the ovarian fossa of the true pelvis, overlying the iliac vessels. It is attached by a mesentery (mesovarium) to the posterior broad ligament and to the pelvic sidewall by a fold of peritoneum called the infundibulopelvic or suspensory ligament.

101. **(A)** The pudendal nerve is derived from the second, third, and fourth sacral nerves and is the major nerve supply to the vulva. It has many complicated nerve endings, including Meissner's corpuscles, especially dense on the prepuce of the clitoris.

102. **(C)** Paracervical blocks take advantage of the autonomic nervous system fibers coursing through the paracervical ganglion. Visceral nerve fibers generally do not discriminate well, and pelvic pain localization is sometimes very difficult. Surgical interruption of the ligaments containing these nerves is used with varying degrees of success to relieve pain.

103. **(A)** The abdominal aorta divides into the two common iliac arteries at about the sacral promontory. The common iliac divides into the internal and external iliac arteries at about the level of the pectineal line. There are anterior and posterior divisions of the internal iliac (hypogastric) artery. The anterior division gives off 7 to 8 branches: the obliterated umbilical, the uterine, the middle hemorrhoidal, the inferior vesical, the inferior gluteal, and the internal pudendal arteries. The posterior division gives off the iliolumbar, the lateral sacral, and the superior gluteal arteries. The ovarian artery arises as a direct branch of the aorta. Ligation of the hypogastric arteries decreases the pulse pressure to the pelvic vessels and can be used as a means to control obstetric bleeding. The superior hemorrhoidal artery arises from the inferior mesenteric.

104. **(E)** After the secondary oocyte is ovulated, fertilization occurs in the tube. It is at this time that the second meiotic division occurs. This is most likely to occur in the fallopian tube. The first polar body is formed at about the time of the LH surge (an often-asked question).

105. **(D)** Group B streptococcus is a pathogen carried in the maternal vagina. When pathologic, it may be associated with an overwhelming sepsis in the first 5 days of life, most commonly in the first 24 hours of life. Mortality can be as high as 10% in term babies and 66% in preterm babies.

106. **(D)** TB was the leading cause of death in the United States in the early 1900s. It has a higher incidence in southeast Asian and Native American populations. Skin tests should be performed routinely during pregnancy in high-risk populations. Only patients with abnormal skin tests or strongly suggestive histories or symptoms (and a negative skin test) should be followed up with chest x-ray. Multidrug therapy can and should be used in pregnancy, with the exception of streptomycin because of its ototoxicity in the fetus. In general, if found and treated in pregnancy, tuberculosis has no adverse effect on mother or child.

107. **(E)** The greatest concern here is that the patient may have hepatitis (hepatitis A, B, C, Delta, or non-A, non-B). The patient is at risk for hepatitis B because of her occupation (handling of blood products). The differential diagnosis should not include preeclampsia because her blood pressure is normal, and the symptoms she has are strongly suggestive of a viral syndrome. Since there is no effective treatment for most causes of hepatitis, the most important task is to establish a diagnosis (measuring liver enzymes) and determine, as well as possible, the cause from the serum markers used for hepatitis screening (after screening elevated liver enzymes).

108. **(C)** This entity, a pelvic infection causing secondary inflammation of the liver with adhesion formation, is called Fitz-Hugh–Curtis syndrome after two Americans who were not the first to describe it. It can cause right upper quadrant pain and elevated liver enzymes, and might be confused with liver or gallbladder disease. No special treatment is needed other than standard treatment of the pelvic infection.

109. **(A)** Passage of a large amount of serosanguinous fluid through the wound on postoperative days 5 to 8 indicates that this wound has dehisced (deep fascial layers are no longer intact). Rather than the fascia just separating, there is more likely a tear of the fascia. About 50% of the time the wound is also infected. The wound must be explored, and in most cases the patient will have to be taken back to the operating room, debrided, and closed again with internal or external retention sutures.

110. **(C)** Sarcoma botryoides (embryonal rhabdomyosarcoma) is a malignant tumor that can involve the vagina, uterus, bladder, and urethra of young girls. It usually begins on the anterior vagina near the cervix and grows to fill the vagina. Eventually, patients experience vaginal discharge and bleeding associated with passage of grape-like lesions. The tumor may also appear as a grape-like mass prolapsing through the vaginal introitus. The combination of surgery, chemotherapy, and radiation therapy offers effective treatment for children with localized disease.

111. **(E)** Informed consent should be initially obtained before physical examination of a sexual assault victim. Physical examination and collection of specimens and blood for various infectious diseases and semen stains must follow informed consent due to legal requirements. Also, the informed consent process allows the victim to regain control of her body without feeling violated by another individual. Certainly, it is important to offer counseling after full evaluation of a sexual assault as well as reporting to the appropriate authorities if there appears to a strong basis for the claim.

112. **(E)** The history of painless, early labors five consecutive times combined with the findings of effacement and dilation make incompetent cervical os the best bet. The history does not make one think of true labor with uterine contractions, although that is a possibility. A mechanical weakness of the cervix is more likely.

113. **(C)** Although bed rest and progesterone may be used, a surgical cerclage procedure, such as the McDonald or Schirodkar, is most apt to be efficacious. The Lash procedure is done in a nonpregnant state. Oxytocin may induce contractions and would certainly be of no help.

114. **(E)** Meticulous repair by layers (i.e., the mucosa, fascia, anal sphincter, perineal muscles, and vaginal mucosa) with interposition of fascia between the rectum and vagina will yield the best results. If a laceration involves the rectal mucosa, it may be called a fourth-degree laceration.

115. **(A)** Rectovaginal fistula is the most common significant early problem. Orders should be written that do not allow enemas after such a repair. Stool softeners should be provided. Later, rectal incompetence may be a problem.

116. **(A, B, C)** Single-gene defects are caused by gene mutations that may produce a major error in the genetic information. Most are rare, with an incidence of about 1 in 2,000 or less. Chromosomal disorders consist of the addition or deletion of whole chromosomes or chromosome segments. They occur in about 7 per 1,000 live births and are present in about 30 to 50% of spontaneous abortion specimens. Multifactorial inheritance is not a single genetic error but a combination of variations, which results in a recognizable defect. They tend to recur in families but do not show the pedigree inheritance of other defects. Teratogens certainly can cause variation, but they are not heritable through the genetic code.

117. **(A, B, C, D)** One of the most important components of early prenatal care is determination of gestational age to establish an estimated date of delivery (EDD). The most accurate means to date a pregnancy include first-trimester ultrasound and/or examination and documentation of when fetal heart tones are first audible. A certain LMP in a woman with normal menstrual cycles is also important. Postterm pregnancy is a pregnancy lasting more than 2 weeks beyond the EDD. Incidence varies, with an average of about 10% of pregnancies. The duration of anencephalic pregnancies may be remarkably long, suggesting that some signal from the fetal brain triggers labor. Twins are likely to deliver early.

118. **(C, D)** Some investigators use 7.20 as the lower limit; serial samples should be obtained if the pH is between 7.20 and 7.25. One should also check maternal pH. If it is high from hyperventilation, it may mask a low fetal value, or if it is low, the fetus may be normal with a low pH.

119. **(D, E)** Shoulder dystocia is a problem of disproportion of fetal shoulders and maternal pelvis. It occurs after the fetal head is delivered. Fundal pressure pushes the shoulders into the symphysis and is contraindicated. The Ritgen maneuver is used for delivery of the head. Correct maneuvers to aid delivery of a baby with shoulder dystocia include McRoberts, flexion of the maternal thighs and knees, and Wood's screw—rotating the fetal shoulders.

120. **(A, B, E)** The vacuum extractor is applied to the fetal scalp. The most common complications involve traumatic injury to the scalp, including tentorial tears, cephalhematomas, and subgaleal hemorrhage. Retinal hemorrhages occur up to 30% of the time. Facial lacerations are very uncommon, and rib fractures are not associated with vacuum extraction.

121. **(A, B, C, D)** The clinical utilization of prolactin measurements should be reserved for situations in which the potential causes of hyperprolactinemia may be suspected. These include galactorrhea, experienced by a woman with significant hyperprolactinemia. The amenorrhea/oligomenorrhea is induced by direct effects of prolactin on inhibiting GnRH secretion from the hypothalamus and gonadotropin secretion from the pituitary gland. If radiographic evidence of an enlarged sella turcica is seen, a pituitary adenoma must be suspected. Pituitary adenomas that elevate prolactin secretion are either prolactinomas (prolactin-secreting adenomas) or nonsecretory adenomas, which increase prolactin via a mass effect inhibiting dopamine secretion to the prolactin-secreting cells. Prolactin is always elevated in normal pregnancy.

122. **(A, B, C, D)** In non-breast-feeding women, circulating prolactin levels decrease to normal by the third to fifth postpartum week. Ovulation occurs approximately 6 weeks after birth. In breast-feeding women, serum prolactin levels decrease 50% during the first postpartum week but continue to remain elevated for at least 6 months. Maintenance of lactation depends on nipple stimulation by suckling, which stimulates prolactin release, thereby perpetuating casein production. Suckling also stimulates oxytocin secretion, which induces myoepithelial cell contraction and milk letdown. Environmental stimuli, such as anticipation of breast-feeding and baby crying, also can initiate oxytocin release and milk letdown. Amenorrhea accompanying lactation reflects suppression of hypothalamic GnRH release. Serum gonadotropin levels are low, and ovulation is delayed beyond the tenth postpartum week. Weaning (absence of suckling) removes the stimulatory signal for prolactin release and milk letdown. Alveolar engorgement by milk further inhibits casein production by a local phenomenon. Circulating gonadotropin levels gradually increase, and ovulation occurs within 2 to 4 weeks of weaning.

123. **(A, B, C, E)** Conditions of inappropriate prolactin secretion cause nongestational lactation, referred to as galactorrhea. The most common cause is a prolactin-secreting pituitary adenoma (prolactinoma). Although one quarter of the general population harbors a pituitary adenoma (most of which are biologically inert), about one half of patients with symptomatic hyperprolactinemia have radiologic evidence of a pituitary adenoma. Prolactinomas cause an elevation in circulating prolactin levels. A concomitant suppression of pulsatile GnRH secretion results in amenorrhea. Prolonged estrogen deficiency under these conditions increases the risk of osteoporosis since estrogen plays a role in inhibiting bone reabsorption. Primary hypothyroidism accounts for about 3 to 5% of patients with symptomatic hyperprolactinemia. The compensatory increase in thyrotropin-releasing hormone (TRH) stimulates prolactin release, causing galactorrhea and/or amenorrhea. These symptoms may be the only manifestation of hypothyroidism. Other conditions associated with hyperprolactinemia include:

- Hypothalamic tumors (e.g., craniopharyngioma), via interruption of dopamine release
- Medication: exogenous estrogen (OCs), dopaminergic antagonists (phenothiazines, tricyclic antidepressants, reserpine, alpha-methyldopa), opiate peptide derivatives (meperidine), histamine (H_2-receptor) antagonists (cimetidine), serotonergic agonists (amphetamines)
- Areolar neural stimulation (prolonged suckling, herpes zoster, chest surgery)
- Renal failure, via reduced metabolic clearance of prolactin
- Ectopic prolactin secretion (bronchogenic carcinoma, hypernephroma)

Intrapartum hemorrhage may cause pituitary necrosis with no estrogen or prolactin secretion

124. **(A, C, D, E)** Masculinization of the female fetus represents either (1) increased fetal androgen production due to an enzymatic defect in the pathway of cortisol synthesis (congenital adrenal hyperplasia [CAH]), or (2) transplacental transfer of excess circulating androgens in the mother (CAH, androgen-producing tumors of the adrenal and ovary, androgenic

medication). The placenta has a large capacity to metabolize androgens so that the fetus is usually protected from androgen excess in the mother. Three forms of CAH cause androgen excess: 3-beta-hydroxysteroid dehydrogenase deficiency, 21-hydroxylase deficiency, and 11-beta hydroxylase deficiency. These individuals do not produce müllerian inhibitory factor and therefore have a uterus, fallopian tubes, and a vagina. Fertility is possible if appropriate therapy is instituted. Deficiency of 20-22 desmolase prevents conversion of cholesterol to pregnenolone so that none of the biologically active steroids are produced. These infants have female external genitalia and usually do not survive.

125. **(A, B, C, E)** In most instances, the urine screen for glucose, Pap smear, and cholesterol are done as a routine part of scheduled health care screening, checking for commonly found abnormalities. Most medical groups recommend mammography either annually or every other year, depending on patient risks. Serum creatinine would generally be reserved only for those patients with suspected renal disease.

126. **(A, B, D, E)** Newer formulations attempt to minimize the effects of dry mouth, urinary hesitancy, blurred vision, and confusion. Constipation is a more common complaint than diarrhea. These side effects often will prevent the patient from being compliant with the medication.

127. **(A, B, C, D)** Predisposing factors for TSS include high-absorbency tampons (which obstruct or ulcerate the vagina), neutral vaginal pH created by vaginal blood, and high vaginal oxygen content (due to tampon insertion). In addition, the longer a tampon is left in place, the greater the risk for developing TSS. Coital frequency is not a factor.

128. **(A, B, C, E)** Most medical professional liability claims represent negligence torts. They require proof of four elements of negligent action: duty, breach of duty, causation, and damage. Duty is the physician's responsibility to act in accordance with a standard of care to prevent or avoid patient injury. Breach of duty involves violation of this standard of care. Causation, or proximate cause, is the essential element of a liability claim. It links the physician's negligent act to actual damages.

129. **(A, B, C, D)** This question serves to illustrate one of the problems common in medicine: Namely, a proliferation of immature squamous cells confined to the surface epithelium is called many names. Dysplasia is graded as moderate to severe. Carcinoma in situ is immaturity of the entire epithelial thickness. Squamous intraepithelial lesion is the identification in the Bethesda system for these lesions found on Pap smears. Many pathologists and colposcopists would like this term to generalize to the interpretation of biopsy specimens also. None are a cancer because they all lack invasion. Metaplasia is a nondysplastic normal change.

130. **(A, B, C, D)** Repair of cell injury with multiple sublethal fractions (many doses) allows tumor cells to be killed and normal cells to survive. Repopulation refers to the fact that the tissues with increased numbers of progenitor cells (normal tissues) have a greater ability to regenerate. Reoxygenation means that hypoxic cells are known to be more resistant to radiation than are well-oxygenated cells. Cells greater than 100 mm from capillaries may not be reached by adequate oxygen. If tumor cells are isolated from oxygenation, they will not respond as well. Synchrony means simply that by killing a large fraction of tumor cells, the remaining cells will often become "synchronized" in the same part of the cell cycle (because rapid growers are killed first). Specific regeneration of T and B cells is not known to be involved.

131. **(B, D)** Necrotizing fasciitis is a life-threatening surgical emergency. Prompt aggressive debridement must be performed to remove the necrotic tissue involving the subcutaneous tissue and fascia. The initial presentation may be consistent with cellulitis, but the patient generally appears toxic with signs of sepsis. Surgical explorations are required to rule out necrotizing fasciitis in such suspicious cases. Broad-spectrum antibiotics are necessary for treatment. Patients with diabetes, malnutrition, obesity, and poor tissue perfusion are more susceptible.

132. **(D)** Osteitis pubis occurs 2.5% of the time following MMK. It probably occurs because of suture placement in the periosteum covering the pubic rami. The condition can be incapacitating. Erythrocyte sedimentation rate is elevated. The treatment is bed rest, pain medications, and anti-inflammatory agents. The condition is self-limiting, although it can last for months.

133. **(B)** Pubovaginal slings can be performed with autologous or synthetic, inorganic materials. Autologous materials have less risk of infection and subsequent poor healing. Given her prior radiation and increased risk of poor healing, Mersilene was probably not a good choice, and urethral erosion is a serious risk.

134. **(A)** The most serious complication from suprapubic catheter placement is bowel perforation. It is more likely to occur if there is anterior pelvis scarring from prior surgery. Bowel contents may be draining from the catheter site. While retropubic abscess is possible, it would be less likely after a Stamey operation, and her symptoms might not be so generalized.

References

Agency for Health Care Policy and Research. *Clinical Handbook of Preventive Services,* 2nd ed. Washington, DC: U.S. Department of Health and Human Services, 1998.

American College of Obstetricians and Gynecologists. *ACOG Criteria Set,* No. 3. Washington, DC: ACOG, January 1995.

American College of Obstetricians and Gynecologists. *ACOG Educational Bulletin,* No. 242. Washington, DC: ACOG, November 1997.

American College of Obstetricians and Gynecologists. *Emergency Oral Contraception.* ACOG Practice Pattern 3. Washington, DC: ACOG, 1996.

Beckman CRB, Ling F, Laube DW, Smith RP, Barzansky BM, Herbert WN. *Obstetrics and Gynecology,* 4th ed. Baltimore, MD: Williams & Wilkins, 2002.

Benson JT. *Female Pelvic Floor Disorders.* New York: Norton Medical Books, 1992.

Carr BR, Blackwell RE. *Textbook of Reproductive Medicine,* 2nd ed. Stamford, CT: Appleton & Lange, 1998.

Chandrasoma, P, Taylor CR. *Concise Pathology,* 3rd ed. New York: McGraw-Hill, 2001.

Copeland LJ, Jarrell JF. *Textbook of Gynecology,* 2nd ed. Philadelphia: WB Saunders, 2000.

Cunningham FG, Gant NF, Leveno KJ, Gilstrap LC, Hauth JC, Wenstrom KD. *Williams Obstetrics,* 21st ed. New York: McGraw-Hill, 2001.

DeCherney AH, Nathan L. *Current Obstetric and Gynecologic Diagnosis and Treatment,* 9th ed. New York: McGraw-Hill, 2003.

DiSaia PJ, Creasman WT. *Clinical Gynecologic Oncology,* 2nd ed. St. Louis, MO: Mosby, 1984.

Emans SJH, Goldstein DP, eds. *Pediatric and Adolescent Gynecology,* 3rd ed. Boston: Little, Brown, 1990.

Gabbe SG, Niebyl JR, Simpson JL. *Obstetrics: Normal and Problem Pregnancies,* 4th ed. New York: Churchill Livingstone, 2002.

Greenspan FS, Strewlar GJ. *Basic and Clinical Endocrinology,* 6th ed. New York: McGraw-Hill, 2001.

Greer BE, Berek JS. *Gynecologic Oncology.* New York: Elsevier, 1991.

Hacker NF, Moore JG. *Essentials of Obstetrics and Gynecology,* 3rd ed. Philadelphia: WB Saunders, 1998.

Hoskins WJ, Perez CA, Young C. *Principles and Practice of Gynecologic Oncology,* 2nd ed. Philadelphia: Lippincott-Raven, 1997.

Lemcke DP, Pattison J, Marshall LA, Cowley DS. *Primary Care of Women.* Norwalk, CT: Appleton & Lange, 1995.

Lentz GM, ed. *Urogynecology.* London: Arnold, 2000.

Manning FA. *Fetal Medicine: Principles and Practice.* Norwalk, CT: Appleton & Lange, 1995.

Moore KL. *The Developing Human—Clinically Oriented Embryology,* 3rd ed. Philadelphia: WB Saunders, 1982.

Ostergard DR, Bent AE. *Urogynecology and Urodynamics,* 3rd ed. Baltimore, MD: Williams & Wilkins, 1991.

Santoso JT, Coleman RL. *Handbook of Gynecologic Oncology.* New York: McGraw-Hill, 2001.

Sciarra JJ, Dooley S, Depp R, et al. *Gynecology and Obstetrics,* Vol. 26. Philadelphia: Lippincott-Williams & Wilkins, 2002.

Scully RE. *Tumors of the Ovary and Maldeveloped Gonads,* 2nd series. Washington, DC: Armed Forces Institute of Pathology, 1993.

Seltzer VL, Pearse WH. *Women's Primary Health Care: Office Practice and Procedures.* New York: McGraw-Hill, 1995.

Smith RP. *Gynecology in Primary Care.* Baltimore, MD: Williams & Wilkins, 1996.

Speroff L, Glass RH, Kase NG. *Clinical Gynecologic Endocrinology and Infertility,* 6th ed. Baltimore, MD: Williams & Wilkins, 1999.

Stenchever MA, Droegmueller W, Herbst AL, Mishell DR. *Comprehensive Gynecology,* 4th ed. St. Louis, MO: Mosby-Year Book, 2001.

Thompson MW, McInnes RR, Willard HF. *Genetics in Medicine,* 6th ed. Philadelphia: WB Saunders, 2002.

Wall LL, Norton PA, DeLancey JO. *Practical Urogynecology.* Baltimore, MD: Williams & Wilkins, 1993.

Yen SSC, Jaffe RB, Barbieri RL. *Reproductive Endocrinology: Physiology, Pathophysiology and Clinical Management,* 4th ed. Philadelphia: WB Saunders, 1999.

NOTES

NOTES

NOTES

NOTES

NOTES

NOTES

NOTES

NOTES

NOTES

NOTES

NOTES

NOTES

NOTES

NOTES